Handbook of Clinical Diagnostics

Xue-Hong Wan • Rui Zeng
Editors

Handbook of Clinical Diagnostics

PMPH PEOPLE'S MEDICAL PUBLISHING HOUSE

Springer

Editors
Xue-Hong Wan
West China Hospital
Sichuan University
Chengdu
China

Rui Zeng
Department of Cardiology
Sichuan University
Chengdu
China

ISBN 978-981-13-7676-4 ISBN 978-981-13-7677-1 (eBook)
https://doi.org/10.1007/978-981-13-7677-1

This Springer imprint is published by the registered company Springer Nature Singapore Pte Ltd.
The registered company address is: 152 Beach Road, #21-01/04 Gateway East, Singapore 189721, Singapore

Preface

While medical education has become increasingly internationalized in China, a systematic textbook written in English, targeting clinical medical students and aimed to be used in bilingual teaching—including that of overseas students—is lacking. To address such a shortage, we compiled *Handbook of Clinical Diagnostics* (1st edition), with support from the National Health and Family Planning Commission and Ministry of Education. The whole compiling process accords with instructions from the National Health and Family Planning Commission on compiling "The 13th Five-Year Plan" textbooks in English. *Handbook of Clinical Diagnostics* (1st edition), as one of the country's 37 planned textbooks in English complied to meet the needs for an elite and internationalized medical education, will also contribute to the country's general goal of promoting sociocultural advancement and medical development, improving bilingual teaching and overseas students teaching in medical universities and schools, and ensuring the quality and homogeneity of medical teaching across China.

The *Handbook of Clinical Diagnostics* serves as not only the foundation of all the other clinical courses but the bond bridging over basic medical knowledge and clinical learning and the key for medical students to grow into high-level clinical talents. For these reasons, it is the very first textbook that paves the way for all the basic training essential for medical students.

The book covers basic theories, basic knowledge, and basic skills on clinical diagnosis and basic requirements for doctors' ethical conduct, clinical reasoning, and documentation of medical records during the process of making a diagnosis. It consists of seven parts.

Part I Symptoms explains the causes, mechanisms, clinical manifestations, and history taking of symptoms of every system, underlying the process in which students familiarize themselves with clinical manifestations and learn history taking. Part II History Taking focuses on the significance, content, methods, and techniques of history taking and introduces special approaches for history taking under unusual conditions. Part III Physical Examination illustrates the importance and basic procedures of physical examination, content and methods used to examine organs and systems, and signs and their clinical significance. This chapter also discusses basic requirements and content for both complete physical examination and focused physical examination. Part IV Auxiliary Examination introduces commonly used clinical supplementary examination procedures including electronic cardiography (ECG), blood gases and acid-base balance, and endoscopy. Part V Common Diagnostic Techniques details indications, contraindications, and operation essentials of common diagnosis and operation skills such as thoracentesis, abdominal paracentesis, lumbar puncture, and bone marrow puncture. Part VI Medical Record stresses the importance and related regulations of documentation of medical records because they are legal documents as well as medical documents. The chapter also elaborates on the basics of medical record documentation. Part VII Clinical Reasoning emphasizes professionalism in the process of diagnosis and explains diagnostic procedures and basic principles and approaches of clinical reasoning. A bilingual vocabulary index is included for easy reference at the end of the book.

It is noteworthy that Clinical Diagnostics, as a discipline, should include at least the following subjects: symptoms diagnosis, physical diagnosis, laboratory diagnosis, clinical radiology, laboratory diagnosis, and functional diagnostics. As part of the curriculum in medical schools, however, Clinical Diagnostics does not include laboratory diagnosis and laboratory diagnosis because they are both independent courses in the curriculum and separate books in this series of textbooks: *Laboratory Diagnosis* and *Medical Imaging*. That justifies the name of our book *Handbook of Clinical Diagnostics*.

Handbook of Clinical Diagnostics is designed for students of clinical medicine mainly. It also helps students majoring in basic medicine, preventive medicine, and stomatology. Readers of other majors and with an interest in diagnostics can benefit as well. This book can be used for teaching overseas students in China as well as teaching Chinese students in a bilingual (English and Chinese) context. Medical students overseas may use it as a reference.

This book is compiled by authors of 14 Chinese medical schools and universities, whose years of experience teaching clinical diagnostics, rich overseas learning or working experiences, proficiency in English and writing, and devotion and dedication have made the book possible. Our gratitude goes to the authors of two books that we use for major reference. Both books are national planned textbooks under The 12th Five-Year Plan: *Diagnostics* (8th edition) by Xuehong Wan and Xuefeng Lu, People's Medical Publishing House, 2013 (in Chinese), and *Clinical Diagnostics* (3rd edition) by Xuehong Wan and Hong Chen, People's Medical Publishing House, 2015 (in Chinese).

The completion of this book has witnessed tremendous enthusiasm and efforts from all authors. Nevertheless, defects or even errors still seem unavoidable for various reasons. The readers' suggestions are welcomed and will be considered for the next edition as appropriate.

Chengdu, China — Xue-Hong Wan
Chengdu, China — Rui Zeng
January 23, 2019

Contents

List of Contributors

Chief Editors

Xuehong Wan Sichuan University, Chengdu, China

Rui Zeng Sichuan University, Chengdu, China

Editors

Xuehong Wan Sichuan University, Chengdu, China

Jianfang Ma Shanghai Jiaotong University, Shanghai, China

Ke Wang Jilin University, Changchun, China

Yi Liu Anhui Medical University, Hefei, China

Shiming Liu Guangzhou Medical University, Guangzhou, China

Fei Chen Wuhan University, Wuhan, Hubei, China

Gang Chen Fujian Medical University, Fuzhou, China

Jialin Chen Peking Union Medical College, Beijing, China

Jianping Zhao Huazhong University of Science and Technology, Wuhan, China

Zhijun Duan Dalian Medical University, Dalian, China

Ling Dong Fudan University, Shanghai, China

Weihong Jiang Central South University, Changsha, China

Rui Zeng Sichuan University, Chengdu, China

Lie Dai Sun Yat-Sen University, Guangzhou, China

Fei Dai Xi'an Jiaotong University, Xi'an, China

Part I

Symptoms

1 Fever

Lie Dai and Rui Zeng

Core body temperature is maintained within a narrow range around 37 °C in normal individual. Hypothalamus acts as the body's thermostat which regulates heat balance. Increased body temperature results from excessive heat production or interference with heat dissipation. Fever is elevation of core body temperature resulting from upward resetting of the hypothalamic thermostatic set-point caused by pyrogens. Hyperthermia is elevation of body temperature beyond the unchanged hypothalamic thermostatic set-point resulting from dysfunction of body temperature center or impairment of heat production and/or heat loss mechanisms.

Body temperature varies slightly with different measurement methods (See Session III, Chap. 2). Many physiological factors can influence the level of body temperature, including age, gender, time of day, ambient temperature and activity level. The body temperature in the elderly is lower than that in the younger individuals. There is a circadian rhythm with lower temperatures in the morning and higher temperatures in the late afternoon with daily variation less than 1 °C. The body temperature may slightly rise after strenuous exercise, work stuff, meal, stress, before menstruation or during pregnancy.

1.1 Etiology and Mechanisms

Many disorders including infectious and noninfectious diseases can cause elevation of body temperature. Infectious fever is more common in clinic than noninfectious fever.

L. Dai
Department of Rheumatology and Immunology, Sun Yat-Sen University, Guangzhou, China

R. Zeng (✉)
Department of Cardiology, Sichuan University, Chengdu, China

1.1.1 Infectious Causes

All pathogens can cause fever, including virus, bacteria, mycoplasma, rickettsia, spirochete, fungi, parasites and other microorganisms. Both localized and systemic infection can induce fever. Microbes and microbial products act as exogenous pyrogens which can stimulate endogenous pyrogen-generating cells to generate and release endogenous pyrogens leading to fever.

1.1.2 Noninfectious Causes

Noninfectious disorders can cause elevation of core body temperature including noninfectious fever and hyperthermia. Noninfectious pyrogenic activators can act as exogenous pyrogens leading to fever, including antigen-antibody complex, components of the complement cascade, noninfectious inflammation-genesis irritants, and certain steroids such as etiocholanolone.

- Neoplasma: such as leukemia, lymphoma, malignant histiocytosis and solid tumors.
- Noninfectious inflammatory and immune diseases: such as Still's disease, gout, inflammatory bowel disease, systemic lupus erythematous, rheumatic fever, systemic vasculitis, sarcoidosis, familial Mediterranean fever and other familial periodic fevers.
- Metabolic and endocrine diseases: such as hyperthyroidism, pheochromocytoma adrenal insufficiency and severe dehydration.
- Tissue necrosis: such as thrombus and embolic diseases (e.g. myocardial infarction, pulmonary infarction), postoperative fever, entorrhagia, large hematoma, extensive empyrosis and hemolysis.
- Allergic diseases: such as drug fever and serum sickness.
- Central thermoregulatory disorders: such as brain tumor, cerebrovascular accident, encephalitis, hypothalamic dysfunction and severe sedative-hypnotic poisoning.

X.-H. Wan, R. Zeng (eds.), *Handbook of Clinical Diagnostics*, https://doi.org/10.1007/978-981-13-7677-1_1

- Hyperthermia: heat overproduction due to status epileptic, malignant hyperthermia induced by anesthetics; heat stroke; impaired heat dissipation due to generalized dermatitis, extensive skin edema caused by heart failure.

1.2 Clinical Manifestations

1.2.1 Grades of Fever

Fever can be divided into four grades according to oral temperature: low grade: 37.3–38 °C, medium grade: 38.1–39 °C, high grade: 39.1–41 °C, very high grade: >41 °C.

1.2.2 Clinical Process and Febrile Phases

The typical process of fever can be divided into three phases as followed:

- Effervescence period: Release of endogenous pyrogens elevates the hypothalamic thermostatic set-point leading to increased body temperature. Onset of fever may be marked by a chill with shivering and cutaneous vasoconstriction as the body begins generating increased heat and decreasing heat loss. Severe chills are called rigors. In this period, body temperature may rise abruptly over 39 °C within a few hours, usually accompanied with rigors or even convulsion in pediatric patients. This can occur in malaria, lobar pneumonia, septicemia, influenza, acute pyelonephritis or infusion reaction. Body temperature may also rise gradually (e.g. for several days) to peak without rigors which usually occurs in typhoid, tuberculosis or brucellosis.
- Persistent febrile period: When the new set-point is reached with heat equipoise at a higher level, the skin becomes warm and flushing caused by cutaneous vasodilation. The new set-point and the pattern of fever reflect dynamics of particular pathophysiologic process. Fever may maintain for several hours as in malaria, for several days as in lobar pneumonia or influenza, or for several weeks as in typhoid.
- Defervescence period: Return of the set-point to normal, either temporarily or permanently, is marked by sweating and moist of skin as the body dissipates the accumulated heat. Intense sweating may cause significant dehydration. Elevated body temperature may decrease to normal or even lower within a few hours, usually accompanying with intense sweating. This sudden defervescence is known as "crisis" which is commonly seen in malaria, acute pyelonephritis, lobar pneumonia or infusion reaction. Elevated body temperature may decrease slowly to normal after several days, called "lysis" which is usually occurred in typhoid fever or rheumatic fever.

1.3 Fever Patterns

The patient's temperatures are recorded at a regular interval and temperature curve is generated by connecting each point. The patterns of temperature fluctuations may be a useful clue for the diagnosis and differential diagnosis of febrile illnesses. It must be noted that fever patterns can be influenced by drug use and individual response. Typical or specific patterns of fever in particular febrile diseases could be changed to atypical or irregular fever by the use of antibiotics, antipyretic drugs or glucocorticoids. Severe pneumonia in elder patients could show low grade fever or even no fever rather than typical pattern of pneumonia fever.

1. **Continuous fever** : The temperature remains above 39–40 °C for days or weeks with diurnal temperature

Fig. 1.1 Continuous fever

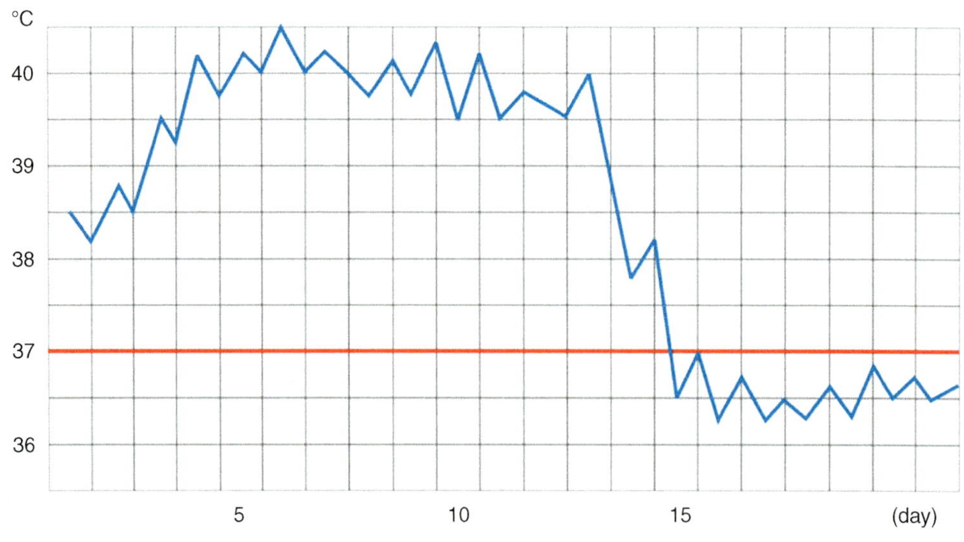

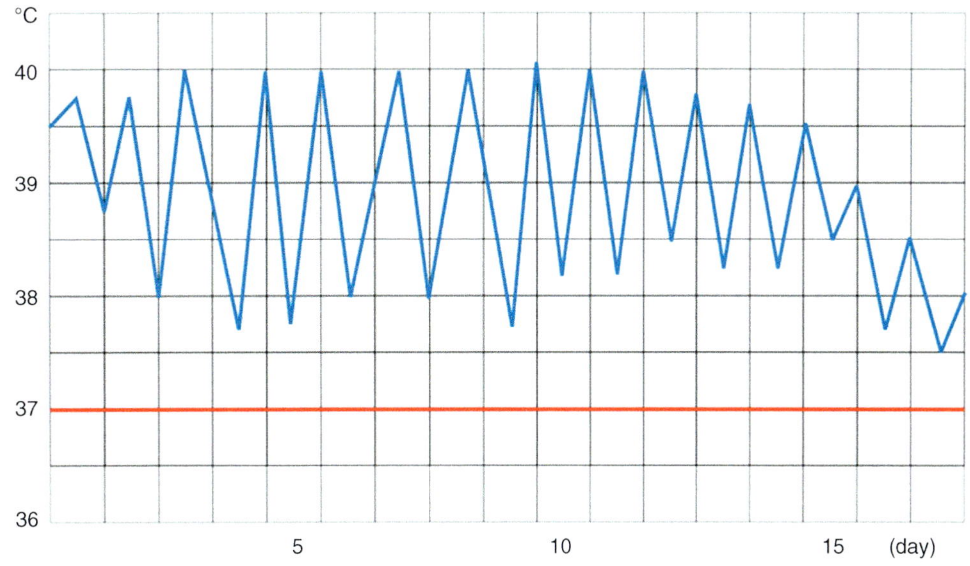

Fig. 1.2 Remittent fever

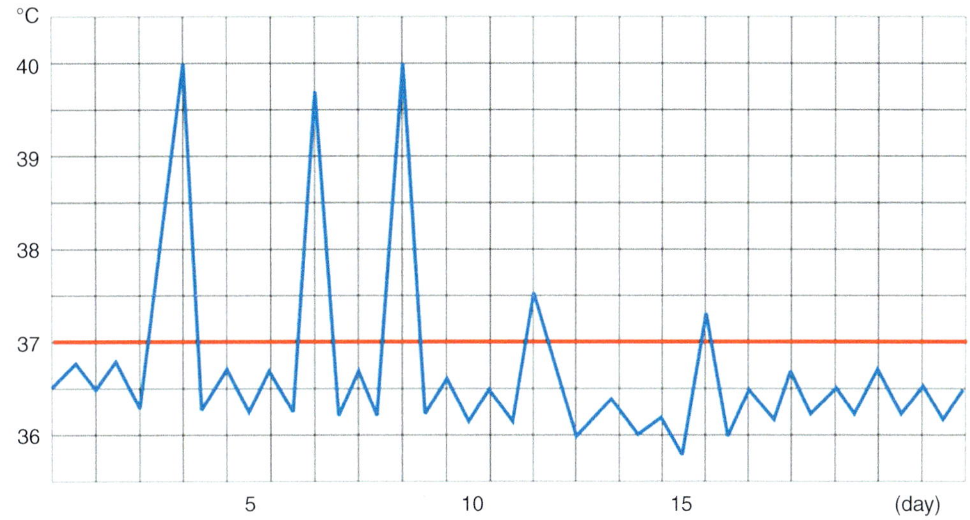

Fig. 1.3 Intermittent fever

fluctuation less than 1 °C (Fig. 1.1). This pattern is commonly seen in the persistent febrile period of lobar pneumonia, typhoid or typhus.

2. **Remittent fever**: The temperature remains above 39 °C with diurnal temperature fluctuation more than 2 °C and without any normal readings (Fig. 1.2). This pattern is commonly seen in septicemia, rheumatic fever, severe tuberculosis, suppurative infection or infectious endocarditis.
3. **Intermittent fever**: The temperature rises abruptly to peak sustained for several hours and then decreases rapidly to normal followed by one or several days of afebrile period (the intermittent period). This pattern of repeated cycles of episodes of fever and afebrile period is commonly seen in malaria, acute pyelonephritis or biliary tract infections (Fig. 1.3).Gram-negative bacilli septicemia may present two episodes of fever within one day, which is known as double quotidian fever. Long lasting intermittent fever is also named hectic fever.
4. **Undulant fever**: The temperature gradually rises up to or above 39 °C for a few days and then gradually decreases to normal for several days. This pattern of repeated cycles of fever is also called relapsing fever which is commonly seen in brucellosis, connective tissue diseases or tumor (Fig. 1.4).
5. **Recurrent fever**: The temperature abruptly rises up to or above 39 °C and sustains high fever for days, then decreases suddenly to normal with several days of afebrile period. This regular alternation of recurrent bouts of high fever and afebrile period is commonly seen in Borreliarecurrentis, Hodgkin's disease or periodic fever (Fig. 1.5).
6. **Irregular fever**: The pattern of temperature curve is irregular which is commonly seen in tuberculosis, rheumatic fever, bronchial pneumonia or exudative pleurisy (Fig. 1.6).

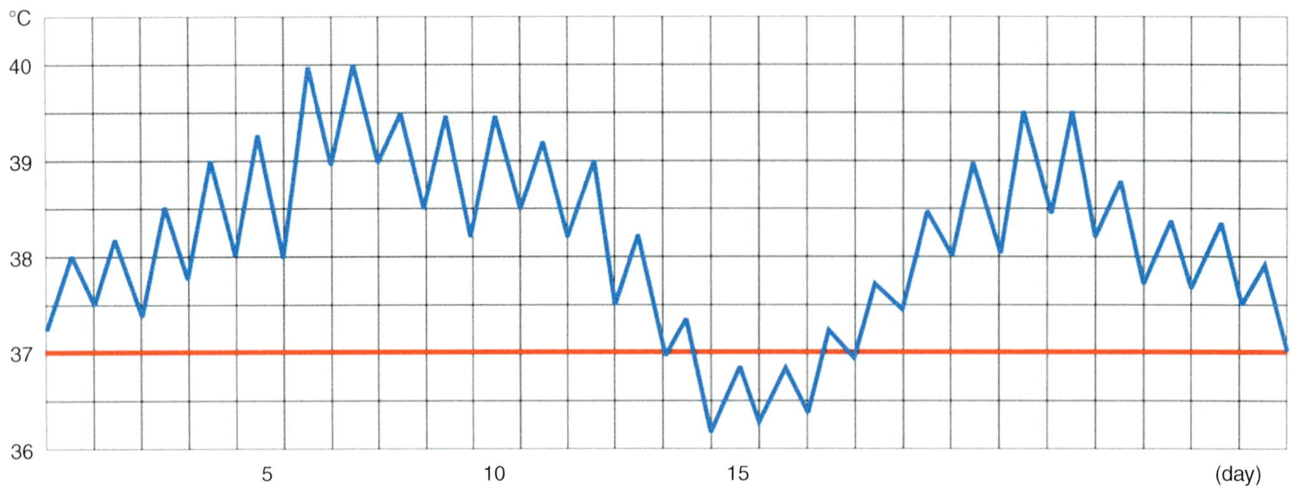

Fig. 1.4 Undulant fever

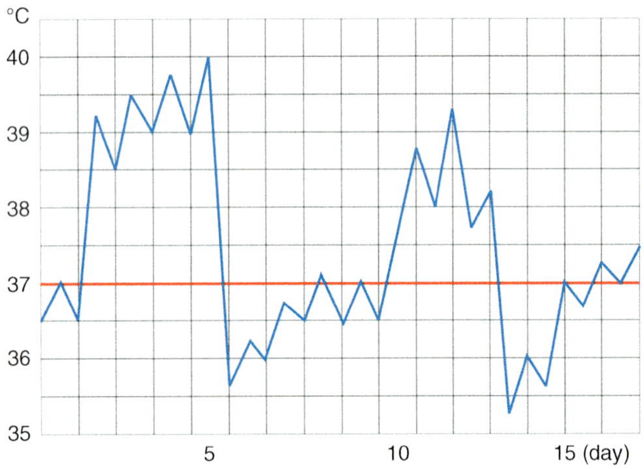

Fig. 1.5 Recurrent fever

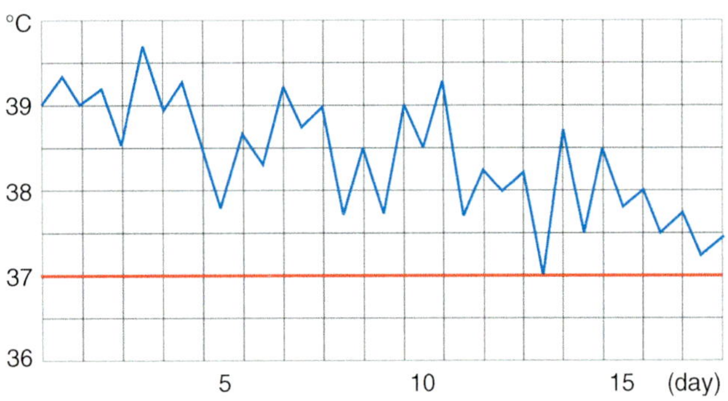

Fig. 1.6 Irregular fever

1.4 Accompanying Symptoms and Signs

1. **Rigor**: Fever with rigor is commonly seen in lobar pneumonia, septicemia, acute cholecystitis, acute pyelonephritis, epidemic cerebrospinal meningitis, malaria, leptospirosis, drug fever, acute hemolysis or transfusion reaction.
2. **Rash**: It presents in measles, scarlet fever, rubella, chicken pox, typhus, rheumatic fever, connective tissue diseases (e.g. adult onset Still's disease, systemic lupus erythematosus), or drug fever.
3. **Mucocutaneous bleeding**: Hemorrhagic fever may present in severe infections, acute infectious diseases(e.g. epidemic hemorrhagic fever, viral hepatitis, typhus, septicemia), or hematological diseases(e.g. acute leukemia, aplastic anemia, malignant histiocytosis).
4. **Arthralgia**: It is commonly seen in acute gout arthritis, infective arthritis, septicemia, scarlet fever, brucellosis, rheumatic fever and connective tissue diseases.
5. **Conjunctival congestion**: It may present in infectious diseases such as measles, epidemic hemorrhagic fever, typhus or leptospirosis.
6. **Herpes labialis**: It is commonly seen in acute febrile illnesses such as lobar pneumonia, meningococcal meningitis, tertian malaria or influenza.
7. **Lymphadenopathy**: Localized enlargement of lymph node is commonly seen in tuberculosis, focal suppurative infection and metastatic cancer. Generalized lymphadenopathy may present in infectious diseases (e.g. infectious mononucleosis, rubella, brucellosis, leptospirosis, filariasis, leishmaniasis), leukemia, lymphoma and connective tissue diseases.
8. **Hepatosplenomegaly**: It may occur in liver and biliary tract infection, acute schistosomiasis, infectious mononucleosis, viral hepatitis, brucellosis, malaria, leishmaniasis, connective tissue diseases, leukemia and lymphoma.
9. **Coma**: If fever is prior to coma, it may reveal encephalitis, typhus, epidemic cerebrospinal meningitis, toxic bacillary dysentery or heat stroke. If coma is prior to fever, it is seen in cerebral hemorrhage or barbiturate poisoning.

Key Points in History Taking

1. The onset of fever (slowly or abruptly), its grade and duration, the pattern of temperature fluctuation, frequency (intermittent or persistent), predisposition factors and season.
2. Whether it occurs with chills, rigors, sweating or night sweats.
3. Review of systemic symptoms, such as cough, sputum, hemoptysis, chest pain; abdominal pain, vomiting and diarrhea; urinary frequency, urgency, dysuria; rash, bleeding, headache, muscle pain and arthralgia.
4. General status including mental status, appetite, any change of weight, sleep, urination and defecation.
5. Detail information about previous treatment, especially medication and their dosage, efficacy including antibiotics, antipyretics, corticosteroids and anti-tuberculosis therapy.
6. History of exposure to infectious diseases and contaminated water, surgical history, history of miscarriage or childbirth.

Headache

2

Jianfang Ma and Rui Zeng

Headache, referred to the pain above the juga connection from frontal, parietal, temporal and occipital skull, is a common symptom. The long-lasting headache, or headache of episodic and recurring condition, is often presented as a clinical signal of the underly neurological and non-neurological disorders needing urgent diagnosis and treatment.

2.1 Etiology

1. **Neurological disorders**
   - Infectious diseases: meningitis, encephalitis, brain abscess, central nervous system tuberculosis, brain parasites infection, toxic encephalopathy, etc.
   - Vascular diseases: subarachnoidhemorrhage, cerebral hemorrhage, cerebral infarction, cerebral embolism, cerebral aneurysm, hypertensive encephalopathy, reversible cerebral vasoconstriction syndrome, cerebral venous sinus thrombosis, primary cerebral vasculitis, etc.
   - Space-occupying lesion: brain tumor, brain metastasis, brain tuberculoma, intracranial leukemia infiltration, neurocysticercosis, and echinococcosis, etc.
   - Trauma: brain concussion, brain contusion, subdural hemorrhage, post-traumatic brain syndrome, etc.
   - Others: migraine, chronic daily headache, intracranial hypotension headache, post-lumber puncture headache, etc.
2. **Extracranial disorders**
   - Bone: basis cranii indentation, cervical spondylosis, chiari malformation, etc.
   - Pericranial inflammation: sinus infection, dental disease, temporal arteritis, etc.
   - Cranial neuralgia: trigeminal neuralgia, occipital neuralgia, etc.
   - Tension-type headache, cluster headache.
   - Others: headache caused by the disorders of eye, ear, nose and teeth.
3. **Systemic disorders**
   - Infection: influenza, pneumonia, etc.
   - Cardiovascular disorders: hypertension, heart failure, etc.
   - Toxin and medication: alcohol, CO, salicylic acids, etc.
   - Others: anemia, systemic lupus erythematosus, heat stroke, etc.
4. **Psychogenic headache**

2.2 Pathogenesis

The main reasons for headache are probably over stimulation of the pain-sensitive structures or psychological-based reaction. The pain-sensitive structures in the brain included: (a) scalp, cervical or pericranial muscle, vascular system, eye, ear and sinus; (b) cranial sinus venous, meningeal artery, trigeminal nerve (V), facial nerve (VIII), glossopharyngeal nerve (IX), vagus (X), cervical nerve (1–3), part of the dura; There are some cranial structures which are insensitive to pain stimulation, including pia mater, arachnoid, most of the dura, brain parenchyma, ependyma ventriculorum and skull.

Several mechanism underlying headache have been hypothesized: (a) neurovascular: constriction or dilation of the cranial vessels caused by different lesions such as brain occupying lesion; (b) stimulation of meninges; (c) hyperactivity of the cranial nerves such as trigeminal nerve, facial nerve, glossopharyngeal nerve, vagus and cervical nerves (I, II, III); (d) increased muscle activity of the cervical muscle; (e) endocrinological or psychological dysfunction.

J. Ma
Department of Neurology, Shanghai Jiaotong University, Shanghai, China

R. Zeng (✉)
Department of Cardiology, Sichuan University, Chengdu, China

X.-H. Wan, R. Zeng (eds.), *Handbook of Clinical Diagnostics*, https://doi.org/10.1007/978-981-13-7677-1_2

2.3 Clinical Manifestations

Headache can be presented as variable symptoms and signs.

1. **Onset of headache**: Acute headache with fever is usually caused by infectious disorders. Thunderclap headache without fever, accompanied by variable changes of consciousness, often suggests a vascular nature (for example, subarachnoid hemorrhage). Long-lastingrecurrent headache, sometimes characterized by throbbing features, usually occurs in migraine or tension-like headache. Chronic progressive headache, accompanied by vomiting or blurred vision, should be treated cautiously because these symptoms in combination indicate a possibility of chronic intracranial hypertension.
2. **Location of headache**: The localization of headache also has a diagnostic value. The symptoms of migraine can be unilateral as well as bilateral. Headache from brain lesion or systemic diseases, is often deep inside without specific location. Subarachnoid hemorrhage or meningitis generally present stiff neck with headache. Headache caused by eye or sinus problems is commonly superficial and localized to the eye, frontal or temporal regions.
3. **Severity of headache**: The severity of headache is not paralleled with the severity of the underlying disease. Sometimes psychosis can be presented as severe headache while subarachnoid hemorrhage show a minor headache. Severe headache are often seen in meningitis, migraine, intracranial hypertension, glaucoma, cranial neuralgia, hypertensive crisis and reversible cerebral vasoconstriction sydrome, etc. In general, headache caused by brain tumor is mild or moderate in severity.
4. **Characteristics of headache**: Throbbing-like headache is mainly seen in hypertension, migrain or infectious diseases. Cranial neuralgia headache is characterized by sudden explosive headache, sometimes described as electric-shock like headache. Tension-type headache is characterized by generalized pressure or a sensation of tightness in the head.
5. **Time of headache attack and duration**: Morning headache is a common symptom of brain occupying lesion or sinus infection. Cluster headache often occurs in the evening. Migraine in women mostly occurs in menstrual period. Headache from brain tumor is usually continuous, with variable time of alleviation.
6. **Factors in relation to aggravating or alleviating headache**: Factors that aggravate headache (intracranial hypertension, migraine, infectious disease or brain tumor) include coughing, sneezing or benting over. Tension headache can be relieved by massage, while migraine can be alleviated by ergotamine.

2.4 Accompanying Symptoms

For headache with vomiting, it should be suspected for intracranial hypertension or migraine. Headache with vertigo may indicate cerebellar tumor or vertebrobasilar insufficiency. Headache with fever is commonly seen in infectious diseases. Chronic progressive headache with psychosis suggests the possibility of brain tumor. Chronic headache with sudden deterioration to inconsciousness indicates the possibility of brain herniation. Headache with blurred vision can be found in glaucoma or brain tumor. Headache with neck stiffness suggests meningitis or subarachnoid hemorrhage. Headache with seizure is common in cerebral vascular malformation, tumor or parasite infection. Headache with insomnia or anxiety should be suspected for psychological diseases.

Key Points in History Taking

1. Onset of headache: acute or chronic, duration, location, nature, severity, frequency for recurrence/episodic headache, provocating or alleviating factors;
2. Accompanying symptoms: insomnia, anxiety, vomitting, dizziness, vertigo, syncope, sweating, seizure, blurred vision, sensory disturbance, weakness, psychosis, somnolence, consciousness changes;
3. Other diseases: infectious disease, hypertension, arteriosclerosis, head injury, tumor, psychological diseases, epilepsy, neurosis, eye or nose problems;
4. Occupations or toxic contaminations;
5. Response to any treatment.

Edema

3

Jialin Chen and Rui Zeng

Edema is a pathological phenomenon of excess fluid to gather in the interstitial space. Mild fluid retention cannot cause edema, you can see the naked eye edema until the body fluid storage capacity is more than 4–5 kg. Edema is divided into systematic and non-systematic. Systemic edema means the liquid distributed diffusely in the body tissue space, shows swell of many parts on body and the skin sunken after a long time press, what also known as depression edema. Pleural effusion, pericardial effusion and ascites are respectively called when the fluid accumulates in pleural, pericardial, peritoneal cavity. In general, systematic edema often means that the body has a serious disease, but local cause or systematic diseases can also causes non-systematic edema.

3.1 Mechanism

All the human body cells are soaked in body fluid. The body water is about 2/3 of the body weight. Distribution of total body water is: which 2/3 in the intracellular fluid, 1/3 in the extracellular fluid. In the extracellular fluid, about 1/4 is distributed in the blood vessels, and 3/4 is in interstitial. Edema is caused by a variety of diseases, there are two basic reasons: firstly, an increase of extracellular fluid volume, much more liquid distributed in the interstitial space can cause edema; secondly, the imbalance of intravascular fluid exchange, the interstitial fluid generates more than reflux and result in edema. Some of factors that make the liquid from a capillary outflow greater than inflow would result in edema, such as congestive heart failure, acute nephritis, renal failure, the amount of fluid more than renal excretion, intravascular fluid volume increased, or thrombosis, thrombophlebitis cause local venous return blocked. Various causes of hypoalbuminemia, such as malnutrition, liver disease, massive proteinuria, severe diarrhea or high decomposition metabolic state, can cause the plasma colloid osmotic pressure reduced, which is lead to another important reason for edema. Capillary endothelial damage can also lead to increased capillary permeability, such as bacterial, physical and chemical factors, allergic reactions or immune damage, etc. Lymphatic obstruction can cause lymphedema, such as filariasis.

3.2 Clinical Manifestations

When edema occurs, patient's skin appears tight and shiny with the original skin wrinkles become shallow, shrink or disappear. Also the skin depress by finger pressing and even liquid exudation. However, in some situation, edema caused by some diseases cannot depress as usual. If necessary, monitor the changes of body weight, and compare with the state before disease.

According to the cause of edema, it can be divided into the following:

1. Systemic Edema
    - *Cardiac edema*: It is result of congestive heart failure. Edema first appears in sagging body parts and associates with other systemic congestion manifestations, such as jugular venous distention, hepatomegaly, elevated venous pressure, or even hydrothorax, ascites, etc.
    - *Nephrogenic edema*: It can be found in various types of nephritis and nephropathy. The characteristic is eyelid and facial edema in early morning, and then develop to the whole body edema. *Nephritic syndrome* is often associated with moderate or severe edema, obvious depression, accompanied with pleural effusion, ascites. Patients often have abnormal urine, blood pressure and renal function impairment. The different features of nephrogenic and cardiogenic edema see follow table (Table 3.1).

J. Chen
Department of Internal medicine, Peking Union Medical College, Beijing, China

R. Zeng (✉)
Department of Cardiology, Sichuan University, Chengdu, China

X.-H. Wan, R. Zeng (eds.), *Handbook of Clinical Diagnostics*, https://doi.org/10.1007/978-981-13-7677-1_3

Table 3.1 Identification of cardiac edema and nephrogenic edema

	Nephrogenic edema	Cardiac edema
The beginning part	The eyelids, facial	Sagging body parts
Development speed	Rapid	Slow
Accompanied symptoms	Abnormal urine, renal function, hypertension	Abnormal cardiac enlargement, heart murmur, hepatomegaly, elevated venous pressure

- *Liver edema*: The patients usually are at decompensation stage of liver cirrhosis. Fluid builds up within the intraperitoneal with massive ascites formed and intra-abdominal pressure increased. As it further impedes venous reflux, lower extremity edema is resulted. Edema appeared on the ankle, can gradually spread upward, but often do not appear in the head, face and upper limbs. Patients often associated with splenomegaly, abdominal wall vein engorgement and esophageal gastric fundal varices and jaundice, liver palms, spider nevus and abnormal liver function.
- *Malnutrition*: The patients with chronic wasting disease or severe burn often have nutritional deficiency, protein loss and malnutrition edema. The malnutrition patients, whom with vitamin B1 deficiency caused heart disease, can experience increase the degree of edema. To patients who experience long period of fasting, edema can become more severe after high salt content meal. Edema is characterized by the beginning of the foot and gradually spread the whole body, often accompanied by body weight loss, emaciation, etc.
- *Mucinous edema*: seen in hypothyroidism. It is non depressed edema (due to high protein content in tissue fluid), appear in the anterior region of the lower limb, but also can occur in the vicinity of the orbit.
- *Premenstrual tension syndrome*: before menstruation 7–14 days, eyelids, ankle and hand appear mild edema, associated with breast pain, pelvic heaviness feeling. After menstruation, edema subsided gradually.
- *Drug-induced edema*: A large number of used drugs can cause edema, included adrenal cortical hormone, androgen, estrogen, insulin, Glycyrrhiza and vasodilators, especially calcium antagonistic agents can cause edema that related to retention of sodium and water.
- *Idiopathic edema*: The syndrome occurs almost exclusively in women. Reasons are unclear, may associated with endocrine function disorders. Clinical characteristics is periodic edema, mainly in the body sagging parts, body weight vary greatly at day and night, up to a few kilograms, especially in the hot weather or before menstruation.
- *Others*: Gestosis, scleroderma, dermatomyositis and serum sickness can also cause edema.

2. Localized Edema
   - Edema is caused by blocked local vein and lymph flow, or increased capillary permeability. For examples: local inflammation and allergy, limb venous thrombosis, thrombophlebitis, inferior vena cava obstruction syndrome, filariasis and so on.

3.3 Accompanying Symptoms

- Edema accompanied with hepatomegaly often caused by cardiogenic, hepatic and dystrophic factors. When edema accompanied with jugular venous distention is usually caused by cardiogenic factor.
- Edema with proteinuria or hematuria is commonly caused by primary disease of the kidney, such as nephritis or nephrotic syndrome. When it accompanied with other manifestations, such as diabetes, may caused by diabetic nephropathy. Edema caused by autoimmune diseases is often associated with arthritis, skin changes, while mild proteinuria also visible in cardiogenic condition.
- Edema with dyspnea and cyanosis often developed due to heart disease, superior vena cava syndrome and so on.
- Myxedema is often associated with other clinical manifestations of thyroid hypofunction, such as apathy, afraid of the cold, hoarseness and appetite lack and so on.
- Edema has a great relationship with menstrual cycle can seen in idiopathic edema.
- Edema with insomnia, irritability and mental anxiety can be seen in the premenstrual tension syndrome.

Key Points in History Taking

1. Time of edema occurs, triggers and precursor symptoms.
2. First symptomatic location and progression order, Whether it is influenced by the body position, whether the patient have edema in face, lower limb and the waist and other parts of the sacral.
3. Progression speed of the edema, nature of edema, whether it can be depressed or have pleural effusion.
4. Whether there are signs of infections and allergic reactions, and malnutrition.
5. Whether have the treatment of adrenal cortical hormones, testosterone, estrogen, and other drugs.
6. Accompanied symptoms: Local: skin color, temperature, tenderness, rash and thickness; systemic: whether there is flustered, shortness of breath, cough and expectoration diseases of the heart and lung; the urine color change, hypertension, urinary and renal function; gastrointestinal manifestations, liver disease, jaundice and bleeding tendency; whether have appetite loss or weight change, afraid of the cold and unresponsive and constipation.
7. Female patients should also be asked about the relationship between edema and menstruation, body position weather influences, and the symptom changes in the daytime and nighttime.

Obesity

4

Chen Jialin and Rui Zeng

Obesity is a symptom that associates with many diseases. When fat, especially the triglyceride, stored up in human body exceeding the average quantity of normal people, thus the condition is recognized as obesity.

Body fat is an active metabolic organ that reserves a large amount of triglyceride. When body lacks physical energy, the triglyceride is broke down into glycerol and fatty acid in order to meet energy demand. When energy supply exceeding the demand, other nutrients will convert into triglyceride and deposited in the adipose tissue of different body parts, especially in the subcutaneous tissue. Formation of fat cells in adipose tissue happens in every period of physical development. Generally, the major proliferation of fat cells happens in the fetal period, after that, a secondary proliferation often happens before or after puberty. However, in adults, especially in the elderly, the change of fat cells is mainly the increase of intracellular fat content quantity and total cell volume, but not number of cells.

4.1 Measurements of Obesity

1. Body fat proportion: The proportion of body fat varies in sex and age. In newborns, fat is about 10% of the body weight. In adult male, it is ranges from 10 to 15%, and in female ranges from 15 to 20%.if the body fat exceeding 25% in male and 30% in female, it is called obesity.
2. Standard-weight for height method: When taking weight measurement, excluding the influence of time, clothes, food-intake and defecation are necessary for yield accurate results. Generally, there are two categories for exceeding body weight: overweight and obesity. According to Chinese weight/height table, exceeding 10% of standard weight is overweight, and exceeding 20% is obesity. [Exceeding rate = (actual weight − normal weight)/normal weight]. Nowadays, WHO considers standard-weight for height method is most applicable for children, and the recommends apply is worldwide. Details are available in relevant documents.
3. Body mass index (BMI): Body mass index or BMI is widely used in weight assessment, BMI = weight(kg)/height(m)^2. The 2003 edition of "*the guideline of preventing and controlling overweight and obesity of Chinese adults (trial implementation)*" recommends that 24–28 in BMI should be the cutting point of overweight and obesity respectively. That means BMI between 18.5 and 23.9 kg/m^2 is normal weight, 24–27.9 kg/m^{2}is overweight, and BMI ≥28 kg/m^{2}is obesity. However, for children, whose body is not fully developed, WHO recommends the age-gender-BMI percentage curve and age-skinfold thickness percentage curve. And if BMI ≥ 85%, it is at risk of overweight. If at the same time, the triceps skinfold thickness and subscapular skinfold thickness ≥ 90%, it is called obesity.
4. Triceps skinfold thickness(TSF): The thickness of triceps skinfold can be used to evaluate the body fat status. An average of 50% fat is stored under the skin. Skinfold thickness is made up of the skin and subcutaneous adipose. Measuring skinfold in different location can estimate body fat storage. Usually we measure the skinfold at subscapular, inferior of thoracic cage, iliac crest and abdomen. The triceps' is very convenient to measure, and usually do not interfered with edema.
5. Waist circumference: In 2003 WHO recommended that, for the Asian-Pacific region adults, if waist circumference is more than 90 cm in men and 80 cm in women, it is called central obesity. Nowadays, it's well acknowledged that there is a causative link between central obesity and cardiovascular diseases.

C. Jialin
Department of Internal Medicine, Peking Union Medical College, Beijing, China

R. Zeng (✉)
Department of Cardiology, Sichuan University, Chengdu, China

X.-H. Wan, R. Zeng (eds.), *Handbook of Clinical Diagnostics*, https://doi.org/10.1007/978-981-13-7677-1_4

4.2 Etiology and Pathogenesis

1. Simple obesity: It is caused by anabolism exceeding catabolism, lead to excessive accumulation of body fat, or take too much food consciousness or unconsciousness, especially eating sweet or greasy food.
2. Obesity caused by nervous system diseases: Tumors, infections and injuries damage subcortical center, which change the diet and exercise habit, consequently causing obesity.
3. Obesity caused by endocrine system diseases: Adrenocortical hyperplasia and adenoma cause hyperadrenocorticism. And excessive production of cortisol leads to series of syndromes. Malfunction of thyroid, gonad and pancreas can cause obesity as well.
4. Drug-induced obesity: Long-term use of chlorpromazine, insulin, glucocorticoid and other protein synthesis-promote medicines can also result in obesity.

4.3 Clinical Manifestations and Accompanying Symptoms

1. Simple obesity: Simple obesity is the most common obesity, which accounts for a majority in outpatients; these people are overweight since childhood and have a good appetite. The features of simple obesity are as follows:
   - Family history of obesity or overnutrition history;
   - Evenly distributed obesity, with excessive fat deposition in abdominal area.
   - History or recent endocrine and metabolism diseases are not found.

   Before making diagnose of simple obesity, endocrine or other internal medicine diseases should be excluded.
2. Hypothalamus related obesity: Hypothalamus diseases may lead to certain endocrine syndromes, with obesity in varying degrees, such as Prader-Willi syndrome. The features of hypothalamus obesity are as follows:
   - Evenly distributed moderate obesity;
   - Abnormal liquid or solid intake, body temperature, sleeping pattern and mental status;
   - Other endocrine diseases.
3. Diencephalon obesity: Diencephalon damage can cause autonomic nerve-endocrine dysfunction, which is called diencephalon syndrome. Diencephalon obesity clinically presents as appetite fluctuations, abnormal sleep rhythm, general obesity, sexual dysfunction, diabetes insipidus, and instability of temperature/pulse/blood pressure.
4. Obesity agenesis syndrome: It is also known as Frohlich syndromes and usually onsets at juveniles. The damage of adjacent tissue of hypothalamus-pituitary leads to disorder of appetite, lipometabolism, and sexual dysfunction. Body parts prone to fat accumulation is neck, chest, belly, buttocks and thigh. Breast fat increases, while arms and calves are not fatter. Malformations like cubitus valgus, genu varum and reproductive organ agenesis is commonly. If it onsets in adult, other from obesity, will present as loss of genital function, azoospermia and lack of libido.
5. Pituitary-induced obesity: Common in Cushing's syndrome (active basophilic adenoma) and acromegaly arose(oncocytoma). The former weight gain is often not obvious, and tends to be central obesity. Patients may present with plethora, purple striae, hypertension, hypokalemia, and alkalosis, may present with complication as diabetes mellitus or osteoporosis at the same time. Owing to hyperplasia of muscle, skeleton and visceral, the latter will have weight gain. Clinical presentation is acromegaly, hypertension and hyperglycemia, accompanied by headache and visual impairment, which is caused by pituitary tumor oppression.
6. Pituitary prolactinoma: It is mostly female patients, presented with amenorrhea, menstrual disorder, lactation, infertility, obesity, edema, hypoplasia etc. It is also more serious when happens to man, with symptom like headache, hypoplasia, visual field defect and sexual dysfunction.
7. Hypothyroidism: The patients with hypothyroidism, who are not experiencing excess body fat, are actually the main reason for over weight which over accumulating of subcutaneous protein and water. Fat accumulation is more obvious in the neck if patient was overweight, and the facial feature resembles moon face. Meanwhile, hypothyroidism patients have symptoms such as dull expression, bradypragia, slow-pronunciation, low-voice, feeling-cold, hypohidrosis, yellowish white coarse skin, nonpitting edema, hair loss and constipation etc.
8. Cortisol-induced obesity: Excess secretion of cortisol caused by hyperadrenalism leads to a set of symptoms, which is called Cushing's syndrome. It presents with central obesity, plethora figure, round face, purple striae skin, hypertension and other associated symptoms, such as, impaired glucose tolerance, sometimes diabetes mellitus, amenorrhea or menstrual disorder, male impotence, female masculinization, osteoporosis, and even fractures.
9. Pancreatic obesity: Weight gain before diabetes mellitus when it onsets in middle age or elderly. The body fat is evenly distributed, with full subcutaneous fat.

10. Gonadal obesity: It usually onset after gonadectomy or radiation related gonad damage. Adipose are mainly distributing below the waist, bottom and thigh. In female, the presentation has no significant difference between amenorrhea or menopause.
11. Obesity-hypoventilation syndrome: It also known as Pickwickian syndrome, whose etiology is not reveal, presented with dwarfism, obesity, hypoventilation, drowsiness, cyanosis, acropachia, secondary polycythemia, periodic respiration and right heart failure.

Key Points in History Taking

1. Dietary habit and diet composition;
2. Family history;
3. For adult, asking about menstruation, sexual function and fertility condition;
4. Occurring time, trigger, changes in particular body parts, and associated symptom.

5 Emaciation

Jialin Chen and Rui Zeng

Nowadays, there are two definitions about emaciation at home and abroad. If body weight is lower than 10% standard weight of normal population, it is called emaciation. Generally, many low-weight people don't have any disease. So a new definition is made: below 10% standard weight of normal population is called emaciation, lower than 20% standard weight can be called as significant weight loss. The other definition is comparing with previous weight. In physiological or pathological condition, weight loss exceeds 5% of previous weight in 6–12 months is called involuntary body weight loss or unintentional body weight loss. Weight is affected by genetic, nutrition, digestion-absorption, consumption and so on. There are low weight children, which is not definitely a pathological state. In clinical practice, most time we should compare with patients' previous weight.

5.1 Etiology and Pathogenesis

Negative balance between absorption and consumption is the main reason of weight loss. Details as follow:

- Nervous-endocrine diseases increases catabolism rate.
- Chronic contagious diseases, infection, connective tissue diseases, tumor, hematopathy and trauma can increase energy consumption.
- Gastrointestinal diseases cause digestive and absorption dysfunction.
- Drugs, to like thyroxine and amphetamine, can significantly promote metabolism. Long-term use of laxative can affect absorption function. Other oral medicines, such as aminophylline, ammonium chloride, aminosalicylic acid and estrogen, can cause anorexia and epigastric discomfort, thus leading to intake and absorption dysfunction, causing emaciation.
- Psychosomatic disease like mental stress, anxiety and depression might cause anorexia

5.2 Clinical Manifestations and Accompanying Symptoms

1. Malnutrition: Such diseases, caused by insufficient calorie intake, are as follows:
   - Oropharynx diseases: include oral ulcer, glossitis, alveolar abscess, toothache, osteomyelitis of mandible, pharyngolaryngeal and esophagus tumor.
   - Gastrointestinal diseases and others: such as nephropathy and pregnancy, which lead to severe vomiting and diarrhea. Those may decrease food intake or digestion and absorption function.
   - Hepatobiliary diseases: usually accompanied with fever, jaundice, epigastric discomfort and stool character change.
   - Pancreatic diseases: may present with epigastric discomfort, abdominal pain, nausea, vomiting, severe pancreatic diarrhea, even cachexia.
2. Chronic consumptive diseases
   - Gastrointestinal diseases: related symptoms and signs.
   - Chronic hepatitis: presented with fatiguemalasia, anorexia, nausea, abdominal distention and hepatalgia. Sometimes, it is accompanied with jaundice and low heat.
   - Tuberculosis: symptoms as low heat, night sweats, cough and hemoptysis.
   - Tumor: may accompanied with cachexia and tumor-relate symptom and sign.
   - Connective tissue diseases: clinical manifestations are arthralgia, rash, hair loss, oral ulcer, Raynaud's phenomenon, amyosthenia and so on.

J. Chen
Department of Internal medicine, Peking Union Medical College, Beijing, China

R. Zeng (✉)
Department of Cardiology, Sichuan University, Chengdu, China

X.-H. Wan, R. Zeng (eds.), *Handbook of Clinical Diagnostics*, https://doi.org/10.1007/978-981-13-7677-1_5

3. Endocrine diseases
   - Hyperthyroidism: may accompany with heat intolerance, hidrosis, anxiety, irritability, tremor, hyperactivity, palpitation, polyphagia, increase defecation, exophthalmos and goiter.
   - Diabetes mellitus: typical manifestations are "three polys and one little", which stands for excessive drink, excessive food, diuresis, and weight loss.
   - Addison's disease: may be accompanied with skin pigmentation, fatigue, anorexia, hypotension, hypoglycemia and suppressed immune system.
   - Sheehan's syndrome: symptoms of hypoadrenocorticism, such as hypogonadism, amenorrhea, agalorrhea, ochrodermia, hair loss and so on.
4. Anorexia nervosa: Anorexia nervosa can presented with severe weight loss, accompanied by vellus hair, amenorrhea, bradycardia, hyperactivity and self-induced vomiting. The features are as follows:
   - Being mostly young females and usually below 25 years old, with eating disorder.
   - Having significant weight loss, usually below 25% of normal weight in population; however, they are in good condition.
   - Presenting usually with amenorrhea; if body weight returns to normal, the menstruation will back.
   - Needing apart from other organic or mental diseases.
5. Psychical and psychological diseases: Such as depression, may lead to severe emaciation for anorexia or apocleisis.

Key Points in History Taking

Basically, they are same with obesity. Attention should be made to inquire personality, work and life pressure.

1. Dietary habit, diet composition, food quantity, exercise;
2. Emaciation onset-time, weight loss rate, trigger, change site of the body and associated symptom;
3. Family history;
4. For adult, ask about menstruation, sexual function and fertility condition;
5. Socio-psychological factors.

6 Anemia

Jialin Chen and Rui Zeng

Anemia is defined as a significant reduction in the mass of circulating red blood cells or the concentration of hemoglobin. Nowadays, we mostly use automated instruments to count the red blood cells and hemoglobin in the peripheral blood. The normal values slightly vary with the age of the individual, with gender and location (especially the altitude above sea level). In general, normal levels is shown in Table 6.1. At present, domestic standard for the diagnosis of anemia is as follows, in adults, Males: Hb < 120 g/L, Females: Hb < 110 g/L, Pregnancy: Hb < 100 g/L. But China is a country with vast expanse of territory, the normal ranges for these values can be slightly varied in different areas.

6.1 Etiology and Pathogenesis

Anemia is not the name of a disease. Due to hypoxia, it has specific signs and symptoms. There are many kinds of classification methods for anemia, and three of which are used widely: (a) According to the morphology of red blood cells, we can divide anemia into normocytic, macrocytic and microcytic anemia (Table 6.2); (b) On the basis of etiology and pathogenesis, anemia can be caused by the underproduction of red cell, increased destruction of red cell and excessive loss of red cell (Table 6.3); (c) According to the hyperplasia of the bone marrow, we can also classify it into hyperplasia anemia and dyshyperplasia anemia. The causes of anemia usually are not single factor, may be several factors at the same time.

6.2 Clinical Manifestation

No matter what causes the anemia, it has the common clinical manifestation. The signs and symptoms are caused by dysfunction of body systems due to the reduction of the oxygen carrying capacity of the blood. The clinical presentation of anemia is depending on the severity, rapidity of the hemorrhage, body's compensatory, adaptive capacity to hypoxia, and conditions of patient's physical activity. The common clinical manifestations of anemia are as follows.

1. General manifestation: Pallor of the skin and mucous membrane is the most commonly and remarkably encountered physical finding in patients with anemia. Observation of the nail beds, wrinkles of palm skins, oral mucous membranes and palpebral conjunctivas is usefulness as a physical finding. Fatigue, weakness, dizziness, tinnitus, memory loss and distraction are the early and common symptoms of anemia. The symptoms of severe anemia often have mild fever, withered skin, Matt's hair and even appear bloated legs.
2. Cardiovascular system: Patients with mild anemia may complain of palpitations and dyspnea after exercise. If the patients have moderate anemia, cardiac output is likely to rise, with an increase in heart rate. Patients with severe anemia may develop complaints due to angina or cardiac failure. Tachycardia, forceful heartbeat, wide pulse pressure are noted in physical finding. Some patients usually have cardiomegaly, and a systolic ejection murmur is often heard over the precordium, particularly at the pulmonic area.
3. Digestive system: Gastrointestinal symptoms such as anorexia, nausea, vomiting, abdominal distension, or even diarrhea is apparent. Some may take obviously glossitis. Apart from the hypoxia of anemia, these presentations may be related to primary digestive system diseases.

J. Chen
Department of Internal medicine, Peking Union Medical College, Beijing, China

R. Zeng (✉)
Department of Cardiology, Sichuan University, Chengdu, China

X.-H. Wan, R. Zeng (eds.), *Handbook of Clinical Diagnostics*, https://doi.org/10.1007/978-981-13-7677-1_6

Table 6.1 Normal values for red blood cell measurements

Measurement	Unit	Normal range
Red blood cell (RBC) count	$\times10^{12}$/L	Males: 4.0–5.5 Females: 3.5–5.0
Hemoglobin	g/L	Males: 120–160 Females: 110–150
Hematocrit(HCT) Mean cell volume (MCV)[a]	% fl	35–50 82–97
Mean cell hemoglobin (MCH)[b]	pg	27–32
Mean cell hemoglobin concentration(MCHC)[c]	g/L	320–360
Reticulocyte percentage	%	0.8–2.0

[a]MCV(fl) = Hct(%) × 10/RBC count($\times10^{12}$/L)
[b]MCH(pg) = Hb(g/L)/RBC count($\times10^{12}$/L)
[c]MCHC = Hb/Hct
*Actual normal ranges for many of these values may vary slightly, depending on factors such as the location and type of laboratory instruments used, altitude above sea level, and patient age

Table 6.2 Anemia due to morphology of red blood cells

Normocytic Anemia (MCV80–100 fl)	Macrocytic Anemia (MCV>100 fl)	Microcytic Anemia (MCV<80 fl)
Acute blood loss Early iron deficiency anemia Anemias of chronic disease Myelosuppression(may be Macrocytic) Aplastic anemia Pure red blood cell aplastic anemia Chronic renal insufficiency	Megaloblastic Myelodysplastic syndrome Hemolytic anemia Liver disease Alcoholism Medications	Iron deficiency anemia Thalassemia Anemias of chronic disease Sideroblastic anemia Lead exposure

Table 6.3 Anemia due to etiology and proliferation of bone marrow

The pathogenesis of anemia	Clinical disease
Underproduction of red cells	
Abnormalities in hemopoietic stem cell and microenvironment	Aplastic anemia, Myelofibrosis, Tumor invasion of the bone marrow
Insufficient hematopoietic raw material	Megaloblastic
Synthesis disorders of red blood cells	Iron deficiency anemia, Thalassemia
Increased destruction of red cell	Autoimmune hemolytic anemia, Hereditary spherocytosis, Hypersplenism
Blood loss	Any conditions that result in the excessive loss of red blood cells

4. Urogenital system: Manifestations include polyuria, low urine specific gravity are attributable to the reduction of the renal function of concentration at early stage. And even proteinuria occurs in severe anemia. Moreover, abnormal menstruation(amenorrhea) and loss of libido is quite common.

6.3 Accompanying Symptom

In addition to the common clinical manifestations of anemia, individuals with different causes of anemia often have different associated symptoms. Common types of anemia are as follows.

1. Iron deficiency anemia: Patients may complain of frizzy, brittle and dry hair, and fingernails (koilonychia), glossitis, dysphagia and pica, together with malnutrition that leads to anemia. Symptoms such as maransis, poor skin elasticity are attributed to malnutrition. Anemia caused by digestive system diseases may accompany with digestive symptoms.
2. Vitamin B12 and folate deficiency: Patients with anemia can have digestive symptoms such as anorexia, abdominal distension, diarrhea and glossitis. Glossitis stands out, atrophic lingual papilla, smooth surface, showing as "beefy tongue". B_{12} deficiency may accompany with combined degeneration of lateral and posterior funiculus of spinal cord, resulting in peripheral polyneuritis, which makes difficulties in walking and loss of sense of touch, topognosis and vibratory. Emotional change can also occur in combination with folate deficiency.
3. Aplastic anemia: Patients with aplastic anemia are often associated with bleeding tendency and infections. The patient's bleeding site is wide. Besides bleeding spots in the skin and ecchymosis, deep position bleeding is common such as hematochezia, hematuria and intracranial hemorrhage. Fever can occur more frequently in patients with infections.
4. Hemolytic anemia: Yellow-color of skin and mucous membrane is one of the important symptoms of hemolysis. Acute hemolysis such as different group blood transfusion may be accompanied by severe aching pain in

lower back and limbs, headache, vomiting, chills and high fever, even peripheral circulatory failure or acute renal failure, following with hemoglobinuria and jaundice. Chronic hemolysis may lead to varying degrees of jaundice, hepatosplenomegaly and bile pigment gallstones.

5. Anemia of blood system tumor diseases: Anemia caused by Lymphoma, acute leukemia and malignant histiocytosis usually accompanies obviously systemic or local lymphadenopathy and hepatosplenomegaly.

In a word, we can find out the etiology of anemia on various concomitant symptoms by the other characteristics linked to diseases.

Key Points in History Taking

1. The occurring time of the anemia, course and various symptoms of anemia.
2. The history of acute or chronic hemorrhage, melena and soy colored urine; If females have menorrhagia.
3. Nutritional status, picky eater or not, weight loss; the history of digestive system diseases such as peptic ulcer, gastric cancer and hemorrhoids.
4. The contact history of chemical toxicant, radioactive materials or special medicaments. If does, you should ask the concentration of toxicant in the environment, contact form, duration, protective measures and the name of the drug, dosage and course in detail.
5. The family history of anemia, consanguineous marriage of parents or not, anemia occurring in infant or not, similar attack in the past or not.
6. Youth and rural patients should ask the history of parasite infection, such as hookworm, roundworm infection.
7. It is also important for the history of chronic inflammation, infection, liver and kidney disease, connective tissue diseases and malignant tumor.

Mucocutaneous Hemorrhage

7

Jialin Chen and Rui Zeng

Mucocutaneous hemorrhage are typically characterized by spontaneous or slightly traumatic bleeding resulting from the coagulopathies and hemostatic disorders, which means that circulating blood infiltrating into the skin or submucosal tissue from the capillaries. This kind of bleeding should be distinguished with the local severe bleeding because of the damage of vascular caused by trauma, surgery, ulcer, tumor necrosis and rupture of varicose veins and hemangioma. The latter type does not belong to the scope of this chapter.

7.1 Etiology and Pathogenesis

The health individual has perfect and complex hemostatic function. When vascular injury hemorrhage, the circulating blood is rapid to be coagulated and is localized to the area of vascular injury, preventing continuous bleeding caused by slightly injuries. Under the pathological circumstances, slightly injuries can appear severe bleeding tendency that leads to the skin, mucosal bleeding because of the hemostasis and coagulation deficiencies, or hyperfunction of anticoagulative system.

Basic causes of skin and mucous membrane bleeding include three aspects: vascular wall abnormalities, abnormal quantity or function of platelet and coagulation dysfunction.

1. Vascular wall abnormalities: Blood vessel can be divided into arteries, veins and capillaries. Normal structure and function of vascular wall are critical factors to ensure the blood fluidity. Artery and vein wall is composed of three layers: the inside membrane, membrane and the outer membrane. Capillary wall is basically a layer of endothelial cells, only basement membrane and thin layer of connective tissue outside the endothelial. Under normal circumstances, injured blood vessel can make the smooth muscle of the middle blood vessel wall reflexive contraction through axon reflex, resulting in the closure of the distal capillary, slowing blood flow to stop bleeding. In addition, some humoral factors such as catecholamines, 5-serotonin, angiotensin, thromboxane A2 (TXA2) after the platelet activation, and endothelin generated by endothelial cells can also make blood vessels constrict. When blood vessels, especially the capillaries, have a structural abnormalities or systolic dysfunction due to hereditary or acquired defects, it can cause skin and mucosal bleeding.

   Hereditary telangiectasia is commonly seen in hereditary defects in the blood vessel wall, while Henoch-Schonlein Purpura, Purpura Simplex, senile Purpura, and Vitamin Deficiency Purpura is common in acquired defects.
2. Abnormalities of blood platelets: Platelets play an important role in the process of hemostasis. When vascular wall injured, platelet is activated at a site of vascular injury through the adhesion of platelets to the local endothelial intimal surface (platelet–vessel wall interaction) and the adhesion is mediated by von Willebrand factor, which sticks circulating platelets to the area of damaged vessel wall. The activated platelets undergo a "release reaction," including adenosine diphosphate (ADP), simultaneously elaborate thromboxane A2 and so on. The factors, such as ADP and thromboxane A2 can activate additional platelets from the circulation to the site of vascular injury. The result is rapid formation of a hemostatic clot that consists of platelets and fibrin, and is localized to the area of vascular injury. Activated platelets can simultaneously release other components like platelet factors, 5-hydroxytryptamine and storage coagulation factors, participating in the process of blood coagulation and making blood clot contraction. Abnormal platelet counts resulting in mucocutaneous hemorrhage can be found in a variety of primary and secondary thrombocytopenia, such as Idiopathic Thrombocytopenic Purpura, secondary immune Thrombocytopenic Purpura, aplastic anemia,

J. Chen
Department of Internal Medicine, Peking Union Medical College, Beijing, China

R. Zeng (✉)
Department of Cardiology, Sichuan University, Chengdu, China

X.-H. Wan, R. Zeng (eds.), *Handbook of Clinical Diagnostics*, https://doi.org/10.1007/978-981-13-7677-1_7

hypersplenism. Platelet dysfunction can be congenital abnormalities, such as thrombasthenia, giant platelet syndrome; can also be acquired abnormalities, such as secondary to drugs, uremia, liver disease, and abnormal immune globulin serum.

3. Coagulation deficiencies: Human blood coagulation process is extremely complex, which is a series of plasma coagulation factors enzyme-activated one after another, resulting the thrombin to form a fibrin clot in order to achieve the purpose of stopping the bleeding. During the process of hemostasis, fibrinolysis system in the body also starts, and its main role is to dissolve the fibrin deposited in the blood vessels to maintain vessel patency, preventing thrombosis. Due to the deficiencies and/or dysfunction of coagulation factors, or fibrinolysis hyperthyroidism, the blood coagulation is going wrong, resulting in mucocutaneous and deep tissue hemorrhage. Common causes include:

(A) The absence or dysfunction of coagulation factors: such as congenital coagulation factor deficiency of hemophilia A, hemophilia B; lack of coagulation factors I, II, V, VII; von Willebrand disease (vWD). Acquired coagulation factor deficiency or dysfunction or dysfunction includes severe liver disease, drug poisoning such as Warfarin overdosage, which is the antagonist of the vitamin K, and Antiphospholipid Antibody Syndrome, etc. (B) During certain conditions of some disease, bleeding caused by the hyperfunction of the fibrinolytic system, such as disseminated intravascular coagulation (DIC).

7.2 Clinical Manifestation

Although various hemorrhagic disorders may appear mucocutaneous and deep tissue hemorrhage, vascular and platelet disorders are the most common.

According to the site, degree and scope of bleeding, there are several common types of mucocutaneous hemorrhage, each hemorrhagic manifestations can appear alone or coexist in one patient.

1. Bleeding spots: Also known as petechiae, referring to that the diameter of the mucocutaneous hemorrhage does not exceed 2 mm, like needle size, which can be found in all parts of the body, especially in the lower torso and limbs. Bleeding spots is usually not higher than skin surface, unfading under pressure, dark red in early stage, and totally absorbed about a week. Small bleeding spots should be identified with the red mole, both of them do not fade under pressure, but the latter has more bright color, and slightly higher than skin surface. Bleeding spot is common in thrombocytopenia and dysfunction.
2. Purpura: Diameter of subcutaneous hemorrhage is in 3–5 mm which is the same characteristics as bleeding spot. Purpura is common in thrombocytopenia, abnormal function of platelet and blood vessel wall defects.
3. Ecchymosis: Diameter of subcutaneous hemorrhage excess 5 mm, which is common seen in limbs easily rubbed and bumped and acupuncture point. It is usually not higher than skin surface, unfading under pressure, dark red or purple in early stage, gradually turning into a tawny, yellow or yellowish-green, and totally absorbed about two weeks. Ecchymosis is suggestive of blood vessel wall defects and dysfunction of blood coagulation. Large areas of ecchymosis can be seen in serious coagulation disorders, hyperfunction of fibrinolysis and severe thrombocytopenia and dysfunction.
4. Deep tissue and subcutaneous hematoma: It is characterized by large areas of subcutaneous hemorrhage and ecchymoses, accompanying with obvious swelling of skin or joint cavity. It is common in serious dysfunction of blood coagulation disorders, inherited such as von Willebrand disease, acquired such as circulating anticoagulant, sweet bean overdose.
5. Hemophysallis: Dark black or purple blister-like bleeding, vary in size; can be often found in the mouth and tongue etc., which is common in severe thrombocytopenia.
6. Hemorrhinia: Hemorrhinia, also known as epistaxis, is bleeding from the nose. In most cases, the amount of bleeding is less, occasionally emergency department visit due to heavy bleeding. In addition to nasal mucosal lesions and inflammation, a vascular abnormality in nasal mucosa (such as Hereditary Telangiectasia), thrombocytopenia and dysfunction, coagulation abnormalities are also common causes of nose bleeding.
7. Bleeding gums: Causes are common in gum inflammation and injury, which can also be thrombocytopenia, severe blood coagulation disorders and vitamin deficiencies.

7.3 Accompanying Symptom

Symmetric purpura in limbs with joint pain, abdominal pain, and hematuria, which is mainly seen in Henoch-Schonlein Purpura; Purpura with generalized bleeding, such as nasal bleeding, gum bleeding, hematuria, and melena, can be found in thrombocytopenic purpura and disseminated intravascular coagulation (DIC); Purpura with jaundice found in liver disease; Sustained bleeding after minor injuries since childhood, with joint swelling and deformity, found in Hemophilia; Bleeding with gum swelling, excessive keratinization of skin and hair follicle should exclude vitamin C deficiency; With symptoms of increased intracranial pressure and compression of central nerve should consider intracranial hemorrhage; Arthritis or multi-system damage should be alert to diffuse connective tissue disease; Bleeding with fever, sterna tenderness, anemia are important signs of acute leukemia, accompanied with skin and mucous membrane pale should think of aplastic anemia.

Key Points in History Taking

1. Onset age: Bleeding of childhood implies congenital bleeding disorder, and adult onset is mainly due to acquired factors.
2. Gender: In the hereditary bleeding disorders, Hemophilia is common in male, and von Willebrand disease (vWD) in both male and female. Young women with repeated ecchymosis in lower limbs should is common in Purpura Simplex.
3. Incentives, location, distribution and characteristics: The location, size, distribution, duration, fading and frequency of mucocutaneous hemorrhage should be focused on asking.
4. Pay attention to the concomitant symptom: Whether there is fever, pain, proteinuria, hematuria, arthritis, rash and multiple system damage.
5. Past history: Pay attention to ask past medical history,diagnosis and treatment.

Cough and Expectoration

8

Ke Wang and Rui Zeng

Cough is a human body's defensive reflex action to clear respiratory secretions and foreign body. But persistent, frequent and severe cough interferes with work and rest, causes sore throat, hoarseness and respiratory muscle pain. Cough is also one of the most common symptoms of respiratory system diseases. A protracted severe cough may result in complications in those people who accompany underlying diseases, such as respiratory infections diffusion, bleeding, spontaneous pneumothorax, angina pectoris, cerebral hemorrhage, etc. Sputum is the trachea, bronchial secretions or exudate of the alveoli. The elimination of sputum from the lungs by coughing is called expectoration.

8.1 Etiology and Mechanism

The cough reflex and expectoration can be initiated by a wide variety of stimuli, especially bronchopulmonary and pleural diseases.

1. **Respiratory diseases**: Irritation to the whole mucous membrane of respiratory tract from nasopharynx to small bronchi can cause cough. The most sensatory points are located in the laryngeal arytenoid gap and tracheal bifurcation. Various parts of the respiratory tract (such as pharynx, larynx, trachea, bronchi, alveoli) stimulated by irritating gas inhalation (such as hot and cold air, chlorine, bromine, ammonia), smoke, dust, airborne fine particulate matter (PM2.5, PM10), foreign body, inflammation, tumor and bleeding may cause cough. It is one of the earliest symptoms of diseases, such as asthma, chronic bronchitis, pneumonia, lung cancer, etc.
2. **Pleural diseases**: Pleurisy, pleural mesothelioma and pleural stimulation (such as spontaneous or traumatic pneumothorax, hemothorax, and pleural puncture) may also cause cough.
3. **Cardiovascular diseases**: Pulmonary hypertension, pulmonary congestion, pulmonary edema and pulmonary embolism may cause cough through transudation or exudation from alveoli and bronchia stimulating alveolar walls and bronchial mucosa.
4. **Gastro-esophageal reflux disease (GERD)**: Reflux content may irritate and damage airway due to the anti-reflux mechanism weakened. A few GERD patients show cough and asthma as the first or main symptom. The reflux of liquid into the lungs may result in aspiration pneumonia and pulmonary fibrosis.
5. **Central nervous mechanisms**: Cough can originate from the cortex (voluntary cough). The impulses are transmitted from cortex to the medulla cough center, which sends impulses to the muscular system of chest and the larynx. Encephalitis and meningitis can also cause cough.

Coughing action is caused by the stimulation from afferent nerve fibers to relative respiratory muscles. The mechanical events involved in a typical cough are rapid successions of: (1) a rapid and short inspiration; (2) the tight closure of the glottis; (3) the quick and forceful contraction of the expiratory muscles; and (4) the sudden opening of the glottis. High velocity of airflow takes the secretions and foreign body away from the airway.

Expectoration is the action that expels respiratory or oral secretions by coughing. Usually, a thin layer of mucus produced by the submucosal bronchial glands and the goblet cells covers the cilium to keep the airway membrane moist. An increase in volume and viscosity of bronchial secretions often occurs in infection or irritation of the lungs, which induce the congestion of membrane, edema, increasing of the permeability of capillary. The exudate, mucus, red blood cells, white blood cells, macrophages, fibrin, fine particles of dust inhaled, pathogens and certain tissue destruction products mix together into sputum.

K. Wang
Department of Respiratory, Jilin University, Changchun, China

R. Zeng (✉)
Department of Cardiology, Sichuan University, Chengdu, China

X.-H. Wan, R. Zeng (eds.), *Handbook of Clinical Diagnostics*, https://doi.org/10.1007/978-981-13-7677-1_8

Therefore, it is important to pay attention to the clinical significance of related examination of the airway deep sputum. For example, tumor cells, virus, bacterial, atypical pathogenic body, ameba and some parasite eggs can be detected through the sputum or bronchoalveolar lavage fluid in patients with lung cancer, respiratory infection and parasitic lung disease. In the pulmonary congestion or edema, the leakage of serosity from pulmonary capillary can initiate expectoration. Frothy, pink secretion is characteristic of pulmonary edema.

8.2 Clinical Manifestation

1. **Cough characteristics**: Cough without sputum is called dry cough or unproductive cough. It is usually caused by acute pharyngitis, early stage of acute bronchitis, lung cancer, pleurisy, laryngeal tuberculosis, mitral stenosis, primary pulmonary hypertension, interstitial pneumonia, etc.

   Cough with sputum is called productive cough. It is caused by chronic obstructive pulmonary disease (COPD), pneumonia, lung abscess, bronchiectasis, cavitary pulmonary tuberculosis, lung cyst infection, bronchial fistula, etc.
2. **The duration and pattern of cough**
   - Cough initiated suddenly is mostly developed by acute laryngitis, trachea-bronchitis, trachea or bronchial foreign body, whooping cough, endobronchial tuberculosis, trachea or bronchial bifurcation oppressed stimuli (such as the lymph nodes tuberculosis, cancer or aortic aneurysm), etc.
   - Chronic cough is often associated with chronic respiratory diseases such as COPD, cellulose bronchitis, bronchiectasis, pulmonary cyst, abscess, tuberculosis, idiopathic pulmonary fibrosis, pneumoconiosis, etc. In addition, cough caused by COPD, upper airway cough syndrome (UACS), bronchiectasis and lung abscess will become worse and with expectoration when changing body position in the early morning or at night.
   - Postprandial, supine, bending or paroxysmal nocturnal cough suggests GERD, having nothing to do with the season.
   - Nocturnal cough particularly associated with left heart failure. It may be related to the exacerbation of pulmonary congestion and increased excitability of the vagus at night.
3. **The tone quality of cough**
   - A "hoarseness" cough is common in laryngitis, laryngeal tuberculosis, laryngocarcinoma, recurrent laryngeal nerve paralysis, etc. Clearing the throat or having the feel of postnasal drip suggests UACS caused by rhinitis, sinusitis.
   - Cough with metal tone may be seen in compression of the trachea by mediastinal tumor, aortic aneurysm, lung cancer, lymphoma and sarcoidosis.
   - Paroxysmal protracted severe cough accompanied by a high-profile inspiratory stridor (cock-like cough) is often caused by whooping cough, epiglottis and larynx disease, and upper airway obstruction.
   - Low sound or silently cough is seen in patients with severe emphysema, extreme weakness, vocal cord paralysis, respiratory muscle weakness and phlegm obstruction.
4. **The character and volume of sputum**: Characteristics of sputum include mucoid, serous, mucopurulent, purulent, blood stained, etc.
   - Less sputum, mostly mucinous or mucopurulent is characteristically present in cases of acute respiratory inflammation.
   - Sputum of COPD is mostly sticky mucoid sputum. An exacerbation of COPD causes increased sputum volume and/or purulence.
   - Bronchiectasis, lung abscess, bronchial fistula often accompany with large amounts of sputum (purulent and yellow-green), especially in the morning and before sleeping. Sputum excretion is often brought on by changes in posture. It can be divided into three layers after placing for a certain length of time (upper layer is frothy, middle layer is serous or purulent serous, lower layer is necrosis substance).
   - Foul-smelling purulent sputum suggests anaerobic infections.
   - Yellow-green or viridis sputum suggests pseudomonas aeruginosa infection.
   - Sputum, being white and sticky, pulling into the wire and difficulty to cough up, suggests candida albicans infection.
   - Bulk thin serofluid sputum containing vermicelli-like material suggests hydatid disease (echinococcosis).
   - Pink frothy sputum is the characteristics of pulmonary edema.
   - It is indicative of cellulose bronchitis when coughing up pink or white flexible, tough quality of dendrimers after repeated severe cough.
   - It should be considered diffuse bronchioloalveolar carcinoma if cough hundreds to thousands milliliter of serofluid, frothy sputum daily.

8.3 Accompanying Symptoms

1. **Fever**: It is more common in respiratory infections, pleurisy, tuberculosis et al.

2. **Chest pain**: It is often present in a variety of pneumonia, pleurisy, lung cancer, pulmonary embolism, and pneumothorax, etc.
3. **Dyspnea**: It may be seen in laryngitis, laryngeal edema, laryngeal cancer, bronchial asthma, severe COPD, severe pneumonia, tuberculosis, massive pleural effusion, pneumothorax and pulmonary congestion, pulmonary edema, tracheal and bronchial foreign body etc.
4. **Large amount of purulent sputum**: It is common noted in bronchiectasis, lung abscess, lung cysts and bronchipleural fistula, etc.
5. **Hemoptysis**: It suggests tuberculosis, bronchiectasis, lung abscess, lung cancer, mitral stenosis, bronchial stones, pulmonary hemosiderosis and pulmonary hemorrhage-nephritic syndrome (Goodpasture syndrome), etc.
6. **Clubbed fingers (toes)**: It is commonly seen in bronchiectasis, lung abscess, bronchial carcinoma, and thoracic empyema, etc.
7. **Wheeze**: It is often seen in bronchial asthma, chronic asthmatic bronchitis, diffuse pan bronchiolitis (mostly expiratory wheezing), cardiac asthma, tracheal and bronchial foreign body and bronchial carcinoma.
8. **Nasal congestion**: Clearing the throat or having the feel of postnasal drip is considered to be UACS.
9. **Burning sensation**: In upper abdomen (under the xiphoid), acid reflux and significantly coughing after meal suggests GERD related cough.

Key Points in History Taking

1. What is the age of onset, duration and pattern of cough? Is it acute or chronic cough? Is it sudden or gradual? Whether there are differences between day and night? What is the relationship between chronic cough and seasonal climate?
2. What is the degree, sound and influence factor of cough? Is it severe or mild? Is it intermittent, continuous or paroxysmal? What is the pitch level and timbre? Does it become worse when stimulated by pungent smell? Whether accompany with wheezing, chest pain and fever?
3. Does the cough produce sputum? How about the amount, color, character of sputum? Does the sputum have any special smell? Whether has bloody sputum? What's the impact on expectoration in different position? Whether stratification will occur after sputum standing for?
4. Is there a history of occupational exposure? Such as occupational dust, fine particulate matter, toxic chemicals, bird droppings and animal contact history. Irritating cough can be considered as interstitial disease, including silicosis, beryllium poisoning, asbestosis or farmer disease, etc.
5. Is there a history of smoking? Cigarette smoke is toxic gas that may increase the risk of bronchitis, COPD and lung cancer in long-term smokers. Passive smoking (especially in children) is also risk factor for cough. More than 40 years old, long-term smokers should take lung cancer screening as early as possible if irritating cough occurs more than one month. The possibility of lung cancer progression, tuberculosis or HIV infection should also be considered when weight loss significantly.
6. Is there any special medication history? Pay attention to the side effects of drugs which can cause coughing, such as angiotensin-converting enzyme inhibitors (such as captopril).

9 Hemoptysis

Wang Ke and Rui Zeng

Hemoptysis refers to the bleeding of trachea, bronchus or lung tissue, the expectoration of blood from the mouth through coughing. The quantity of blood is not completely consistent with severity of disease. Small amount of bleeding sometimes only shows blood-tinged sputum, but blood effused from nose and mouth could block respiratory tract, and even cause suffocation in massive hemoptysis.

It sometimes has to be searched carefully using nasopharyngoscope to rule out the circumstance that blood may come from nose, mouth, upper gastrointestinal or respiratory tract, or the blood is expectorated from mouth exclusively. Firstly, check mouth and nasopharynx to observe whether there is local hemorrhagic foci. Nosebleed mostly flows from anterior naris, and hemorrhagic foci often are found below the front of nasal septum; nosebleed in posterior nasal cavity is easily confused with hemoptysis, especially when hemaorrhage volume is large. Blood flows through posterior naris along the soft palate and the posterior pharyngeal wall, making patients have foreign body sensation in the throat; checking with nasopharyngoscopy can make diagnosis more reliable. Hematemesis refers to the upper gastrointestinal bleeding disgorged through mouth. The distinction between hemoptysis and hematemesis is shown in Table 9.1.

Table 9.1 The distinction between hemoptysis and hematemesis

	Hemoptysis	Hematemesis
History	T.B, bronchiectasis	Ulcer, cihrrosis
Presymptom	Cough, chest uncomfortable	Vomit, nausea, epigastric uncomfortable
Mode of expectoration	Blood spitting	Vomiting
Color of blood	Bright red	Dark red and black
Material mixed with blood	Air bubble and sputum	Food debris and gastric juice
pH	Alkaline	Acid
Melena	No, occasionally swallowed	Yes, may continue for several days
Sputum character after bleeding	Bloody sputum for several days	Generally no sputum

9.1 Etiology and Mechanism

Hemoptysis is a clinical manifestation related to multidisciplinary diseases, which is common in bronchial and lung diseases, cardiovascular and hematological diseases, and acute infectious diseases.

1. **Bronchial disease**: Bronchial disease is often seen in bronchiectasis, bronchogenic carcinoma, bronchial tuberculosis and COPD, etc.; bronchial stones, benign bronchial tumors, non-specific bronchial mucosa ulcers are rarely seen. It is mainly due to inflammation, tumor or stones which damage bronchial mucosa, or increase capillary permeability or lead to rupture of submucosal vessels in lesions.
2. **Lung diseases**: Lung diseases such as tuberculosis, pneumonia, pulmonary abscess, pulmonary congestion, pulmonary embolism, pulmonary fungal disease, lung fluke disease, pulmonary amebiasis, pulmonary cysts, alveolitis, pulmonary hemosiderosis disease, malignant tumors lung metastasis. Lung diseases cause the increase of capillary permeability, blood exuding, or eroding small vessels to bleed.
3. **Cardiovascular diseases**: Cardiovascular diseases such as acute left ventricular failure, primary pulmonary hypertension, certain congenital heart diseases (such as atrial septal defect, patent ductus arteriosus causing pulmonary hypertension), pulmonary vasculitis, pulmonary arteriovenous fistula, etc. The mechanism is that pulmonary congestion leading to rupture of alveolar wall or endobronchial capillaries, or bronchi submucosal veins varices.
4. **Hematological diseases**: Hematological diseases such as idiopathic thrombocytopenic purpura, leukemia,

W. Ke
Department of Respiratory, Jilin University, Changchun, China

R. Zeng (✉)
Department of Cardiology, Sichuan University, Chengdu, China

X.-H. Wan, R. Zeng (eds.), *Handbook of Clinical Diagnostics*, https://doi.org/10.1007/978-981-13-7677-1_9

hemophilia, aplastic anemia; acute infectious diseases, such as epidemic hemorrhagic fever, lung hemorrhagic leptospirosis; rheumatic diseases such as Wegener granuloma swollen, Behcet's disease, systemic lupus erythematosus (SLE) and so on; bronchial endometriosis, etc. The mechanism is coagulation disorder, intimae of tracheal and bronchial endometriosis cyclical spalling causing bleed.

9.2 Clinical Manifestation

1. **Age of onset**: Young adults hemoptysis is common in tuberculosis, bronchiectasis, mitral stenosis and so on, people over 40 years old with a long history of heavy smoking should be considered to lung cancer; the elderly with chronic underlying diseases such as diabetes, tuberculosis, cerebrovascular disease with bulbar paralysis, presence of brick red gelatinous bloody sputum is often considered to be Klebsiella pneumonia, drinking water with bucking reaction should be thought of aspiration pneumonia.
2. **Signs and symptoms**: Minimal hemoptysis(less than 100 mL/d) is usually asymptomatic; moderate hemoptysis may show chest tightness, itchy throat, cough and other aura symptoms; massive hemoptysis(more than 500 mL/d or 100–500 mL once) presents coughing up a mouthful of blood or hemoptysis within a short time without stopping, often accompanied with bucking, fast pulse, cold sweats, polypnea, pale, nervous or fear, even drop in blood pressure, oliguria, cold limbs and other signs of shock.
3. **Color and character**: (a) brisk bleeding is commonly associated with tuberculosis, bronchiectasis, lung abscess, bleeding disorders, endobronchial tuberculosis; (b) ferruginous bleeding is seen in pneumococcal pneumonia; (c) brick red gelatinous bloody sputum suggests Klebsiella pneumoniae; (d) hemoptysis caused by mitral stenosis and pulmonary congestion is mostly dark red; (e) serous pink foamy bloody sputum is seen in pulmonary edema caused by left ventricular failure, severe pneumonia, ARDS; (f); hemoptysis caused by pulmonary infarction is viscous dark red.

9.3 Accompanying Symptoms

(a) hemoptysis with fever: It is seen in tuberculosis, pneumonia, lung abscess, epidemic hemorrhagic fever, etc. (b) hemoptysis with chest pain: It is more common in lobar pneumonia, tuberculosis, pulmonary embolism, bronchogenic carcinoma and so on. (c) hemoptysis with purulent sputum: It is commonly noted in bronchiectasis, lung abscess, tuberculous cavity and pulmonary cyst complicated with infection, purulent pneumonia. Bronchiectasis patients that show repeated hemoptysis without purulent sputum are called dry bronchiectasis. (d) hemoptysis with mucocutaneous hemorrhage: It is often present in blood diseases, epidemic hemorrhagic fever, leptospirosis hemorrhagic lung, rheumatic diseases. (e) hemoptysis with clubbing fingers (toes): It is commonly seen in bronchiectasis, lung abscess, bronchogenic carcinoma. (f) hemoptysis with jaundice: It suggests leptospirosis, lobar pneumonia, pulmonary infarction, etc.

Key Points in History Taking

1. Make sure if it is hemoptysis. Where does blood come from, respiratory tract, digestive tract, nose or oropharynx? Find out if there are apparent cause and prodromal symptoms? Observe the color of blood and the mixture in blood.
2. Color and characters of hemoptysis. Bright red blood is seen in a large amount of bleeding, faster bleeding or bronchial artery bleeding, but dark red blood is mostly found in bronchial venous bleeding.
3. The volume, character and odor of sputum. Serous pink foam sputum is the feature of pulmonary edema.A large number of serous water sputum is commonly associated with bronchioloalveolar carcinoma, in which cancer cells are easily found. Rusty sputum is mainly seen in lobar pneumonia.
4. Simultaneous phenomenon. If it is accompanied with fever, chest pain, dyspnea or other associated symptoms? Make sure if the severity of symptoms has the relationship with hemoptysis?
5. Personal life history. Find out if the patient has history of exposure to tuberculosis, smoking, occupational dust exposure history, history of eating raw seafood? Pay attention to menstrual history, hemoptysis caused by parasitic disease of lung or endometriosis.
6. Medication history. Check whether the drug can cause bleeding, especially anticoagulants.

Chest Pain

10

Shiming Liu and Rui Zeng

Chest pain is a common symptom in clinical practice, commonly caused by chest diseases. The level of chest pain varies based on individual pain thresholds and is not completely consistent with the severity of diseases.

10.1 Etiology

Chest pain can be caused by many diseases and is commonly found in chest diseases. Heart diseases are the most common causes of chest pain. Its causes include:

1. **Chest wall disease**: Subcutaneous cellulites, herpes zoster, intercostal neuritis, rib fracture, acute leukemia, multiple myeloma, ankylosing spondylitis, etc. Precordial pain can be caused by cervical spondylosis, namely, cervical angina pectoris.
2. **Cardiovascular disease**: Angina pectoris, acute coronary syndrome (ACS), myocarditis, acute pericarditis, aortic dissecting aneurysm, pulmonary embolism, hypertrophic obstructive cardiomyopathy, cardiovascular neurosis, etc.
3. **Respiratory disease**: Pleuritis, spontaneous pneumothorax, hemothorax, hemopneumothorax, pneumonia, acute bronchitis, pulmonary carcinoma, etc.
4. **Mediastinum disease**: Mediastinitis, mediastinal emphysema, mediastinal tumor, reflux esophagitis, esophageal hiatus hernia, esophageal carcinoma, etc.
5. **Others**: Subdiaphragmatic abscess, liver abscess, splenic infarction, hepatocellular carcinoma, etc. Sometimes, the diseased organ, with its local pain, may induce the pain of certain body surface or internal organ far away from the original lesion, namely, radiating pain or referred pain.

S. Liu
Department of Cardiology, Guangzhou Medical University, Guangzhou, China

R. Zeng (✉)
Department of Cardiology, Sichuan University, Chengdu, China

10.2 Clinical Manifestations

1. **Age of onset**: Chest pain in young adults should be considered as a symptom of tuberculous pleuritis, spontaneous pneumothorax, lobar pneumonia, myocarditis, cardiomyopathy, or rheumatic valvular disease. If the chest pain occurs in patients older than 40 years of age, diseases like angina pectoris, ACS, or pulmonary carcinoma should be considered first.
2. **Sites and radiation of chest pain**: (a) Chest pain related to the diseases of chest wall occurs in a confined space with localized tenderness. Inflammatory diseases can cause chest pain accompanied by red, swelling, and fever in a limited area. (b) Herpes zoster presents a seriously painful skin rash with blisters along one side of the intercostal nerve that are not beyond the front midline of the body surface. (c) Diseases of the esophagus and mediastinum cause retrosternal pain, which gets worse when eating or swallowing. (d) Hepatic and gall bladder diseases can cause chest pain in the lower right chest. (e) Chest pain resulting from angina pectoris or myocardial infarction is commonly located at the precordial, retrosternal, or subxiphoid area, which can radiate to the left shoulder, left arm inside, or even to the ring and little fingers, and sometimes to the left neck, pharynx, or cheek. (f) Chest pain resulting from acute pericarditis is commonly located at the retrosternal or precordial area, which may radiate to the neck, left shoulder, left arm, or left scapula, sometimes even to the upper abdomen. (g) Aortic dissection can cause thoracic and dorsal pain, radiating down to the lower abdomen, waist, both sides of the groin, and lower limbs. (h) Chest pain resulting from spontaneous pneumothorax, pleuritis, or pulmonary embolism is commonly located near the anterior axillary or midaxillary lines of the diseased side. (i) Chest pain resulting from pulmonary apex carcinoma, such as Pancoast cancer, is commonly located at the shoulder or the axilla, radiating to the interior of upper limbs.

X.-H. Wan, R. Zeng (eds.), *Handbook of Clinical Diagnostics*, https://doi.org/10.1007/978-981-13-7677-1_10

3. **Nature of chest pain**: Herpes zoster causes unbearable cutting or burning pain. Esophagitis causes burning pain. The pain resulting from Angina pectoris is a rushing type with sensation of asphyxia, while that of myocardial infarction is more severe with fear and dying sensation. Acute pericarditis causes sharp or crushing pain, the location and sites of radiation of which are similar to those of acute myocardial infarction. Dry pleuritis causes sharp, blunt, or tearing pain. Pulmonary carcinoma commonly causes chest tightness, while Pancoast cancer causes burning pain, especially during the nighttime. A dissecting aneurysm causes a sudden and unbearable tearing pain in the thorax and dorsum. Pulmonary infarction can also cause sudden and severe pricking pain or colic pain, usually accompanied by dyspnea and cyanosis.
4. **Duration of chest pain**: The pain caused by stenosis of vessels related to smooth muscle spasm is paroxysmal, while that of the inflammation, carcinomas, embolism, or infarction is continuous. For example, the pain only lasts for 1–5 min in angina pectoris, while it lasts for more than 30 min or several hours in myocardial infarction.
5. **Influencing factors of chest pain**: Multiple factors can induce, increase, or relieve the pain. The pain in angina pectoris can be induced by physical activity or mental stress. It can be relieved after resting or 1–2 min after the administration of sublingual nitroglycerin or isosorbide dinitrate. However, this treatment has no effect on the pain related to myocardial infarction. The pain resulting from esophageal diseases commonly occurs or worsens when eating, while it can be reduced or relieved by oral antacids or prokinetics. Chest pain resulting from pleuritis and pericarditis maybe worse by coughing or forced breathing.

10.3 Accompanying Symptoms

(a) Chest pain accompanied by cough, sputum, and/or fever is commonly seen in diseases of trachea, bronchus or lungs, especially in infectious diseases. (b) Chest pain accompanied by dyspnea may suggest a large-scope lesion, such as lobar pneumonia, spontaneous pneumothorax, pulmonary embolism, etc. (c) Chest pain accompanied by hemoptysis is commonly seen in pulmonary embolism, bronchogenic carcinoma, pulmonary tuberculosis, bronchiectasis, etc. (d) Chest pain accompanied by a pale complexion, hypotension, or shock is commonly seen in myocardial infarction, dissecting aneurysm, massive pulmonary embolism, etc. (e) Chest pain accompanied by dysphagia is commonly seen in esophageal diseases, such as reflux esophagitis, esophageal carcinoma, mediastinal diseases, etc.

Key Points in History Taking

Much attention should be paid in recording the following characteristics of the pain: onset time, nature, position, frequency, duration, precipitating factors, accompanying symptoms, etc. High incident diseases and their risk factors should also be noted, such as coronary heart disease with its risk factors including hypertension, hypercholesteremia, diabetes, etc., acute pulmonary embolism, dissecting aneurysm, anorexia, etc. Based on their characteristics, the most possible etiologies may be found and the necessary examinations can be prescribed further. The following characteristics of the pain should be noted and recorded:

1. Slow or rapid onset, position, area and radiation, and its effect on the patient.
2. Nature, degree, duration, precipitating factors, factors that worsen or relieve the pain, such as effects of coughing and deep breath, relationship with physical activity, food intake, emotion, etc.
3. With or without accompanying symptoms, such as fever, cough, sputum, hemoptysis, palpitation, cyanosis, dyspnea and their severity.
4. Others, such as occupation, hobbies, precipitating factors, relieving factors etc.

11 Dyspnea

Ke Wang and Rui Zeng

Dyspnea is usually described subjectively by the patient as "shortness of breath" or "out of breath", objectively manifests as overexertion in breathing motion. If the symptom becomes worse, it is always accompanied by mouth breathing, dilatation of nares, orthopnea, cyanosis, using of accessory muscles of respiration and abnormalities of respiratory rate such as depths or rhythms.

11.1 Etiology and Mechanism

Dyspnea can be caused by many reasons, especially respiratory and circulatory system diseases. Asthma, COPD, congestive heart failure and pulmonary edema are the main reasons, in addition, obesity, interstitial lung diseases, ischemic heart diseases can also lead to dyspnea.

11.1.1 Respiratory Dyspnea

The main manifestations: (a) Airway obstruction: laryngeal and airway diseases, such as acute epiglottitis, acute laryngitis, laryngeal edema, diphtheria, foreign body of larynx, trachea tumor, tracheal compression (goiter, mediastinal tumor, etc.), bronchial asthma, COPD, lung cancer and so on. (b) Pulmonary diseases: lobar or bronchial pneumonia, lung abscess, pulmonary edema, atelectasis, pneumoconiosis, diffuse interstitial lung disease, SARS (severe acute respiratory syndrome) and ARDS (acute respiratory distress syndrome), pneumocystis carinii pneumonia (PC), etc. (c) Chest wall, thoracic and pleural diseases: pneumothorax, large pleural effusion, widely significant pleural adhesion and thickening, severe chest trauma, and thoracic or spinal malformations, etc. (d) Nerve-muscle diseases and adverse drug reactions: poliomyelitis and motor neurone disease, including the cervical spinal cord and acute multiple nerve root neuritis, myasthenia gravis, drugs (muscle relaxants, aminoglycoside antibiotics, clindamycin) which lead to respiratory muscle paralysis, etc. (e) Diaphragm diseases and movement limitation: diaphragmatic paralysis, severe intestinal tympanites, massive ascites, abdominal huge tumor, gastric dilatation and late pregnancy, etc.

The mechanisms: (a) airway obstruction, chest and diaphragm movement dysfunction, respiratory muscles weakness and limited mobility induce pulmonary ventilation reduction and alveolar oxygen partial pressure (PaO_2) decrease. (b) The dyspnea of pulmonary parenchymal diseases are mainly due to pulmonary ventilation/perfusion (V/Q) imbalance. (c) The dyspnea of pulmonary edema, interstitial lung diseases are mainly because of oxygen diffusion dysfunction, resulting in arterial oxygen tension (PaO_2) decreased, causing breathing difficulties.

11.1.2 Cardiac Dyspnea

There are various reasons which can result in heart failure, such as cardiac tamponade, constrictive pericarditis, primary pulmonary hypertension and pulmonary embolism (mainly thromboembolism, amniotic fluid embolism and fat embolism), etc. Left heart failure is common in hypertensive heart diseases, coronary heart diseases, rheumatic heart diseases, myocarditis, cardiomyopathy, too much and too fast transfusion, etc.

The main mechanisms of left heart failure causing dyspnea include: myocardial contractility decreases or ventricular afterload (systolic and diastolic) increases, heart dysfunction, and left cardiac output decrease, which can result in end-diastolic hypertension (mitral stenosis is short of this process), leading to left atrial pressure, pulmonary venous pressure and capillary pressure increase in succession. The above pathophysiological process can cause that: (a) lung congestion leads to interstitial pulmonary edema,

K. Wang
Department of Respiratory, Jilin University, Changchun, China

R. Zeng (✉)
Department of Cardiology, Sichuan University, Chengdu, China

X.-H. Wan, R. Zeng (eds.), *Handbook of Clinical Diagnostics*, https://doi.org/10.1007/978-981-13-7677-1_11

blood vessel wall thickening, diffusion dysfunction; (b) increased alveolar tension irritates lung tension receptors, then excites respiratory center through vagus nerve; (c) decreased alveolar elasticity results in alveolar ventilation reduction; (d) increased pulmonary circulation pressure stimulates the respiratory center.

The main mechanisms of right heart failure that causes dyspnea are: (a) Increased pressure of right atrium and the superior vena cava can stimulate baroreceptor and reflexively excite the respiratory center; (b) oxygen content decrease, and acidic metabolites such as lactic acid, pyruvic acid increase, stimulating respiratory center; (c) congestive hepatomegalia, ascites and pleural effusion can lead to a limited respiratory movement, and pulmonary gas exchange area reduction.

11.1.3 Toxic Dyspnea

The main manifestations of toxic dyspnea as follows: (a) acidosis caused by various reasons, such as acute and chronic renal failure, diabetic ketoacidosis, renal tubular acidosis, etc. (b) acute infection and infectious diseases; (c) drugs and chemicals poisoning, such as morphine, barbiturates, benzodiazepines drugs, organophosphate insecticide poisoning and carbon monoxide, nitrites, aniline, cyanides (including almond, cassava that contain more hydride) poisoning, etc.

The main mechanisms of dyspnea are slightly different, which can be probably divided into: (a) the excitability of respiratory center increased when it is stimulated. Acidosis increases alveolar ventilation to exhaust CO_2 through indirect stimulation of the carotid sinus and aortic body chemical receptor or act directly on the respiratory center. (b) various intoxication have different influences on respiratory center. Carbon monoxide and hemoglobin form carboxyhemoglobin, nitrite and aniline can make hemoglobin into methemoglobin, resulting in the loss of oxygenation; cyanide restrains the activity of cytochrome oxidase so that cellular respiration is inhibited (asphyxia), leading to tissue hypoxia and dyspnea. Above kinds of dyspnea are not accompanied by hypoxemia, but alveolar hyperventilation can cause a lot of CO_2 excretion, resulting in $PaCO_2$ decreased. Morphine and sedative hypnotics poisoning have direct inhibition on respiratory center, causing breathing weakened and slow and alveolar ventilation reduced, if getting worse, it will not only cause hypoxemia but also CO_2 retention.

11.1.4 Neuropsychiatric Dyspnea

Neuropsychiatric dyspnea mainly manifests as follows: (a) organic brain diseases, such as traumatic brain injury, cerebrovascular diseases, encephalitis, meningitis, brain abscess and brain tumors, etc. (b) mental or psychological disorders, such as hysteria, depression, etc. The main mechanisms are: the former is due to the decrease of respiratory center excitability induced by increased intracranial pressure and decreased blood supplement; the latter is due to the effect of mental or psychological factors that lead to respiratory rate increasing significantly, hyperventilation causes respiratory alkalosis, respiratory inhibition even convulsion and unconsciousness.

11.1.5 Hematogenic Dyspnea

Hematogenic dyspnea is seen in severe anemia. It is because oxygen-carrying red blood cells are reduced, oxygen content is decreased and oxygen is insufficient for tissues. When bleeding or shock, rapid breathing is related to the stimulation to the respiratory center by ischemic and drop of blood pressure.

11.2 Clinical Manifestation

11.2.1 Respiratory Dyspnea

- Inspiratory dyspnea: hard to breathe, severe cases have visible indrawing of the suprasternal notch, the supraclavicular spaces and the intercostal spaces in the inspiratory process, which is called "three depression signs", Three depressions are due to the extreme effort of inspiratory muscles and increased chest negative pressure, always accompanied by dry cough and high pitched inspiratory wheezing, suggesting larynx, trachea or large bronchial stenosis and obstruction, which are common in endobronchial tuberculosis, upper airway mass, surgery and postoperative tracheotomy, etc.; It should be considered as foreign body obstruction (particularly in children), laryngospasm or laryngeal edema, if happen suddenly; If older, gradual emergence and get worse progressively, it should be considered as larynx, trachea or mediastinal malignancies; sudden fever is considered to be laryngitis, diphtheria, etc.
- Expiratory dyspnea: laborious expiration, expiratory time is obviously prolonged and slow, expiratory rhonchi by lung auscultation are mainly found in the obstruction of lower respiratory tract. Obstruction of lower respiratory tract, paroxysmal dyspnea with extensive wheezing can be relieved by bronchodilator, suggesting the acute exacerbation of bronchial asthma.
- Mixed dyspnea: breathing is extremely difficult during both inspiration and expiration, respiration is quick and shallow, and often accompanied by abnormal respiratory sounds (weakened or lost), pathologic respiratory sounds also can be heard. It is mainly seen in the extensive lung

parenchyma, interstitial lung disease and severe chest, diaphragm, pleura and nerve-muscle diseases, such as ARDS, severe pneumonia, myasthenia gravis, dermatomyositis, etc. Mixed dyspnea can also manifests significantly prolonged expiratory phase, the shape of chest is like barrel and pulmonary alveolar respiratory sounds are weakened, suggesting obstructive pulmonary emphysema.

11.2.2 Cardiac Dyspnea

Manifestations of dyspnea caused by left heart failure: (a) dyspnea happens or becomes worse on exertion, taking a rest can relieve or reduce. (b) It is exacerbated by supine position and relieved by sitting . Severe patients are often forced to take a half sitting or orthopnea. It is mainly because that cardiac load and body oxygen consumption increases when in activity, and venous return reduces and the degree of lung congestion mitigates when sitting, diaphragm becomes lower and mobility increases, vital capacity increases by 10–30% at the same time.

Paroxysmal dyspnea tends to occur primarily in acute left ventricular failure, often occurs in sleeping during the night, called paroxysmal nocturnal dyspnea. The reasons are: (a) excitability of vagus nerve increases during sleeping, leading to coronary vasoconstriction, reducing myocardial blood supplement, decreasing cardiac function subsequently; Bronchiole constricts, which further reduces alveolar ventilation. (b) supine position reduces lung capacity, increases venous return, which makes the original pulmonary congestion worse. (c) susceptibility of respiratory center becomes lower at night, slowly in response to mild hypoxia caused by lung congestion, only when congestion significantly increased, it will "wake up" the respiratory center to make response.

Patients often suddenly feel oppression in chest and suffocation when sleeping, and wake up with a start, forced to sit, disturbed with fear, accompanied by cough. The mild one can gradually relieve after a few minutes to tens of minutes; dyspnea is aggravated in the severe cases, with facial cyanotic, profuse sweating and wheeze, even cough up a large number of serous bloody sputum or pink foamy sputum. The base of lungs have much moist rales, with heart rate increased. Gallop rhythm also exists in auscultation. Such dyspnea is also known as "cardiac asthma". It is common in the elderly hypertensive heart disease, coronary heart disease, rheumatic heart disease, myocarditis, cardiomyopathy and acute left ventricular dysfunction caused by congenital heart disease, etc. Right heart failure patients also take semi-sitting position to relieve dyspnea. Dyspnea caused by chronic pulmonary heart disease is related to the primary diseases; patients with pericardial diseases prefer to take forward position to relieve the heart oppression on the left lung.

11.2.3 Toxic Dyspnea

Patients with various acidosis performance regular big and deep breath (Kussmaul breathing), fast or slow, exhaled air can has urine (ammonia) taste (uremia) or rotten apple (diabetic ketoacidosis poisoning) because of different causes. Tachypnea is seen in acute febrile disease. Respiratory becomes deep and rapid, caused by abnormal hemoglobin derivatives (methemoglobinemia, vulcanization hemoglobinemia) in the blood or cyanide poisoning, the severe cases with cerebral edema can depress respiratory center then result in superficial and slow respiration, it may also have rhythm abnormalities, such as Cheyne-Stokes respiration and Biot breathing.

11.2.4 Neuro-Psychogenic Dyspnea

The respiration becomes deep and slow in patients suffering from craniocerebral diseases, often accompanied by snoring and severe breathing rhythm abnormalities, such as breathing containment (inspiratory abruptly terminated), suction (sobbing like breathing), etc. The respiration of hysterical patients are often superficial, frequency up to 60–100/min, and often with respiratory alkalosis that lead to perioral and acral numbness or tetany because of hyperventilation. Neurosis patients often feel chest tightness and shortness of breath, but there is no objective performance of dyspnea, occasionally with sighing breath after a deep inspiration, then consciously relaxed and comfortable.

11.2.5 Hematogenic Dyspnea

Hematogenic dyspnea shows superficial respiration, tachypnea and tachycardia, associated with blood circulation disorders, thrombosis, coagulopathy, bleeding, anemia and hemoglobin oxygen-carrying dysfunction.

11.3 Accompanying Symptoms

(a) Dyspnea with diffuse pulmonary wheeze is present in bronchial asthma and cardiac asthma. (b) paroxysmal severe dyspnea is common in acute larynx edema, foreign body in bronchi, massive pulmonary embolism, spontaneous pneumothorax, ARDS, etc. The latter is accompanied by obvious cyanosis. (c) slow progressive dyspnea is often seen in COPD, diffuse interstitial pulmonary fibrosis, pneumocystis carinii pneumonia. (d) dyspnea with one side chest pain is frequently observed in lobar pneumonia, acute exudative pleurisy, pulmonary embolism, spontaneous pneumothorax, acute myocardial infarction and bronchial carcinoma, etc. (e) dyspnea with fever is commonly noted in pneumonia, lung abscess, caseous pneumonia, pleurisy, acute pericarditis, etc. (f) dyspnea with cough and purulent sputum is often seen in chronic bronchitis, obstructive pulmonary emphysema with infection, purulent pneumonia, lung abscess, bronchiectasis complicated with infection. (g) dyspnea with large amount of foamy sputum is found in acute left ventricular heart failure and organophosphorus pesticide poisoning or bronchioloalveolar carcinoma. (h) dyspnea with disturbance of consciousness is seen in the cerebral hemorrhage, meningitis, uremia, diabetic ketoacidosis, pulmonary encephalopathy, acute poisoning, etc.

Key Points in History Taking

1. Onset of urgency, sudden or gradual, reasons and incentives, the exposure history of drugs and poisons (kind of drug/poison, the name, dosage, administration and contact time) and various situations that lead to immune dysfunction.
2. Specific performance of dyspnea: inspiratory, expiratory, or mixed dyspnea?
3. Whether there is urination and dietary disorders, and high blood pressure, kidney disease and history of metabolic diseases?
4. Whether there is headache, unconsciousness or brain trauma history?

Cyanosis

12

Ke Wang and Rui Zeng

Cyanosis refers to a bluish color of the skin and mucous membranes resulting from an increased quantity of reduced hemoglobin (>50 g/L). It may also due to the rise of sulfhemoglobin (SHb), methemoglobin (MetHb) and carboxyhemoglobin (HbCO). Cyanosis can be not only systemic but also limited to peripheral, often seen in the thinner skin, less pigment and capillary-rich parts, such as tongue, lips, nose, earlobes, cheek and finger (toe) nail bed, etc.

12.1 Etiology and Mechanism

1. **Increase of reduced hemoglobin in the blood is mainly due to cardiopulmonary diseases**
   - Respiratory diseases: It is often seen in airway obstruction, pulmonary parenchyma and interstitial disease, such as pneumonia, COPD, pulmonary heart disease, diffuse interstitial pulmonary fibrosis, pulmonary congestion, pulmonary edema, ARDS, SARS and pulmonary vascular diseases (such as pulmonary embolism, primary pulmonary hypertension, pulmonary movement fistula etc.) Such diseases can lead to increase of reduced hemoglobin in systemic circulation because of dysfunction of ventilation and inadequate oxygenation.
   - Cardiovascular diseases: It is more common in heart failure and cyanotic congenital heart diseases, such as tetralogy of Fallot, Eisenmenger syndrome. The former is mainly owing to dysfunction of pulmonary gas exchange, and the latter is mainly due to abnormal passage between heart and the great vessels. A part of venous blood is out of oxygenation by lungs and then enters arterial blood systemic circulation through abnormal channels. Cyanosis will occur if sub-flow is more than 1/3 of the left cardiac output.
   - Peripheral circulation disorders: (a) local venous diseases, such as thrombophlebitis, varicose veins, superior vena cava syndrome, due to local hyperemia, surrounding slow blood flow, excessive oxygen uptake by tissue; (b) arterial insufficiency, found in shock, thrombosis obliterans, peripheral arterial occlusive atherosclerosis, Raynaud's disease, peripheral cyanosis disease, severe chills, livedo, vibration disease and hyperlipidemia agglutinin, cryoglobulinemia, etc.; (c) Shock caused by lack of circulating blood volume, reduced stroke volume and peripheral vessel spasm and shrink, slow blood flow, surrounding tissue hypoperfusion and hypoxia, leading to cyanosis; (d) Cold agglutinemia (common in mycoplasma pneumonia) and cryoglobulinemia, due to agglutination of red blood cells in the acral capillary and cryoglobulins agglutinate automatically blocking peripheral vascular caused by cold; (e) Cyanosis caused by polycythemia vera because of too many red blood cells, and high blood viscosity, resulting in slow blood flow, excessive oxygen uptake by tissue and increase of reduced hemoglobin.
   - Low oxygen partial pressure in inspiratory gas: at high altitude (>3500 m) areas with too low partial pressure of oxygen in the atmosphere leading to decreased alveolar oxygen partial pressure (PAO_2) and arterial oxygen saturation (SaO_2) decline, tissue hypoxia, even if without original cardiopulmonary disease, can also cause cyanosis, severe cases could happen in those with high altitude heart disease.
2. **Abnormal hemoglobin derivatives in blood**
   - Methemoglobinemia: caused by drug or chemical poisoning, such as primaquine, nitrite, perchlorate, sulfonamides, phenacetin, styrene alum, nitrobenzene aniline poisonings. Cyanosis presents when methemoglobin content in blood up to 30 g/L. Toxic methemoglobinemia caused by eating a large number of vegetables which containing nitrites deterioration, can also cause cyanosis, called "enterogenic cyanosis".

K. Wang
Department of Respiratory, Jilin University, Changchun, China

R. Zeng (✉)
Department of Cardiology, Sichuan University, Chengdu, China

X.-H. Wan, R. Zeng (eds.), *Handbook of Clinical Diagnostics*, https://doi.org/10.1007/978-981-13-7677-1_12

- Sulfhemoglobinemia: hydrogen sulfide is formed in the intestines of patients with constipation or after taking sulfide, acting on hemoglobin and forming the sulfthemoglobin. When the blood content up to 5 g/L, cyanosis appears.

12.2 Clinical Manifestation

1. **Increase of reduced hemoglobin.**
   - Central cyanosis: systemic cyanosis, in addition to the limbs and face, also found in the mucous membranes (including the tongue and oral mucosa) and trunk, with warm skin. It is mainly seen in cardiopulmonary insufficiency diseases and right-left shunt congenital heart diseases, often accompanied with palpitations, cough and asthma.
   - Peripheral cyanosis: cyanosis is most common in the peripheral limbs and sagging parts, such as extremities, earlobes and apex nasi. It appears when local skin temperature is low and cold due to poor peripheral circulation. Cyanosis may disappear when local skin becomes warm by massage or heat. This is helpful to distinguish from central cyanosis which will not disappear through massage or heat. In addition, it also could be caused by vein drainage disturbance, systemic venous congestion or tortuous veins, engorgement or tenderness in the parts of local drainage cyanosis, and local cold, pale or cyanosis coexist in patients caused by limb or peripheral arterial obstruction and spasm, with weakened or disappeared arterial pulse. For polycythemia vera, in addition to the cyanosis of extremities and lips, the face and thenar, hypothenar present fuchsia, conjunctival congestion, peripheral red blood cells and hemoglobin significantly increase.
   - Mixed cyanosis: both of the two types exist, seen in heart failure (left heart, right heart and whole heart failure) or the aforementioned cardiopulmonary diseases combining with peripheral circulatory failure.
2. **Abnormal hemoglobin derivatives exist in blood**
   - Methemoglobinemia caused by drug or chemical poisonings. Cyanosis can appear abruptly and temporarily with serious illness. Oxygen therapy can't diminish cyanosis. Blood appears dark brown and can't be transformed into bright red when exposure to air. Black absorption band is seen in 618–630 nm examined by spectroscope. Methylene blue, sodium thiosulfate or large doses of vitamin C by intravenous infusion can also make cyanosis subside.
   - Congenital methemoglobinemia: cyanosis appears since childhood has family history, without cardiopulmonary disease or other disorders causing abnormal hemoglobin, the body is generally healthy.
   - Idiopathic methemoglobinemia: seen in women, cyanosis is related to menstrual cycle, paroxysmal, the mechanism is not clear.
   - Sulfthemoglobinemia: cyanosis lasts for a long time, up to several months or longer. Because sulfthemoglobin can't be restored to hemoglobin no matter in vivo or in vitro, erythrocyte life are still normal; patients' blood is blue brown, absorption band is seen in 630 nm examined by spectroscope. Sometimes it is difficult to distinguish from methemoglobinemia. The presence of sulfthemoglobin can be ensured if absorption band disappear after adding potassium cyanide.

12.3 Accompanying Symptom

1. **Dyspnea** common in severe cardiopulmonary diseases and acute respiratory obstruction, pneumothorax, etc. Although congenital methemoglobinemia and sulfthemoglobinemia come with obvious cyanosis, but it generally is mild or no dyspnea.
2. **Clubbing fingers (toes)** mainly seen in cyanotic congenital heart diseases and certain chronic lung diseases such as diffuse interstitial lung disease, bronchiectasis, etc., with longer course.
3. **Acute onset with disoriented and weak performance** found in certain drugs or chemicals acute poisonings, shock, acute lung infection, etc.

Key Points in History Taking

1. **Inducement and performance of cyanosis**: It suggests congenital heart disease if cyanosis present since birth and with a history of squatting in the childhood; If cyanosis appeared since childhood, and no history of cardiopulmonary and abnormal hemoglobin is seen in congenital methemoglobinemia, consider whether children have wheeze laryngeal spasm, laryngeal tracheitis and acute subglottic laryngitis.
2. **Degree of cyanosis urgency**: Acute or subacute onset of cyanosis is seen in acute myocardial infarction, pneumothorax, pulmonary embolism, and pneumonia or airway obstruction. Chronic diseases are found in methemoglobinemia, COPD, pulmonary fibrosis or pulmonary arterio-venous fistula.
3. **Whether accompanied with dyspnea**: Obvious dyspnea suggests pulmonary or cardiac cyanosis (such as cyanotic congenital heart disease, emphysema, pulmonary fibrosis or pulmonary embolism). Note body temperature.
4. **Whether patients have relevant medical history**: Relevant medical history or intake history of drugs, chemicals, metamorphic vegetable associated with cyanosis, potassium chloride, sulfa drugs and coal tar products can cause methemoglobinemia and sulfthemoglobinemia.
5. **Systemic, localized or single limb cyanosis**: Profound shock can result in systemic cyanosis; circulatory disorder. Raynaud's disease can cause limbs cyanosis. Arterial thrombosis or venous thrombosis can caused single limb cyanosis.

13 Palpitation

Shiming Liu and Rui Zeng

Palpitation is defined as an uncomfortable sensation of a forceful, rapid or irregular beating of the heart. The sensation may be described as "fluttering" "flip-flopping" "pounding" or "jumping". Heart rate may be fast, slow, regular, or irregular. As palpitation is an occasional manifestation of potentially life-threatening arrhythmias, Detailed medical histories and physical examinations, followed by targeted diagnostic tests, are necessary to distinguish cardiac causes from others.

13.1 Etiology

The mechanism of palpitation is not clear yet. It may be related to the heart rate, rhythm, abnormal contraction, or sometimes only cardiovascular neurosis. Palpitation is a common and unspecific symptom, which can be seen in the heart diseases, systemic diseases, or healthy persons. There are different classifications for palpitation: pathological or physiological, cardiac or non-cardiac, and arrhythmic or non-arrhythmic. In this section, the arrhythmic and non-arrhythmic classifications are used by clinical preferences. All kinds of arrhythmias, including both bradyarrhythmias and tachyarrhythmias, may lead to palpitation, but the sensation is not completely consistent with severity of arrhythmias. The common causes of palpitation are summarized in Table 13.1.

Table 13.1 Common causes of palpitation

Classification	Common causes	
Arrhythmic	All kinds of arrhythmias	
Non-arrhythmic	Drugs	Aminophylline, atropine, adrenaline, thyroxine, hormones, caffeine, etc.
	Illness	All kinds of cardiac diseases, pheochromocytoma, anemia, fever, hyperthyroidism, hypoglycemia, severe insomnia, etc.
	Others	Exercise, anxiety, smoking, alcohol drinking, depression, cardiac neurosis, etc.

13.2 Accompanying Symptoms

1. **Palpitation with dizziness, syncope, or dyspnea**: It indicates that palpitation is caused by serious or emergent situations, such as ventricular tachycardia, ventricular fibrillation, third degree atrioventricular block, sinus arrest, etc.
2. **Palpitation with fever**: It can be seen in infectious and non-infectious diseases, especially for the former. Acute or chronic infections with bacteria, virus, rickettsia, chlamydia, or fungi, all can lead to palpitation. Non-infectious fever, such as rheumatic autoimmune disease, drug-induced fever, etc., can also lead to palpitation.
3. **Palpitation with chest pain**: It may suggest coronary heart disease (such as angina and myocardial infaction), aortic stenosis or incompetence, hypertrophic obstructive cardiomyopathy, pericarditis, etc.
4. **Palpitation with anemia**: It can be seen in all kinds of acute blood loss, often accompanied with abnormal sweating, weak pulse, hypotension, or even shock. Patients with chronic anemia may experience palpitation on exertion.
5. **Palpitation with dyspnea**: It can be seen in acute myocardial infaction, pericarditis, myocarditis, heart failure, pulmonary heart disease, pulmonary embolism, severe anemia, etc.
6. **Palpitation with weight loss, irritability, sweating**: It can be seen in hyperthyroidism.
7. **Palpitation with cyanosis**: It can be seen in congenital heart diseases, right heart failure, shock, etc.

S. Liu
Department of Cardiology, Guangzhou Medical University, Guangzhou, China

R. Zeng (✉)
Department of Cardiology, Sichuan University, Chengdu, China

X.-H. Wan, R. Zeng (eds.), *Handbook of Clinical Diagnostics*, https://doi.org/10.1007/978-981-13-7677-1_13

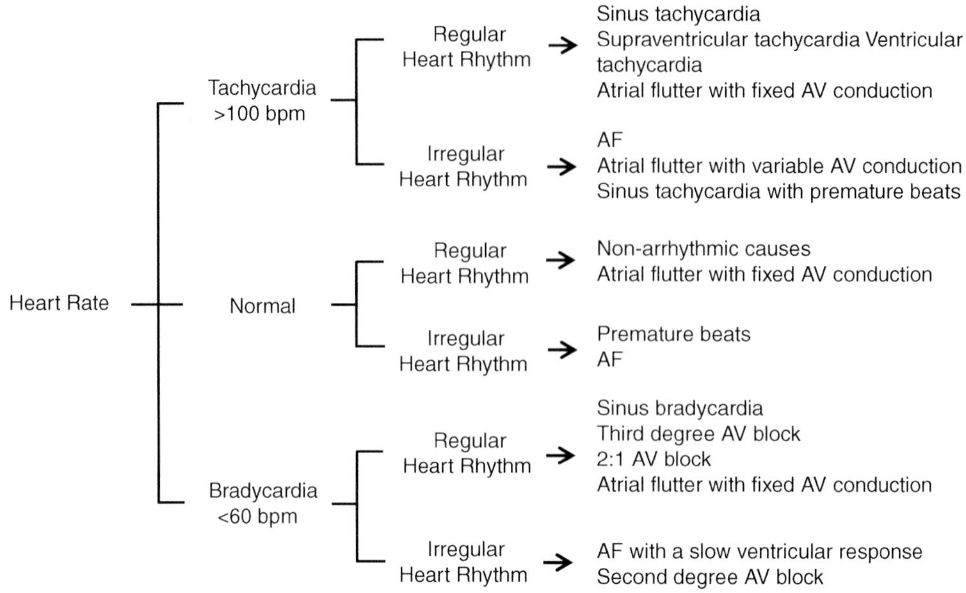

Fig. 13.1 Differential diagnosis of palpitation. *AV* atrioventricular, *AF* atrial fibrillation

Key Points in History Taking

1. Precipitating factors of palpitation. These may include exercise, taking food, sleep, use of medicine, mental state, etc.
2. Characteristics of palpitation. These includes duration of onset, heart (pulse) rate and rhythm when onset, as well as their accompanying symptoms, especially for some manifestations of abnormal hemodynamics, such as dizziness, amaurosis, syncope, chest pain, dyspnea, etc. Heart (pulse) rate and rhythm can help to evaluate palpitation from arrhythmic or non-arrhythmic diseases, and preliminarily estimate types of arrhythmias (Fig. 13.1).
3. Onset and termination of palpitation. These help to evaluate its etiology. Palpitation described as "attacks beginning and ending abruptly" may suggest arrhythmias. Palpitation, relieved 3–5 min after the administration of sublingual nitroglycerin, may strongly suggest ischemic heart disease.
4. Past medical histories related to palpitation. These include previous treatment process of palpitation, possible diagnosis, as well as their auxiliary examinations.

Nausea and Vomiting

14

Ling Dong and Rui Zeng

Nausea, retching, and vomiting are common symptoms encountered in clinical practice, which can appear individually or consecutively. Vomiting is a complex reaction regulated by the vomiting center while nausea and retching are not involved in this complex mechanism.

14.1 Mechanism

The vomiting center is located in the outer medullary dorsal reticular formation, which receives signals from the following three pathways, (a) afferent impulse from organs such as pharynx, gastrointestinal tract, heart, testicles, etc. (b) efferent signals released from the cerebral cortex, brain stem, labyrinthine system and cerebellum. (c) the chemoreceptor trigger zone located at the base of the fourth ventricle medulla which detects endogenous and exogenous vomiting triggers outside the blood-brain barrier. Stimulants such as drugs (morphine, digitalis, etc.) and endogenous metabolites (infection, ketoacidosis, uremia, etc.) release afferent impulses towards the vomiting center.

Vomiting reflex involves various receptors: (a) 5-hydroxytryptamine 3 receptor releases dopamine upon activation, which binds with dopamine 2 receptors located in the vomiting center, activating the vomiting reflex series. (b) histamine-1 and hydroxycholine-1 receptor are rich in the vestibular center and nucleus of solitary tract. These receptors are therapeutic targets for motion sickness, vestibular dysfunction, and hyperemesis gravidarum. (c) the cannabinoid-1 receptor located at the dorsal vagal complex which can inhibit vomiting reflex. (d) the combined complex of neurokinin 1 receptor and substance P located at the ventral side of the fourth ventricle area postrema, constitutes the terminal of the vomiting reflex circuit. Neurokinin 1 receptor antagonist is more efficient in counteracting emesis triggered by peripheral and central stimulation, in comparison to 5-HT_3 receptor inhibitors and other antiemetic drugs.

L. Dong
Department of Gastroenterology, Fudan University, Shanghai, China

R. Zeng (✉)
Department of Cardiology, Sichuan University, Chengdu, China

14.2 Etiology

Etiologies for nausea and vomiting could be seen in Table 14.1.

Table 14.1 Etiologies for nausea and vomiting

Abdominal etiologies
Mechanical obstruction
Gastric outlet, intestinal tract, biliary tract, urinary tract
Motility dysfunction
Intestinal pseudo-obstruction, functional gastrointestinal disease, gastroparesis
Abdominal cavity infection
GI ulcer, appendicitis, cholecystitis, hepatitis, mesenteric ischemia, Crohn's disease, pancreatitis, peritonitis, etc.
Medications
NSAID, anti gout agents, oral hypoglycemic drugs, certain antibiotics, cytostatic agents, digitalis, morphine, anesthetics, CNS drugs.
Infections
Infection of digestive and non-digestive organs
Metabolic and endocrine etiologies
Porphyria, Addison disease, diabetic ketoacidosis, hyperparathyroidism, hyponatremia, pregnancy, etc.
CNS
Intracranial hypertension, intracranial hypotension, demyelinating disease, hydrocephalus, various encephalitis, meningitis, cerebral hemorrhage, cerebral ischemia, cerebral trauma, cerebral edema, seizures, etc.
Vestibular dysfunction
Labyrinthitis, motion sickness, etc.
Others
Pharyngeal stimulation or disease; glaucoma; refractive disorder; anxiety; depression, heart disease; severe pain; post-operative status; alcohol abuse; hunger; radiotherapy, etc.

X.-H. Wan, R. Zeng (eds.), *Handbook of Clinical Diagnostics*, https://doi.org/10.1007/978-981-13-7677-1_14

14.3 Clinical Manifestation

Nausea is a subjective uncomfortable, purging sensation, often accompanied by symptoms of vagal excitation, such as skin pallor, perspiration, hygrostomia, hypotension and bradycardia, etc. Retching, a symptom that follows nausea, is characterized by closing of the glottis, short apnea, contraction of the gastric antrum and abdominal wall muscle, increase in abdominal pressure, opening of the esophagus and pharynx, but without expulsion of stomach content. Vomiting is a conscious act of forcibility expelling contents of the stomach and (or) small intestines through the esophagus and oral cavity. Different from regurgitation, the latter is not an act of forcible expulsion of stomach and (or) small intestinal content through the esophagus and oral cavity.

Clinical features of nausea and vomiting:

1. **Digestive tract obstruction**: Vomitus from secondary esophageal obstruction due to conditions such as esophageal achalasia, stenosis or large diverticulum is usually non-acidic and absent of bile fluid. Vomitus from gastric retention is characterized by a fermented and rotten smell, or presence of undigested food, which is suggestive of gastric outlet obstruction and gastroparesis. Intestinal obstruction results in a large volume vomitus. If the vomitus does not contain bile fluid, the obstruction is most likely located above the duodenal papilla. On the contrary if large amount of bile fluid is observed, the obstruction is most likely located below the papilla. If the vomitus is tainted with a fecal odor, it is suggestive of a low-level obstruction. Other than prominent, recurrent, severe nausea and vomiting, without alleviation of abdominal pain after vomiting, patients suffering from intestinal obstruction often experience cessation of flatulence and defecation. Superior mesenteric artery syndrome is prone in patients who experience recent weight loss, are bedridden or have lordoma.
2. **Acute gastroenteritis or food poisoning**: Postprandial vomiting accompanied by abdominal pain and diarrhea, similar symptoms experienced by dining companion, or history of consuming contaminated food. Mild cases are usually self-limited, while severe cases may result in circulatory failure.
3. **Acute appendicitis**: Referred pain in the right lower abdomen.
4. **Acute pancreatitis**: Severe and persistent upper abdominal pain, which often prompts patients to seek emergency care. Often experienced after consuming large amounts of alcohol or meat. Some patients may have a prior history of choledocholithiasis or cholecystectomy.
5. **Acute biliary tract infection or cholelithiasis**: Right upper abdominal pain, fever and chills, and jaundice.
6. **Peptic ulcer**: Chronic, periodic upper epigastric pain, which can be exacerbated by anxiety, emotional stress, fatigue, and weather changes. Some patients report familial history, while others have no prominent symptoms. Long-term use of NSAIDs and corticosteroids puts patients at high risk for peptic ulcer.
7. **Renal colic and urinary tract infection**: Symptoms include gross hematuria, severe lower back pain, lower abdominal pain, frequent and urgent micturition, and odynuria.
8. **Acute myocardial infarction**: History of hypertension and angina pectoris. Vomiting is usually accompanied by chest pain, palpitations or epigastric pain.
9. **Diseases of central nervous system**: Patients with intracranial hypertension experience projectile vomiting, with severe headache, and varying degrees of consciousness. Headache is not alleviated after vomiting. Patients with cerebral infection may present with fever and chills, while shock may be observed in severe cases. Vomiting secondary to intracranial tumor usually occurs concurrently with severe headaches and often presents symptoms of cranial nerve damage. Cerebral vascular accidents are usually characterized by a rapid onset of headache, paralysis, dysphonia and changes in consciousness.
10. **Early stages of pregnancy, drugs and metabolic diseases**: Diabetes mellitus, uremia, liver decompensation, etc. may present as morning sickness, secondary to CTZ activation of the vomiting center. The vomitus does not usually contain stomach contents, but mainly saliva and gastric fluid. A history of menstrual cycle for women of child-bearing age must be noted upon admission. History of medication usage, past history of hepatorenal diseases, and history of diabetes are significant in all patients presenting with nausea and vomiting.
11. **Vestibular diseases**: Vomiting in labyrinthitis, Meniere's Diseases, etc., is characterized by a rapid onset and severe symptoms. Some cases may present as projectile vomiting, usually accompanied by vertigo, headache, tinnitus, hearing loss and nystagmus.
12. **Glaucoma and refractive disorder**: Accompanying symptoms include headache, vertigo, changes in vision or visual field. A physician must complete tonometry tests and fundus examination.
13. **Psychological factor**: Usually presents as morning sickness. Symptoms can be affected by environmental and psychological factors.
14. **Nasosinusitis**: Nausea and vomiting are triggered by pharyngeal stimulation secondary to the outflow of pus from the sinus cavity. Symptoms are prominent in the morning.

Key Points in History Taking

1. Disease onset: Rapid or chronic onset; Do dining companions have similar symptoms during rapid onset?
2. Characteristics of vomiting: Time of occurrence, environment, psychological state; The time, environment, mental state, way of vomiting, relationship between food consumption and vomiting; characteristic of vomitus.
3. Associated symptoms: Abdominal pain, diarrhea, fever, jaundice, dysphagia; hematuria, severe lower back pain, lower abdominal pain, frequent and urgent micturition, odynuria; headache, paralysis, dysphonia, changes in consciousness; vertigo, tinnitus, hearing loss, nystagmus; chest pain, palpitations, dyspnea, hypertension; hematemesis, melena, anemia.
4. Past history: Chronic hepato-renal diseases, diabetes mellitus, tumor, etc.; long-term medication usage; trauma, surgical procedure, menstrual cycle, alcohol consumption and cigarette smoking, etc.
5. Diagnosis and treatment: (a) routine lab exams: blood, urine routine, liver and renal function, blood glucose, blood electrolytes, pH, viral hepatitis markers, thyroid function, pregnancy test (women of child-bearing age). (b) endoscopy exams, abdominal ultrasound, abdominal x-ray, esophageal contrast x-ray. (c) response to treatment.

15 Dysphagia

Ling Dong and Rui Zeng

Dysphagia is a series of symptoms characterized by the difficult passing of food through the esophagus and cardiac orifice, commonly due to motility disorder or stricture of the oropharynx and esophagus. Emotional factors may exacerbate the symptoms of dysphagia.

15.1 Etiology

Dysphagia can be classified based on different etiologies: inflammatory, obstructive, neuromuscular, psychological, etc.; based on location: oropharynx, esophageal, extraluminal esophageal compression, neuromuscular diseases; or based on pathogenesis: mechanical or motility (Table 15.1).

15.2 Mechanism

15.2.1 Mechanical Dysphagia

Secondary to esophageal luminal stricture. Normal esophagus is flexible and can expand up to 4 cm. When the diameter of lumen is less than 2.5 cm, dysphagia may be present. When lumen is less than 1.3 cm, dysphagia is prominent. Pan-esophageal luminal stricture due to esophageal wall lesions is more severe compared to eccentric luminal stricture caused by localized lesions, including compressive strictures, which often presents with milder, later onset symptoms.

Table 15.1 Etiology of dysphagia

Mechanical	Motility
Intraluminal factor: large bolus or esophageal foreign object Luminal stricture: • Inflammation, pharyngitis, tonsillitis, oropharyngeal injury, esophagitis • Benign esophageal stricture: benign tumors (e.g. leiomyoma, lipoma, hemangioma and polyps); esophagitis (e.g. reflux esophagitis, radiation esophagitis, erosive esophagitis, tuberculosis and fungal infection) • Malignant tumor: esophageal cancer, cardiac cancer, sarcoma, lymphoma, etc. • Esophageal web: Plummer-Vinson Syndrome (iron deficiency dysphagia) • Mucosal Ring: Lower esophagus mucosal ring (Schatzki's ring) Compressive stricture • Retropharyngeal mass or abscess • Severe thyromegaly • Mediastinal lesions: mediastinal tumor, abscess, left atrial enlargement and aortic aneurysm Hiatal hernia	Oral Phase Myasthenia gravis Parkinson's disease, bulbar poliomyelitis, motor neuron disease and syringomyelia Chewing pain Oral pharynx inflammation, abscess, tumor, trauma Aptyalism: e.g. Sjogren's syndrome Pharyngeal Phase Weakness of pharyngeal muscles Bulbar paralysis, Parkinson's disease, cerebral vascular accident, Wilson's disease, motor neuron disease, syringomyelia, myasthenia gravis, scleroderma, muscle atrophy and polymyositis UES[a] insufficient opening Cricopharyngeal muscle achalasia, Zenker's diverticulum Esophageal phase: Primary esophageal smooth muscle and neurological diseases Gastroesophageal reflux, achalasia, diffuse esophageal spasm and systemic diseases Scleroderma, diabetes, and alcoholic myopathy

[a]*UES* upper esophageal sphincter

15.2.2 Motility Dysphagia

- Oral phase: (a) neurological disease causes muscle rigidity, paralysis or asthenia, in which swallowing cannot be initiated. (b) Oral cavity pain causes reluctance to chew and inability for the bolus to form an appropriate shape for swallowing. (c) Aptyalism.

L. Dong
Department of Gastroenterology, Fudan University, Shanghai, China

R. Zeng (✉)
Department of Cardiology, Sichuan University, Chengdu, China

X.-H. Wan, R. Zeng (eds.), *Handbook of Clinical Diagnostics*, https://doi.org/10.1007/978-981-13-7677-1_15

- Pharyngeal phase: Pharyngeal muscle weakness secondary to bilateral upper motor neuron lesion, medulla injury and striated muscle diseases. Insufficient opening of the upper esophageal sphincter or uncoordinated movements of the pharyngeal muscles.
- Esophageal phase: (a) Gastroesophageal reflux disease may be caused by lower esophageal stenosis secondary to severe inflammation, or hypersensitivity towards the food bolus during peristalsis. (b) Achalasia is due to a state of smooth muscle segmental denervation, in which the esophageal body and lower esophageal sphincter are desensitized to methacholine, absent propulsion and contraction of the esophageal body and inability of the lower esophageal sphincter to relax. (c) Diffuse esophageal spasm may be caused by neuromuscular degeneration or esophageal hypercontraction due to methacholine stimulation. (d) Scleroderma and other systemic diseases may cause weakness of smooth muscle contraction and irregular contraction of the esophagus.

15.3 Clinical Manifestations

15.3.1 Oropharyngeal Dysphagia (Swallowing)

Difficulty of passing of food bolus from the mouth to the pharynx. The location of dysphagia is explicit, may accompany bucking, fluid reflux to the nasal cavity, or aspiration pneumonia.

15.3.2 Esophageal Dysphagia

The location of dysphagia is ambiguous, accompanied with a choking sensation, food stagnation, or slow passing of food. Dysphagia can be presented with sore throat, post-sternal chest pain, vomiting, hematemesis, ingestion disorders and malnutrition. If the lesion is located in the lower esophagus, patients may not experience dysphagia, but the food bolus is unable to pass through the cardia and is stagnated in the lower esophagus. The vomitus is not acidic. Pseudo dysphagia has no esophageal stricture, but merely a sensation of laryngopharyngeal obstruction and discomfort. Does not affect normal uptake of food and in some cases symptoms may be alleviated with ingestion.

15.3.3 Points of Clinical Symptoms of Common Diseases

- Esophageal foreign bodies: Can cause varying degrees of dysphagia and odynophagia. Patient history is crucial.
- Acute tonsillitis and peripheral abscess: Acute onset, common in adolescents. Usually accompanied by fever, pharyngalgia, odynophagia, tonsillar enlargement and purulent discharge.
- Retropharyngeal abscess: Common in children, accompanied with fever, pharyngalgia, retropharyngeal congestion, swelling and purulent discharge.
- Reflux esophagitis: Typical symptoms include heartburn, acid reflux, dysphagia and chest pain.
- Erosive esophagitis: History of ingesting strong acidic or alkali corrosive agents. Early stages present as odynophagia, chest pain, dysphagia, nausea, vomiting, fever, ingestion disorder, and malnutrition due to oropharyngeal, esophageal mucosal edema, ulcers or perforation; Late stages may present as dysphagia due to esophageal stenosis.
- Candida esophagitis: Common in the elderly and infirm. Long-term use of antibiotics and immunosuppressant. Can result in varying degrees of dysphagia and chest pain.
- Tongue cancer, laryngeal cancer, nasopharyngeal cancer: Can present as different degrees of dysphagia, tongue pain, motility dysfunction; hoarseness, dyspnea, coughing; epistaxis, nasal congestion and headache.
- Esophageal cancer: Common in elderly male patients. Progressive dysphagia of solid food to semi-liquid and liquid food usually within six months.
- Esophageal Compression: Severe pericardial effusion, left atrial enlargement, aortic aneurysm, thyroid goiter and spinal lesions can cause dysphagia, along with symptoms of the primary disease.
- Achalasia: Chronic onset with intermittent dysphagia, often presents with gastroesophageal reflux and nighttime bucking. Onset of disease can be related with psychological factors.
- Diffuse esophageal spasm: Common in the elderly patients, presents with post-sternal chest pain and intermittent dysphagia.
- Scleroderma: Common in 20–50 years old female patients. Scleroderma skin lesions and Raynaud's phenomenon are often observed.
- Myasthenia gravis: Initial symptoms often present as ocular myasthenia gravis. Dysphagia, chewing weakness, and bucking can occur when the medullary muscles are affected.
- Paralysis: Caused by medullary degeneration, brainstem tumor and vascular diseases. Symptoms include dysphagia, dysarthria, bucking, tongue muscle atrophy and fremitus.
- Hysteria: Common in young or middle-aged female; related to emotional factors.

Key Points in History Taking

1. Onset condition: Progressive or intermittent.

2. Associated symptoms: Fever, hygrostomia, pharyngalgia, hoarseness; heartburn, acid reflux and chest pain; headache, paralysis, dysarthria and changes in consciousness; xerostomia, swelling and thickening of skin; chewing weakness, bucking, dyspnea, verbal dysfunction; anemia, weight loss
3. Other history: History of swallowing foreign objects; ingestion of strong acidic or alkali agents; long-term use of antibiotics or immunosuppressant; heart diseases, hyperthyroidism, cerebral diseases; Past esophageal or stomach surgeries.
4. Diagnosis and treatment: (a) Routine tests: blood routine, liver and kidney function, thyroid function. (b) Laryngoscopy, gastroscopy, abdominal X-ray and esophageal barium swallow test. (c) Response to treatment.

Dyspepsia

16

Ling Dong and Rui Zeng

Dyspepsia is a series of symptoms presenting primarily as epigastric pain or discomfort, including postprandial fullness, early satiation, epigastric burning, bloating, nausea, vomiting, belching and other upper gastrointestinal symptoms. These symptoms can originate from organic diseases, but most are functional in nature, which is defined as absence of an organic etiology. Dyspepsia is a common clinical symptom, incidence ranges from 20 to 50%. Approximately 1/3 patients reported interference with their normal daily activities and quality of life.

16.1 Etiology

Etiologies for dyspepsia could be seen in Table 16.1.

Table 16.1 Dyspepsia etiologies

Gastrointestinal Tract Lesion
GI Ulcer
Stomach or Esophageal Tumor
Intolerance to Food
Chronic Gastrointestinal Ischemia
Gastroparesis
Infiltrative Inflammatory Disease (Crohn's Disease, Eosinophilic Gastroenteritis, Sarcoidosis, Amyloidosis)
Ménétrier Disease
Gastric Infection (*H. pylori*, Cytomegalovirus, Fungal Infection, Tuberculosis)
Hepatobiliary and Pancreatic Diseases
Chronic Hepatitis, Cirrhosis, Intrahepatic Cholestasis
Chronic Cholecystitis, Cholelithiasis
Sphincter of Oddi Dysfunction
Chronic Pancreatitis
Hepatobiliary and Pancreatic Tumor
Gestation
Functional Indigestion
Gastroesophageal Reflux
Medication
Ethanol
Iron Supplements
Potassium Chloride (KCl)
Nonsteroidal Anti-inflammatory Drugs (NSAIDs)
Antibiotics
Anti-tuberculosis Drugs
Digitalis Drugs
Theophylline
Nitrate Drugs
Calcium Channel Blockers (CCB)
Chemotherapy Drugs
Immunosuppressant
Systemic Diseases
Diabetes Mellitus
Chronic Obstructive Pulmonary Disease
Cardiac, Pulmonary, Renal Insufficiency
Cardiac Ischemia
Thyroid Disease
Hyperparathyroidism
Adrenal Insufficiency
Intraabdominal Non-GI Tumor

16.2 Clinical Manifestations

Postprandial fullness, early satiation, epigastric pain and burning are specific symptoms of gastric and duodenal diseases or functional disorders. Along with upper abdominal bloating, nausea, vomiting, and belching, various clinical syndromes can be formed (Table 16.2).

Dyspeptic symptoms are usually chronic in nature and can be persistent or intermittently exacerbated, with or without triggering factors. Symptoms related to ingestion are suggestive of an organic disease. For example, pain relived after ingestion suggests gastric acid hypersecretion, typically observed in peptic ulcer or ulcer-like dyspepsia; on the contrary, if pain is exacerbated after ingestion, it is suggestive of a decrease in gastrointestinal secretory function and motility, commonly observed in atrophic gastritis, gastric cancer, or

L. Dong
Department of Gastroenterology, Fudan University, Shanghai, China

R. Zeng (✉)
Department of Cardiology, Sichuan University, Chengdu, China

X.-H. Wan, R. Zeng (eds.), *Handbook of Clinical Diagnostics*, https://doi.org/10.1007/978-981-13-7677-1_16

Table 16.2 Symptoms of dyspepsia (Rome III Consensus)

Symptoms	Definition
Postprandial Fullness	Persistent discomfort due to intragastric food stagnation.
Early satiation	Fullness experienced after ingestion of a small amount of food.
Epigastric pain	Localized abdominal pain between the xiphoid process, umbilicus, and bilateral midclavicular line. Epigastric pain is usually subjective with varying descriptions.
Epigastric Burning	Burning sensation located between the xiphoid process, umbilicus, and bilateral midclavicular line.
Bloating in the Upper Abdomen	Bloating sensation in the upper abdomen without observed bulging.
Nausea	Subjective feeling of discomfort and an urge to vomit.
Vomiting	Forcible emptying of stomach and (or) intestinal contents through the esophagus and mouth.
Belching	Emission of gas from the stomach and esophagus through the mouth or nose.

motility disorder dyspepsia. While, pain exacerbation experienced after ingestion of meat or greasy food is suggestive of hepatobiliary and pancreatic diseases. Association of symptoms and the use of antacids or acid inhibitory drugs can help determine the relationship between disease and stomach acid secretion.

If a patient over 45 years old complains of newly onset prominent symptoms, with progressive exacerbation, a physician must cautiously screen for all possible organic etiologies. The effect of drug usage and life event on dyspeptic symptoms should also be recognized. If the patient has concurrent alerting symptoms, such as anemia, jaundice, dysphagia, odynophagia, hematemesis, melena, upper abdominal mass, significant decrease in appetite and weight loss, one must consider the presence of an organic disease and promptly provide routine exams to differentiate between benign or malignant diseases and assess for hepatobiliary and pancreatic involvement.

Key Points in History Taking

1. Ask for a patient's exact symptom or syndrome: Patients from different regions, different ethnicities, and different cultural levels may have varying descriptions of a symptom. A physician should fully understand the patient's experience before categorizing it into a dyspeptic symptom. For example, if a patient complains of upper abdominal "stuffiness", "stomach-turning", or "stomach churning", then symptom confirmation can only be achieved through completely understanding the patient's experience.
2. Onset of symptoms and persistence: Useful in differentiating between organic or functional, benign or malignant diseases.
3. Triggering and alleviating factors: Food or medication, Psychological or work-related stress, living environment.
4. Other history: History of smoking or alcohol consumption, history of chest or abdominal surgery.
5. Concurrent alerting symptoms: Anemia, jaundice, dysphagia, odynophagia, hematemesis, melena, upper abdominal mass, significant decrease in appetite, and weight loss.
6. Diagnosis and Treatment: (a) routine exams: blood, urine, stool routine, liver and renal function, blood glucose and lipids, viral hepatitis markers, thyroid function. (b) Endoscopy exam, abdominal ultrasound, electrocardiogram. (c) Treatments received.

Abdominal Pain

17

Ling Dong and Rui Zeng

Abdominal pain is a particularly common clinical symptom, which is also an important factor that prompts patients to seek medical attention. Abdominal pain is commonly caused by abdominal visceral diseases, but extra-abdominal diseases and systemic diseases can also result in abdominal pain. Pathological changes can be visceral or functional. Some abdominal pain presents as a severe acute pain, while other might be chronic and mild. Due to complex etiologies and different disease mechanisms, a detailed patient history, full physical exam and necessary supplementary tests (including laboratory and instrumental examinations) must be completed when diagnosing a patient with abdominal pain. An accurate diagnosis can only be made on the basis of examination results and the possible pathophysiological association. Clinically, abdominal pain can be categorized into acute or chronic according to the onset and duration of the symptom.

17.1 Etiology

Etiologies for abdominal pain could be seen in Table 17.1.

17.2 Mechanism

Abdominal pain can be divided into three categories according to characteristics of the afferent nerve and clinical presentation:

1. **Visceral Pain:** Stimulation of sensory afferent nerve distributed in the hollow organ mucosa and muscularis mucosa, visceral peritoneum, mesentery, is known as visceral pain. The physical stimulation results in traction and distention of hollow organs. Inflammation, trauma, ischemia and necrosis release bradykinin, substance P, calcitonin gene-related peptide, prostaglandin, vasoactive amine and intragastric H^+, which are all chemical stimulators of visceral pain. The scarce distribution of visceral sensory nerve endings, thin sensory afferent nerves, absent myelin sheath, and a relatively slow transmission of nervous impulse, result in the following characteristics of visceral pain: (a) unable to localize pain, usually around mid-abdominal line; (b) vague pain, usually presents as spasms, discomforts, dull pain, or burning sensation; (c) progressive and prolonged pain; d. can occur concurrently with dysautonomia symptoms, such as nausea, vomiting, sweating, and bradycardia, etc.
2. **Somatic Pain:** Stimulation of sensory afferent nerves distributed along the abdominal wall and diaphragm is known as somatic pain. The dense distribution of somatic nerve endings, thick afferent nerves, presence of myelin sheath, and rapid nervous impulse transmission result in the following characteristics of somatic pain: (a) clear localization of pain; (b) severe pain, acute onset and alleviation; (c) can occur with localized abdominal muscle rigidity; (d) abdominal pain may be exacerbated by cough or change in position.
3. **Referred Pain:** Different visceral and somatic sensory afferent nerve unite into the same spinal dorsal root segment, causing the cerebral cortex to depict the visceral sensory afferent nervous impulse as a superficial or deep somatic stimulation, which is also known as referred pain. Characteristics include: (a) clear localization of pain; (b) severe pain. Understanding the mechanism of referred pain can be valuable in clinical settings. For example, dyspptic pain can present as backaches; angina is not limited to the precordium, but can involve the ulnar side of the left arm; splenic rupture can present as left neck and shoulder pain, known as Saegesser's sign; cholecystitis pain can extend to the subscapular angle (Table 17.2).

L. Dong
Department of Gastroenterology, Fudan University, Shanghai, China

R. Zeng (✉)
Department of Cardiology, Sichuan University, Chengdu, China

X.-H. Wan, R. Zeng (eds.), *Handbook of Clinical Diagnostics*, https://doi.org/10.1007/978-981-13-7677-1_17

Table 17.1 Etiologies of abdominal pain

Acute abdominal pain	Chronic abdominal pain
Acute Abdominal Visceral Inflammation Acute gastritis, acute enteritis, acute pancreatitis, acute hemorrhagic necrotic enteritis, acute cholecystitis, etc.	Chronic Abdominal Visceral Inflammation Reflux esophagitis, chronic gastritis, chronic cholecystitis and cholangitis, chronic pancreatitis, tuberculous peritonitis, ulcerative colitis, Crohn's disease, etc.
Hollow Visceral Obstruction or Distension Intestinal obstruction, choledocholelithiasis, biliary ascariasis, urolithiasis obstruction, etc.	Changes in Hollow Visceral Compliance Gastrointestinal spasm, distention or gastrointestinal or biliary tract dysmotility, etc.
Visceral Torsion or Rupture Volvulus, intestinal strangulation, mesenteric or omental torsion, ovarian torsion, hepatic rupture, splenic rupture, ectopic pregnancy rupture, etc.	Peptic or Duodenal Ulcer
Peritonitis Mainly due to gastrointestinal perforation or spreading of an infection. Spontaneous peritonitis is rare.	Visceral Torsion or Obstruction Chronic stomach or intestinal torsion.
Intraabdominal Vascular Obstruction Ischemic enteropathy, abdominal aortic dissection or aneurysm, etc.	Stretching of Visceral Membrane Pathological swelling of a solid organ can cause an increase in visceral membrane tension resulting in abdominal pain, as in hepatic congestion, hepatitis, liver abscess, hepatocellular carcinoma, etc.
Abdominal Wall Disease Abdominal wall contusion, abscess, or herpes-zoster infection, etc.	Toxicity and Metabolic Disorders Lead poisoning, uremia, etc.
Referred pain induced by Thoracic Disease Pneumonia, pulmonary infarction, angina, myocardial infarction, acute pericarditis, pleuritis, hiatal hernia, thoracic vertebral tuberculosis or tumor, etc.	Tumor Compression or Infiltration Mostly due to malignant tumors; as tumors increase in size, sensory nerves may be compressed or infiltrated.
Abdominal pain secondary to Systemic Disease Abdominal Henoch-Schönlein purpura, uremia, lead poisoning, hematoporphyria, etc.	Gastrointestinal Neurosis Functional gastrointestinal disorders.

Table 17.2 Common referred pain

Viscera involved	Referred pain	Viscera involved	Referred pain
Stomach, Pancreas	Left upper abdomen, interscapular region	Appendicitis	Upper abdomen or umbilical region
Liver, Gallbladder	Right shoulder	Uterus and Rectal Disease	Lumbosacral region
Peptic ulcer peroration	Top of the shoulder	Acute Myocardial Infarction	Left arm, neck or lower mandible
Urolithiasis	Inner thigh, perineum		

Table 17.3 Location of abdominal pain of common disease

Disease	Location of pain
Stomach, duodenum, hepatobiliary, and pancreatic disease	Upper middle abdomen
Cholecystitis, cholelithiasis, liver abscess	Right upper abdomen
Acute appendicitis	Right lower abdomen
Small intestinal disease	Umbilical region
Colon disease	Left or right lower abdomen
Cystitis, pelvic inflammatory disease, and ectopic pregnancy rupture	Lower abdomen
Acute diffuse peritonitis (primary or secondary), mechanical bowel obstruction, acute hemorrhagic necrotic enteritis, hematoporphyria, lead poisoning, abdominal Henoch-Schönlein purpura, etc.	Unable to localize

17.3 Clinical Manifestations

1. **Location of Abdominal Pain:** Pain is usually localized to the viscera involved (Table 17.3).The location of pain may diverge as disease progresses, for instance, a typical acute appendicitis may present as right lower abdominal referred pain. During the initial stages, abdominal pain can present as a vague visceral pain, usually located around the umbilical region, with or without nausea or vomiting. As the disease continues to progress, inflammation is spread to the peritoneum and is depicted as referred pain to right lower abdomen or McBurney's point. The somatic pain is clearly localized, severe, usually accompanied with abdominal muscle rigidity, tenderness and rebound tenderness.

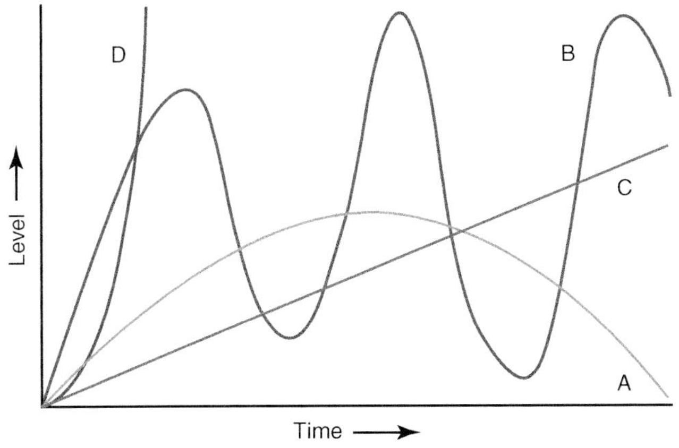

Fig. 17.1 Acute abdominal pain disease duration

2. **Common disease onset and duration** (Fig. 17.1): (a) acute onset, self-limited duration, commonly seen in acute gastroenteritis; (b) colicky pain from hallow organ obstruction, intermittent pain; (c) progressive abdominal pain, such as acute appendicitis, pancreatitis; (d) fatal disease, such as abdominal aortic aneurysm rupture.
3. **Degree and characteristic of abdominal pain:** Degree of abdominal pain may be influenced by a patient's physical and mental status, which can be difficult to evaluate. The degree of pain is not necessarily an accurate reflection of disease severity. Description of pain characteristics is affected by a patient's cultural level and language habits. Colicky pain secondary to hollow organ obstruction can be intermittent and severe, causing restlessness and concern. Abdominal pain from acute diffuse peritonitis can be exacerbated with breathing, raising one's voice, and changing positions. Patients are often quite and sometimes accompanying hydroids or tachycardia, which should be paid attention to.
4. **Triggering and alleviating factors:** Ingestion of greasy food often precedes cholecystitis or choleliathiasis, while alcohol consumption or excessive eating may cause acute pancreatitis. Some cases of mechanical bowel obstruction are related to a prior history of abdominal surgery. Severe abdominal pain accompanied with shock and a history of brutal impact can be secondary to hepatic or splenic rupture; abdominal pain relived after ingestion or use of acid inhibitory drugs suggests an association with stomach acid hypersecretion; symptoms relieved after use of antispasmodic drugs suggests smooth muscle spasm; pain alleviated after vomiting is commonly seen in stomach and duodenal diseases.
5. **Time of onset and postural relations:** Postprandial pain can be secondary to biliary and pancreatic diseases, gastric tumors or dyspepsia; periodic preprandial pain is commonly seen in gastric antrum or duodenal ulcer. Abdominal pain from endometriosis is associated with menstrual cycle, while follicular rupture is common during menses. Pain exacerbated or alleviated with the change of posture may provide clinical evidence for diagnosis. For instance, pain and vomiting from duodenal stasis can be relieved if the patient is in a knee chest or prone position. Abdominal pain secondary to pancreatic cancer is prominent in a supine position, but alleviated in a leaning forward or prone position. Burning pain from reflux esophagitis is exacerbated in a leaning forward or supine position, while reduced in an upright stance.
6. **Accompanying symptoms:** Abdominal pain with concurrent fever and chills may indicate probable inflammation, as seen in acute cholangitis, cholecystitis, liver abscess, abdominal cavity abscess, or extra-abdominal disease. Abdominal pain along with jaundice is suggestive of hepatobiliary and pancreatic disease. Acute hemolytic anemia can also present as abdominal pain and jaundice. Abdominal pain accompanied with shock and anemia may be due to abdominal visceral rupture (e.g. hepatic, splenic or ectopic pregnancy rupture); while those without anemia are observed in gastrointestinal perforation, strangulated bowel obstruction, and acute hemorrhagic necrotic pancreatitis. Extra-abdominal disease such as myocardial infarction or pneumonia may also present as abdominal pain along with shock. Concurrent vomiting is suggestive of esophageal or gastrointestinal disease. Large volume vomit is observed in gastrointestinal obstruction, while acid reflux and belching are commonly seen in gastroduodenal ulcers, gastritis, or ulcer-like dyspepsia; abdominal pain accompanied with fullness and loss of appetite may be secondary to an organic etiology, while pain with diarrhea is suggestive of malabsorption or enteritis, ulcer or tumor. Abdominal pain with hematuria can be due to urinary tract disease (e.g., urolithiasis).

Key Points in History Taking

1. Onset of abdominal pain, symptom progression, location, degree, characteristics, trigger and alleviating factors, duration, and relations with postural changes.
2. Trauma or surgical history.
3. Lifestyle and occupation history, medication history, travel history, history of contact with animals, and past medical history.
4. Diagnosis and Treatment: (a) routine exams: blood, urine, stool routine, amylase and lipase, liver and renal function, blood glucose and lipids, and viral hepatitis markers; (b) endoscopy exam, abdominal ultrasound, abdominal CT, and electrocardiogram. (c) Treatments received.

Hematemesis

18

Dong Ling and Rui Zeng

Hematemesis, or vomiting of blood, is a presentation of upper gastrointestinal tract bleeding. Upper gastrointestinal tract is commonly defined as organs located above the ligament of Treitz, including esophagus, stomach, duodenum, liver, gallbladder and pancreas.

18.1 Etiology and Mechanism

18.1.1 Common Causes

- GI ulcers: Gastric ulcer and duodenal ulcers
- Acute erosive gastritis: Commonly due to NSAIDs usage (including aspirin and indomethacin, etc.) and stress-induction.
- Hemorrhage due to gastroesophageal variceal rupture: Portal hypertension secondary to liver cirrhosis.
- Esophageal or gastric carcinoma:Tumor vasculature rupture.

18.1.2 Other Causes

- Esophagus: Esophagitis, esophageal diverticulitis, esophageal foreign object, Mallory-Weiss Syndrome, esophageal hiatal hernia, etc. Puncture of the aorta from a esophageal foreign object can cause life-threatening massive hematemesis.
- Stomach and duodenum: Vascular malformation such as Dieulafoy Syndrome and other life-threatening hematemesis.
- Bile duct: Blood entering the duodenum from the bile duct can originate from: (a) malignant hepatic tumor (e.g., hepatocellular carcinoma), liver abscess or rupture of liver aneurysm; (b) cholelithiasis or cholangilithiasis, parasitic infection of the bile duct (commonly roundworms), gallbladder cancer, cholangiocarcinoma, periampullarycarcinoma are all potential sources of bleeding. Hemorrhage through the bile duct can enter the duodenum causing hematemesis or melena.
- Pancreas: Acute pancreatitis with concurrent abscess or cyst, and pancreatic tumor rupture can hemorrhage through the pancreatic duct into the upper gastrointestinal tract.
- Hematological disease:Idiopathic thrombocytopenic purpura, Henoch-Schönlein purpura, leukemia, hemophilia, Hodgkin lymphoma, hereditary hemorrhagic telangiectasia, disseminated intravascular coagulation and other clotting factor deficiencies (e.g., overdose of anticoagulation drugs), etc.
- Others: Uremia, epidemic hemorrhagic fever, leptospirosis, etc.

18.2 Clinical Manifestations

Hematemesis is often preceded by upper abdominal discomfort and nausea, followed by vomiting of hemorrhagic stomach contents. The color of the blood is dependent on the volume of blood loss, stasis duration in the stomach, and source of bleeding. Large volume of blood loss usually has a short stasis duration and if the source of bleeding is from the esophagus, then the blood can be bright or dark red in color. However, if blood loss is minimal or stomach stasis is prolonged, the effect of stomach acid on hemoglobin will result in acidified methemoglobin, presenting as coffee grain-like dark brown vomit. Portions of the blood may be eliminated through the lower GI tract, as evident by hematochezia or melena.

When a patient complains of hematemesis, a physician must differentiate between mouth, nose, throat, respiratory tract and upper GI bleeding. If vomiting of blood is bright

D. Ling
Department of Gastroenterology, Fudan University, Shanghai, China

R. Zeng (✉)
Department of Cardiology, Sichuan University, Chengdu, China

X.-H. Wan, R. Zeng (eds.), *Handbook of Clinical Diagnostics*, https://doi.org/10.1007/978-981-13-7677-1_18

red, accompanied with coughing, it is more likely hemoptysis.

A 10–15% loss of blood volume may present as dizziness, but seldom affect blood pressure or pulse; Loss of over 20% blood volume can present as cold sweat, cold extremities, palpitations, tachycardia and other circulatory compensation symptoms. Over 30% loss of blood volume will present as acute circulatory failure, which includes weak pulse, drop in blood pressure, rapid breathing and shock. Other than continuous hematemesis and melena, active bowel sounds, profuse sweating, and tachycardia are all suggestive of active bleeding.

Different etiologies may present as different symptoms: (a) concurrent abdominal pain: young or middle-aged patients: chronic recurrent epigastric pain, with certain regularity, are commonly seen in GI ulcers; elderly patients: chronic epigastric pain accompanied with decrease in appetite, weight loss, without regularity, may indicate stomach cancer. (b) concurrent hepatosplenomegaly: splenomegaly, spider nevus, liver palm, abdominal wall varicose vein or ascites, is suggestive of portal hypertension secondary to liver cirrhosis; hepatic region pain, solid liver, and uneven or nodular liver surface are suggestive of liver cancer. (c) concurrent jaundice, chills, fever, and upper right abdominal colicky pain, may indicate purulent cholangitis; jaundice, fever, skin and mucosal petechiae are observed in some infectious diseases, such as sepsis and leptospirosis, etc. (d) Skin and mucosal petechiae: suggestive of hematological disease and blood coagulation dysfunction.

Key Points in History Taking

1. Whether coughing or vomiting preceded hematemesis; color of vomit; presence of stomach content; whether bleeding came from the nose; volume of hematemesis.
2. Triggering factors History of ingesting unsanitary food, excessive alcohol consumption, prior contact with toxic or special medication.
3. Accompanying dizziness, palpitations, sweating, syncope, etc.; change in posture induces palpitations or heart rate changes.
4. Previous surgical or medical history.
5. Treatment and Diagnosis (a) routine exams blood, urine, stool routine, liver and renal function, blood glucose and lipids, and viral hepatitis markers. (b) endoscopy exam, abdominal ultrasound, and abdominal CT. (c) treatments received.

Hematochezia

19

Ling Dong and Rui Zeng

Hematochezia and melena are common symptoms of gastrointestinal bleeding. Passage for bright or dark red blood per annum is known as hematochezia while tar-like stool is known as melena. Stool color is dependent on the source of bleeding.

19.1 Etiology and Mechanism

Different etiologies and source of gastrointestinal bleeding have varying clinical presentations. Proximal to the ligament of Treitz is known as the upper gastrointestinal tract, while middle gastrointestinal tract starts from the ligament of Treitz to ileocecal valve, and from the ileocecal valve onwards is known as the lower gastrointestinal tract. Lower GI tract bleeding usually passes through the anus rapidly as bright or dark red bloody stool, therefore, hematochezia is usually indicative of lower GI bleeding. However fatal torrential hemorrhage from the upper GI tract (>1000 mL) may present as both hematemesis and hematochezia. Under normal circumstances, hemoglobin from an upper or middle GI bleed will acidify into methemoglobin, then conjugates with intestinal sulfide to form iron sulfide, which presents as black tar-like stool. Melena is commonly seen in upper and middle GI bleeding with an average volume of blood loss. However lower GI tract bleeding can also present as melena if intestinal stasis is prolonged. From a high probability perspective, hematochezia and melena can reflect upper or lower GI bleeding (Table 19.1), but the pathogenesis of low probability incidence should not be neglected.

Table 19.1 Etiology and source of bleeding for hematochezia and melena

Upper GI Tract		Probability of hematochezia or melena based on source of bleeding	Refer to Chap. 18
Middle GI Tract			Small intestine diverticulosis, vascular malformation, polyps, Crohn's disease, intestinal typhoid, acute hemorrhagic necrotic enteritis, ancylostomiasis, tumor, small intestinal ulcer, Meckel's diverticulitis or ulcer, intestinal intussusception
Lower GI Tract			Hemorrhoids, anal fissure, polyp, colorectal tumor, ulcerative colitis, anal fistula, ischemic enteropathy, bacteria dysentery, amebic dysentery, schistosomiasis, etc.

19.2 Clinical Manifestations

1. **Hematochezia:** Minimal loss of blood may appear as blood stains on tissue, or lining of blood on yellow stool; some patients reported dripping of blood per annum When blood is mixed with stool before defecation, it can appear as brick red or brown stool. Massive hemorrhage

L. Dong
Department of Gastroenterology, Fudan University, Shanghai, China

R. Zeng (✉)
Department of Cardiology, Sichuan University, Chengdu, China

X.-H. Wan, R. Zeng (eds.), *Handbook of Clinical Diagnostics*, https://doi.org/10.1007/978-981-13-7677-1_19

can present as large volume of blood loss from the anus with minimal stool content.

2. **Melena:** Melena secondary to gastrointestinal bleeding is usually covered in mucus and may appear glossy, or tar-like with a bloody odor. Unlike stool from the use of bithmus, iron, charcoal powder or Chinese Traditional Medicine, which is usually dark gray or black in color without glare. Stool from ingesting animal blood or pig liver can also appear black, but lacks a bloody scent. Occult blood is helpful for differential diagnosis.
3. **Occult blood:** Blood loss less than 5 mL per day, difficult to distinguish with naked-eye, is known as occult blood, which is determined by a fecal occult blood test.
4. **Common diseases and clinical presentations**
   - Gastrointestinal ulcer: Usually located in the upper GI tract, presents as melena when active bleeding occurs; mostly chronic with periodic epigastric pain, which is relieved after GI bleeding.
   - Dieulafoy Syndrome: Commonly seen in the upper GI tract, due to Dieulafoy artery rupture; can present as hematemesis and large volume melena.
   - Biliary tract bleeding: Accompanied with epigastric colicky pain and jaundice. Jaundice is prominent during active bleeding.
   - Bacterial dysentery: Hematochezia or purulent hematochezia is observed along with abdominal pain, which is relieved after defecation. Mucus-like purulent bloody stool and fever are common.
   - Ulcerative colitis: Patients with mild conditions may have mucus bloody stool, while severe patients can have brick red or brown hematochezia.
   - Amebic dysentery: Dark red jelly-like purulent hematochezia, accompanied with abdominal pain
   - Acute hemorrhagic necrotic enteritis: Defection of bloody water, without peculiar odor.
   - Colorectal Cancer:Hematochezia, constipation, abdominal pain, lower GI obstruction, anemia, weight loss, abdominal mass.
   - Colorectal polyp: Hematochezia, melena, anemia, rarely have abdominal pain
   - Hemorrhoids, anal fissure: Fresh blood is not mixed with stool; bloody lining on fecal surface. Bleeding before and after defecation or dripping of blood is suggestive of anus or anal canal disease.
5. **Accompanying symptoms**
   - Abdominal pain: Other than gastrointestinal ulcers, bile duct hemorrhage, bacterial dysentery, amebic dysentery, ulcerative colitis, acute hemorrhagic necrotic enteritis, colorectal cancer, hematochezia or melena can also be observed in intestinal intussusception, mesenteric thrombus formation or thrombosis, etc.
   - Tenesmus: Feeling of incomplete defection or increase bowel movement frequencies, but minimal feces is defecated. Suggestive of anal or rectal diseases; seen in dysentery, rectitis, and rectal cancer.
   - Fever: Commonly seen in infectious disease, such as bacteria dysentery, typhoid fever, sepsis, hemorrhagic fever, leptospirosis, and some malignant tumors, such as intestinal lymphoma and leukemia, etc.
   - Hemorrhagic tendencies: Skin and mucosal petechiae is seen in acute infectious disease and hematological diseases, such as severe hepatitis, hemorrhagic fever, leukemia, Henoch-Schönlein purpura, hemophilia, etc.
   - Skin changes: Spider nevus and liver palm are suggestive of portal hypertension secondary to liver cirrhosis. Web of dilated capillaries observed on skin and mucosa is suggestive of hereditary telangiectasia.
   - Abdominal mass: Probable intestinal malignant lymphoma, colon cancer, intestinal tuberculosis, intestinal intussusception and Crohn's disease, etc.

Key Points in History Taking

1. History of ingesting unsanitary, raw, spicy food, or animal blood. Dining with other patients.
2. History of alcohol consumption, medication use, past medical history, prior endoscopic or surgical treatment.
3. Color of melena or hematochezia relative to other stool samples.
4. Volume of melena and C
5. Accompanying symptoms abdominal pain, tenesmus, jaundice, fever, abdominal mass, obstruction, hemorrhagic tendencies, etc.
6. General condition of a patient (dizziness, palpitations, sweating, syncope).
7. Treatment and Diagnosis (a) routine exams: blood, urine, stool routine, liver and renal function, blood glucose and lipids, and viral hepatitis markers; (b) endoscopy exam, capsule endoscopy, abdominal ultrasound, and abdominal CT. (c) Treatments received.

Diarrhea

20

Ling Dong and Rui Zeng

Diarrhea is defined as an increase in defecation frequency (more than 3 times per day), stool volume(more than 200 g per day), and stool liquidity (water content more than 85%). A high fiber diet can increase the amount of daily fecal excretion, thus fecal volume is an insufficient representation of diarrhea. Frequent defecation is also observed in fecal incontinence, secondary to ano-rectal neuromuscular diseases or pelvic diseases. Although loose stool can be observed in such conditions, but the underlying mechanism disregards intestinal water, electrolyte absorption and motility dysfunction, therefore cannot be defined as diarrhea.

20.1 Etiology

1. **Acute diarrhea:** Approximately 80% of acute diarrhea is caused by infections and the remaining 20% is secondary to dyspepsia, drugs, toxins, hypersensitivity, and acute intestinal ischemia, etc.
2. **Chronic diarrhea:** Different from acute diarrhea, majority of chronic diarrhea are due to non-infectious (Table 20.1), and multifactorial etiologies. Chronic diarrhea can be subdivided into secretary, osmotic, and mixed diarrhea according to its pathophysiological characteristics.

Table 20.1 Chronic diarrhea etiology

Etiology	Pathogenesis	Disease
Secretary diarrhea	Exogenous factors in promoting secretion	Various intestinal toxins
	Endogenous factors in promoting secretion	Neuroendocrine neoplasm
	Lack of ion transporter	Congenital chloride diarrhea
	Decrease in intestinal surface area	Large segment bowel resection, diffuse intestinal disease
	Intestinal ischemia	Diffuse mesenteric atherosclerosis
	Rapid intestinal motility	Post-vagotomy
Osmotic diarrhea	Ingestion of food that is difficult to absorb	Intake of magnesium preparation
	Nutrient transport deficiency	Lactase deficiency
Mixed diarrhea	Polypeptide released by intestinal endocrine cells	Cholera, inflammatory bowel disease, irritable bowel syndrome, malabsorption
	Inflammatory mediators released by immune cells	
	Activation of the enteric nervous system	
	Secretion of hormones by the endocrine system	

20.2 Mechanism

Under physiological conditions, the intestinal tract absorbs majority of the ingested fluid and gastrointestinal secretions, ranging from 9 to 10 L per day. When the absorption ability is reduced by 1%, due to various pathogenic factors, diarrhea may occur. Peristalsis provides a suitable environment optimal for the absorption of water, electrolytes and nutrients. Increase in intestinal secretion and acceleration of peristalsis can promote expulsion of intestinal infection and toxins.

1. **Secretory diarrhea:** Water is absorbed along with water soluble particles in the intestinal tract. The osmotic gradient resulting from active absorption of NaCl plays a key role in water absorption. The tight gap junction between cellular membrane and intracellular matrix also has a high permeability for water. A variety of enterotoxin secondary to intestinal infections can interfere with epithelial reabsorption of sodium ions, by increasing secretion of

L. Dong
Department of Gastroenterology, Fudan University, Shanghai, China

R. Zeng (✉)
Department of Cardiology, Sichuan University, Chengdu, China

X.-H. Wan, R. Zeng (eds.), *Handbook of Clinical Diagnostics*, https://doi.org/10.1007/978-981-13-7677-1_20

anions (Cl^- and HCO_3^-)or by inhibiting Na^+-H^+ exchange of the epithelial cells, which in turn hinders intestinal electrolytes and water reabsorption. Severe watery diarrhea caused by the exotoxin of vibrio cholera is a typical example of secretory diarrhea. The exotoxin stimulates the intracellular adenyl cyclase of intestinal mucosal cells, increasing the amount cAMP, which results in a large volume secretion of water and electrolytes into the intestinal tract, causing diarrhea. Infection of toxigenic E. coli, gastrointestinal endocrine tumors, such as gastrinoma and vasoactive intestinal peptide tumor can also result in secretory diarrhea.

In addition, decrease in surface area of the intestinal lumen can restrict the reabsorption of sodium and other electrolytes, as well as reabsorption of water. This condition is commonly observed after large segment bowel resection and diffuse intestinal diseases.

2. **Osmotic diarrhea:** As the enteral osmolality increases, large amount of body fluid enters the hypertonic intestinal lumen. For instance, the inability to hydrolyze lactose in lactase deficiency results in a hypertonic enteral environment. Similarly, ingestion of saline laxative and mannitol also results in osmotic diarrhea.
3. **Mixed diarrhea:** The above mentioned classification depicts an easily understandable mechanism behind diarrhea. However, most cases involve more than one pathogenesis (Fig. 20.1), in which one particular mechanism dominates. For example, as an agonist, prostaglandin stimulates intestinal epithelial function, smooth muscle contraction, and paracellular pathways, which affects ion transportation, intestinal motility, mucosal permeability, and often results in diarrhea.

PINE: paracrine, immune, neural, endocrine. Acute diarrhea is a protective mechanism of the intestinal tract to expel toxins through secreting body fluid and increasing motility; Chronic diarrhea lacks normal coping mechanism.

20.3 Clinical Manifestations

1. **Onset and course of disease:** Acute diarrhea is characterized by a rapid onset, with over 10 or more defecations of large volume, watery stool, often accompanied with stomach rumble, colicky pain or tenesmus. The course of disease is generally less than 3 weeks. Symptoms that lasts more than a month is considered chronic diarrhea.
2. **Secretory and osmotic diarrhea:** Secretory diarrhea has the following features: (a) Volume of feces per day exceeds 1 L (can reach 10 L in severe cases). (b) Watery stool without pus, blood and foul smell. (c) Fecal pH value is mostly neutral or alkaline. (d) Diarrhea remains persistent even after fasting for 48 h, with a fecal volume of more than 500 mL/d. (e) Secretory diarrhea is rarely accompanied by abdominal pain.Osmotic diarrhea is characterized by the relief or cessation of diarrhea after fasting for 48 h.
3. **Pathological lesion:** Small intestinal and colonic diarrhea differ in presentation (Table 20.2).
4. **Diarrhea caused by intestinal inflammation:** Diarrhea caused by intestinal inflammation damages the integrity of the intestinal mucosa, resulting in lesions like hyperemia, edema, erosion, ulcer and hyperplasia. Gross bloody purulent stool are often seen in colonic inflammation, especially left colonic inflammation. Feces of intes-

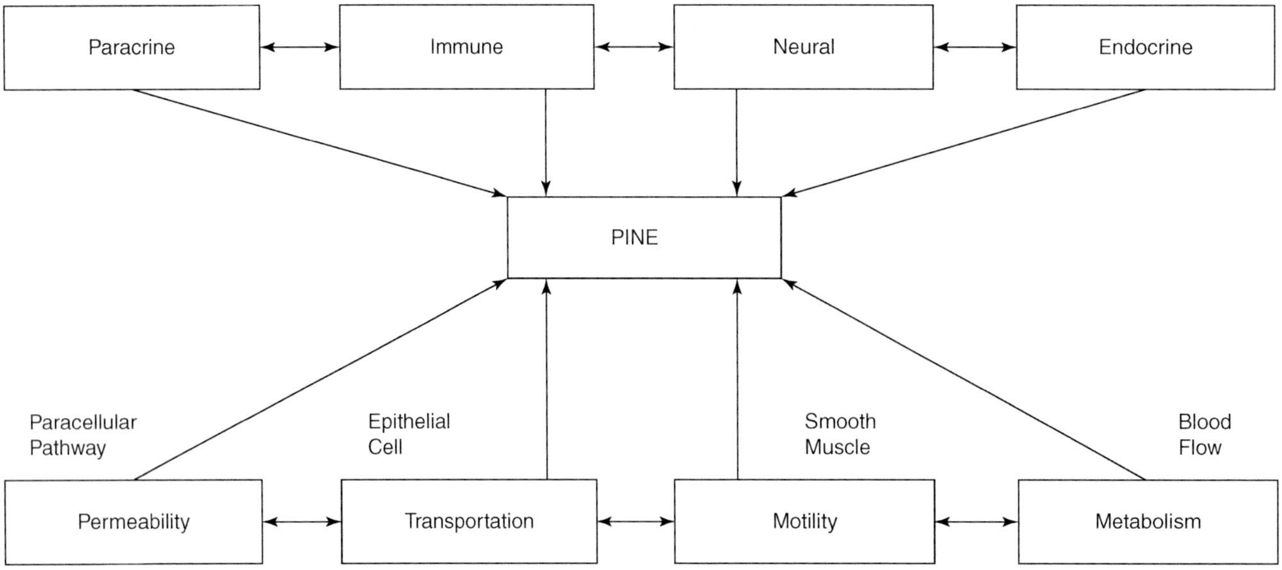

Fig. 20.1 Intestinal PINE network regulatory system

Table 20.2 Diarrhea characteristics of small intestine and colon

	Intestinal diarrhea	Colonic diarrhea
Abdominal pain	Umbilical region	Lower abdomen or left lower quadrant
Feces	Large in volume Loose stool Steatorrhea Few mucus Foul Smell	Less in volume Bloody and purulent With mucus
Frequency	2–10 times per day	Could exceed 10 times per day
Tenesmus	None	May be present
Weight loss	Often	Rare

tinal inflammation often contain an even mixture of exudates and blood, only visible under the microscope. Gross bloody and purulent stool are rare, unless there is a large amount of exudates or rapid peristalsis.Feces in amebic dysentery is dark red in color or jelly-like. While cholera presents as rice-water stool. For vibrio parahemolyticus infection, the stool could be bloody or pink watery stool. Rotavirus enteritis in infants presents as egg drop like watery stool. For intestinal toxigenic E. coli enteritis in children, the stool is usually green watery stool.

5. **Diarrhea caused by other abnormal intestinal motility:** Patients with diarrhea caused by other abnormal intestinal motility usually suffer from urgency of defecation. Feces tends to be loose or watery, without exudates or blood. Hyperactive bowel sounds and abdominal pain could also be observed in these patients. When diarrhea is caused by dyspepsia, the stool usually has a foul smell, grease-like and viscous. If the stool only has mucus without other pathological signs, the patients most likely suffer from IBS(irritable bowel syndrome).
6. **Accompanying Symptoms:** (a) Fever could be seen in patients suffering from acute bacillary dysentery, typhoid fever, paratyphoid fever, intestinal tuberculosis, intestinal malignant lymphoma, active ulcerative colitis and sepsis. (b) Tenesmus could be observed in patients with colorectal lesions, such as acute dysentery, rectal inflammation and rectal tumor. (c) Obvious weight loss could be seen in patients with small intestinal lesions, such as gastrointestinal malignant tumor and malabsorption syndrome. (d) Skin lesions such as rash and subcutaneous hemorrhage could be seen in patients suffering from sepsis, typhoid fever, paratyphoid fever, measles, Henoch-Schönlein Purpura, pellagra, etc. (e) Abdominal mass could be palpable in patients with gastrointestinal malignant tumor, intestinal tuberculosis, Crohn's disease and schistosomiasis granuloma. (f) Severe dehydration is common in patients suffering from secretory diarrhea, such as in cholera, bacterial food poisoning, uremia, etc. (g) Arthralgia and arthrocele could be observed in patients with Crohn's disease, ulcerative colitis and systemic lupus erythematosus.

Key Points in History Taking

1. The onset and course of diarrhea. For elderly patients, presence of fecal incontinence is important.
2. Prior history of consuming contaminated, uncooked, spicy or greasy food before experiencing diarrhea? Whether dining companions suffer from similar symptoms?
3. History of drug use, alcohol abuse, traveling, surgical procedures, past medical history or similar symptoms within the patient's community or family.
4. Frequency of defecation, volume, characteristics, fecal odor Presence of steatorrhea or bloody purulent stool. General condition of the patient (dizziness, palpitation, cold sweat, syncope, etc).
5. Factors of alleviation or exacerbation Ingestion of food, consuming greasy food, fasting, or antibiotic usage, etc.
6. Is the occurrence of diarrhea related to tension or anxiety?
7. Accompanying symptoms Abdominal pain, fever, tenesmus, dehydration, weight loss, anemia, edema and malnutrition, etc.
8. Diagnosis and treatment
   - Laboratory tests: blood routine, urine routine, stool routine, liver and kidney function, blood glucose, blood lipid, blood electrolytes, viral hepatitis markers, etc.
   - Gastroscopy, colonoscopy, capsule endoscopy, abdominal ultrasound and abdominal CT scan.
   - Response to treatment.

Constipation

21

Zhijun Duan and Rui Zeng

Constipation is defined as difficult defecation, straining of stool passage, reduced frequency of bowel movements and lumpy or hard stools. About 2–28% of the population suffer from constipation, which is more common in females than males. The incidence of constipation increases with age, and the prevalence in the elderly population ranges from 15 to 20%.

21.1 Etiology

Constipation may have various etiologies (Table 21.1). According to different pathogenesis, constipation can be divided into two categories, organic constipation and functional constipation. Functional constipation can be induced by a lack of fibrous diet or water intake, changes in living environment, disturbed bowel habits, laxative abuse, irritable bowel syndrome, etc. Risk factors for constipation include female, old age, low income, lack of education, decreased activity and frequent drug use.

21.2 Mechanism

After food is digested and absorbed in the digestive tract, the remaining chyme is transported from the small intestine to the colon, where water and electrolytes inside the chyme are further absorbed, and then feces is formed and moved to the proctosigmoid, and ultimately excreted. Each part of this process could be impaired by abnormal neurological activity, intestinal smooth muscle diseases and anal sphincter dysfunction, resulting in constipation. The physical activities of bowel movements include: (a) The mechanical irritation induced by increasing fecal matter in the rectum creates the urge of defecation and defecation reflex followed by a series of muscle activities; (b) Contraction of rectal smooth muscle; (c) Relaxation of internal and external anal sphincter; (d) Contractions of the diaphragm and abdominal muscles increase abdominal pressure, which may lead to excretion. If any kind of disorder occurs in the above mentioned process, constipation may occur.

According to pathophysiology, functional constipation can be classified as: Normal transmission, Slow transmission, Outlet obstruction, and Mixed constipation (Table 21.2).

Table 21.1 Pathogenesis of organic constipation

Mechanical obstruction	Metabolic and endocrine diseases
Archostegnosis Colorectal cancer Colorectal compression Intestinal stenosis	Diabetes, Heavy metal poisoning Hypercalcemia, Hypothyroidism Hypokalemia, Hypopituitarism Pheochromocytoma, Pregnancy Porphyria, Gestation
Drugs	**Nerve and muscle disease**
Antiacid, Anticholinergic, Antispastic Antitumor drug Calcium channel blocker Diuretic, Serotonin blocker Iron supplements Non-steroidal anti-inflammatory drugs Opioid agonist	Amyloidosis, Autonomic neuropathy Dermatomyositis Intestinal pseudo-obstruction Multiple sclerosis, Parkinson's Disease Spinal cord injury, Stroke Others Redundant colon

Table 21.2 Pathophysiological classification of functional constipation

Normal transmission	Lack of food, fiber or water intake causes insufficient chyme and fecal volume to stimulate the intestinal peristalsis.
Slow transmission	Reduction of colonic motility, extension of transit time and decrease of rectal filling speed will weaken rectal response. Excessive water absorption in the bowel results in hard stools and aggravates constipation.
Outlet obstruction	Abnormal rectum sensitivity, reduction of inhibitory reflex or dyssynergic bowel movements.
Mixed constipation	Slow transmission + Outlet obstruction.

Z. Duan
Department of Gastroenterology, Dalian Medical University, Dalian, China

R. Zeng (✉)
Department of Cardiology, Sichuan University, Chengdu, China

X.-H. Wan, R. Zeng (eds.), *Handbook of Clinical Diagnostics*, https://doi.org/10.1007/978-981-13-7677-1_21

21.3 Clinical Manifestations

Healthy people usually defecate once or twice per day, or once every other day with formed or soft stools, and some can defecate three times per day or once every three days with half-formed or sausage-like stool. Therefore we cannot regard defecation of once per day as a standard for normal bowel movement. Instead, we should focus on the presence of difficult defecation or changes in stool characteristics. Anxious patients often seek medical attention for the inability to defecate every day, thus thorough explanation is necessary.

The common symptoms of constipation include difficult defecation, lumpy or hard stools, a sensation of incomplete excretion and decreased bowel movements, with the respective incidence of each symptom at 80, 72, 54 and 40%. Decrease in frequency of defecation (less than 2–3 times per week) is only experienced in 35% of patients.

Patients with mild symptoms that have no impact on their daily lives can usually self-adjust or receive drug treatment for a short period of time. Those patients with serious and continuous symptoms which severely affect their daily lives rely on laxatives, or sometimes lack an effective treatment.

Acute constipation can be accompanied with clinical symptoms of primary diseases. Symptoms are often accompanied by abdominal pain, abdominal distension, nausea and vomitingS secondary to intestinal obstruction of various etiologies. Chronic constipation is atypical and some patients may have mild symptoms such as a bitter sensation, decrease in appetite, abdominal distension, discomfort in the lower abdomen, dizziness, headaches and fatigue. Other patients excrete 'sheep-dung' stools and may have cramping and a straining sensation in the left or lower abdomen while defecating. Spasmodic sigmoid colon can often be palpated in the left lower abdomen. Patients suffering from serious difficult defecation may become nervous and anxious due to bleeding of hemorrhoids or anal fissure. Different types of functional constipation may present as different symptoms (Table 21.3).

Table 21.3 Characteristics of functional constipation

Normal transmission	Incomplete evacuation, present/absent abdominal pain.
Slow transmission	Defecation less than once a week; defecation hypesthesia, poor reaction to fiber and laxatives, general malaise, fatigue, more common in young women.
Outlet obstruction	nervous, incomplete evacuation, manual facilitation.

21.4 Accompanying Symptoms

The accompanying symptoms of constipation can be mild or severe. (a) Vomit, abdominal distention and intestinal colic attribute to various causes of intestinal obstruction. (b) Patients with abdominal mass should be screened for colon cancer. However, the spasmodic sigmoid colon in the left lower abdominal quadrant should not be mistaken for a tumor. The sausage-shaped sigmoid colon can be palpated and may disappear after defecation. In intestinal tuberculosis and Crohn's disease, a mass can also form due to intestinal adhesions, which requires differentiation. (c) Alternation between constipation and diarrhea are common in intestinal tuberculosis and irritable bowel syndrome. (d) Changes in living conditions and heavy stress can lead to functional constipation.

Key Points in History Taking

1. Whether defecation is difficult with or without straining of stool passage? Inquire as to frequency of bowel movement, fecal characteristics, stool volume, and frequency of manual facilitation.
2. Whether constipation follows diarrhea, is continuous or intermittent? Whether anxiety or stress leads to constipation. Whether the dietary or living habits have changed.
3. Whether the patient has long-term use of laxatives, whether he/she is addicted to laxatives.
4. Current use of medication, course of treatment and effectiveness, as well as past abdominal or pelvic surgeries.
5. Accompanying symptoms. Nausea, vomiting, abdominal distension, cramps, abdominal mass, intestinal pattern, anemia, hematochezia and general physical condition including diet, weight, mental state and sleep.
6. Diagnosis and treatment. (a) Routine tests: routine blood test, routine stool test, occult blood test, blood glucose, blood calcium, and carcino-embryonic antigen (CEA). (b) Colonoscopy, barium meal, abdominal ultrasound, and abdominal computed tomography(CT). (c) Treatment response.

Jaundice

22

Zhijun Duan and Rui Zeng

Jaundice is a symptom or a physical sign of yellow pigmentation of skin, sclera and mucous membranes resulting from high bilirubin in the plasma. The highest value of normal serum bilirubin is 17.1 μmol/L (1.0 mg/dl), in which conjugated bilirubin is 3.42 μmol/L, and unconjugated bilirubin is 13.68 μmol/L. Jaundice is not prominent when serum bilirubin level is between 17.1 and 34.2 μmol/L, also known as recessive jaundice. The jaundice becomes apparent when bilirubin level reaches 34.2 μmol/L (2.0 mg/dl) or more. Normally, there is a dynamic balance between bilirubin "entering" and "leaving" the blood circulation, which keeps its concentration in the blood relatively constant.

22.1 Formation, Metabolism and Transport of Bilirubin

About 7.5 g of hemoglobin is produced daily from destroyed red blood cells, which generates 4275 μmol (250 mg) bilirubin in adults, accounting for 80–85% of total bilirubin. About 171–513 μmol (10–30 mg) bilirubin is derived from the hemoglobin in immature red blood cells of bone marrow and the proteins containing ferroheme in the liver (e.g., catalase, peroxidase, cytochrome oxidase and myoglobin), all of which are called bypass bilirubin, accounting for 15–20% of total bilirubin.

The formation of bilirubin mentioned above is known as non-combined bilirubin or unconjugated bilirubin. Unconjugated bilirubin binds with albumin, is water-insoluble, and cannot be filtrated by the glomerulus, therefore it does not appear in the urine. Unconjugated bilirubin is transported to the liver through circulation and is separated from albumin, before being absorbed by hepatic cells via the Disse Space (Fig. 22.1). Bilirubin may be transferred to the endoplasmic reticulum, where conjugation occurs. Formation of bilirubin glucuronide, or conjugated bilirubin, is catalyzed by microsomal glucuronyltransferase. The conjugated bilirubin is transported to the microvilli of bile canaliculus, bile duct, and eventually enters the intestinal tract. The majority of the bilirubin drained from bile is diester bilirubin. Water soluble conjugated bilirubin is filtered mainly through the glomerulus and can be detected in the urine. In the terminal ileum and colon, conjugated bilirubin is dehydrogenated by bacterial enzymes to form urobilinogen (total amount of 68–473 μmol), the majority of which is oxidized into urobilin and ultimately defecated, thus urobilin is also called stercobilin. A small portion (10–20%) of urobilinogen is absorbed by the intestine and returned to the liver through the hepatic portal vein, where most of the urobilinogen is converted into conjugated bilirubin and re-excreted into the intestine. This phenomenon is known as the "enterohepatic circulation of bilirubin ". Less than 6.8 μmol(4 mg) of the urobilinogen that is reabsorbed to the liver is excreted through the kidneys per day (Fig. 22.1).

22.2 Classification

According to the etiological and pathophysiological mechanism, jaundice can be divided into hemolytic, hepatocellular, obstructive and congenital non-hemolytic jaundice. Depending on the nature of the increased bilirubin, jaundice may be further defined as two major pathophysiologic categories: increased unconjugated bilirubin(UCB) and increased conjugated bilirubin(CB) jaundice.

22.3 Etiology and Mechanism

1. **Hemolytic jaundice:** Many disorders may cause hemolytic jaundice, including congenital hemolytic anemia (e.g., globin thalassemia or genetic spherical red cell

Z. Duan
Department of Gastroenterology, Dalian Medical University, Dalian, China

R. Zeng (✉)
Department of Cardiology, Sichuan University, Chengdu, China

X.-H. Wan, R. Zeng (eds.), *Handbook of Clinical Diagnostics*, https://doi.org/10.1007/978-981-13-7677-1_22

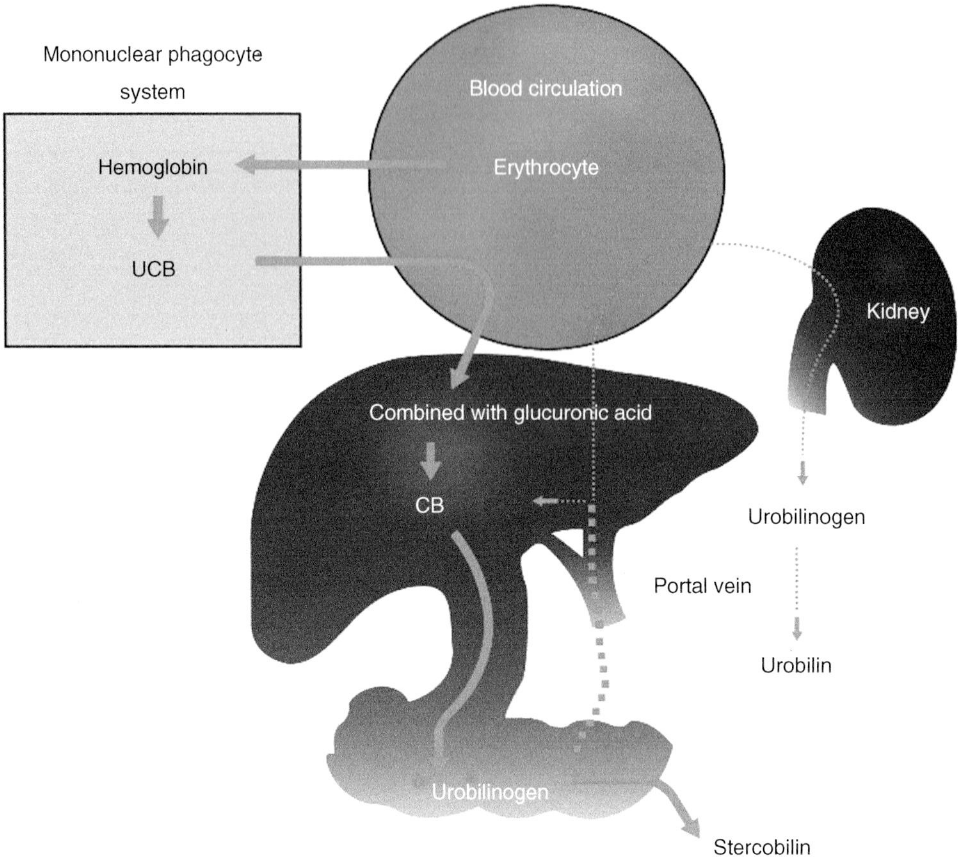

Fig. 22.1 The formation, metabolism and transport of bilirubin

histiocytosis) and acquired hemolytic anemia (autoimmune hemolytic anemia; hemolytic disease of the newborn; hemolysis due to different blood type transfusion, favism, snake venom or mushroom; primaquine and paroxysmal nocturnal hemoglobinuria; etc.). The dramatic increase in circulation of UCB caused by destruction of a large number of red blood cells exceeds the capacity of bilirubin uptake, as well as conjugation and excretion of liver cells, resulting in retention of UCB in the blood and therefore jaundice.

2. **Hepatocellular jaundice:** Hepatocellular jaundice may be caused by all types of hepatitis viruses, alcohol, drugs, poisons, bacterial toxins and proinflammatory cytokines, autoantibodies, graft-versus-host disease, lymphoma, parasites, disorders of copper or iron metabolism, hepatic ischemia reperfusion, sepsis, pregnancy, full enteral parenteral nutrition, etc. The injured liver cells are incapable of bilirubin uptake, combination and excretion. In some pathological conditions, damage of the capillary bile duct may lead to impaired bile formation and/or bile flow, which may cause CB reflux to the blood. Therefore, both high serum UCB and CB can be detected in hepatocellular jaundice.
3. **Cholestatic jaundice:** Cholestasis is a clinical and biochemical syndrome caused by the disorder of bile formation and/or bile flow. It can be subdivided into two types, intrahepatic and extrahepatic cholestatic jaundice. Intrahepatic cholestatic jaundice is also known as cholestatic liver disease, so its common causes are the same as those of hepatocellular jaundice. Extrahepatic cholestatic jaundice is the other major cause of cholestasis, most commonly due to gallstones, stenosis, inflammatory edema, cancer embolus, parasitic diseases (e.g., Clonorchis sinensis disease) occurring in the extrahepatic bile duct. These disorders may cause biliary obstruction, increase in bile duct pressure, cholangiectasis, and may ultimately result in rupture of the small bile duct and capillaries, causing the reentrance of bilirubin into the blood circulation. Thus, for diagnosis of cholestatic jaundice, marked CB increase in serum is necessary.
4. **Congenital non-hemolytic jaundice:** The hereditary disorders of hepatic bilirubin metabolism are characterized by the inability of the liver to perform bilirubin uptake, conjugation and excretion, leading to hyperbilirubinemia. This condition is relatively rare in clinical settings.

- Gilbert's syndrome Mild unconjugated hyperbilirubinemia is recognized most commonly during the second and third decades of life. Gilbert's syndrome results from a decrease in hepatic UCB uptake and a lack of glucuronyl transferase.
- Crigler-Najiar syndrome Serum UCB level increases due to deficiency of glucuronyl transferase in hepatocellular microsomes, impairing conjugation of bilirubin. Crigler-Najiar syndrome occurs in the newborn and is called kernicterus newborn. This condition has a poor prognosis.
- Rotor's syndrome Unconjugated hyperbilirubinemia is caused by congenital defects of liver cells to uptake UCB and excrete CB.
- Dubin-Johnson syndrome Hyperbilirubinemia results from the dysfunction of liver cells to excrete CB and certain anions (such as indocyanine green, X-ray contrast agent) into the bile capillaries, resulting in increase of CB and jaundice.

22.4 Clinical Manifestations

Different types of jaundice are distinctive in aspects of skin color, pruritus, feces and urine color, liver function and urine routine test, etc. (Table 22.1).

Table 22.1 Differential diagnosis of three common jaundices

	Hemolytic	Hepatocellular	Cholestatic
Skin color	light yellow	pale yellow to deep yellow	dark yellow to dark green
Cutaneous pruritus	negative	slight	obvious
Urine color	tawny	dark	dark
Stool color	darker	darker	lighter
Other symptoms	fever, shiver, headache, vomiting, osphyalgia; anemia, splenomegaly	fatigue, anorexia, diarrhea, edema, (bleeding tendency in severe cases)	Abdominal pain, fever, bradycardia
Bilirubin	UCB↑	UCB↑ CB↑	CB↑
CB/TB	<20%	>30%	>60%
Urobilirubin	(−)	(+)	(++)
Urobilinogen	↑	↑↑	↓
ALT, AST	normal	↑↑	↑
ALP	normal	↑	↑↑
GGT	normal	↑	↑↑

Abbreviation: *TB* total bilirubin, *UCB* unconjugated bilirubin, *CB* conjugated bilirubin, *ALT* alanine aminotransferase, *AST* aspartate transferase, *ALP* alkaline phosphatase, *GGT* glutamyltranspeptidase

22.5 Specific Examinations

1. **Color doppler ultrasonography**: Ultrasonography is often preferred over CT as the first diagnostic modality. It is useful for evaluating liver size and shape, liver lesions, and gallstone and gallbladder size; allows differentiation between intra- and/or extrahepatic biliary system dilation; and can detect splenomegaly and pancreatic lesion.
2. **Electronic computed tomography(CT):** The upper abdominal scan plays an essential role in detection and identification of the jaundice caused by liver, gallbladder, pancreas or other lesions. It also provides valuable assessment for bile duct dilation and intraabdominal mass.
3. **Magnetic resonance imaging (MRI)**: MRI has high resolution for soft tissue and is able to show multi-direction, multi-sequence imaging. MRI is superior to CT in detecting and identifying benign and malignant liver tumors. It can also be used to detect metabolic and inflammatory liver diseases. Magnetic resonance cholangiopancreatography (MRCP) can better display the diameter of the bile duct and pancreatic duct, which provides superior value to ultrasound and CT for detecting stones in the middle and lower portions of the bile duct.
4. **Endoscopic retrograde cholangiopancreatography (ERCP)**: ERCP provides direct observation of lesions in the ampulla and papilla, and allows determination between intrahepatic or extrahepatic obstruction. Meanwhile, it can be applied in detecting pancreatic lesions.
5. **Radionuclide examination**: Radionuclide ^{198}Au or ^{99m}Tc scanning can help to identify liver masses. The application of ^{131}iodine rose bengal in liver scanning is useful in identifying cholestatic jaundice and hepatocellular jaundice.
6. **Percutaneous transhepatic cholangiography (PTC)**: PTC can clearly display the whole biliary system, distinguish between extrahepatic and intrahepatic obstruction of the bile duct, and show the location, extent and scope of the obstruction.
7. **Liver biopsy and laparoscopy**: The principal role of a liver biopsy and laparoscopy is in the differential diagnosis of difficult or confusing cases with intrahepatic cholestasis. Liver biopsy is an invasive procedure and is not recommended in routine workup of suspected obstruction. The procedure can result in peritonitis caused by the overflow of bile in cases of cholestatic jaundice. Internal bleeding may also occur due to disturbance of blood coagulation in patients with hepatic insufficiency.

Key Points in History Taking

1. To determine whether it is jaundice Jaundice should be distinguished from ochrodermia, fat below the bulbar conjunctiva, and carotenemia. (see detail in eye examination). Urine color is key in verification.
2. The onset of jaundice Acute or chronic onset, duration, and development of the finding may provide important clues.
3. Ask about potential etiologic or predisposing factors Epidemic onsets, traveling experiences, drug use, long-term alcohol consumption, parasitic infections, liver or gallbladder diseases and past surgery history must be reviewed in detail.
4. Accompanying symptoms of jaundice Some nonspecific symptoms may be important evidence, including gastrointestinal symptoms, skin itching, vision disorders, fever, abdominal pain, etc.
5. The effects of jaundice on systemic health There is a positive correlation between the degree of hepatocellular jaundice and severity of liver function damage. Generally, patients with congenital disorders of bilirubin metabolism have little discomfort.
6. Diagnosis and treatment (a) Routine laboratory tests: routine blood, urine, and stool tests, fecal occult blood test, liver function, renal function, blood glucose, blood lipids and alpha-fetoglobulin(AFP); (b) Abdominalultrasonography, CT and MRCP; (c) Treatment response.

Hematuria

23

Jialin Chen and Rui Zeng

Hematuria (haematuria) is a common symptom of urinary system diseases. Normal people's urine has a small amount of red blood cells. The definition of hematuria is: (a) red blood cell of fresh urine is more than three per high-power field in microscopic examination after centrifugation (10 mL of urine to 1500 rpm for 5 min), (b) direct counting red blood cells of fresh urine is more than 8000/mL, (c) per hour of red blood cell discharge number more than 30,000 for male and more than 40,000 for women in 3 h urine cell counting, (d) 12 h urine Addis count red cell more than 5 × 10^6. Mild hematuria is only seen blood cell increased under the microscope, called microscopic hematuria. Bleeding bulls' urine color is usually like water of wash the meat, tea colored or red, called as the naked eye hematuria. Hematuria first need to rule out false hematuria caused by menstruation, vaginal or rectal bleeding, in addition to the normal human after strenuous exercise, urine red blood cells can be increased temporarily to 10,000–60,000/mL.

23.1 Etiology

The hematuria is mainly caused by the urinary system itself, also can be caused by systemic diseases and urinary tract adjacent organ disease. The common causes of the disease are as follows.

1. Urinary system diseases
   - Primary glomerular diseases: IgA nephropathy, crescent nephritis, focal segmental glomerular sclerosis, etc...
   - Secondary glomerular diseases, such as systemic lupus erythematosus, allergic purpora, and post infectious glomerulonephritis;
   - Infection: pyelonephritis, cystitis, urethritis, prostatitis, kidney and bladder tuberculosis;
   - Stones: kidney, ureter, bladder and urethral stones, etc...
   - Tumors: kidney, ureter, bladder and prostate tumors, etc...
   - Genetic diseases: hereditary nephritis, polycystic kidney, kidney and urinary tract abnormalities, etc...
   - Vascular diseases: renal artery thrombosis and embolism, renal vein thrombosis, renal arteriovenous malformations, etc...
   - Other reasons such as interstitial nephritis, renal papillary necrosis and urinary system trauma.
2. The disease of adjacent organs: Acute appendicitis, pelvic inflammation, inflammation of the fallopian tube or adjacent organs tumor stimulation or invasion to the bladder and ureter, can cause hematuria.
3. Systemic disease
   - Blood disease: thrombocytopenia purpura, regeneration barrier anemia, leukemia, blood coagulation factor deficiency, the use of anticoagulant therapy.
   - Infectious diseases: such as infective endocarditis, sepsis, epidemic hemorrhagic fever, epidemic meningitis, etc...
   - Vascular diseases: such as malignant hypertension, congestive heart failure, etc...
   - Endocrine and metabolic diseases: diabetic nephropathy, renal amyloidosis, etc...
4. Physical, chemical factors and drug: Radiation nephritis, cystitis; chemicals mercury, lead and cadmium heavy metals; animal and plant toxins; sulfa drugs, non steroidal anti-inflammatory drugs, mannitol and other drugs on the kidney injury; cyclophosphamide induced hemorrhagic cystitis; anticoagulation with heparin and Warfarin overdose.
5. Functional: Healthy people with a sudden increase in the amount of exercise may appear hematuria.
6. Idiopathic: After a comprehensive careful examination, we are failed to clear the cause of hematuria.

J. Chen
Department of Internal Medicine, Peking Union Medical College, Beijing, China

R. Zeng (✉)
Department of Cardiology, Sichuan University, Chengdu, China

X.-H. Wan, R. Zeng (eds.), *Handbook of Clinical Diagnostics*, https://doi.org/10.1007/978-981-13-7677-1_23

23.2 Mechanism

According to the source of red blood cells in the urine, hematuria is divided into: (A) Renal hematuria: refers to red blood cells in the urine from the kidney parenchyma; its characteristics is abnormal erythrocyte morphological; (B) Non renal hematuria: refers to red blood cells in the urine from the urinary system, including renal pelvis, ureter, bladder and urethra, red blood cells rarely occur deformation. The occurrence mechanism of hematuria is mainly in the following aspects.

1. Immune abnormal

   Under the effects of some pathogenic factors, body produce autoimmune reaction and form the immune complex deposition in the glomerular basement membrane, some auto-antibodies produce direct immune response to glomerular basement membrane as a target antigen. These immune responses disrupt the function of the glomerular basement membrane, which cause red blood cells enter to the urine fluid and form hematuria. The kidney damage of glomerular nephritis and connective tissue disease are often caused by the mechanism. The Immune response makes small renal vascular produce inflammatory reaction, necrosis, expansion, stenosis, occlusion, also can cause hematuria, such as: polyarteritis nodosa, microscopic polyangiitis and Wegener's granulomatosis.
2. Inflammatory reaction caused by infection

   The urinary system infection, which mainly is urethral infection, results in urinary tract mucosal inflammatory reaction, edema, congestion and small vessel damage.
3. Urinary system diseases

   The urinary system tumors, stones and trauma can cause urinary tissue damage and result in hematuria.
4. Sports injury

   Excessive sports make the kidney excessive movement, extrusion, ischemia, blood vessels pulled or distorted, etc...
5. Other reasons of hematuria

   Including toxic, allergic, renal vascular malformations and so on, they all can cause hematuria.

23.3 Clinical Manifestations and Accompanying Symptoms

According to the time of hematuria in urination, it can be divided into initial, terminal and total hematuria. Three cups of urine test can distinguish the three kinds of circumstances. The urine is developed in three cups when micturition namely, if hematuria appear in the beginning stage of urination (at the beginning of 10–15 mL), then the first cup has the blood, and the remaining two cup out of blood, the lesion site may be urethral; if hematuria appear in end stage of urine(the end of 10–30 mL), the third cup has the blood, hematuria called terminal hematuria, the lesion site may be the bladder neck and bladder carotid triangle or Posterior urethra; as whole are hematuria; if hematuria appear in the whole stage of urination, three cups of urine test can see blood cells, the lesion site may be the upper urinary tract or bladder. Hematuria of different causes can appear corresponding symptoms.

1. Hematuria with pain

   Basic characteristic of kidney stones is mainly waist pain with hematuria. Ureteral calculus is mainly colic and have radiation down ward abdominal and perineal; bladder and urethral stones have dysuria, micturition interrupts, often accompanied with urinary frequency and urgency. In addition, the tumor of urinary tract, renal tuberculosis and pyelonephritis can also have pain.
2. Hematuria accompanied with bladder irritation symptoms (urinary frequency, urgency, dysuria)

   Showed lesions in the bladder or posterior urethra, acute cystitis is the most common. It can also be seen in acute pyelonephritis, acute prostatitis, bladder cancer, tuberculosis.
3. Hematuria accompanied with abdominal mass

   Are commonly seen in kidney neoplasms, polycystic kidney, kidney prolapse, ectopic kidney, etc..
4. Hematuria with bleeding tendency

   Usually seen in the blood disorders, such as leukemia, hemophilia, thrombocytopenic purpura, etc.…
5. Hematuria with fever

   Can be seen in acute pyelonephritis, renal tuberculosis, epidemic hemorrhagic fever, leptospirosis etc...
6. Hematuria with high blood pressure, edema, and proteinuria

   Can be found in glomerular nephritis, etc...
7. Hematuria with chyluria

   Can be found in filariasis or chronic pyelonephritis, etc...
8. Asymptomatic hematuria

   It only has hematuria without any other discomfort, is commonly seen in IgA nephropathy, basement membrane nephropathy, and renal tumor, etc...
9. The relationship between hematuria and age or sex

   Hematuria in children may be found in glomerulonephritis, Wilms or congenital hydronephrosis. When the adult below 40 years old have hematuria, the female are more commonly caused by the urinary tract infections; the male are commonly caused by stones, prostatitis, tuberculosis and urethritis. When the adult over 40 years old have hematuria, it needs to consider tumors, benign prostatic hyperplasia and infection.

Key Points in History Taking

1. We first clear whether false hematuria caused by the following reasons: (A) Food factors: such as pepper, sugar beet, artificial colors, etc..; (B) Drug: rifampicin, phenol sulfonephthalein, Macau phenolphthalein sodium, rhubarb etc.; (C) Myoglobinuria caused by metabolic disorder of porphyrin or injury; (D) Vaginal or rectal bleeding.
2. Once determine the true hematuria: You need ask when patients presented with hematuria, at initial voiding, middle, or end of hematuria and whether there is a blood clot. Whether it is associated with other parts of the bleeding, such as hemoptysis, gastrointestinal bleeding, skin bleeding and excessive menstruation, it often suggests that there is a primary or secondary coagulation dysfunction.
3. We must clear whether the patients have history of kidney, urinary tract and prostate, including hypertension, edema, proteinuria and renal dysfunction.
4. Whether it is associated with urinary tract irritation, urinary interruption, renal colic, and abnormal urine volume.
5. Drug: whether it have a long-term or a large number of applications of sulfa drugs and antibiotics (such as aminoglycosides), antipyretic analgesic drugs, anti-cancer drugs and anticoagulants.
6. Whether it has excessive exercise recently, abdominal or lumbar trauma or urinary tract equipment inspection history.
7. Whether it has kidney disease, hematuria, deafness and family history of polycystic kidney disease.

Frequency, Urgency and Dysuria

24

Jialin Chen and Rui Zeng

Adult averagely have to urinate about 3–5 times daily, and most twice at night. An average output of urine every time is 200–400 mL. Frequency means voiding at frequent intervals. Urgency is an exaggerated sense of needing to urinate. Dysuria refers to pain or a burning sensation during urination. Frequency, urgency and dysuria are known as vesical irritability.

24.1 Etiology and Pathogenesis

1. Infection

   Infection is the commonest cause to produce irritative signs of the bladder and urethra, including:

   - Urinary-tract infection: These infection diseases, including pyonephrosis, nephropyelitis, renal tuberculosis, ureteritis are often concomitant with lower urinary tract infection and have the symptoms of frequency, urgency and dysuria.
   - Cystitis and urethritis: Including tuberculosis, fungi, chlamydia and gonorrhea result in the infection.
   - Infection of the adjacent organs of the bladder and urethra: The irritation signs of bladder can be also caused as follow: endometritis, salpingitis, coleitis, skenitis, prostatitis, balanitis, condyloma acuminatum and herpes simplex genitalis. The inflammation or abscessus of intestinal tract and appendix can cause same symptom as well.

2. Tumor

   The tumor that adjacent organs of the bladder and urethra, such as bladder cancer, prostate cancer, cervical and rectal cancer etc., could decrease bladder capacity by pressing down on the bladder and cause irritation signs of the bladder and urethra. The presence of tumor mass is often accompanied by dysuria

3. Stones and other stimulates

   Bladder and urethra calculi are usually reason of irritation signs. The symptoms of frequency, urgency and dysuria are produced by chronic bladder fibrosis, interstitial cystitis, urethra caruncle, bladder diverticula, foreign matter in urethra, that can caused by radioactive or chronic inflammatory injury. Pregnant woman that always suffers from a small bladder in late pregnancy because of bladder pressed also appears the similar symptoms

4. Chemical irritation

   The symptoms of frequency, urgency and dysuria may be presented because urine concentration during dehydration, highly acidic urine, medicine (cyclophosphamide).

5. Neurogenic bladder

   It is a series of symptoms that nervous system disease, including Lesions of the cerebral cortex or basal ganglia, Parkinson's disease, multiple sclerosis, present dysfunction of bladder urination and reserve.

6. Frequency by Polyuria

   Frequency is caused by drinking lots of water, diuretics, kidney disease, endocrine and metabolic diseases (diabetes insipidus, diabetes mellitus), these diseases often do not associate with dysuria, urgency.

7. Psychological factor

   Patients with psychentonia, dysphoria and anxiety can display urgency when they heard or see water.

24.2 Clinical Manifestations and Accompanying Symptoms

1. Acute Pyelonephritis

   Symptoms of this disease include a high fever, shaking chills and renal percussive pain, can accompany with or without frequency, urgency and odynuria. Acute cystitis

J. Chen
Department of Internal Medicine, Peking Union Medical College, Beijing, China

R. Zeng (✉)
Department of Cardiology, Sichuan University, Chengdu, China

X.-H. Wan, R. Zeng (eds.), *Handbook of Clinical Diagnostics*, https://doi.org/10.1007/978-981-13-7677-1_24

and urethritis usually present with frequency, urgency and odynuria, but rarely with body symptom because infection on mucosal surface.

2. Renal Tuberculosis

   Frequency, urgency and dysuria are common symptoms in early stage of the patient with renal tuberculosis because pyuria containing tuberculosis stimulates bladder and urinary tract. More serious of frequency is presented due to reduce the volume of bladder caused by bladder contracture. Few patients with renal tuberculosis do not have frequency, urgency and dysuria because of urinary tract obstruction in late period, but usually with other symptoms of tuberculosis infection such as fatigue, night sweats and hot flashes.

3. Urinary-tract infection

   The irritation signs of the bladder accompany with pus discharge and swollen of urethra often indicate infection of Neisseria gonorrhoeae and Chlamydia trachomatis through sexual transmitted.

4. Prostatitis

   Acute prostatitis is acute onset, with the symptoms of infective intoxication. Digital palpation examination can find swollen tenderness of prostate. Patient with chronic prostatitis feels perineum swollen and suprapubic pain, some patients develop in obstruction symptoms and sexual dysfunction.

5. Prostate Hypertrophy

   The patient is usually more than 50 years old, with progressive dysuria. On examination, there are bladder filling, enlarged prostate with smooth surface and springy.

6. Cystic Calculus

   Cystic Calculus often presets dysuria, interrupted urination or bifurcation of urination.

7. Neurogenic bladder

   The patient usually has a history of neurologic disease and often are accompanied by sensory and motion dysfunction of lower limbs.

Key Points in History Taking

1. When did frequency, urgency dysuria happen?
2. Frequency and numbers of urination, times in night urination and urinary volume of every time;
3. Location, nature, duration and radiation of dysuria;
4. Accompanying signs, such as fever, lumbago, hematuria, pyuria, dysuria and pus discharge from the urethral;
5. History of catheterization, urinary tract instrument examinations, and abortion;
6. Past history such as tuberculosis infection of urinary system, stones, pelvic disease, pelvic operation, CNS injury, and psychiatric history;
7. Personal history We should ask the patients or their spouses about history of sexual intercourse.

Oliguria, Anuria and Polyuria

25

Jialin Chen and Rui Zeng

The 24 h urine amount of the normal person is about 1000–2000 mL. Oliguria is defined as a urine output that is less than 400 mL/24 h or less than 17 mL/h in adults. Anuria is defined as urine output that is less than 100 mL/24 h or 0 mL/12 h. Polyuria is a condition characterized that there is large volumes of urine (at least 3000 mL over 24 h). Many factors affect the urine volume.

25.1 Etiology and Pathogenesis

The formation of urine requires glomerular filtration and tubular secretion and reabsorption. Glomerular filtration rate (GFR) depends upon renal blood perfusion, glomerular filtration membrane permeability, effect filtration area and pressure. Reabsorption and secretion of tubule depend upon structure and function of renal interstitial and tubule, are also influenced by factors of endocrine and metabolism. Urination needs ureter, bladder and urethra to keep unobstructed.

There are three different reasons often cause oliguria and anuria.

25.1.1 Oliguria and Anuria

- Prerenal: It is caused by decrease renal perfusion and effect filtration pressure. (A) Hypovolemia, such as massive bleeding, serious dehydration, hypoproteinemia, cirrhosis and nephritic syndrome; (B) Cardiovascular disease, including shock, heart failure, pericardial tamponade, acute coronary syndromes (ACS), pulmonary embolism (PE), and serious arrhythmia; (C) Renal vascular disease, including renal artery stenosis, polyarteritis, renal artery thrombosis, hypertensive crisis.
- Renal parenchymal: The site of injury can cause oliguria and anuria due to reduce glomerular filtration permeability and glomerular filtration area. (A) glomerular diseases: such as acute glomerulonephritis, rapidly progressive glomerulonephritis, chronic nephritis with acute at-tack, Goodpasture syndrome, lupus nephritis(LN), Wegener granulomatosis, thrombotic thrombocytopenic purpura (TTP), accelerated hypertension; (B) tubular and interstitial disease: such as acute tubular necrosis, necrotic renal papillitis, acute hyperuricemia, Hematosepsis; (C) renal vascular disease: such as malignant arteriolar nephrosclerosis, renal vein thrombosis; (D) others: such as acute rejection after renal transplantation.
- Postrenal**:** It is always caused by obstruction of the urine flow however produce of urine is normal. (A) Ureteral obstruction: mechanical blockade (such as calculi, tumor, blood clots, pus or Chylous block) or adhesions narrowing (such as tuberculosis chronic infection) are both result oliguria and anuria. Other causes include renal torsion, ureteral injure and edema or external pressure. (B) Urethra blockage such as ureteral calculus and vesical calculus, urethral stricture, prostatic hyperplasia or tumor, vesical rupture, nervous bladder.

25.1.2 Polyuria

There are four different reasons often cause polyuria.

- Renal disease: Including chronic nephritis, chronic pyelonephritis, dysfunction of proximal tubule (for example renal glycosuria, Fanconi syndrome), distal tubule diseases (renal diabetes insipidus and Bartter' syndrome).There is other disease of solute diuresis, including hypokalemia, hypercalcemia and medullary cystic diseases and so on.
- Endocrine- metabolism diseases: Such as idiopathic or second diabetes insipidus, diabetes mellitus, primary

J. Chen
Department of Internal Medicine, Peking Union Medical College, Beijing, China

R. Zeng (✉)
Department of Cardiology, Sichuan University, Chengdu, China

X.-H. Wan, R. Zeng (eds.), *Handbook of Clinical Diagnostics*, https://doi.org/10.1007/978-981-13-7677-1_25

hyperparathyroidism, and primary aldosteronism. These diseases result to inhibit tubule reabsorption for water or result solute dieresis.

- Urinary Polyuria: It could be caused by compulsive water drinking, such as high sodium diet, hyperglycemia, polydipsia in patient with Sjogren's syndrome. It is sure to cause polyuria by diuretic drugs.
- Psychogenic polyuria: Such as habit, psychiatric disorders, neurologic lesions.

25.2 Clinical Manifestations and Accompany Symptoms

25.2.1 Oliguria and Anuria

Oliguria and anuria may be related with relevant diseases when accompanied as follows symptoms and singe.

- Cardiac failure: with palpitation, shortness of breath, and difficult to lie flat at night;
- Renal arterial thrombosis: with renal colic;
- Kidney or ureteral calculi: with lumbago, the pain may radiate to umbilicus, hematuria;
- Bladder or urinary tract stones: usually accompany with dysuria, hematuria, urinary interruption, urinary bifurcation;
- Acute pyelonephritis: with fever, lumbago, frequency, urgency;
- Nephrotic syndrome: with severe edema, hypoproteinemia, proteinuria;
- Acute nephritis or rapidly progressive glomerulonephritis: with hypertension, hematuria, edema, proteinuria;
- Hepatorenal syndrome: with skin yellowness, spider, ascites, weakness, anorexia;
- Goodpasture syndrome: with oliguria or anuria, hemoptysis;
- Prostatic hypertrophy: with frequency, dysuria, and even odynuria;
- Acute tubular necrosis, initially little or no urine, then the obvious Polyuria.

25.2.2 Polyuria

Polyuria may be related with relevant diseases when accompanied as follows symptoms and singe.

- Diabetes: with polydipsia, polyphagia, marasmus;
- Diabetes insipidus: with thirst, polydipsia, nocturia, low specific gravity of urine;
- Primary hyperparathyroidism: with hypercalcemia, renal calculus, osteodynia, pathologic fracture;
- Primary aldosteronism: with hypertension, hypernatremia, hypokalemia, metabolic alkalosis;
- Renal tubule acidosis: with osteodynia, hypokalemia, paradoxical aciduria;
- Acute tubular necrosis: with oliguria or anuria before polyuria;
- Psychogenic Polyuria: with mental symptom.

Key Points in History Taking

1. Oliguria and Anuria
   - When does oliguria occur? Total volumes of urine in 24 h, color of urine.
   - Accompanying symptoms, including frequency, urgency, urinary interruption, and dysuria.
   - Special food or drugs such as nephrotoxic drugs, chemicals, used to eat raw fish guts or toadstool;
   - History of relevant diseases, such as hemorrhoea, shock, heart failure, renal percussive pain, high fever, etc.;
   - Past history; including respiratory infection, angina, chronic nephritis, urinary calculus, prostate hyperplasia;
   - Travelling history, such as epidemic hemorrhagic fever or Leptospirosis epidemic area should be pay attention.
2. Polyuria
   - When does polyuria occur? Total volumes of urine in 24 h, and times of nocturia;
   - Accompanying symptoms, such as Polydipsia (water intake in 24 h), bone pain, easy to fracture, periodic paralysis, hypertension and weight loss.
   - With or without oliguria and anuria;
   - Taking diuretics or not;
   - Food habits, such as high salt diet or not;
   - Family history of chronic kidney disease(e.g. Fanconi syndrome, Bartter syndrome, etc..).

Urinary Incontinence

26

Rui Zeng

The normal urine collection function of bladder involves the balance between the following two factors: the compliance of detrusor muscles maintains a low pressure within the bladder when it collects urine and the tension in sphincter muscles as well as the surrounding tissue is high enough to avoid involuntary urine leakage, which is also referred to as urinary incontinence.

26.1 Etiology and Mechanism

Urinary incontinence can occur due to various reasons leading to abnormal contraction of detrusor muscles or overfilling of the urinary bladder, which lead to an elevation in bladder pressure greater than the normal urethral pressure. It can also occur due to relaxation or paralysis of sphincter muscles, which lead to an decrease in urethral pressure. These factors result in inability of voluntary urination, with manifests as drips or continuous urine leakage from the urethral orifice. Urinary incontinence can occur in patients at different age groups, but is more commonly seen in the elderly.

26.2 Clinical Manifestations and Accompanying Symptoms

There are four main types of incontinence in terms of clinical manifestation.

1. **Urge incontinence.** It is caused by the weakened inhibition effects of cerebral cortex on spinal micturition center, which leads to involuntary detrusor muscle contraction or hyperreflexia and subsequently uncontrolled bladder contraction. It can also be caused by focal bladder inflammation or orifice obstruction. Urge incontinence is characterized by involuntary urination with a small amount of recurrent urine leakage and is often accompanied by urinary urgency and frequency. The diagnosis is made primarily on history. Physical examination on pelvis, rectum and nervous system can reveal positive findings.

   Main causes include:
   - CNS disorders: cerebrovascular accident, tumor, multiple sclerosis, Parkinson's disease, etc.
   - Bladder dysfunction caused by focal bladder inflammation or irritation: Lower urinary tract infection, fecal impaction, atrophic vaginitis, prostate hyperplasia, uterus prolapse, etc.
2. **Overflow incontinence** is characterized by continuous involuntary urine leakage. It occurs in the setting of bladder outlet blockage or when the detrusor muscles are too weak to empty the bladder, which lead to subsequent urine retention and over filling of bladder. Physical examination often reveals bladder filling, signs of spinal cord disorder peripheral neuritis. Residual urine volume is often elevated after micturition.

   Common causes:
   - Lower urinary tract obstruction: prostatic hyperplasia, bladder neck obstruction, congenital verumontanum hyperplasia, narrowing of the urethra, etc.
   - Neurological diseases: spinal shock at the early stage of spinal cord injury, spinal cord tumor, myelophthisis and diabetes-related bladder paralysis, etc.
3. **Stress incontinence:** Detrusor muscles function normally, but the urethral resistance is decreased due to reduced tension of sphincter muscles as well as the muscles or ligaments surrounding the urethra. Generally, patients are able to control urination. However, when abdominal pressure increases due to coughing, laughing, sneezing, running, weight lifting or body position change, intra-bladder pressure elevates and exceeds urethral pressure, with subsequent leakage of urine from the urethra. It is more often seen in middle aged multiparas and patients

R. Zeng (✉)
Department of Cardiology, Sichuan University, Chengdu, China

X.-H. Wan, R. Zeng (eds.), *Handbook of Clinical Diagnostics*, https://doi.org/10.1007/978-981-13-7677-1_26

with a history of pelvic or urethral surgery. Medical history is important to make the diagnosis of stress incontinence and physical examination may reveal bladder fistula, rectal fistula or uterus prolapse.

4. **Functional incontinence:** It is a temporary state in which patients are aware of the need to urinate, but are not able to micturate due to physical, mental or medical reasons. It is commonly seen in patients with severe arthritis, cerebrovascular diseases, dementia, abrupt changes of urination environment or habit, as well as administration of diuretics or anticholinergic drugs.

The above four types of incontinence may coexist. For instance, patients can suffer from both urge and stress urinary incontinence, which is also referred to as mixed incontinence caused by over stimulation of detrusor muscles and weakness of sphincter muscles.

26.3 Accompanying Symptoms

1. Urinary incontinence accompanied with progressive difficulty in micturition is most commonly seen in male patients over 50 years old with prostatic hyperplasia or prostate cancer. Among middle-aged female patients with stress incontinence, physical examination can reveal vaginal relaxation, cystocele, urethrocele and urine leakage when coughing.
2. Urinary incontinence accompanied by neurological symptoms and signs indicates neurogenic bladder.
3. Urge incontinence caused by acute cystitis is often accompanied by frequent and urgent urination, dysuria, hematuria and pyuria.

Key Points in History Taking

1. The time that urinary incontinence occurs, whether it's intermittent or persistent.
2. Precipitating factors of each episode.
3. The severity of incontinence, the frequency and the amount of urine leakage each time.
4. History of trauma, pelvic or perineum surgery, recurrent urinary infection; History of diabetes, benign prostatic hyperplasia, neurological diseases, pelvic or urinary diseases.
5. Abrupt changes in urination habit or environment; medications that may cause functional urinary incontinence.

Dysuria

27

Rui Zeng

Dysuria happens when the patient cannot void urine due to various reasons, which manifest as hesitancy and difficulty in urination, extended time, shortened range, weak urine stream, interrupted voiding and dribbling after urination, etc. With progression of the disease, failure to empty urine from the bladder results in urinary retention or ischuria. These patients always exhibit frequency and urgency on urination, urinary incontinence and dribbling after urination.

27.1 Etiology and Mechanism

1. **Mechanical obstruction:** The function of muscles and nerves which participate in urination is normal, but there are obstructive lesions between the bladder neck and external urethral orifice.

   Common causes of mechanical obstruction:

   - Bladder-neck obstruction: Internal organs lesions which are adjacent to bladder neck, such as benign prostatic hyperplasia, fibrosis and tumor, bladder calculus, blood clot and foreign bodies, uterine myoma, or uterine incarceration.
   - Urethral obstruction: Stricture of the urethra caused by inflammation or trauma, urethral calculus, foreign bodies, tuberculosis, tumor and diverticulum. Phimosis and posterior urethral valve are common causes of urethral obstruction in male infants.
2. **Dynamic obstruction:** There is no mechanical obstruction in the urinary tract. The cause of difficulty in urination is injury of the central or peripheral nerves, which leads to paralysis of detrusor muscle or spasm of the urethral internal sphincter. Some medications can also lead to the same finding.

   Common causes:

   - Neurological: congenital deformity such as rachischisis, spinal meningocele and meningomyelocele, cerebral or spinal cord tumors, stroke, encephalitis, poliomyelitis and myelophthisis, diabetes, radiation, multiple sclerosis and peripheral neuritis, which can damage peripheral nerves that control urination.
   - Surgical: injury of pelvic nerves during anesthesia, surgery of the central nervous system, pelvic surgery which can injure pelvic nerves or cause dysfunction
   - Medications: anticholinergic agents (atropine, 654-2 etc.), antidepressant, antihistamine and opiates.
   - Psychological: mental stress, unfamiliar environment or habit of urination.

27.2 Clinical Manifestations and Accompanying Symptoms

1. **Benign prostatic hyperplasia or prostatic cancer:** commonly seen in male patients over the age of 50 with progressive difficulty in urination, accompanied by urinary frequency and urgency. Patients with terminal cancer may have tumor related clinical manifestations.
2. **Stricture of urethra:** Theses patients have the history of urethral injury, gonorrheal urethritis or lower abdominal radiotherapy. Purulent secretion near urethral orifice is usually seen in gonorrheal urethritis.
3. **Bladder or urethral calculus, foreign bodies:** Interruption of urinary stream or bifurcation of flow can be found in these patients, some may manifest dysuria and hematuria.
4. **Neurogenic bladder:** Diabetic peripheral neuropathy, neurological diseases or injuries are commonly found in these patients, usually accompanied with laxitas of anal sphincter and absent anal reflex, lower abdominal distention, frequent micturition and urinary incontinence.
5. **Lower urinary tract infection:** These patients typically have symptoms of urinary irritation including frequent

R. Zeng (✉)
Department of Cardiology, Sichuan University, Chengdu, China

X.-H. Wan, R. Zeng (eds.), *Handbook of Clinical Diagnostics*, https://doi.org/10.1007/978-981-13-7677-1_27

and urgent urination, dysuria, also systemic symptoms of infection, such as fatigue and fever.

Key Points in History Taking

1. Duration and severity of difficulty in streaming (such as the trajectory, force and the duration of micturition), the frequency of urination (including the nocturnal polyuria) and urine volume.
2. Whether difficulty in streaming is combined with frequent micturition and urgent urination, dysuria, interruption of urinary stream and systemic symptoms (such as fever, fatigue and emaciation).
3. History of trauma, surgery or infection of cerebrum, spinal cord and urinary tract.
4. History of diabetes, peripheral neuritis and radiation of pelvic area.
5. Medications that can lead to difficulty in streaming, such as anticholinergic agent, antidepressant, antihistamine and opiates.

Low Back Pain

28

Lie Dai and Rui Zeng

Low back pain is the pain that occurs in the area between the lowest ribs and the crease of the buttocks. It is extremely common which affects about 80% of the population at least once in lifetime. It is also one of the most common causes of disability and the history is used to highlight potentially serious or treatable causes of the pain.

28.1 Etiology

Low back pain can be caused by a large number of underlying disorders which may originate from damage of spinal or its surrounding structure. However, the majority of low back pain does not have a clear cause and nonspecific terms of diagnosis such as lumber strain, sprain, or degenerative process are commonly used, indicating non-serious musculoskeletal disorders.

1. **Trauma:** such as lumber sprain or strain, vertebral or rib fractures.
2. **Spinal degenerative diseases:** such as age-related degenerative process in the intervertebral disks and facet joints, lumbar spinal stenosis with or without neurogenic claudication.
3. **Metabolic and endocrine diseases:** such as osteoporosis and hyperparathyroidism.
4. **Destructive bone diseases:** including neoplasia (such as primary vertebral tumors, metastatic or hematologic malignancy) and infection (such as vertebral osteomyelitis, vertebral tuberculosis, paraspinous abscess, epidural abscess, septic diskitis).
5. **Congenital malformations of spine:** such as severe scoliosis or kyphosis, spinal bifida, sacralization of fifth lumbar vertebra.
6. **Spondyloarthritis:** HLA-B27 related inflammatory diseases, mainly affect sacroiliac joints and spine, including ankylosing spondylitis, psoriatic arthritis, reactive arthritis/Reiter's syndrome and inflammatory bowel disease arthritis.
7. **Referred pain from visceral diseases:** such as diseases of pelvic organs (e.g. prostatitis, endometriosis, chronic pelvic inflammatory disease), renal diseases (e.g. nephrolithiasis, pyelonephritis, perinephric abscess), abdominal aortic aneurysm, and gastrointestinal diseases (e.g. pancreatitis, cholecystitis, posterior duodenal ulcer).
8. **Miscellaneous disorders:** such as psychogenic diseases, improper posture.

28.2 Mechanism

The mechanism of low back pain varies in different causes. There are three general types of low back pain by cause: mechanical back pain, non-mechanical back pain (including neoplasia, infection, inflammatory back pain, and others such as osteochondrosis, Paget's disease of bone), and referred pain.

1. **Mechanical back pain** Mechanical back pain is caused by structural injury, such as strain of muscle, ligament or tendon, discogenic disorder, spinal stenosis, osteoporotic compression fracture, spondylisthesis, traumatic fracture, and congenital diseases. Mechanical disorders underlie most cases of low back pain (around 90% or more).
2. **Neoplasia** Primary or metastatic bone tumors cause bone destruction, such as multiple myeloma, metastatic carcinoma, lymphoma and leukemia, spinal cord tumors, retroperitoneal tumors, primary vertebral tumors.
3. **Infection** Infectious diseases may cause back pain by tissue injury.

L. Dai
Department of Rheumatology and Immunology, Sun Yat-Sen University, Guangzhou, China

R. Zeng (✉)
Department of Cardiology, Sichuan University, Chengdu, China

X.-H. Wan, R. Zeng (eds.), *Handbook of Clinical Diagnostics*, https://doi.org/10.1007/978-981-13-7677-1_28

4. **Inflammatory back pain** Inflammatory back pain, mainly seen in spondyloarthritis, is caused by inflammation through accumulation of large amount of pro-inflammatory cytokines such as interleukins and tumor necrosis factor.
5. **Referred pain** For example, cholecystitis and kidney stones may present back pain.

28.3 Clinical Manifestations

1. **Low back pain** Low back pain is the first complaint in patients with lumbodorsal diseases which is mostly prominent at the site of lesions. It can be classified by duration as acute, subacute or chronic back pain showing different management and prognosis. Pain lasting less than six weeks is classified as acute, pain lasting 6–12 weeks is subacute, and more than 12 weeks is chronic.
2. **Dysfunction** The range of spinal motion or even the movement of limbs and respiration are restricted.
3. **Deformity** Deformities are caused by permanent structural destruction, such as vertebral compression fracture, vertebral tuberculosis, ankylosing spondylitis, congenital scoliosis and scar contracture secondary to soft tissue injury.

28.4 Accompanying Symptoms

The accompanying symptoms of low back pain are complicated varying in different underlying disorders. It is important to find red flags symptoms which should trigger further investigation.

1. **Constitutional symptoms** Constitutional symptoms, such as listlessness, appetite loss, weight loss, fever and anemia, may reveal systemic diseases such as infection (e.g. tuberculosis), rheumatic diseases (e.g. spondyloarthritis) or tumor.
2. **Morning stiffness** The presence of morning stiffness indicates inflammatory arthropathy such as spondyloarthritis. Stiffness lasting more than 30 min in the morning helps to distinguish inflammatory back pain from mechanical back pain.
3. **Relationship with exercise or rest** Mechanical back pain is often exacerbated by exercise but relieved after rest. Inflammatory back pain is often worse after a period of rest or inactivity and improves with exercise. Worsening night pain or rest pain are red flags.
4. **Arthritis and/or enthesitis** Spondyloarthritis may affect large joints at lower extremities such as hip, knee and ankle, characterized by non-symmetrical and recurrent involvement pattern.
5. **Radicular pain** Lumbar disk herniation presses the nerve root and results in pain, numbness, or a tingling sensation at the served distribution of the nerve. Presence of cauda equina syndrome or progressive neurologic deficit require surgical management.
6. **Other red flags** Other red flags include history of trauma, previous history of cancer and long-term steroid usage.

28.5 Differentiation of Inflammatory and Mechanical Back Pain (Table 28.1)

Key Points in History Taking

1. Age at the onset of low back pain, the speed of onset (abrupt or insidious), nature of pain (sharp or dull, colicky or tearing, radiating and shooting), precipitating and relieving factors, location and rhythm of pain (persistent or intermittent).
2. Whether the pain is exacerbated after rest or at night, or ameliorated with exercise or inactivity.
3. Whether the pain is accompanied with systemic symptoms such as fever, fatigue, weight loss, rash, or neurologic deficit.
4. Whether back pain is accompanied with joint pain, swelling, deformity or dysfunction.
5. Previous episode, past history, results of laboratory test and response to previous treatment.
6. Family history of similar diseases, any social or psychological distress that may amplify or prolong the pain.

Table 28.1 Differentiation of inflammatory and mechanical back pain

	Inflammatory back pain	Mechanical back pain
Age	<40 years	At any age
Onset	Chronic, insidious	Abrupt
Duration of symptoms	>3 months	<4 weeks
Morning stiffness	>1 h	<30 min
Nocturnal pain	Common	No
Pain after exercise	Ameliorated	Exacerbated
Sacroiliac joint tenderness	Common	No
Spinal motion	Limited in all directions	limited in flexion
Chest expansion	usually reduced	Normal
Abnormal neurological examination	Rare	Common

29 Arthralgia

Lie Dai and Rui Zeng

Arthralgia is the pain in the area of joints which is a subjective symptom of patient with or without joint tenderness. Arthralgia could be a result of articular or periarticular disorders and also be a part of systemic diseases with joint involvement.

29.1 Etiology

Many disorders may cause arthralgia, or even normal persons especially women may have arthralgia.

1. **Diffuse connective tissue diseases**, associated with autoantibodies, such as rheumatoid arthritis, systemic lupus erythematosus, Sjögren's syndrome, systemic sclerosis, and vasculitis.
2. **Spondyloarthritis**, associated with HLA-B27 gene, such as ankylosing spondylitis, psoriatic arthritis, reactive arthritis/Reiter's syndrome and inflammatory bowel disease arthritis.
3. **Degenerative joint disease**, mainly osteoarthritis.
4. **Infection**, including infectious arthritis (such as bacterial, viral, fungal and parasitic arthritis), osteomyelitis.
5. **Crystal arthritis**, such as gout, pseudo-gout.
6. **Tumors**, such as primary synovium neoplasm, primary bone tumors or bone metastases.
7. **Neuropathy**, such as radiculopathy, spinal stenosis and Charcot's joint.
8. **Bone diseases** with joint involvement, such as osteoporosis, osteomalacia.
9. **Non-articular soft tissue rheumatism**, such as tenosynovitis, bursitis, fibromyalgia.
10. **Other disorders**, such as trauma, hemophilia, drug-induced rheumatic syndrome.

29.2 Mechanism

The pathophysiology of arthralgia varies in different diseases.

1. **Intra-articular structural damage** Damage of structures within the joint can cause pain, including joint capsule, periosteum, ligaments, subchondral bone or synovium. Large amounts of pro-inflammatory mediators and autoantibodies are produced in inflammatory arthritis which cause inflammation in synovium, cartilage, ligaments or enthesis through complex immune response. Joint pain also can be seen in non-inflammatory arthritis without typical inflammatory manifestations.
2. **Periarticular soft tissue disorders** Joint pain can arise from structures around or adjacent to the joint. Tendons and bursa are commonly affected causing tendonitis, tenosynovitis, bursitis, fasciitis, epicondylitis or fibromyalgia. These disorders are also known as soft tissue rheumatism, peri-arthritis or non-articular rheumatism.
3. **Referred pain** Referred pain from more distant sites can also cause joint pain, such as angina radiating to the left shoulder, biliary colic radiating to the right shoulder.

29.3 Clinical Manifestations

1. **Joint pain** Arthralgia is always the first complaint of patients with joint diseases. The perceived sensation of pain varies from patient to patient because of different threshold of pain. However, the severity of pain is generally parallel to the severity of the disease. Arthralgia caused by different disorders shows different characters of joint pain, for example, joint pain caused by intra-articular structural damage is often deep and diffuse,

L. Dai
Department of Rheumatology and Immunology, Sun Yat-Sen University, Guangzhou, China

R. Zeng (✉)
Department of Cardiology, Sichuan University, Chengdu, China

X.-H. Wan, R. Zeng (eds.), *Handbook of Clinical Diagnostics*, https://doi.org/10.1007/978-981-13-7677-1_29

while joint pain caused by periarticular soft tissue disorders is often limited with local tenderness.

2. **Joint Swelling** Joint swelling is related to synovial hypertrophy, joint effusion and/or inflammation of para-articular soft tissue, which indicates the presence of inflammatory arthritis. The formation of osteophytes in patients with non-inflammatory arthritis (such as hands or knee osteoarthritis) can lead to bony swelling which can be identified and differentiated by palpation.
3. **Redness and heat in the joint** Redness and heat suggest prominent inflammation, commonly seen in acute arthritis, such as infectious arthritis or gouty arthritis. Periarticular soft tissue lesions usually do not cause heat or elevation of skin temperature.
4. **Stiffness or morning stiffness** Stiffness is a perceived sensation of tightness when attempting to move joints after a period of inactivity and it will subside over time or after activity. This symptom often occurs upon waking in the morning, so called morning stiffness. Its duration tends to be correlated with the degree of inflammation and prolonged morning stiffness is a symptom of inflammation. In rheumatoid arthritis, the duration of morning stiffness often maintains for more than 30 min and is positively associated with disease activity. While in non-inflammatory arthritis, the duration is usually less than 30 min.
5. **Joint deformity** Internal derangement of destructed joint structures can lead to joint deformities such as flexion, subluxation or dislocation. Periarticular soft tissue lesions usually do not cause joint deformity.
6. **Joint dysfunction** Pain or structural damage can cause limitation of joint motion.
7. **Joint crepitus** When the affected joint is actively or passively moved, the hand placed on the joint will feel the crepitus. Crepitus is most commonly palpated in knee osteoarthritis, suggesting cartilage damage.
8. **Muscle atrophy** Muscle atrophy around the affected joints is mostly caused by disused atrophy.

29.4 Accompanying Symptoms

Systemic diseases with joint involved may manifest not only constitutional symptoms (e. g, fatigue, malaise, fever, poor appetite, weight loss), but also corresponding extra-articular symptoms. For example, systemic lupus erythematosus may present facial butterfly rash, photosensitivity, Raynaud's phenomenon and serositis. Behçet's syndrome is characterized by recurrent oral aphthae, genital aphthae and skin lesions. Sjögren's syndrome manifests dry mouth and eyes. Rheumatoid arthritis may accompany with subcutaneous nodules and pulmonary fibrosis. Spondyloarthritismay present back pain, skin rash, urethritis, enteritis and ophthalmia. Fibromyalgia may accompany with diffuse pain of the whole body, sleep and emotional disorders.

Key Points in History Taking

1. Speed of onset (abrupt or insidious), any predisposition factors or premonitory symptoms.
2. Distribution and number of involved joints: large joints, small joints or both involved; mono-articular, oligo-articular or poly-articular; symmetric or asymmetric.
3. Severity of pain.
4. Rhythm of joint involvement: migratory, persistent or intermittent.
5. Inflammatory manifestations (such as redness, swelling or heat in joint), morning stiffness, its relationship with activity, joint deformity.
6. Accompanying systemic symptoms, such as fever, fatigue, malaise, weight loss, skin rash and optic lesions.
7. Family history and previous treatment.

30 Vertigo

Jianfang Ma and Rui Zeng

Vertigo is a sensation of environment spinning, often caused by lesion in the vestibular pathway (also termed as true vertigo). Dizziness is usually a sensation of lightheadedness, presyncope or imbalance. It is sometimes misdiagnosed as vertigo and also called as pseudovertigo.

30.1 Etiology

Based on neuroanatomy of the lesion, vertigo can be classified into: (a) vertigo caused by lesion in vestibular pathway, either peripheral or central; (b) vertigo caused by lesion out of vestibular pathway.

1. **Peripheral vertigo** This type of peripheral vertigo is often caused by lesions in the inner ear or cranial nerve (VIII), such as external auditory canal cerumen, middle ear infection, vestibular neuritis, benign paroxysmal positional vertigo, Meniere's disease, vestibular paroxysm or perilymph fistula, etc.
2. **Central vertigo** It is often caused by lesions in vestibular nuclei or associated connecting nerve fibers, such as stroke, multiple sclerosis, migraine, acoustic neuroma, transient ischemic attack (vertebral-basilar artery), epilepsy, migraine, etc.
3. **Others** (a) systemic diseases: hypotensionS, hypertension, severe arrhythmia, acute infectious diseases, uremia, diabetes mellitus, ophthalmological diseases, etc.; (b) Medication: aminoglycoside antibodies, anti-epileptics, anti-hypertensive or sedatives, etc.; (c). Physiological conditions: carsickness, seasickness, or airsickness, etc.

30.2 Pathogenesis

Information from visual, positional and vestibular system is collected by the sensory afferent nerves and transmitted into central nerve system to be integrated and then regulates the efferent nerve fibers to maintain the balance. Any disturbance within these pathways can result in occurrence of vertigo.

1. **Visual dysfunction** Visual disturbance can cause vertigo, resulted from disturbance in localizing the position of the body. Ophthalmological problems associated with vertigo include diplopia, ametropia, watching fast-moving or rotating objects, etc.
2. **Deep sensory dysfunction** Lesions in deep sensory pathway may result in localization problems of the body and cause position related sensory vertigo. This type of vertigo can be compensated by visual input.
3. **Vestibular dysfunction** The peripheral vestibular system is the main system associated with vertigo. It is composed of three semicircular canals, the utricle and saccule, and the vestibular component of cranial nerve VIII. The mismatch between the stimuli from the vestibular system and the deep sensation from the joints and muscles or the spatial orientation impulse from the visual receptor, which is caused by the lesion in the vestibular system, eventually results in the motion illusion which is usually accompanied by nystagmus, imbalance, nausea, vomit, diarrhea, etc.

30.3 Clinical Manifestations

1. **Peripheral vertigo** The symptoms occur abruptly and severe in intensity, sometimes accompanied by autonomic symptoms and lasting for several minutes or days. Vertigo patients describe the feeling of environment spinning or turning around of the body, and they need to hold on something tightly, close their eyes to prevent themselves falling down. They tend to lean to one side and have

J. Ma
Department of Neurology, Shanghai Jiaotong University, Shanghai, China

R. Zeng (✉)
Department of Cardiology, Sichuan University, Chengdu, China

X.-H. Wan, R. Zeng (eds.), *Handbook of Clinical Diagnostics*, https://doi.org/10.1007/978-981-13-7677-1_30

Table 30.1 Clinical manifestation of peripheral vertigo

Disease	Clinical manifestations
Meniere's disease	Sudden onset of vertigo with hearing loss, ear fullness, tinnitus and nystagmus, accompanied by nausea, vomiting, sweating, bradycardia, hypotension, without impairment of consciousness; Recurrent attacks that usually last for several minutes or hours;
Vestibular neuritis	Often with a history of otitis media or surgery on middle ear; Single prolonged attack lasting for several days or weeks, accompanied by nausea, vomit or imbalance; Positive head thrust test;
Benign paroxysmal positional vertigo	Positional triggered episodic vertigo lasting for less than 1 min, accompanied by nausea, vomit, positional triggered nystagmus but often without hearing loss;
Vertigo associated with medication	Chronic onset but get worse gradually, accompanied by hearing loss, tinnitus;

unsteady gait. Physical examination finds unidirectional spontaneous nystagmus which never changes direction, either horizontal or torsional pattern. The nystagmus can be suppressed by visual fixation. Romberg's test can be positive in some patients. Differential diagnosis of vertigo is listed in Table 30.1.

2. **Central vertigo** Central vertigo often has a sub-acute onset and moderate severity. Symptoms can be worse in certain position but never only occur after position changes. It is less common to have simultaneous autonomic dysfunction, hearing loss or tinnitus. These symptoms usually last for at least several days and are accompanied by other focal neurological deficits such as pyramidal signs, ataxia or diplopia, etc. The central nystagmus can be horizontal, vertical or torsional pattern. The direction of gaze-evoked nystagmus can be changed sometimes.
3. **Physiological vertigo** It is more common in women than men and can occur in travel by boat, car or airplane, sometimes accompanied by nausea, vomiting with negative neurological signs. Medication such as Dramamine can alleviate the symptoms.
4. **Vertigo caused by systemic diseases** Various clinical pictures can be presented, such as floating sensation or numbness. Sensation of environment spinning is rare.

30.4 Accompanying Symptoms

1. Autonomic dysfunction: nausea, vomit, pale face, sometimes hypotension, bradycardia, sweating, etc.
2. Hearing dysfunction: tinnitus, hearing loss, common in vestibular lesions or tumor.
3. Visual disturbance: diplopia, common in brain stem lesion.
4. Other neurological dysfunction: ataxia, common in cerebellum lesion.

Key Points in History Taking

1. Condition when vertigo occurs, any position that triggers vertigo;
2. More detail description about the symptoms, such as spinning of the environment, lightheadedness, syncope, imbalance, etc.;
3. Hearing loss or tinnitus accompanied by vertigo, unilateral or bilateral;
4. History of other long-lasting medical conditions;
5. Recurrent or any treatments for vertigo.

Syncope

31

Jianfang Ma and Rui Zeng

Syncope is defined as a transient loss of consciousness associated with cerebral hypoperfusion that can be improved by recumbent posture without any residual deficits. Presyncope, which is a prodrome of syncope, often presents with symptoms like dizziness, lightheadedness, tremulousness, sweating, nausea, imbalance, vertigo and palpitations. On certain circumstance, syncope can be presented as urinary incontinence and abnormal movements during the state of unconsciousness, such as convulsion, etc.

31.1 Etiology

Currently, there are several known causes resulting in syncope, which include vasovagal reflex, cardiac diseases, neurological diseases and other conditions:

1. **Vasovagal syncope:** It includes neurocardiogenic syncope (sometimes termed as vasodepressor syncope) which can be triggered by cough or laughing, carotid sinus syndrome, orthostatic hypotension, etc.
2. **Cardiac diseases:** Severe cardiac arrhythmias can cause syncope, such as bradyarrhythmias or tachyarrhythmias, cardiac left or right ventricular outflow obstruction such as aortic stenosis or pulmonary embolus, atrial myxoma, myocardial ischemia or infarction, etc.
3. **Neurological diseases:** Syncope can be caused by cerebral hypotension due to cerebral vascular diseases including vertebral-basilar insufficiency, migraine, subclavian steal syndrome, etc.
4. **Others:** Hyperventilation, hypoglycemia, hypoxia, several anemia, etc.

J. Ma
Department of Neurology, Shanghai Jiaotong University, Shanghai, China

R. Zeng (✉)
Department of Cardiology, Sichuan University, Chengdu, China

31.2 Pathogenesis

The autonomic system plays an important role in maintaining hemodynamic stability. When a person stands, the gravity pools the blood in the lower extremities and leads to reduced venous return to the heart and decreased blood pressure afterwards. On that condition, the activity of sympathetic nerve system increases and parasympathetic decreases, resulting in the elevation of the heart rate and constriction of the vessel to maintain the blood pressure. The falling of blood pressure can cause vascular insufficiency or brain hypoxia which leads to syncope clinically. Therefore, any lesion within these systems can cause syncope. For example, vasovagal reflex can cause decreased sympathetic and increased parasympathetic activities to reduce blood pressure. Micturition, cough or pain can trigger the vasovagal reflex to produce syncope. Carotid sinus syndrome shows a hypersensitivity to baroreceptors and can cause overstimulation of vagal reflex. Orthostatic hypotension can reduce the venous return to the heart, which in combination with sympathetic dysfunction, leads to decreased cardiac outflow and blood pressure. Heart diseases can directly decrease the blood output to the brain resulting in syncope consequently. In neurological diseases, especially cerebral vascular diseases, syncope can be caused by vascular insufficiency and hypoxia in the brain. Hypoglycemia, severe anemia, hyperventilation can cause brain hypoxia which lead to syncope clinically.

31.3 Clinical Manifestations

Syncope is often presented as a sudden loss of consciousness within a short duration from seconds to minutes. In the presyncope stage, patients always feel fatigue, dizziness, nausea or fainted and have vomiting, sweating, blurred vision or palpitation. Then patients collapse suddenly with loss of consciousness, decreased blood pressure, bradycardia or tachycardia, urinary incontinence, pupil dilation or even

X.-H. Wan, R. Zeng (eds.), *Handbook of Clinical Diagnostics*, https://doi.org/10.1007/978-981-13-7677-1_31

seizure. After a few seconds or minutes, patient starts to recover without any residual deficits. Sometimes it takes several days to be completely normal.

31.4 Accompanying Symptoms

1. Autonomic dysfunction: Patients can show paled face, sweating, nausea, vomiting, which are common in vasovagal syncope and hypoglycemia.
2. Cyanosis, dyspnea, palpitation, arrhythmias, common in heart diseases.
3. Seizure, common in neurological or cardiac diseases.
4. Fever, edema or clubbing fingers, common in cardiac or pulmonary diseases.
5. Increased breathing rate, numbness, common in hyperventilation.
6. Facial pain, common in neuralgia.

Key Points in History Taking

1. The age of the onset, any syncope associated features such as gender, trigger factors, position changes, micturition, cough or pain, etc.
2. The characteristics of syncope: acute or chronic onset, duration, accompanied symptoms, blood pressure, pulse rate, etc.
3. Family history, any heart, pulmonary, brain diseases, etc.

32 Tics and Convulsion

Jianfang Ma and Rui Zeng

Tics and convulsion differ in etiology, but can be confused sometimes. Tics are one of extrapyramidal symptoms, characterized by sudden, intermittent, repetitive, involuntary or semi-voluntary movements. Convulsion is abnormal involuntary contraction of the muscles. Sometimes convulsion is epileptic in nature, but not all epilepsy presents with convulsion.

32.1 Etiology

Following diseases can cause tics or convulsion:

1. **Cerebral diseases:**
   - Infection: encephalitis, meningitis, brain abscess, brain tuberculosis infection, brain parasites infection, etc.;
   - Trauma: birth trauma, brain trauma, etc.;
   - Tumor: primary cerebral tumor, cerebral metastasis, glioma, astrocytoma, meningioma, etc.;
   - Cerebral vascular diseases: cerebral hemorrhage, subarachnoid hemorrhage, hypertensive encephalopathy, cerebral infarction, arteriovenous malformation, etc.;
   - Others: congenital brain diseases, tuberous sclerosis, kernicterus, etc.
2. **Systemic diseases:**
   - Infection: acute gastroenteritis, toxic bacillary dysentery, sepsis, otitis media, etc.;
   - Toxicity: hepatoencephalopathy, uremia, alcohol, benzene, lead, arsenic, mercury, chloroquine, atropine, camphor, ginkgo, organophosphorus insecticides, etc.;
   - Heart and vascular diseases: hypertension, Adams-Stokes syndrome, etc.;
   - Metabolic disorders: hypoglycemia, hypocalcemia, hypomagnesemia, hyper-osmotic state, acute intermittent porphyria, eclampsia, etc.;
   - Rheumatic diseases: systemic lupus erythematosus, vasculitis, etc.;
   - Others: sudden stop of medication such as anti-epileptics or hypnotics, heatstroke, asphyxia, etc.
3. **Psychogenic diseases:** Hysteria, pseudoseizure, etc.
4. **Infantile convulsion:** only in children and sometimes accompanied by fever.

32.2 Pathogenesis

Disruption of the depolarization and repolarization of the neuron caused by genetics, immune or endocrinological deficits lead to abnormal neuronal excitability. The abnormal excitability of neuron then propagates and synchronizes the firing of a group of neurons which result in convulsion occurrence. However, abnormal neural circuits in basal ganglion account for the occurrence of various involuntary movement including tics.

32.3 Clinical Manifestations

Tics and convulsion can present with different presentation, commonly classified into generalized or focal types.

1. **Generalized types:**
   - Generalized seizure: it typically starts with a tonic phase of sudden contraction of the axial and limb musculature, accompanied by upward eye deviation, papillary dilation and cyanosis, followed by a clonic phase of fast jerks with deep breathing. After the jerks, patient remains lethargic for a while before coming back to normal condition with complaints of headache and muscle soreness.

J. Ma
Department of Neurology, Shanghai Jiaotong University, Shanghai, China

R. Zeng (✉)
Department of Cardiology, Sichuan University, Chengdu, China

X.-H. Wan, R. Zeng (eds.), *Handbook of Clinical Diagnostics*, https://doi.org/10.1007/978-981-13-7677-1_32

Table 32.1 The clinical characteristics of simple or complex infantile convulsion

	Simple infantile convulsion	Complex infantile convulsion
Percentage in total infantile convulsion	70%	30%
Age of onset	6 months to 5 years	Sometimes ≤6 months or ≥5 years
Seizure type	generalized seizure	Generalized or partial seizure
Duration	<10 min	>10 min
Frequency	≤2 during 24 h	multiple during 24 h
Focal neurological signs	No	Usually have
Status epileptic	Rare	Common

- Hysterical convulsion: Sometimes it is difficult to be differentiated from epileptic seizure. It is often triggered by emotional events, having a varied presentation and lasting longer than epileptic seizure, accompanied by different psychiatric symptoms.
- Infantile convulsion: It occurs in children aged from 6 months to 5 years, accompanied by fever usually higher than 39 °C. Simple infantile convulsion is usually managed by antipyretic treatment without antiepileptic medication. The differentiation of simple and complex infantile convulsion is listed in Table 32.1.
- Breath-holding syndrome: It often occurs in children between 6 and 18 months and presents with crying, episodic apnea with loss of consciousness and changes in posture, lasting for about 1–2 min and thus can be confused as a seizure sometimes.

2. **Focal types:**
   - Partial seizure: It is characterized by muscle contraction of eyelid or facial muscle or limbs, without consciousness changes. Epileptic discharge can be found in electroencephalogram (EEG) which is associated with clinical attacks.
   - Tourette's syndrome: It usually occurs in children aged between 2 and 10 years old with a male predominance in boys (3–4:1). Clinically, it presents with tics involving cranial, neck and upper limbs, including eye blinks, stretching of the face, head shaking, sniffing, grunting or whistling. A great majority of patients have behavioral problems such as attention deficit hyperactivity disorders (ADHD) and obsessive-compulsive disorder.
   - Hypocalcaemia: It is clinically characterized by tetany or paresthesias, numbness of the fingertips and perioral area, or spontaneous muscle cramps, sometimes it can be confused with partial seizure or tics. Hypocalcaemia can have two positive signs, Chvostek's sign or Trousseau's sign.

32.4 Accompanying Symptoms

1. **Fever:** common in infectious diseases, severe dehydration, gastrointestinal disturbance, etc. However, convulsion itself may cause fever during the attack.
2. **Hypertension:** common in hypertension, nephritis, eclampsia, lead poisoning, etc.
3. **Meningeal irritation:** Seen in meningitis, encephalitis, subarachnoid hemorrhage, etc.
4. **Dilated pupil and tongue injury:** Seen in generalized seizure but not in hysterical convulsion.
5. **Severe headache:** common in hypertension, acute infection, subarachnoid hemorrhage, brain occupying lesion, etc.
6. **Loss of consciousness:** Seen in generalized seizure, severe brain trauma, etc.

Key Points in History Taking

1. Basic information: Age of onset, duration, any trigger factors or aura, any relationship with activity, pregnancy, etc.
2. Characteristics of convulsion: Generalized or focal, tonic or clonic, etc.
3. Accompanied symptoms: consciousness, incontinency, tongue injury, muscle pain, the posture in attack, etc.
4. Manifestation before and after seizure: consciousness, any muscle twitch, any Problems in orientation, etc.
5. History: brain diseases, systemic diseases, psychological diseases, toxicant exposure, trauma, birth state of newborn, developmental problems, etc.

Disturbance of Consciousness

33

Jianfang Ma and Rui Zeng

Consciousness is a state of awareness of self and the surroundings. Alternation in this awareness is defined as disturbance of consciousness which is classified into different types based on the involvement in the level of arousal or the content of mental function.

33.1 Etiology

Disturbance of consciousness is always caused by brain dysfunction, either brainstem or bilateral cerebral cortex.

1. **Systemic causes**
   - Multiple or diffuse metabolic encephalopathy: metabolic or osmotic changes, vitamin deficiency, hyperthermia or hypothermia, overdose of medication or drug, intoxication, trauma, etc.
   - Hypoxic-ischemic encephalopathy: myocardial infarction, arrhythmia, hemorrhage, shock, asphyxia, respiratory failure, etc.
   - Systemic diseases: systemic lupus erythematosus, disseminated intravascular coagulation (DIC), etc.
2. **Focal brain lesions**
   - Diffuse cerebral diseases: cerebral vascular diseases, brain tumor, intoxication, trauma or cerebral demyelinating diseases, etc.
   - Brain stem diseases: brain stem or cerebellar infarction, hemorrhage, inflammation or tumor, etc.

J. Ma
Department of Neurology, Shanghai Jiaotong University, Shanghai, China

R. Zeng (✉)
Department of Cardiology, Sichuan University, Chengdu, China

33.2 Pathogenesis

Pathological causes such as hypoxia, ischemia, hypoglycemia and other changes can induce metabolic disturbance which leads to brainstem reticular activating system damage and cerebral dysfunction, resulting in consciousness impairment.

As shown before, consciousness consists of two parts: arousal and content. The content of consciousness includes cognitive and affective mental functions which include memory, orientation and visual spatial ability, etc. Disturbance in anterior cingulated cortex, right prefrontal cortex, or thalamus will result in consciousness impairment. Arousal system consists of classical sensory projection system (specific projection system) and brainstem reticular activating system (non-specific projection system). Altered level of arousal will lead to altered level of consciousness.

33.3 Clinical Manifestations

1. **Arousal system related consciousness impairment**
   - Somnolence (or lethargy): It is referred to a state of baseline unresponsiveness that requires mild stimuli such as calling name to restore arousal. Patient usually cooperates during the physical examination and becomes asleep as soon as the stimuli stops.
   - Stupor: It is referred to a state of baseline unresponsiveness that requires vigorous stimuli such as yelling or shaking to restore arousal and the patient usually cannot cooperate during the physical examination.
   - Coma: It is referred to a state of complete unresponsiveness and cannot achieve arousal. This can be further classified into three subtypes. (a) Mild coma: patients can still have some spontaneous movements. In painful stimuli, patients can have expression changes or withdraw of the limbs. Vital signs are within normal range. Corneal reflex, papillary reflex and swallow function can be preserved. (b) Moderate coma: less spontaneous movements than mild coma.

X.-H. Wan, R. Zeng (eds.), *Handbook of Clinical Diagnostics*, https://doi.org/10.1007/978-981-13-7677-1_33

Patients can only present expression changes or limbs withdraw after vigorous stimuli. Vital signs are not stable. Reduced reflex are seen in corneal reflex, papillary reflex. Bladder and bowel function are abnormal. (c) Severe coma: no response to any stimuli, no spontaneous movements, and no reflex can be induced. Vital signs are abnormal and muscle tone is reduced or increased with urinary and bowel incontinence.

2. **Mental content related consciousness impairment**
   - Confusion: It is referred to a state of inability to maintain normal thought, but still retain simple mental function.
   - Delirium: It is referred to an acute mental disturbance characterized by abnormal and fluctuating attention including disorganized thinking, sleep–wake cycle changes, disorientation and memory impairment, agitation or behavioral abnormalities. Some patients are restored without any residual deficits. However, some patients deteriorate into coma.
3. **Certain types of consciousness impairment**
   - Decorticate syndrome: It is referred to a state of loss of consciousness while preserving sleep–wake cycle. Thus patient can open or close eyes, or move eyes unconsciously, but cannot produce any response to external stimuli. The corneal reflex, papillary reflex and swallow or chewing function are preserved. No spontaneous movements can be found. Patients have decorticated posturing in which elbows and wrists are flexed bilaterally, with shoulder adduction and extension of the lower extremities.
   - Persistent vegetative state (PVS): In this condition, patients lose cognitive function but retain other cerebral function such as sleep–wake cycle, regulation of cardiac, respiratory function, and maintenance of blood pressure. Spontaneous movements may occur such as crying or chewing. Eyes may open in response to external stimuli, but the patient does not speak or obey commands.

33.4 Accompanying Symptoms

1. **Fever:** seen in severe infectious disease, or subarachnoid hemorrhage, barbiturate intoxication, etc.
2. **Slow breathing rate:** a sign of respiratory center inhibition, common intoxication of morphine, barbiturates, organophosphorus insecticides, or coral snake poisoning, etc.
3. **Pupil dilation:** belladonna intoxication, alcohol intoxication, cyanide intoxication, epilepsy, hypoglycemia, etc.
4. **Miosis:** morphine, barbiturates, organophosphorus insecticides intoxication, etc.
5. **Bradycardia:** intracranial hypertension, atrioventricular block, morphine or toadstool intoxication, etc.
6. **Hypertension:** hypertensive encephalopathy, stroke, nephritis, etc.
7. **Hypotension:** shock with different causes.
8. **Skin or mucous changes:** bleeding, ecchymosis and purpura (severe infection or hematological diseases). Cherry-like lips indicate carbon monoxide poisoning, etc.
9. **Meningitis irritation:** seen in meningitis, subarachnoid hemorrhage, etc.
10. **Paralysis:** seen in cerebral hemorrhage, infarction or brain occupying lesions, etc.

Key Points in History Taking

1. Onset: time of onset, pre- and post stage condition, any trigger factors, duration or severity. Pay attention to environment, season, location and situation when people lose consciousness.
2. Accompanying symptoms: any fever, headache, vomiting, diarrhea, bleeding, sensory or motor dysfunction, etc.
3. History: infection, hypertension, arteriosclerosis, diabetes mellitus, hepatic or renal diseases, pulmonary-cardiac diseases, epilepsy, head trauma and tumor, addiction or toxic exposure, etc.

34 Affective Disorders

Xuehong Wan and Rui Zeng

Affective disorders refer to extra paranormal, long-lasting and manifest emotional reaction, which features extensive affective disorder, psychomotor dysfunction and autonomic symptoms. When judging whether an affective reaction is normal, the doctor needs to consider three conditions: the intensity of affective reaction, the duration of it and its conformity to its surrounding. Normal affections, such as joy, anger, sadness and euphoria are parts of people's daily life, and they should differ from abnormal affections of affective disorders which last longer.

In psychiatry, "affection" and "emotion" are usually considered synonyms collectively known as "feeling", including both the attitude towards objective things and the inner experience gained accordingly by an individual. The two terms differ in that an affection is usually closely related to sociality, featuring greater stability, persistence, implicitness and profundity; whereas an emotion is closely related to naturalness, featuring more situationality, instability, impulsiveness and explicit behavior. Emotions are the outward manifestations of affection, while affection is the intrinsic nature of emotions. A mood is a weak, calm, dispersed and persistent emotional status. An affective disorder is inevitably related to emotions and moods.

There are extensive inner associations between affective disorders and physical maladies. An affective disorder may be a direct or indirect cause to certain physical diseases; it may also be the direct manifestation of impacts of pathological damages on the neural system caused by certain physical diseases, or a reaction to some physical diseases.

X. Wan
Department of Internal Medicine, Sichuan University, Chengdu, China

R. Zeng (✉)
Department of Cardiology, Sichuan University, Chengdu, China

34.1 Clinical Manifestations

Generally, affective disorders are presented in three forms, namely, changes in affective nature, changes in affective fluctuation and changes in affective coordination.

1. Disorders of an affective nature refer to the disproportionate intensity and duration of affective reactions to the stimulation of reality. It is true that under certain circumstances, normal people may also manifest affective reactions such as depression, mania, phobia and anxiety; however, only when such reactions have exceeded the normal degree of stress response to life events and thus cannot be interpreted according to the individual's situation and moods, may they be deemed as psychiatric symptoms. Main changes of affective nature are as the following:
   - Elation: Affective activities see apparent enhancement, featuring morbid gladness, excessively positive self-perception, exorbitant exhilaration incompatible with the surrounding, loud speech, variant facial expressions and exultation, etc. Elation is manifested as a high-spiritedness that is understandable, appealing and easily resonant. It is commonly seen in patients with mania. The high-spiritedness that is not easily understood and features self-content is known as euphoria, which is commonly seen in patients with cerebral organic diseases or drunkenness.
   - Hypothymergasia: People with hypothymergasia show sad facial expressions and sorrow, and consider their future as bleak. Severe cases of hypothymergasia may experience despair and pessimism that often initiate suicidal thoughts and attempts. There are usually accompanying symptoms, such as retardation of thought, movement decrease, and certain inhibitions of physical functions such as anorexia and amenorrhea. Hypothymergasia is a major symptom of depression.
   - Anxiety: Anxiety refers to an expectant status accompanied with extreme restlessness in absence of corre-

X.-H. Wan, R. Zeng (eds.), *Handbook of Clinical Diagnostics*, https://doi.org/10.1007/978-981-13-7677-1_34

sponding objective factors. The patient has a number of manifestations, including excessive worries, a state of nervousness, uneasiness, a feeling of misfortune and constant panic, with a series of autonomic dysfunction symptoms such as palpitation, perspiration, cold hands and feet, quivers and frequent urination. Severe acute anxiety is also known as a panic attack, where the patient often has near-death and out-of-control experiences, accompanied with autonomic dysfunction symptoms such as difficulty in breathing and tachycardia. A panic attack usually lasts a few or tens of minutes.

- Phobia: Phobia refers to the emotional reaction to adverse or dangerous situations. It manifests nervousness, fear and panic, along with evident autonomic dysfunction symptoms such as palpitation, tachypnea, perspiration, trembling limbs and even incontinence. Phobia usually leads to a desire to escape. The fears for certain specific matters are main symptoms of phobia.

2. An affection fluctuation disorder refers to an affective trigger dysfunction, which manifests dramatic affective fluctuations. Normally the disorder lasts a relatively short period of time. The main changes in affection fluctuation are as the following:
   - Labile affect: Patients with labile affect manifest extremely changeable affective responses, going from one extreme to another, which are totally unpredictable. While mild labile affect triggered by external surroundings may be a "character" thing, the labile affect irrelevant to external surroundings is a sign of mental illnesses. Labile affect is commonly seen in cerebral organic mental disorders.
   - Apathy: Apathy refers to the absence of affective responses to external stimulations, even to those the patients own a stake for. The patients are indifferent to what happens around them. They do not have much facial expression, have very few words and lack inner experiences. This manifestation is commonly seen in mental disorders and dementia that accompany schizophrenia and certain physical diseases.
   - Affective fragility: Manifestations of affective fragility include extreme liability to sadness. People who have affective fragility are very likely to be moved by and cry for very trivial matters. Although they may feel such sentiment unnecessary sometimes, they fail to exert self-control. This problem is commonly seen in depression, neurasthenia and dissociative disorders.
   - Emotional stupor: Emotional stupor refers to a status of brief and deep affective inhibition triggered by exceedingly strong mental stimuli. Overwhelmed by extreme grief or panic, the patients lack the corresponding affective experience or facial expressions as an appropriate reaction. This problem is commonly seen in acute stress disorder and dissociative disorder.
   - Irritability: Irritability is manifested as strong affective reactions triggered by mild stimulation. Its manifestations include agitation and anger that often lead to behaviors of bodily harm and/or vandalism. This state is usually transient and is commonly seen in fatigue, personality disorder, neurosis and paranoiac psychosis.
   - Pathological passion: Pathological passion refers to an intense but brief affective eruption. It is usually accompanied by impulsiveness and acts of sabotage, which the patient can only partially recall afterwards. The problem can be seen in cerebral organic mental disorders, mental disorders accompanying physical diseases, schizophrenia, reactive psychosis, and mental disorders accompanying mental retardation.
3. Affective coordination disorder refers to the discordance between affective experiences and environmental stimulation that trigger them, or the contradiction between inner experience and facial expressions. The main changes in affective coordination are as the following:
   - Parathymia: Parathymia refers to inappropriate affective manifestations to inner experience and the surroundings. For instance, the patient may appear sad in a joyous occasion but happy over misfortunes. It is commonly seen in schizophrenia.
   - Affective infantility: Affective infantility means a status in which an adult's affective reaction resembles that of children. The adult becomes naïve, lacks rational control and reacts fast and intense without moderation or concealing. This problem is usually seen in hysteria and dementia.
   - Affective ambivalence: Affective ambivalence is manifested as two opposing affective reactions towards the same person or matter at the same time by the patient, who feels neither painful nor uneasy because he does not see any contradiction or contrast between these two opposing affective reactions. This problem is mostly seen in schizophrenia.

Key Points in History Taking

1. Age of onset, pre-morbid personality, acuteness and chronicity, characteristics of the surroundings and the scene, periodicity and seasonality, and time and location;
2. Exact symptoms and syndrome, the intensity of affective reaction and duration;

3. Inducing factors, pathogenesis, presence or absence of alarming symptoms, and factors for relief or exacerbation;
4. The process of affective disorder;
5. Presence or absence of accompanying symptoms, such as abnormal cognition and psychological state, psychotic symptoms, or psychomotor and autonomic dysfunctions, etc.;
6. Presence or absence of signs of fever, convulsions, coma, and allergic history; presence or absence of signs of infection, craniocerebral traumas, physical disease history, and history of poisoning and medication, etc.; presence or absence of family members with mental disorders, alcohol or drug dependency and history of consanguineous marriage, etc.
7. General conditions during the disease course.

Part II

History Taking

History Taking

The main goal of history taking is to collect all disease-related information of a patient, including symptoms, signs and past history, to help physicians make appropriate decisions for the patient. During inquiry, physicians should encourage patients to express their most important feelings and listen to them attentively, as well as observe for changes in countenance and language. History taking plays a necessary and irreplaceable role in the process of diagnosis, despite the continuous development of various new and cutting edge medical technologies. It remains a basic and one of the most important clinical skills required for physicians.

35 Necessity and Ethics of History Taking

Xuehong Wan and Rui Zeng

History taking is the first step of seeing a patient and serves as an important way to build up rapport between patients and doctors, through which doctors can help relieve patients from fear or misunderstanding of the disease, build up patients' trust in doctors to cure the disease, and enhance the patients' medical compliance.

Medical ethic belongs to professional ethics and involves many facets of clinical medicine. Regarding clinical diagnosis and treatment, it requires doctors to give the safest, least painful and most economical treatment for patients, no matter they are undergoing medical treatment, surgery or clinical trials.

1. Being serious and meticulous is a basic and key requirement, since only such attitude can build up confidence in patients to ensure good cooperation for acquiring a complete and accurate medical history. Doctors should be patient and attentive when listening to the patients.
2. Respect for the patient's privacy and ensuring confidentiality of all inquiry is an act of professionalism. Any information provided by the patient can only be used as scientific evidence for medical purposes. Doctors cannot disclose such information to others nor use it to embarrass or mock the patient.
3. Special attention should be given to the children and the elderly, considering they may not be able to report history fluently or respond properly to physicians as adults.
4. All patients should be treated equally, regardless of their economic, social or political status, education background, sex, age and race. Moreover, doctors should show more sympathy and consideration for the patients in difficult conditions. Discriminating against patients with disability is strictly prohibited.
5. Doctors should not criticize their colleagues at free will in front of patients, or show doubt and dissatisfaction toward past medical care the patient received. When other doctors are taking medical history, we should not make careless comments or evaluation, especially without knowledge of the full scope.
6. Doctors should also give the patients and their families as much health guidance and education as possible, which is part of the doctors' responsibility to the society.

X. Wan
Department of Internal medicine, Sichuan University, Chengdu, China

R. Zeng (✉)
Department of Cardiology, Sichuan University, Chengdu, China

X.-H. Wan, R. Zeng (eds.), *Handbook of Clinical Diagnostics*, https://doi.org/10.1007/978-981-13-7677-1_35

Contents of History Taking

36

Xuehong Wan and Rui Zeng

Basic contents of history taking include: General data, chief complaint, history of present illness, past medical history, review of systems, personal history, menstrual history, marital history, childbearing history and family history.

36.1 General Data

General data include: Name, Sex, Age, Nationality, Domicile of origin, Address, Occupation, Marriage, Admission date, Record date, History presentor (Oneself/Others. If others are the history presentors, should be annotated with the relationship to the patient), Reliability.

36.2 Chief Complaint

Chief complaint briefly state symptoms or signs and duration. The exact Chief complaint could preliminarily reflect Priorities of diseases, and also provide clues to the diagnosis of systematic diseases. Chief complaint is a medical term, which is one sentence extracted from the history of present illness after history taking. For example, "Fever, cough for 1 weeks, palpitation for 2 days".

36.3 History of Present Illness

History of present illness is detailed documentation of patient's current problem. Basic contents of history of present illness include: Onset (sudden or insidious) and duration of chief symptom or signs, features of chief symptom (including location, radiation, quality, frequency, duration intensity, alleviating and aggravating factors), causes of illness and inducements/precipitating factors, progression (chronology of the illness, including the development of main symptom and appearance of other symptoms), associated symptoms and significant negative symptoms, previous studies and treatment (medication, dosage, effects, etc.)

General condition after illness (mental state, appetite, body weight, sleeping, urine, bowel movement, etc.) should also been collected.

36.4 Past Medical History

Basic contents of history of past illness include: Past health status, past illness (mainly indicate any illnesses which may be relevant to present illness), infection, operations, injuries, accidents and vaccinations (document), allergies (medications, foods, environmental agents). For example, a patient who has chronic coronary atherosclerotic heart disease and cerebrovascular accident should be asked whether there is hypertension before. Record history of past illness as the chronological order.

36.5 Review of Systems

1. **General** Fever, changes in body weight, sleep pattern, appetite, malaise, weakness, fatigue and loss of energy.
2. **Skin** Skin lesions or other abnormal changes, changes in color, texture, moisture, temperature, pain and itching previously diagnosed and treated skin disease.
3. **Hematopoietic** Abnormal bleeding, enlarged or tender lymph nodes, anemia, bone pain, and transfusion reactions, contact with drugs, poisons, radioactive material.
4. **Head** Trauma, headache, dizziness, lightheadedness, vertigo.

X. Wan
Department of Internal medicine, Sichuan University, Chengdu, China

R. Zeng (✉)
Department of Cardiology, Sichuan University, Chengdu, China

X.-H. Wan, R. Zeng (eds.), *Handbook of Clinical Diagnostics*, https://doi.org/10.1007/978-981-13-7677-1_36

5. **Eyes** Disturbances of vision, diplopia, photophobia, itching, excess or decreased tearing, previous diagnosis of glaucoma or cataracts:
6. **Ears** Deafness, pain, discharge, vertigo, tinnitus.
7. **Nose** Nasal discharge, epistaxis, obstruction, frequent colds, and sense of smell.
8. **Mouth** Soreness of mouth and tongue, bleeding gums, lesions in mouth, tongue or lips, change in taste, condition of teeth.
9. **Pharynx and larynx** Sore throat, hoarseness, dysphagia
10. **Breast** Pain, swelling, tenderness, discharge, masses, date and result of last mammogram, self-examination pattern.
11. **Respiratory system** Dyspnea, cough, sputum, hemoptysis, pain, wheezing, cyanosis fever, night sweats, date and result of last chest X-ray.
12. **Cardiovascular system** Dyspnea, orthopnea, paroxysmal nocturnal dyspnea, chest pain, edema, palpitations syncope, known hypertension or heart disease, (murmur, heart attack, rheumatic heart disease).
13. **Gastrointestinal system** Appetite, change in bowel habits, diarrhea, constipation, nausea, vomiting, hematemesis, abdominal pain, jaundice, dysphagia, indigestion, eructation, flatulence, rectal tenesmus, character of stools, hemorrhoids, hernia.
14. **Urinary system** Hematuria, frequency, pain, urgency, nocturia, hesitancy, dribbling or incontinence color change oliguria, edema.
15. **Genital system** Sex habits, satisfaction, frequency of intercourse, deviation, recent change in pattern, previous history of venereal disease. Male: genital lesions, ureteral discharge, testicular pain or swelling, impotence and self-exam pattern. Female: vaginal discharge, dyspareunias, genital lesions, date and result of last Pap Smear.
16. **Menstrual-reproductive system** Age of onset, menstrual flow, interval between periods, duration, amount and character of flow, dysmenorrhea, metrorrhagia menorrhagia, postcoital bleeding, pregnancy and childbirth menopause, and contraception.
17. **Endocrine system** Polyuria, polydipsia, polyphagia, intolerance to heat or cold, weakness, tremor, sweating edema change of weight, behavior, bone, skin, facial features, hair, faintness, hunger, history of bleeding after injury, operation, or delivery, hormone therapy
18. **Bones, muscles and joints** Muscular or bone pain, swelling, deformity, or disability of any joint, cramping, weakness, and previous injuries.
19. **Neurological system** Dizziness, convulsions, syncope, vertigo, paresthesia, headache, numbness, paralysis, paresis, ataxia, tremor aphasia, difficulty with bladder or bowel control.
20. **Psychiatric** Hallucinations, disorientation, mood change, delusions, previous emotional illness and treatment.

36.6 Personal History

1. Place of birth, current residence and duration at current residence, educational background, economic status, living conditions. Different contagious diseases have different latencies, ask whether go to somewhere at a certain period of time according to the disease.
2. Professional and working conditions, includes types of work, work environment, exposure to chemical, radioactive materials or industrial poison and exposure, time (if suspected as causative).
3. Habits and hobbies : Such as sleeping, eating, recreation, tea or coffee drinking, smoking and alcohol consumption (amount, duration), other drugs (including sedatives or narcotics) or ingestion of unusual substances (dirt, hair, etc.).
4. History of venereal excursion and sexual intercourse, whether had gonorrhea urethritis, condyloma acuminatum, chancre.

36.7 Menstrual History

Basic contents of menstrual history include: Age of onset, interval between periods, duration, amount and character of flow concomitant symptoms, date of last menstruation, age of menopause Record menstrual history as follows:

Date of last menstruation

$$\text{Age of onset} = \frac{\text{Menstrual duration}}{\text{interval between periods}}$$

or age of menopause

$$\text{Example}: 14\frac{3 \sim 7\,\text{days}}{28 \sim 30\,\text{days}}04/15/2016$$

36.8 Marital History

Basic contents of marital history include: Married or unmarried, marriage age, health status of spouse. If spouse was dead, need to clarify the cause of death, relations of couple.

36.9 Childbearing History

Basic contents of childbearing history include: Age and frequency of pregnancy (ies) and childbirth (s). Number of artificial or natural abortions; stillbirths, operative delivery, puerperal fever. Ask if there are any diseases or drugs which could influence fertility.

36.10 Family History

Basic contents of family history include: Ages, health and disease status of immediate family members (parents, spouse, siblings and children). Family history of illness similar to patient's. Family incidence of infectious diseases (tuberculosis, hepatitis), allergy, cancer, diabetes, etc. Any other (genetic) illness that runs in the family. If any immediate family members are dead, ask cause of death, age at death.

After history taking, doctors should analyze contents of inquisition and write medical records, includes the description of patient's statement, doctor's diagnosis and treatment plan. Medical record is legal documentation, which should be truthfully record. Accurate content, legible handwriting, manual signature and the record date are also very important. Keep privacy of patients, both the medical history and medical record are all confidential.

Skills of History Taking

37

Xuehong Wan and Rui Zeng

Skills of history taking are closely related to the quality and quantity of information doctors obtains from the patient. The inquisition will directly influence the medical care the patient receives and his compliance with treatment.

37.1 Organization

The organization category refers to the structure and organization of the entire inquisition. This encompasses the information gathered in the introduction (during which the student introduces himself and explains his role), the body of history taking (chief complaint, history of present illness, history of past illness, review of systems, personal history, family history), and the closure (or the end of history taking).

The inquisitor imposes structure by systematically following a series of topics. The purpose, agenda, and expectation for today's meeting is made clear as the inquisition progresses. The structure and flow of the inquisition should be the responsibility of doctors.

37.2 Timeline

The timeline pertains to the information contained in the chief complaint and history of present illness. To obtain a timeline, inquisitor should inquire when the patient was last free of this problem, and then follow the progression of the first signs and symptoms to the present. By carefully following the chronological progression of the complaint, inquisitor will avoid missing important information. For example, there may have been environmental changes or the use of drugs which may have alleviated or aggravated the patient's problem. By following a careful timeline, doctors will obtain this information most efficiently. It may be suggested to the inquisitor that a line of questioning might include statements such as, "… then-what happened?" and "…and then what?". This will allow a careful sequencing of events while simultaneously documenting the information obtained. If several symptoms are reported, it is important that their chronological relationship to each other be determined.

Example: a 56 year old male presents with progressive substernal chest pain for the past 2 h. The patient's chest pain first occurred 2 years ago but only upon exertion and disappeared after a few minutes. One year ago the pain increased and was diagnosed as angina pectoris. Nitroglycerin tablets (0.5 mg p.r.n) was taken and the pain disappeared later. The patient continued to take imdur (isosorbide mononitrate, 60 mg qd) and is currently doing so. Two hours ago the patient experienced substernal chest pain and one hour ago the patient experienced sweating, faintness, palpitations and the pain radiated to the left shoulder.

37.3 Transitional Statements

Transitional statements are two part statements used between subsections of history taking to inform the patient that a new topic is going to be discussed and why. For example, "we have been talking about why you came to see me today. Now I'd like to get some information about your own past medical history to see if it has and bearing on your present problem. We will begin with your earliest recollections of what you have been told about your childhood health and progress to the present time." (Pause) "How was your health as a child?" With this type of transition, the patient is not confused about why you are changing the subject and why you are seeking this information

Transitional statements are also important for good communication skills. Poor quality or complete lack of transitional statements can hinder the development of rapport

X. Wan
Department of Internal Medicine, Sichuan University, Chengdu, China

R. Zeng (✉)
Department of Cardiology, Sichuan University, Chengdu, China

X.-H. Wan, R. Zeng (eds.), *Handbook of Clinical Diagnostics*, https://doi.org/10.1007/978-981-13-7677-1_37

between patient and doctor, and can even result in the creation of a hostile or uncooperative patient, Examples of transitional statements that would meet a standard of excellence are: (a) transition to family history: "Now I'd like to talk to you about your family's history. As you know, there are some diseases that tend to run among blood relatives, and in order to have, as complete a picture of your medical history as possible and be able to anticipate and treat future problems, it is important that we have this information Let's begin with your parents. Are they both living? (or "How is the health of your parents ?")" (b) Transition to review of systems: "I've already asked you a lot of questions, and you have been very cooperative. Now, I'm going to ask questions about the parts of your body that we haven't talked about yet, just to be sure we haven't missed anything. This will be very important information to give me a complete picture of your health."

37.4 Pacing of Inquisition

The progression of history taking should flow in a smooth and comfortable manner, The inquisitor should be attentive to the patient and allow him ample time to complete his answers without interruption. Some delays, however, are necessary (such as in reflective thinking) and are an indication of good inquisition skills. A well-placed period of silence may encourage the patient or provide additional relevant data or to talk about sensitive issues that he might otherwise omit. Silence is a double-edged sword, It can be detrimental or a powerful inquisition technique, depending on how it is used. A helpful way to assess pauses in history taking is to judge your feeling for that pause. If you feel embarrassed for the patient, he probably has lost his train of thought. If you feel that you should be giving more information, the pause should be considered an effective technique.

A good technique to help the doctor recover from an awkward pause is to summarize the information previously obtained from the patient, or have some stock questions available, i.e., "Can you tell me about a typical day for you?" It is also important to note that a good inquisitor does not fire questions at the patient so rapidly that the patient has little or no time to consider his answers.

37.5 Questioning Skills-Type of Question

An open-ended question is a general question that allows the inquisitor to obtain a large amount of information about a particular area, It allows the patient to tell the inquisitor "his story". This type of question should be used to begin a line of history taking, (For example, "What brings you here today?" or "Tell me about your general health",) After the inquisitor has obtained information, he should follow up with more focused questions.

Focused, direct, specific of forced choice questions are used to gather specific pertinent information. For example, "How old were you when you had your tonsils removed?", "When did your abdominal pain begin?", "How long have you had abdominal pain?". These questions are used to focus on specific pertinent information. Other types of direct questions typically elicit a "yes" or "no" answer from the patient, or a response to a choice that the inquisitor has provided. Example: "Have you ever had severe headaches? Is your pain sharp or dull?", but a better question to start this line of inquiry would be the open-ended question, "Tell me about your headaches".

To gain accurate information in an organized and efficient manner, the inquisitor should follow a line of history taking that progresses from the general to the specific (e.g., starting with, "Tell me about things that are stressful to you," rather than "Does your job make you anxious?").

Here is an example of a line of history taking utilizing the various types of questions which begins with general questions arid then focuses on more specific questions.

- Inquisitor (I): "Tell me about your problem" (open-ended)
- Patient (P): "For two weeks, I've been having a constant pain m my stomach, right here (patient points) above my navel."
- I: "Tell me about the pain." (focused)
- P: "Well, it's really bad."
- I: "What does the pain feel like?" (focused)
- P: "It's a burning sensation."
- I: "Is it a deep pain or does it feel like it's on-the surface?" (focused)
- P: "It's a very deep one."
- I: "Does the pain seem to travel around?" (focused)
- P: "No"
- I: "What makes the pain feel worse?" (focused)

The inquisitor should avoid using direct or (particularly) forced choice questions in beginning a line of inquiry because it restricts the possible flow of information and makes obtaining the necessary information a tedious task. Furthermore, poor questioning skills may result in erroneous information or omission of pertinent data.

The following three kinds of questions should be avoided by the inquisitor.

1. **Leading questions** Leading questions are questions that tend to imply a particular answer for the patient. They should be avoided because acquiescent respondents may tend to agree with the leading questions rather than contradicting the inquisitor. (e.g., "Your chest pains, have radiated to left arm. correct?").

2. **"Why" questions** "Why" questions often put the patient on the defensive and should be avoided. (e.g., "Why did you eat unclean food?").
3. **Multiple questions** Multiple questions are a series of short questions asked in succession without allowing the patient to answer each individually. The patient can then become confused about which questions to answer, (e.g., "What does the pain feel like after dinner? Is it different than before dinner? Is it sharp? Is it dull?"). Multiple questions can also be one question listing many options (e.g., "Has anyone in your family ever had cancer, diabetes, heart disease, or high blood pressure?"). This is often referred to as a multiple part question.

37.6 Questioning Skills-Duplication

Sometimes it is necessary to ask the patient the same question several times, often rephrasing the main point to clarify data. Example: "You told me your stool was full of blood. This is very important information for your health. I want to make sure that this information is correct. Please describe your stool again for me".

However, unplanned duplication of questions may result in a loss of rapport and loss of faith in the inquisitor's competency. For example, if the inquisitor asks the patient if she has any brothers and sisters after having discovered in the HPI that one sister and two brothers also suffer from similar headaches, this suggests that the inquisitor has not been listening attentively.

37.7 Questioning Skills-Summarizing

Summarizing data at the end of each subsection of history taking serves several communication purposes. (a) It can be a way for the inquisitor to "Jog" his memory in case he has forgotten to ask a question. (b) It allows the patient to hear how the inquisitor understands the information. (c) It provides an opportunity to verify what the patient has told the inquisitor (e.g., "You've also stated the pain in your lower back is a deep, nagging pain, while the pain on the outside of your leg seems more superficial, Is that correct?"

When summarizing the chief complaint and history of present illness, it is important to provide a detailed summarization to the patient, it is important to provide as much detail as possible.

When summarizing the family history, a brief general statement may be sufficient, especially for a negative or non-complex positive family history.

When summarizing the review of systems, it is appropriate to summarize only the positives (e.g., "Other than a few headaches each month and the constipation that you treat by' increasing the roughage in your diet, you appear to be fairly healthy. So it seems that our main task is to clear up the problem you're having with your back. Is this correct?").

37.8 Questioning Skills-Lack of Medical Terms and Jargon

Jargon is defined as "the technical or secret vocabulary of a profession." Since one of the skills of an interviewer is the ability to communicate with the patient, it is necessary to substitute jargon or difficult. Medical terms are terms known to lay persons. The interviewer often makes erroneous assumptions about the patient's level of sophistication on the basis of one or two medical terms that the patient uses during history taking. For example, a patient may be familiar with "otitis media" if he has had problems with his ears, but may know nothing about what the term "palpitations" means. However, because the patient used the term "otitis media", the interviewer may assume that it is safe to use medical terminology in questioning the patient. Jargon may also be misleading to a patient who does not want to admit to the doctor that he doesn't understand the question, (e.g., "productive cough"). Therefore, the interviewer should define questionable terms.

37.9 Questioning Skills-Documentation

In the interest of gaining as accurate a case history as possible, the interviewer must document the information given to him by the patient. If responses from the patient, include specific diagnoses or medications, it is the task of the interviewer to ascertain if the patient knows how the diagnosis was made or to determine the quantity of medication, It is also important to document other information which the patient gives. This includes, but is not limited to, alcohol consumption, smoking history, recreational drugs, caffeine consumption, and allergies. Information about habits should include: what, how much, and how long. For example, pertaining to alcohol consumption, the interviewer should find out what the patient drinks, how much the patient drinks, and how long he has been drinking. The interviewer might also inquire about the pattern of drinking. Documentation also provides an opportunity to clarify information

Example: "I'm not sure I understand how much your problem has been interfering with your attendance at school. Could you tell me how many days of school you've missed since your problem began?".

Also, if, in the course of the interview, the patient utilizes jargon or a specific diagnosis, it is important for the interviewer to verify that the diagnosis is accurate.

Example 1

Patient: "Both my parents have peptic ulcers."

Interviewer: "Are they under a doctor's care fox peptic ulcers?" or "Did they have any tests to find our it they had peptic ulcers?" or "How did they know that they had ulcers ?"

Example 2

Patient: "I had tuberculosis five years ago."

Interviewer: "Who made the diagnosis?"

Patient: "My regular doctor, Dr. Yang."

Interviewer: "Did you have a chest X-ray?"

Patient: "Yes."

Interviewer: "were you treated for tuberculosis?"

Patient: "Yes, I was given medication"

Interviewer: "What kind of medication?"

Patient: "A white tablet"

Interviewer: "Do you know the name of the medication?"

37.10 Appearance and Courtesy

Good appearance may be helpful to develop rapport with the patient. Approaching the patient in a courteous manner may enhance the patient's confidence to talk about sensitive issues that he might otherwise hide. Courtesy may encourage the patient to provide additional relevant data. On the contrary, rudeness and arrogance may result in loss of faith in the interviewer's competency.

37.11 Rapport-Facilitative Behavior

Facilitative behavior can be defined as how comfortable the interviewer makes the patient feel. Eye contact is one element of facilitative behavior. This is a key issue to good interviewing skills. As with any other mannerisms or traits, there is a fine balance between too much and too little eye contact. "Good" eye contact should mean that amount of eye contact that is comfortable for the patient. In other words, the interviewer should be paying attention to the patient, while avoiding staring or conducting the interview as if it were an interrogation. The same is true for non-verbal facilitative behavior and body language. The interviewer should smile and shake his head approvingly when it is appropriate. The interviewer should not place a physical barrier between himself and the patient. He should lean forward in a listening posture when the conversation becomes intense. On the other hand, if the interviewer crosses his arms and legs while the patient relates his sexual history, this suggests something about the interviewer's receptivity to the patient and his problem. Likewise, it is sometimes appropriate for the interviewer to pat the patient on the arm. However, if this is done consistently, it becomes inappropriate. Other important elements that constitute good facilitative behavior include tone of voice, facial expression and neutral verbal cueing (not to be confused with positive verbal reinforcement). This includes short statements that encourage the patient to continue speaking, For example, "I see", "Go on", "Uh-huh", "Tell me more". This may also include echoing a few words of the patient's last sentence.

37.12 Rapport-Positive Verbal Reinforcement

This item is designed to evaluate how well the interviewer is able to use certain verbal reinforcement behaviors to motivate the patient toward a cooperative relationship throughout the interview. By providing intermittent positive verbal reinforcement, the interviewer is responding to the patient's statements in such a way that the patient feels encouraged to provide information to the interviewer. Some examples of such responses might include comments such as "That must have been very difficult for you", or "That's understandable". Occasional social praise such as: "You've quit smoking?, that's excellent, I bet it certainly took will power on your part!" or "I'm glad you're doing a breast self-exam every month-it's very important as most women detect lumps themselves at home…", go a long way towards increasing rapport with the patient.

37.13 Patient's Perspective

It is very important for the interviewer to elicit the patient's perspective on his illness in order for it to be effectively diagnosed and treated. The patient's beliefs and concerns about the etiology of his illness may affect his ability to talk about his symptoms or to understand the diagnosis. For example, the patient may think that his sweet tooth and eating too much sugar has caused his diabetes, The interviewer also needs to discover what the patient knows about the treatment of his disease in order, to effectively educate the patient. The patient might feel that cutting out all desserts and candies will cure his diabetes. The patient's understanding about his prognosis also plays a role in treatment, someone whose uncle died from gastric cancer may well see a diagnosis of peptic ulcer as far more life threatening than the interviewer.

Example:

Patient: "I have stomach pain."

Interviewer: "What do you think is going on?"

Patient: "I think I may have cancer."

Interviewer: "What makes you 'think it may be cancer?"

Patient: "My uncle died of gastric cancer one year ago."

The interviewer should also question the patient about concerns other than those expressed about the chief complaint. Many patients may have hidden concerns which can also be barriers to effective treatment if they are not exposed and understood. For example, a patient with a sexually transmitted disease may be open about his symptoms and anxious for treatment, but may be secretly concerned that the disease will cause impotence.

37.14 Impact on Patient, Family and Self Image

Depending on the diagnosis, as well as the information obtained during the personal history, there could be a tremendous impact of the patient's illness on the patient, his family and the family's lifestyle. An example of this would be a patient with a diagnosis of cancer. This would certainly impact on the patient and effect family members and family lifestyle because of the need for frequent treatment, side effects of drugs, potentially decreased family income, etc.

The interviewer must address the impact on self-image that certain illnesses may have, For example, a patient who has had a mastectomy may have a different self-image after this surgical procedure. Immediately after a heart attack, a patient may need to change his sexual and physical activity. This could certainly affect the way he views himself. The interviewer must explore these issues in depth to the satisfaction of the patient.

37.15 Support Systems

This item is designed to encourage the patient to explore means of financial and emotional support. These support systems might include other family members, friends, and the organization in which he works. These are current resources which could be used immediately. The interviewer may suggest other community resources including charitable organizations, self-help groups, etc., not yet thought of or known to the patient.

37.16 Patient's Expectations

The patient's expectations must be elicited and addressed by the interviewer. It is important to discover what the patient hopes to get from the visit (a prescription, a back to work form). Where there is a need for a continuing or long term relationship, goals may also need to be established over issues such as medications and life style changes. These may require negotiation between the patient and the interviewer.

In many instances, patient education may be necessary for a successful therapeutic relationship or education may be an end in itself. The interviewer should determine how much information the patient would like, how much he needs, and perhaps, how much the patient can comprehend at each visit. The interviewer then needs to provide appropriate information or instruction and educational materials (when available).

37.17 Patient's Understanding

Many times, patients who are labeled non-compliant may in fact not understand the information that is given to them. There are several ways to check the patient's understanding, the interviewer can ask the patient to repeat the information directly back to him, demonstrate techniques, or the interviewer may pose hypothetical situations to see if the patient will react appropriately. It is viral when the patient must continue therapy on his own without direct supervision that he understand how to successfully carry out that task. For example, when prescribing medications, it is important that the patient understand what the medication is for, the schedule that should be followed, and what effect it will have on his body. This is also true if the interviewer must communicate certain findings to the patient.

If the patient does not fully understand, or understands the information incorrectly, this must be clarified immediately.

37.18 Admitting Lack of Experience

The interviewer must be aware of his own level of experience as related to the information he is able to give to the patient. When asked for information or advice that he is not equipped to provide, he admits his lack of experience in that area. For example, a physician referring a patient to a cardiologist may lack knowledge about specialized cardiovascular testing. When questioned by the patient, he must admit lack of experience and immediately offer to seek a resource to answer the patient's questions.

37.19 Rapport-Encouragement of Questions

It is important that the interviewer allow the patient an adequate opportunity to express questions during the interview. Oftentimes during an interview, a patient may think of pertinent information that was not obtained by the interviewer during a specific line of history taking, or the patient may have questions that still need to be addressed by the interviewer.

The interviewer should encourage the patient to discuss these additional points and ask questions by clearly providing an opportunity to do this. For example, the interviewer should state that if the patient has a question or is able to offer additional information that may be pertinent to the topic being discussed, he should do so. This is usually done at the end of a major subsection of history taking, and repeated at the end of the interview.

37.20 Closure of History Taking

It is important that the patient feel that there is some closure at the end of history taking. This closure should include describing future plans, making clear the doctor's and patient's role and obligations, explaining what the doctor expects the patient to do, or planning for the next interview or follow-up communication.

38 Guide for Focused History Taking

Xuehong Wan and Rui Zeng

Focused history taking is focusing on one main complaint of the patient in history of present illness, and attempting to collect all related details in other parts of history. This requires mastering the skill and content for complete health history taking in the previous chapters and abundant knowledge of pathophysiology of disease, as well as capacity to classify and propose the possible diagnosis according to what is known. Usually such focused history taking is required when seeing patients during outpatient service or at emergency department.

Focused health history taking differs from complete health history in that it depends on the specific problem and its degree of emergency. Doctors should inquire selectively to grasp the key information for diagnosis, so the process of history taking is rearranged and simplified in terms of content and order. However, doctors should include the following information: development and progression of the disease, include the onset, development, quality, severity, frequency, aggravating or alleviating factors and associated symptoms. Usually the chief complaints suggest the area for focused inquiry. Therefore, as doctors are taking medical history, they gradually form a hypothesis for diagnosis and determine the involved organ system, where they dig in for focused history taking. From here, they can consider the next step in collecting the associated past, personal, family history and review of systems, skipping the irrelevant contents.

Once the main problem is clear, doctors can quickly determine the involved organ system and form a clinical hypothesis. The rest of history taking then can be focused on the specific organ for a complete understanding of the problem. Direct inquiries are often used to collect further information. Positive answers should be further investigated according to methods mentioned in the previous chapter, whereas negative symptoms which indicate lack of evidence for specific organ system involvement should also be recorded.

For example, a patient with dyspnea might be suspected of circulatory or respiratory diseases, so related symptoms and signs of these two systems should be included in history taking, such as dyspnea at exertion, orthopnea, paroxysmal nocturnal dyspnea, chest pain, palpitations and lower extremity edema, or cough, wheezing, hemoptysis, expectoration and fever. Also, history of asthma or other pulmonary diseases should be noted. All the positive symptoms should be recorded in chronological order and negative symptoms should be written down in separate categories, which can be very helpful for making the final diagnosis.

The reason for taking the history of past illness is to help explain the patient's present problem or further confirm the diagnosis. For example, doctors can focus on one system and ask about related diseases, past surgical procedures, and associated symptoms. If the answer is yes, then we will proceed to inquiring about the patient's related condition, past diagnoses and prognosis. A complete history of past illness is not necessary unless it is considered helpful for solving the present problem. Generally, history of past medication and allergy should be asked on a routine basis.

Whether detailed contents family and personal history are asked depends on the doctor's assumption for diagnosis. For example, if a patient presents with dyspnea, he or she should be asked about history of smoking and exposure to toxic substances, which proves to be helpful regardless of a positive or negative answer. General information in the personal history should be acquired from every patient, including their age, occupation, living condition, mental status and activity. The data collected though review of systems can help support or verify the hypothesis based on history of present illness.

X. Wan
Department of Internal medicine, Sichuan University, Chengdu, China

R. Zeng (✉)
Department of Cardiology, Sichuan University, Chengdu, China

X.-H. Wan, R. Zeng (eds.), *Handbook of Clinical Diagnostics*, https://doi.org/10.1007/978-981-13-7677-1_38

Making a diagnostic hypothesis isn't relying arbitrarily on first impression, but an interactive process between objective data and subjective analysis. The process of creating, testing and revising the diagnosis entails the physicians' active thinking instead of the simple action of collecting answers. It is a challenge for doctors but can also be rewarding after exploring the essence of the disease. Thus the quality of focused history taking depends on the doctor's ability to piece together the information and make reasonable hypothesis. Only when the history is properly taken, will the doctor be able to inquire key components in symptoms and signs for confirming, revising or denying a hypothesis.

History Taking in Special Situations

39

Xuehong Wan and Rui Zeng

1. **Silence and sadness:** Sometimes patients will refuse to talk about their history, which doesn't necessarily indicate lack of incentive in seeking medical help. It might be caused by loss of faith in medical treatment. Physicians should pay more attention to the patients' facial expression, eye contact and body language to find clues for possible diagnoses. On the other hand, physicians should show respect and sympathy and use proper language and gestures to build up trust, encouraging patients to talk about their disease. Sometimes, questions might touch sensitive topics and cause patients to feel unpleasant. Questions that seem irrelevant or are asked in a criticizing manner may lead to silence or anger. Also, throwing out numerous questions at one time or asking at too fast a pace can create fear and anxiety. So physicians should notice if they have made such mistakes and avoid them. If the patients become emotional because of their disease, doctors should stop the inquiry, show compassion, wait until they recover and restart at a slower pace.
2. **Anxiety and depression:** Doctors should encourage these patients to express their feelings and collect verbal or non-verbal information to understand the problem. Any form of comfort and guarantee should be carefully thought over. For example, before telling the patient "everything will be better", doctors should be aware of the main concern and determine the correct way of care to prevent unwanted and usually opposite effects, which may result in resistance and difficulty in communication.
3. **Talkative patients:** Such patients talk incessantly, making it difficult for doctors to cut in and ask questions. Usually one question is ensued by redundantly long answers, making the health history taking process unsuccessful due to limited time and irrelevant content. Doctors should remember the following skills: firstly, the inquiry should be focused on the main problem; Secondly, doctors can interrupt tactfully according to experience when the patient is digressing from the topic; thirdly, doctors can advise the patient to take a break to observe if the patients have thought disorders and conduct the remaining inquiry according to psychiatric requirements; fourthly, doctors can inform the patients of the limited time, and cut the inquiry into several phases. Be sure to do so in a polite and honest manner, and avoid being impatient which may result in loss of rapport.
4. **Anger and hostility:** Patients without sense of security may be angry and unsatisfied and sometimes no specific reasons or targets can be identified for their animosity. It can be directed at doctors, caused by unpleasant feelings incited during the inquiry process. Patients tend to express their anger in front of younger doctors. Impertinent behavior, blunt attitude or verbal conflict may aggravate the situation. Regardless of the cause, doctors should always be sincere, considerate and try their best to explain the problem to the patient to avoid complications in other departments or with other medical workers.
5. **Patients with multiple coexisting symptoms:** Patients with comorbidities are likely to have positive answers for a variety of symptoms, especially those with chronic diseases and no focused manifestation. Doctors should grasp the main problem and true nature of the disease among multiple symptoms.
6. **Patients are fearful of some diagnoses and associated invasive examinations**: As well as the uncertainties in the progression of the disease. Such emotion will change the behavior of the patients, causing them to cast doubt upon their surrounding. When faced with such patients, frankly exposing their lies are not necessary, but doctors

X. Wan
Department of Internal medicine, Sichuan University, Chengdu, China

R. Zeng (✉)
Department of Cardiology, Sichuan University, Chengdu, China

X.-H. Wan, R. Zeng (eds.), *Handbook of Clinical Diagnostics*, https://doi.org/10.1007/978-981-13-7677-1_39

should be aware of the dishonesty in patients and retake history when patients are emotionally stable. When encountered with patients who are factitious or malingering, doctors should analyze comprehensively based on medical knowledge.

7. **Patients with low level of education or speech impairment:** Patients with minimal education are still able to provide certain health history, but their lack of understanding and medical background may affect their response and compliance. So doctors should slow down and use simple words to conduct the inquiry and repeat for confirmation when necessary. For those with language barriers, translators are needed for accurate and objective translation avoiding simple explanations or summaries. Occasionally, body language and hand gestures combined with influent language can help doctors find the key problem. Reaffirming is very important under such circumstance.
8. **Critical and end-stage patients:** doctors should conduct highly focused health history taking and physical examination, which can be carried out simultaneously. Understanding of the slower response in critical patients and avoiding rushing or urging them is necessary. After initial management and stabilizing the condition, doctors can proceed to a more detailed history taking.

   End-stage patients can develop feelings of rejection, loneliness, resistance, regret and depression due to loss of hope in treatment. Doctors should give particular care and encourage the expression of their feelings. Response to questions concerning the diagnosis and prognosis should be as pertinent as possible to minimize harm, not to mention any form of conflict with medical peers on previously received treatment. If the patient cannot understand what is said, proper explanation and appropriate promises should be made, postponing in depth explanation to a later stage. Applying amiable tone and sincere care, such as spending more time bedside are all immense comfort and encouragement for patients, and more beneficial for acquiring a comprehensive health history.
9. **Disabled patients:** For patients with disability, building rapport and acquiring health history is more difficult. Beside giving more sympathy, care and patience, doctors should also spend more time in collecting information using the following skills.

   Patients with loss or impairment of hearing can present with difficulty in communication. Doctors can use simple hand gesture or other body language, and a louder and clear voice without sounding rude or unfriendly. We can also ask families and friends for explanation and details, and at the same time pay attention to the patient's complexion. Written communication can also be adopted when necessary.

   For blind patients, more console should be paid by self-introduction as well as description of the environment. Helping the patient sit down and providing a comfortable environment is beneficial for minimizing fear and gaining trust. Informing the patient of medical staff and equipment present in the room, listening attentively and responding timely can ease the patient's concern to achieve better cooperation.
10. **Elderly patients:** They usually have no obstacle in providing basic information, but the quality of history taking can be affected due to impaired physical strength, vision, hearing and additional mental disorders. Doctors should ask simple and generic questions first, slowing down and reiterating key areas while allowing patients enough time to remember and gather their thoughts. Attention should be paid to the patient's response to determine the presence of impaired thinking and psychological disorders. Refer to family members and friends for additional information when needed.
11. **Children:** Most children cannot independently report their health history and require caregivers in history taking. Credibility of history depends on their careful observation and intimate contact with the patient, therefore the level of credibility should be mentioned in medical records. When facing parents, doctors should try to understand their anxiety and pay particular attention to each described symptom as parents are usually most informed of the circumstance and the first ones to observe associated changes. For the children over 5 or 6 years old, doctors can encourage them to provide additional details of the disease while keeping a critical mind on its accuracy. Some children are reluctant to report the truth due to fear of the hospital and treatment. Doctors should comprehensively analyze the situation during the conversation.
12. **Patients with psychological disorders:** Self-awareness is the ability to understand one's own mental and physiological condition, as well as one's disease under the medical context. For those with retained self-awareness, doctors can rely on the patient to provide the history, but for those without self-awareness, history should be acquired from the patient's family. Since history isn't provided by the patients themselves and limited understanding of family members, the history provided may seem redundant and unorganized. Doctors should analyze the collected information with their professional medical knowledge to draw conclusions.

40 Examples of History Taking

Xuehong Wan and Rui Zeng

40.1 Written Record

The patient is a 38 year old male researcher, coming to West China hospital. He complains about having abdominal pain for 4 years, He says that it has been getting worse over the past 3 months.

Four years ago, the patient has noticed a dull, burning pain in the upper abdominal region. It is usually caused by fatigue, irregular mealtimes, and occurs mostly after a meat or at midnight. The patient can relieve the pain by eating or drinking hot liquids. The pain radiates to the patient's back. There is no regurgitation or belching and the pain usually lasts about 15 days each time and occurs 4–5 times per year. The pain also seems to decrease if he rests or takes regular, mild meals.

Two years ago, the patient visited the outpatient clinic and antacid tablets were prescribed, three tablets (Forgot the name and dose of these drugs), three times per day. After about 1 month, the patient felt well enough to discontinue the medication.

One year ago, the pain recurred and was accompanied by black stools once a day for 1 week. The stool was about 250 g each time. He was admitted to West China hospital. A diagnosis of upper GI bleeding was made. The therapy with antacid complex and infusion fluid was initiated. Afterwards he followed the physician's orders to take the medication for another 2 months with good response.

Three months ago, he experienced a recurrence of the tipper abdominal pain associated with fullness. He attributed this to a heavy load of research work. He felt he stayed up too late and ate irregular meals. He also experienced nausea and black stools for 3 days and vomited twice. The vomit contained residual food. He was admitted to West China hospital again and recovered after 1 week.

Since then, he has continued to have intermittent vomiting, which occurs mostly in the evenings one to two times a week. It contains a large amount of food and has an offending odor. He has used bismuth powder four times a day without any effect on the symptoms, He visits us because he is worried about a possible malignancy or the need for surgery. He has lost approximately 5 kilos over the past 4 years and feels a little tired. He can only eat half the amount of food he used to consume. He is able to work.

Prior to this problem, the patient was in good health. Twenty-two years ago he suffered from an acute hepatitis with jaundice and was admitted to the Chengdu Infectious Hospital. He recovered in one month and his liver function was checked for three years, with normal results. Four years ago, he had acute appendicitis and underwent surgery. He is allergic to sulfa which is manifested by a fixed rash and itching on his left hand. He was vaccinated with type B hepatitis 6 years ago. The patient wears glasses because of near-sightedness with astigmatism for 20 years. He has occasional diarrhea because of reactions to food. A diagnosis of hemorrhoids was made 8 years ago and was treated with traditional Chinese binding methods. The patient fully recovered.

The patient was born and studied in Chengdu. After he graduated from Sichuan University with a master's degree 12 years ago, he came to work in the biology department of the Provincial Science Institute, There is no toxicity in the lab but the work is stressful. He has smoked 10 cigarettes a day for the past 10 years. The patient used to drink a little alcohol but stopped three years ago. He has been married for 10 years and has a 9-year old daughter who is in good health. His father suffers from hypotension and his mother has CHD and was treated at West China hospital. Otherwise she is in good health.

X. Wan
Department of Internal Medicine, Sichuan University, Chengdu, China

R. Zeng (✉)
Department of Cardiology, Sichuan University, Chengdu, China

X.-H. Wan, R. Zeng (eds.), *Handbook of Clinical Diagnostics*, https://doi.org/10.1007/978-981-13-7677-1_40

40.2 Checklist of Content

Introduction

——1. Introduce yourself
——2. Define your role and position
——3. Ask the patient's name and address him correctly
——4. Ask the patient's age and address

Chief Complaints and History of Present Illness

——5. Upper abdominal pain
——6. Onset and durations 4 years and increasing over the past 3 months
——7. Features: burning like, dullness and fullness
——8. Location: upper part of abdomen
——9. Radiation: to back
——10. ——10. Frequency: half a month each time—4–5 times per year
——11. Rhythmicity: after meals or midnight
——12. Alleviating factors: rest, diet or hot drinks
——13. Aggravating factors: tiredness, irregular meals
——14. Progression of the illness: has become more serious, over the previous 3 months
——15. Associated symptoms: Black stools, 1 year ago and 3 months ago, vomiting in past 3 months
——16. Previous diagnostic studies and medications: presumptive diagnosis of upper GI bleeding, antacid and bismuth were used
——17. General condition after illness: loss of weight and appetite

History of Past Illness

——18. General condition: good
——19. Acute hepatitis with jaundice 22 years ago, recovered 1 month later
——20. Acute appendicitis 4 years ago, operated on in 3rd municipal Hospital
——21. Allergic to sulfa, fixed drug rash on left hand
——22. Vaccinated with type B-hepatitis 6 years ago

Review of Systems

——23. Wears glasses for nearsightedness and astigmatism for past 10 years
——24. Diarrhea occasionally because of irregular meals for 20 years
——25. Hemorrhoids. 8 years before and treated with traditional Chinese method

Personal History

——26. Born and studied in Chengdu
——27. Cultured background. Postgraduate degree. 12 years ago.
——28. Occupation: Scientific researcher in Provincial Science Institute.
——29. No toxic exposure
——30. Smokes 10 cigarettes per day for 10 years
——31. Stopped drinking alcohol 3 years ago
——32. Married for 10 years. Wife is 36 years old and works at the same Institute
——33. Normal family life
——34. Good living conditions

Family History

——35. Father-66 years old, hypotensive, treated at West China hospital
——36. Mother-60 years old CHD-treated at West China hospital
——37. Wife-36 years old, occasional insomnia, otherwise normal.
——38. Daughter-9 years old in good health.

Other Problems and Concerns

——39. That the illness may influence his work and his future.
——40. Does he need gastroscopy and surgery?

Key Terms

1	History taking	问诊
2	General data	一般情况
3	Chief complaint	主诉
4	History of present illness	现病史
5	Past medical history	过去史
6	Review of systems	系统回顾
7	Personal history	个人史
8	Menstrual history	月经史
9	Marital history	婚姻史
10	Childbearing history	生育史
11	Family history	家族史

Study Questions

1. What are the whole contents of history taking?
2. How to use basic skills to complete history taking?
3. How to complete focused history taking?
4. How to complete history taking in special situations?

Suggested Readings

Bickley LS. Bates' guide to physical examination and history taking. 10th ed. Philadelphia: Lippincott Williams & Wilkins; 2009.

Swartz MH. Textbook of physical diagnosis. 7th ed. Amsterdam: Elsevier; 2014.

Part III

Physical Examination

41 Basic Skills of Physical Examination

Xuehong Wan and Rui Zeng

There are five basic methods of evxamination: inspection, palpation, percussion, auscultation, and olfactory examination. In addition to using our own perception in physical examination, we also utilize a variety of simple instruments (Table 41.1, Fig. 41.1).

41.1 Inspection

Inspection is a diagnostic method in which we use our eyes to observe the patient's whole body or regional parts. Inspection reflects the doctor's ability of observation and judgment. Through the combination of careful visual inspection and clinical knowledge, the doctor is able to decide whether there is a illness, the potential diagnosis and severity of the disease.

Inspection can be divided into whole body inspection and local inspection.

- Whole body inspection can be applied in assessing the patient's general condition and signs, such as age, development, nutrition, consciousness, mental status, complexion, facial expression, body position, posture, gait and etc. Some diseases can be uncovered upon key features during first inspection. For example, wheezing of the patient in severe asthma, exertional dyspnea in congestive heart failure and cyanosis of the extremities in circulatory collapse are all indicative signs.
- Local inspection can help us discover changes in different parts of the patient's body, such as the skin, mucosa, eyes, ears, nose, mouth, tongue, head and neck, chest, abdomen, muscle, bones and joints. Inspection of some parts including the fundus, tympanic membrane, pharynx and bronchi may require the help of instruments such the ophthalmoscope, otoscope or different kinds of endoscopes.

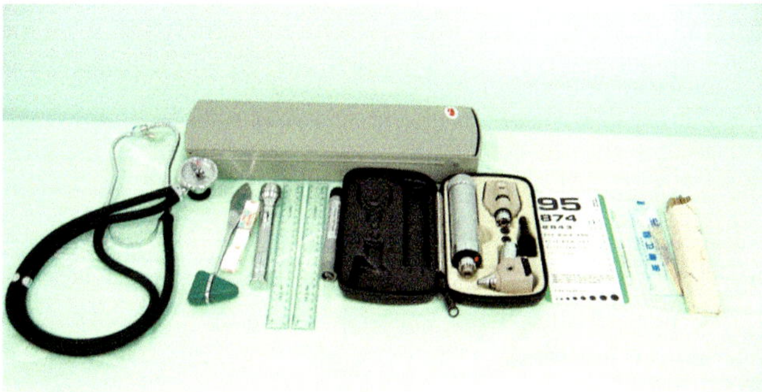

Fig. 41.1 Common instruments and material used during physical examination

Table 41.1 Common instruments and material used during physical examination

Necessary		Elective	
Thermometer	Reflex hammer	Near Vision Card	Slit lamp
Stethoscope	Ophthalmoscope	Otoscope	Gauze
Hamnatodynamometer	Ruler, measuring tape	Rhinoscope	Tape
Spatula	Pins	Gooseneck lamp	Sterile gloves
Pen light	Cotton swab, marker	Tuning fork 128 Hz, 12 Hz	Lubricating oil

X. Wan
Department of Internal Medicine, Sichuan University, Chengdu, China

R. Zeng (✉)
Department of Cardiology, Sichuan University, Chengdu, China

X.-H. Wan, R. Zeng (eds.), *Handbook of Clinical Diagnostics*, https://doi.org/10.1007/978-981-13-7677-1_41

41.2 Palpation

Palpation is a method where the doctor examines the patient by feeling of the hand. Palpation can help us find additional abnormal signs on top of inspection, such as the body temperature, moisture, tenderness, fluctuation, thrills, friction as well as the location, size, outline, surface, hardness and mobility of a mass. Palpation can be applied in a variety of settings. All parts of the body can be examined using palpation, especially the abdomen. The skin of fingertip and the palmer side of the metacarpophalangeal joint are most sensitive. The fingertip is more sensitive in tactile sense and the metacarpophalangeal joint is more sensitive to vibration. The back of the hand is sensitive to temperature. Therefore, different parts of the hand are used during palpation.

Palpation can be divided into light and deep palpation.

41.2.1 Light Palpation

Light palpation is indicated for superficial lesions and examination of the joint, soft tissue as well as superficial arteries, veins, nerves, the scrotum and spermatic cord. The depth of light palpation is around 1–2 cm. During light palpation, the fingers are held together and we put the ulnar side or finger pulps, instead of the finger tip on the site of palpation. By moving our metacarpophalangeal joint or wrist in synchrony, we palpate lightly with a spinning or sliding motion (Fig. 41.2). Jabbing the abdomen with the finger tips should be avoided. After inspection of one site, the hand should be lifted off the skin. Light palpation usually elicit little pain, if any, nor does it cause tension of the muscle. Therefore it is useful in determination of tenderness, resistance, pulsation, mass or enlarged organs. It is carried out before deep palpation to prepare the patient for the next step.

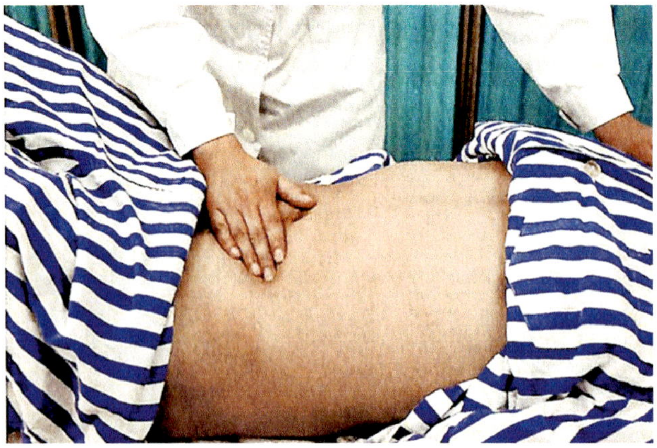

Fig. 41.2 Light palpation

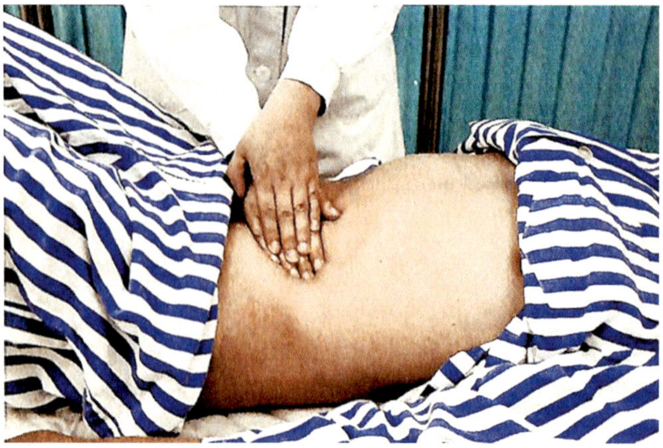

Fig. 41.3 Deep Palpation

41.2.2 Deep Palpation

Deep palpation is used to inspect and evaluate abdominal lesions and organs. The depth of palpation often exceeds 2 cm, reaching 4–5 cm. We can use one hand or stack both hands together during palpation, slowly increasing depth and pressure to meet the purpose of deep palpation (Fig. 41.3). According to different goals and methods, deep palpation can be categorized into the following:

1. **Deep slipping palpation:** Before the examination, tell the patient to breathe through his or her mouth calmly, or carry out a conversation to distract their attention, ensuring the abdominal muscles are relaxed. The doctor then adducts the index, middle and ring finger and begin palpation from the surface of the abdomen to deeper organs or masses. Move in four directions after feeling the mass. If the mass is a segment of the intestine or is cord like, palpation should be carried out perpendicular to the long axis of the segment. This method is used for palpation of deep masses and intestinal lesions.
2. **Bimanual palpation:** The doctor adducts the middle three fingers of the right hand while using the left hand to hold up the mass from the back. The mass is then lifted between the doctor's both hands and closer to body surface. In cooperation with abdominal breathing, bimanual palpation can be used for examining the liver, spleen, kidneys and abdominal masses.
3. **Deep press palpation:** This method requires pressing two or three fingers deeply into the desired site in the abdomen. It is used for detecting lesions deep within the abdomen or determining the site of tenderness, such as McBurney's point, checking Murphy's sign or ureter tenderness point. When checking for rebound tenderness, press the fingers deeply and stay for 2–3 s then quickly withdraw the fingers to see if the patient feels more pain or demonstrates a painful complexion.

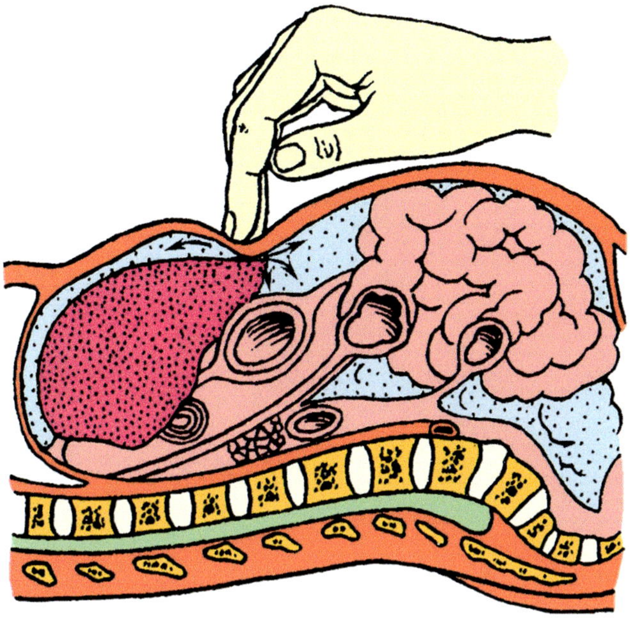

Fig. 41.4 Ballottement

4. **Ballottement:** Holding the index, middle and ring fingers together and making a 70°–90° angle with the abdominal surface, the examiner makes a jabbing motion in the abdomen and can feel visceral organs or masses with his or her fingers (Fig. 41.4). This method is typically used in patients with ascites when it's difficult to palpate the liver, spleen and abdominal masses. The quick jabbing motion can temporarily remove fluid and expose visceral organs, making them possible for palpation. Ballottement can cause discomfort in patients therefore the examiner should avoid using too much force.

41.3 Percussion

Percussion is striking part of the patient's body using one's fingers and determining the underlying disease according to the quality of the sound obtained.

Percussion is particularly important to examination of the chest and abdomen. The resonance from percussion of the chest can help determine lesions up to 5–7 cm in depth. Percussion is typically used to measure the width of lung apex, locate lower border of lung, determine pleural diseases, pleural effusion, presence and quantity of air, quality and extent of pulmonary lesion, thickness of pleura, size and shape of the heart, outline of the liver and spleen, presence of ascites, size of uterus and ovaries, and volume of the bladder. Using fingers or reflex hammers in examining reflexes and evaluating pain on percussion in the chest, abdomen or back is also considered part of percussion.

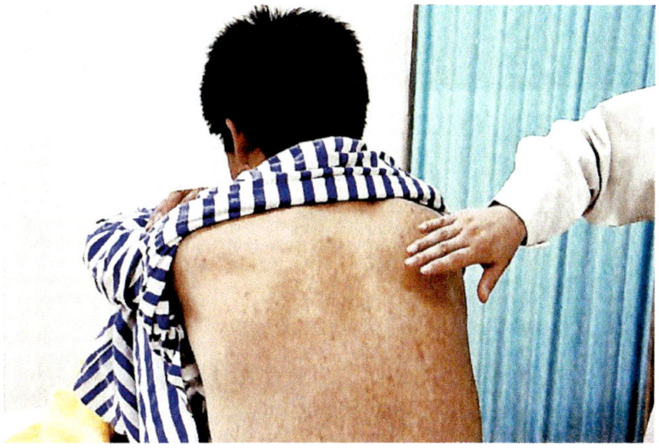

Fig. 41.5 Direct percussion

41.3.1 Methods of Percussion

According to different purpose and method, percussion can be divided into direct and indirect percussion.

41.3.1.1 Direct percussion

In direct percussion, the doctor adducts the middle three fingers of the right hand and directly tap the examined area, determining the lesion by the resonating sound (Fig. 41.5). This method is indicated for extensive pulmonary or abdominal lesions such as pleural adhesion or thickening, massive pleural effusion, ascites or pneumothorax.

41.3.1.2 Indirect Percussion

Indirect percussion is a percussion method commonly used under clinical setting. The doctor places the middle finger (also called the pleximeter finger) of the left hand on the site of percussion, while hyperextending the other fingers to avoid contact with the patient's body surface.

The fingers of the right hand are flexed naturally, and examiner uses the middle finger to strike the proximal or distal interphalangeal joint of the pleximeter finger of the left hand because it's closely placed on the percussion site and sensitive to resonance. The direction of the striking motion should be perpendicular to the body surface of the examined site (Fig. 41.6). The motion of percussion should be oriented by the movement of the wrist and metacarpophalangeal joint, and not the elbow or shoulder joint. The striking movements should be quick, agile and flexible. The pleximeter finger should be elevated immediately after percussion to mitigate the effect on the amplitude and frequency of the percussion note. Two or three taps can be made at each percussion site and if needed, additional percussions can be made to assist in diagnosis. Continuously striking of the same site should be avoided because of difficulty in discerning the quality of the note.

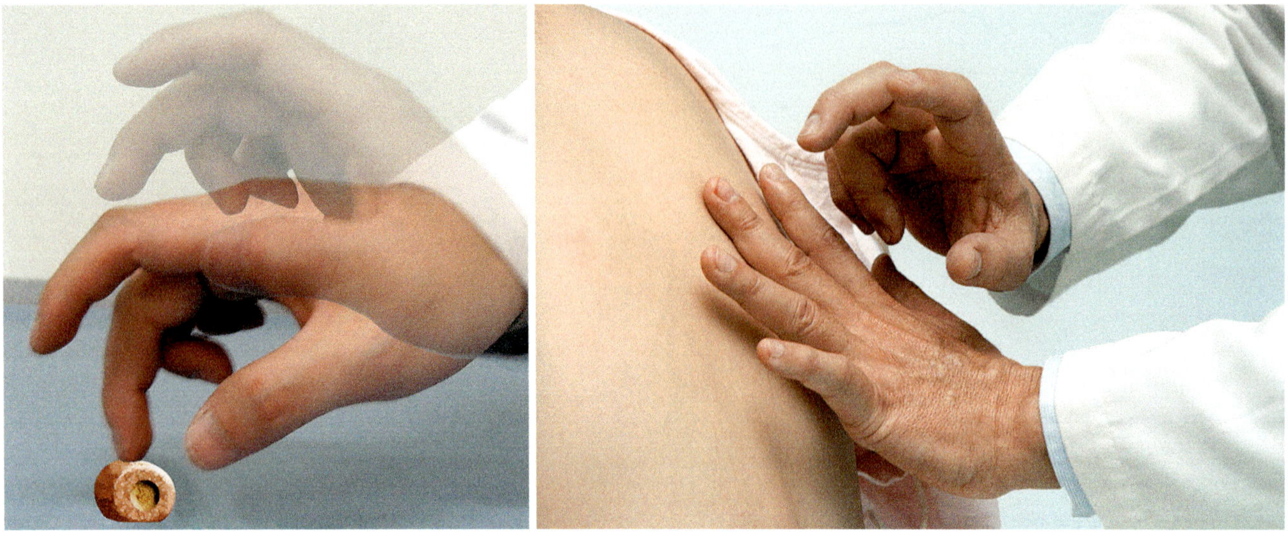

Fig. 41.6 Indirect percussion

Table 41.2 Features of different percussion sounds

Percussion Notes	Intensity	Relative pitch	Relative duration	Normal distribution	Pathological distribution
Resonance	High	Low	Long	Lungs	Bronchitis
Tympany	Highest	High	Longer	Abdomen, gastric air bubble	Severe pneumothorax, lung cavity, pneumoperitoneum
Hyperresonance	Higher	Lowest	Longest	None normally	Emphysema, increased air content in lungs
Dullness	Lower	Highest	Shorter	Part of the heart and liver covered by lungs	Lobar pneumonia
Flatness	Lowest	Higher	Short	Solid visceral organs	Massive pleural effusion, lung consolidation

In determining pain on percussion of the liver or renal span, the doctor can place the palm of the left hand on the desired site while making a fist with the right hand. Strike the back of the left hand with the ulnar side of the fist to evaluate for potential feelings of pain.

41.3.2 Percussion Sounds

Percussion note is the sound produced by the striking of the examined site by fingers. The quality of the sound is dependent on the density, flexibility, gas content, and depth of the tissue or organ. According to the frequency (high frequency high tone, low frequency low tone), amplitude (big amplitude louder sound, small amplitude lower sound), and tune (melodious), percussion notes can be divided into resonant, tympanic, hyper-resonant, dull and flat sounds (Table 41.2).

1. **Resonance:** This is the normal percussion note of the lung, with a frequency of 100–128/s, longer duration of vibration and absence of musical tone. It indicates normal findings in elasticity, gas content and density of the lung.
2. **Tympany:** This sound is similar to drumbeats, with a harmonious musical quality. It is louder and lasts longer than resonance, present during percussion of visceral organs containing a lot of air, normally found at the abdomen. Under pathological conditions, it can be heard on examination of lung cavities, pneumothorax and pneumoperitoneum etc.
3. **Hyper-resonance:** This is a sound with characteristics in between resonance and tympany, which can be considered a variation of tympany with a lower tone and louder sound than resonance. It can be found during percussion of the chest in healthy children because of a thinner chest wall. Under clinical settings, it is commonly found in lung tissue with excessive air content, reduced elasticity such as in cases of emphysema.
4. **Dullness:** This note has a comparatively higher tone, smaller sound and shorter duration. The vibration felt by the pleximeter finger is also weaker. Normally, solid organs with low air content such as the heart or the section of liver covered by the lower lungs (also called relative dull region) can produce dull percussion notes. Pathologically it is found on examination of patients with pneumonia (due to decreased air content).

5. **Flatness:** Compared to dullness, this is a unmelodious note with a higher tone, smaller sound and shorter vibration. It is typically present during percussion of regions of the heart and liver not clouded by lung tissue (also called absolute dull region). Under pathological conditions, it is found in patients with massive pleural effusion or consolidation of the lung.

41.4 Auscultation

Auscultation is the process during which the doctor determines the presence of disease by the sound produced in the patient's different body parts. It is especially important in diagnosis of cardiac and pulmonary illnesses.

Auscultation can be divided into direct and indirect auscultation.

41.4.1 Direct Auscultation

Direct auscultation is directly attaching one's ear to the site being examined. The sound produced is usually very weak. Currently this method is only used during emergencies or other special circumstances.

41.4.2 Indirect Auscultation

Indirect auscultation is auscultating using a stethoscope. This is a convenient technique suitable for all parts of the body because the stethoscope can magnify the sound produced by moving organs and filter noise from the environment. This method can be extensively applied to examination of the heart, lungs, abdomen as well as in auscultating murmurs of the blood vessel, subcutaneous emphysema, muscle tremor, joint movement, friction of the fracture surface.

The stethoscope is composed of an earpiece, a chest piece and tubing (Fig. 41.7). The chest piece can be divided into the bell and the diaphragm. The bell is used to auscultate low pitched sounds (Fig. 41.8) such as the rumbling murmur of mitral stenosis. It should be lightly placed on the site being examined, while avoiding additional sounds caused by friction with the skin surface. The diaphragm is designed for hearing sounds with a higher pitch (Fig. 41.9), such as the murmur of aortic insufficiency, breath sounds and bowel sounds. It should be tightly placed against the examining site during auscultation.

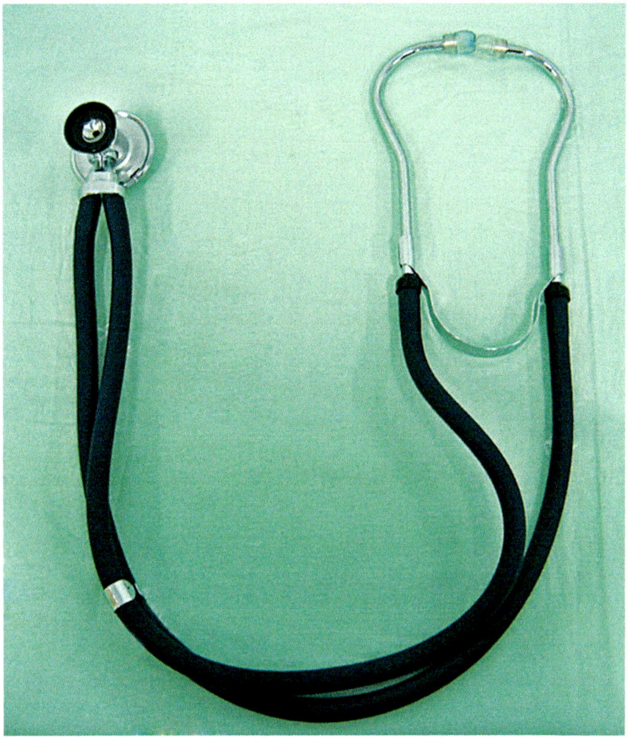

Fig. 41.7 Stethoscope

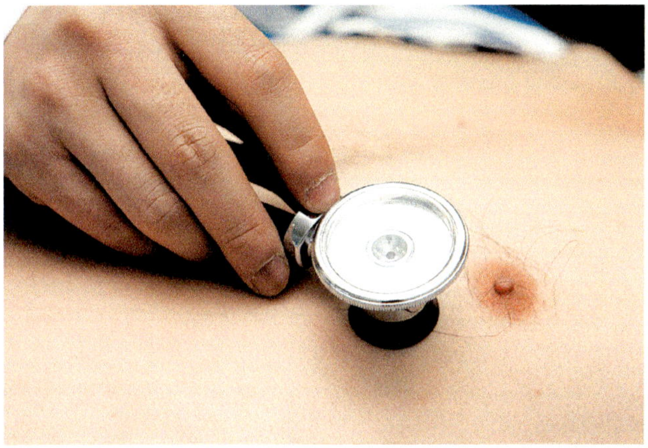

Fig. 41.8 Auscultation with the bell

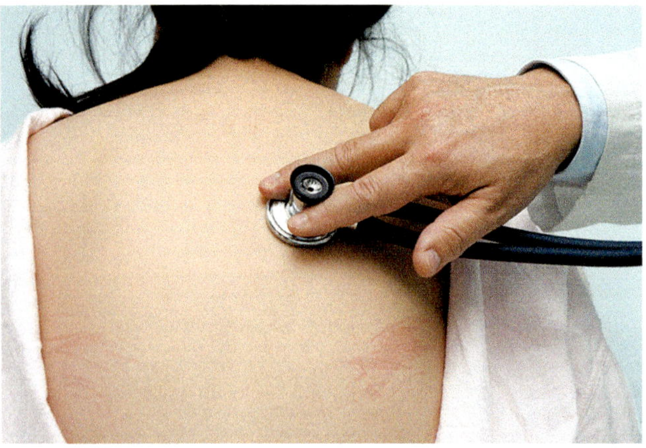

Fig. 41.9 Auscultation with the diaphragm

41.5 Olfactory Examination

Olfactory examination is using one's sense of smell to establish the association between an abnormal odor with a certain disease. Different odors can be emitted by the patient's skin, mucosa, respiratory tract, gastrointestinal tract, vomit, feces, secretion, pus and blood, possessing unique characteristics that belong to different diseases. During this examination, the doctor uses the hands to propagate the smell toward his or her nose for discerning the feature and quality of the odor.

- Normal perspiration is not pungent. Acidic perspiration is often present in patients with rheumatic fever and those on long-term use of salicylate acid, aspirin and other NSAIDs. The body odor from patients with bromhidrosis is due to bacterial processing of sebum secreted by underarm sebaceous glands.
- Normal sputum is scentless. Foul smelling sputum indicates anaerobic infection, typically seen in patients with bronchiectasis or pulmonary abscess. Foul smelling pus can be associated with gas gangrene. Bloody smelling sputum is often found in those with mass hemoptysis.
- Garlic breath is present in organophosphate poisoning. Fruity odor is commonly associated with diabetic ketoacidosis, where large amounts of fatty acids are converted into ketone bodies in the liver and release into blood, resulting in increased acetones in the patient's breath. Ammonia smell is found in uremia. Hepatic encephalopathy causes a fishy smell because dimethyl disulphides and methanethiol cannot be metabolized by the liver and accumulate in the body, resulting in a characteristic odor in the patient's breath or urine.
- Halitosis is commonly called bad breath, and seen in oral infection, gastritis and other gastrointestinal diseases.
- Sour smelling vomit indicates retention of food in the stomach, frequently found in patients with pyloric stenosis or pyloric achalasia. Fecal odor in vomit is present in those with severe vomiting or ileus. Vomit with pus and a smell of rotten apples can be found in gastric gangrene.
- Rotten smell in feces are associated with dyspepsia or pancreatic insufficiency. Foul smell is found in dysentery. Fishy smell is typically found in amoebic dysentery.
- A strong ammonia smell can be found in cystitis, caused by fermentation of the urine by bacteria in the bladder.
- Some diseases have special smells. For example, the smell of freshly baked bread can be found in typhoid fever. The scent of poultry feather can be smelt in patients with leprosy. Honey odor is present in bubonic plague and smell of rats can be found in patients with psychological disorders.
- Working under clinical setting, olfactory examination can quickly provide doctors with important clues. However, it must be used in synergy with other exams to determine the correct diagnosis.

Key Terms

1	Physical examination	体格检查
2	Inspection	视诊
3	Palpation	触诊
4	Percussion	叩诊
5	Auscultation	听诊
6	Olfactory examination	嗅诊

Study Questions

1. What are the whole contents of physical examination?
2. How to use basic skills to complete physical examination?
3. What are the differences between light and deep palpation?
4. What are the differences between direct and indirect percussion?

Suggested Readings and Websites

Bickley LS. Bates' guide to physical examination and history taking. 10th ed: Lippincott Williams & Wilkins; 2009.
Swartz MH. Textbook of physical diagnosis. 7th ed: Elsevier; 2014.

42 General Examination

Fei Chen and Rui Zeng

General examination is the first step in the whole process of physical examination, which is essential to know patient's general condition, evaluate the severity of disease and finally establish the correct diagnosis. The main contents of general examination include: sex, age, temperature, pulse, respiration, blood pressure, development and habitus, state of nutrition, consciousness, facial features and expression, position, skin and lymph nodes.

42.1 Section 1: General State Examination

42.1.1 Sex

The occurrence and differentiation of sex comprise three aspects: chromosomal sex (also known as genetic sex), gonadal sex and phenotypic sex. Sex determination is a continuous process of differentiation and development, and any disorders in this process may lead to sexual differentiation diseases.

1. **Determination of sex:** Normal individual's sexual characteristics are obvious and the sex is easy to be determined. However, sexual characteristics may alter in patients who have certain diseases.
2. **Sexual characteristics affected by certain diseases:** Adrenocortical tumor, or long-term use of adrenocorticotropic hormone may cause female masculinization.
3. **The incidence of certain diseases is related to sex:** Thyroid disease and systemic lupus erythematosus are mainly observed in females. The majority of hemophilia A are males, occasionally occurs in females.

F. Chen
Department of Hematology, Wuhan University, Wuhan, Hubei, China

R. Zeng (✉)
Department of Cardiology, Sichuan University, Chengdu, China

42.1.2 Age

Age is closely related to the occurrence and prognosis of certain diseases, for example, rickets, measles and diphtheria mainly occur in infants and children; Rheumatic fever, tuberculosis are common in teenagers; Atherosclerosis and coronary artery disease are mainly observed in elder patients. Judgment of age is generally based on skin elasticity, hair, wrinkles and teeth.

42.1.3 Vital Sign

Vital sign is of essential to evaluate the existence and quality of life activity, which includes temperature, pulse, respiration and blood pressure. Vital sign is one of the important indicators to observe patient's disease developing, and must be examined and recorded timely and accurately.

42.1.3.1 Temperature

Temperature refers to internal body temperature, which is usually represented by oral, rectal or axillary temperature in clinic.

1. Measurement and normal range of temperature
   Temperature is usually recorded using degrees Celsius (°C). Three conventional methods of temperature measurement are adopted: mouth, axilla and rectum measurement, using mercury or electronic thermometer. The followings are three commonly used methods of temperature measurement with mercury thermometer:
   (a) Oral measurement: The head end of sterilized thermometer is put under the tongue for 5 min, and the normal value of temperature with oral measurement is 36.3–37.2 °C.
   (b) Axillary measurement: The head end of thermometer is put in the top central of patient's armpit, clamping with upper arm, taking out after 10 min and reading

X.-H. Wan, R. Zeng (eds.), *Handbook of Clinical Diagnostics*, https://doi.org/10.1007/978-981-13-7677-1_42

the result. The normal axillary temperature is 36.0–37.0 °C.

(c) Anal measurement: Patient takes lateral position, the head end of thermometer is coated with lubricant and slowly inserted into the rectum to half length of the thermometer for 5 min. The normal rectal temperature is 36.5–37.7 °C, which is 0.2–0.5 °C higher than oral temperature. This method is usually used in children or patients with unconsciousness.

- Taking oral temperature as the standard, fever refers to the temperature is higher than normal. Hypothermia refers to the temperature is lower than normal (<35 °C), which is seen in patients with shock, frail elderly, severe malnutrition, or hypothyroidism.

2. Temperature recording method

Temperature curve refers to temperature results drawn on the recording sheet. Most febrile diseases have certain shapes of temperature curve, which is called fever type.

42.1.3.2 Pulse

Pulse is usually examined by palpation of the radial artery, and the alternative artery may be carotid artery, brachial artery, femoral artery, or dorsalis pedis artery. The rate, rhythm and strength of the pulse should be noticed. Pulse examination method: Putting the index, middle and ring fingers closely together, the finger pulp is placed on the radial artery closing to wrist, and touch the radial artery pulse with proper pressure for at least 30 s (Fig. 42.1).

The normal pulse rate for adults is 60–100 beats per minute (bpm). The pulse rate is usually slower in elderly people, while faster in children.

42.1.3.3 Respiration

Respiratory examination should focus on breathing type, frequency, depth and rhythm. Examination method: After examination of pulse, the physician should still put the finger on the radial artery, and observe the movement of patient's chest or abdomen along with breathing, counting breathing for 1 min.

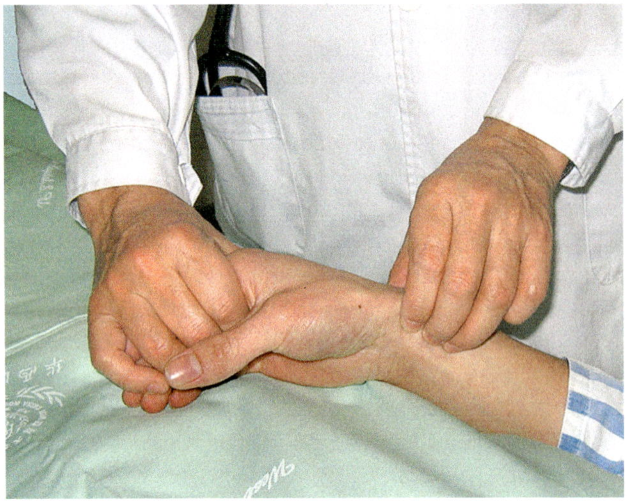

Fig. 42.1 Palpation of the radial artery

42.1.3.4 Blood Pressure

Blood pressure (BP) refers to the arterial blood pressure of the systemic circulation, which is one of the most important vital signs. Blood pressure is classified as systolic blood pressure (SBP) and diastolic blood pressure (DBP). The value of systolic blood pressure minus diastolic blood pressure is called pulse pressure (PP). Mean arterial pressure refers to diastolic blood pressure plus 1/3 pulse pressure.

1. Measurement methods

There are two methods for blood pressure measurement: direct measurement method and indirect measurement method.

(a) Direct measurement method: A catheter is placed in the peripheral artery (such as radial artery) with percutaneous puncture and the blood pressure is automatically displayed on the monitor screen. This method is accurate, real-time, but it is an invasive examination, requiring special equipment, therefore it is only used in critical and surgical patients.

(b) Indirect measurement method: Also known as blood pressure cuff method, measured with a sphygmomanometer. Three kinds of sphygmomanometer are used in clinic: mercury column, spring (meter) type and electronic sphygmomanometer. This is a noninvasive, easy to operate method, and can be applied to any patients.

(c) The following describes the measurement of brachial artery blood pressure (BP) using mercury sphygmomanometer (Fig. 42.2). Specific operating procedures and requirements are as follows:

(d) Sphygmomanometer selection: (a) Regularly calibrated mercury sphygmomanometer, meeting the standards of measurement. (b) Blood pressure cuff with appropriate size.

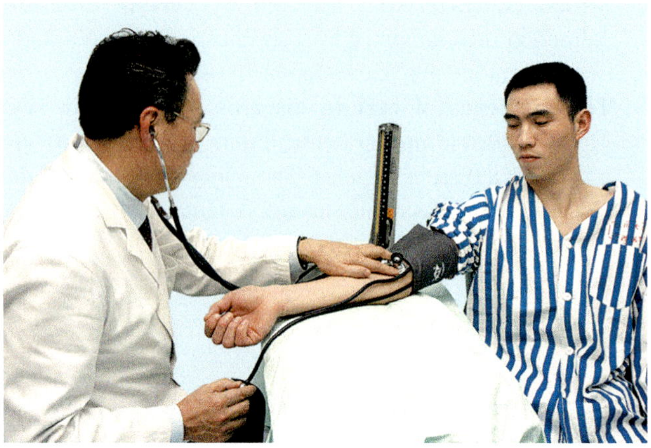

Fig. 42.2 Blood pressure measurement

(e) Preparation of individual being examined: 30 min before measurement, one should not smoke or drink coffee, and rest for 5–10 min.

(f) Measurement procedures: (a) Check the sphygmomanometer: Switch on the mercury column button, and the convex surface of mercury column is at zero-scale. (b) Elbow position: taking sitting or supine position, the upper arm is exposed. The elbow and sphygmomanometer are at the same level with heart. (c) Wrap the blood pressure cuff: The cuff should be evenly tight around the upper arm and the lower edge of the cuff is around 2–3 cm above the bend of elbow. The central part of cuff airbag should be placed on the surface of brachial artery. (d) Position of the stethoscope's diaphragm: Gently press and put the stethoscope's bell on the brachial artery in antecubital fossa (the bell should not be placed in between the cuff and upper arm). (e) Inflate the cuff: Tighten the knob, rapidly squeeze the pump bulb to inflate the airbag. At the same time, listening to the sound of brachial artery beating, watching the rise of mercury column and increasing additional 30–40 mm after the sounds of pulse disappear. f. Deflate the cuff: Release the knob and gradually deflate the cuff at a constant speed (descending speed is 2–6 mmHg/s). The deflating speed should be slower in patients with bradycardia. The cuff should be deflated rapidly to zero-scale after obtaining the diastolic blood pressure reading.

(g) Determination of blood pressure values: Determination of blood pressure values is according to the Korotkoff 5 phases method. The value of mercury column, which corresponds to the first resounding flop (brachial artery beating sound), is the systolic pressure (first phase). With the falling of mercury column, the sound is weakened and accompanied by soft blowing murmur (second phase). When deflation continues and arterial blood flow increases, the sounds are replaced by loud noises (third phase), and then suddenly weakened (fourth phase). The value displayed on the mercury column gauge when the sound disappears, is the diastolic pressure (fifth phase).

(h) After measurement: Deflating the airbag, rolling up the cuff and putting it into the sphygmomanometer. After the mercury in the glass tube is completely flowed back into the mercury tank, switching off the mercury column button and closing the sphygmomanometer.

- Measurement of lower limbs blood pressure: The measurement method of popliteal artery blood pressure is basically the same as upper limbs. In normal conditions, lower limb blood pressure is 20–40 mmHg higher than that of the upper limb in the same side. In certain patients such as aorta coarctation, thoracoabdominal aortic arteritis, lower limb blood pressure may be lower than that of upper limb.

Table 42.1 Definition and categories of adult blood pressure (mmHg)

Category	Systolic		Diastolic
Normal	<120	and	<80
Prehypertension	120–139	And (or)	80–89
Hypertension	≥140	And (or)	≥90
Stage 1 (mild)	140–159	And (or)	90–99
Stage 2 (moderate)	160–179	And (or)	100–109
Stage 3 (severe)	≥180	And (or)	≥110
Isolated systolic hypertension	≥140	And	<90

Note: 1 mmHg = 0.133 kPa. If the systolic or diastolic blood pressure belongs to different categories, the higher category is used for blood pressure classification. Isolated systolic hypertension can be classified as stage 1, 2 and 3 as well according to the systolic blood pressure level

2. Reference values of blood pressure

The average blood pressure of the newborn is 50–60/30–40 mmHg; for adults it is 90–130/60–85 mmHg, and the pulse pressure is about 30–40 mmHg. The systolic pressure increases linearly with age, while the diastolic pressure increases gradually. After the age of 55, diastolic pressure enters the plateau stage and slowly decreases after 60 years old, meanwhile, the pulse pressure gradually increases. In adults, blood pressure in males is slightly higher than that of the females. The blood pressure of two upper limbs may has a variation of 5–10 mmHg in healthy people. Since blood pressure is affected by many conditions, a single measurement is not sufficient to determine whether it is normal or not. Multiple measurements in different occasions are recommended to assess the blood pressure.

The diagnostic standard of hypertension in adults has been revised for several times, which is in consistent with epidemiology and clinical research. Classification standard of blood pressure in Chinese Guidelines for the Management of Hypertension (2010) is shown in Table 42.1.

42.1.4 Development and Habitus

42.1.4.1 Development

Development is determined by comprehensive evaluation of age, intelligence and physical growth status (including height, weight, secondary sexual characteristics). For well-developed individuals, the age, intelligence and physical growth status are well balanced.

Indicators for normal development in adults: (a) Head length is about 1/7 of the height; (b) Chest circumference is approximately half of the height; (c) The length between two middle fingers after horizontal expansion of the upper limbs is approximately equal to the height. (d) Sitting height is approximately equal to the length of the lower limb; (e) The ratio between upper part of the body (from head to the upper edge of pubic symphysis) and lower part of the body (from upper edge of the pubic symphysis to plantar) is about 1:1.

Development is affected by many factors, such as race, heredity, age, gender, endocrine, nutrition, metabolism, environment condition and physical exercise, etc. In addition to height growth in puberty, physique and certain parts of the body change as well. For example, boys show widened shoulder, increased muscle cells, and male sexual characteristics development, etc.; while girls appear hip enlargement, fat cells proliferation, and female sexual characteristics development, etc.

42.1.4.2 Habitus

Habitus is the appearance of physical development of the body, including fat distribution, the growth of bones and muscles.

1. Three types of adult habitus
   (a) Asthenic type: also called leptosomic type. Tall and thin, with slim neck, narrow and drooping shoulders, flat chest, epigastric angle <90°.
   (b) Sthenic type: also known as pyknic type. Thick and strong, with short neck, broad flattened shoulders, epigastric angle >90°.
   (c) Ortho-sthenic type: also known as symmetrical type. All parts of the body are well balanced, epigastric angle is about 90°, and most normal individuals are belongs to this type.
2. Common abnormal habitus
   Abnormal habitus refers to significant differences of habitus when compared with individuals who have the same race, age and sex in the same region.
   (a) Short stature: Referring to adult males whose height is lower than 145 cm, or lower than 135 cm for females. Short stature results from physical growth retardation, which may be observed in delayed puberty, endocrine disorders (such as pituitary dwarfism, cretinism, precocious puberty), malnutrition, metabolic disorders and systemic diseases (such as tuberculosis, tumors, heart disease, congenital or acquired bone disease, hypothalamic lesions).
   (b) Tall stature
      - Constitution tall stature: The height and weight are significantly higher than that of normal individuals. The well-proportioned tall stature is accompanied by good physical strength and normal fertility, without endocrine dysfunction and advanced puberty. As a normal variation, constitutional tall stature is usually related to genetic background.
      - Advanced puberty: Advanced puberty refers to sexual development occurs before the age of 9 in female, and before 10 for male, which is often accompanied with growth acceleration and tall stature.
      - Tall stature caused by diseases: Tall stature may occur in endocrine diseases, such as gigantism and acromegaly.

42.1.5 State of Nutrition

State of nutrition is related to food intake, digestion and absorption, metabolism, which is one of the criteria for identifying the state of health and disease. Abnormal state of nutrition is usually described as obesity and emaciation.

42.1.5.1 Commonly Used Assessment Indicators

State of nutrition is usually determined by comprehensive analysis of skin, hair, subcutaneous fat and muscles, etc. The most convenient and rapid way to assess nutritional status is to observe the subcutaneous fat enrichment. Here are some physical indexes that are applied to assess the state of nutrition:

1. Height and weight
   Height and weight are the most commonly used indicators for body measurements. The following formula is a rough estimate of ideal body weight (IBW, also called standard body weight): IBW (kg) = height (cm) − 105, or IBW (kg) = [height (cm) − 100] × 0.9 (male) or × 0.85 (female). Generally, one's weight in the range of IBW ± 10% is considered as normal weight; overweight refers to the weight is 10–20% higher than IBW; obesity refers to the weight is more than 20% higher than IBW. Emaciation refers to the weight is 10–20% lower than IBW; obvious emaciation refers to the weight is more than 20% lower than IBW; extremely emaciation is called cachexia.
2. Body mass index (BMI)
   BMI is another indicator for weight assessment. Calculation method: BMI = weight (kg)/[height (meters^2)]. BMI is the most important indicator for the diagnosis of obesity. According to WHO standard, a person with a BMI between 18.5 and 24.9 is considered to have a healthy weight; a person with a BMI between 25.0 and 29.9 is considered as overweight; and a person with a BMI of 30 or above is considered as obese.
3. Waist circumstance or waist-to-hip ratio
   Waist circumstance (WC) or waist-to-hip ratio (WHR) represents fat distribution. Waist circumstance refers to the circumferential length measured at the midpoint between anterior superior iliac spine and lower edge of the twelfth rib. Hip circumference refers to the circumfer-

ence measured at the most prominent point of the pelvis around the hips.

4. Arm circumstance
   In some children, the left upper arm circumference may be used to evaluate the nutrition state. Generally, upper arm circumference above 13.5 cm is considered as well nutrition for children of 1–5 years old; 12.5–13.5 cm is considered as fairly nutrition; under 12.5 cm is considered as innutrition.
5. Skinfold thickness
   More than 50% of fat is distributed at subcutaneous. In clinic, subcutaneous fat thickness measured by skinfold caliper is used to estimate the fat accumulation. Measurement position: upper arm, scapular region and abdomen. Commonly used measurement position is triceps skinfold of upper arm. The normal skinfold thickness is generally 13.1 ± 6.6 mm (median 11.4 mm) for adult males, and 21.5 ± 6.9 mm (median 20.8 mm) for females.

42.1.5.2 Nutrition State Levels

Nutrition state is generally categorized as well, fairly or poorly.

1. Well Ruddy mucosa, glossy skin with good elasticity, rich subcutaneous fat, normal or increased skinfold thickness, strong muscles, smooth nails and hair, full scapular and abdominal muscles. IBW and BMI are in the normal range or slightly higher than normal.
2. Poorly Dry skin and mucosa with poor elasticity, thin subcutaneous fat, lower skinfold thickness, weakened muscles, rough nails, thin dull hair, protruding scapula and ribs. IBW and BMI are significantly lower than normal.
3. Fairly Nutrition state is between well and poorly mentioned above.

42.1.5.3 Common Abnormal Nutrition States

1. Innutrition
   Innutrition manifests as weight loss, characterized by emaciation, IBW < 10%, adult BMI <18.5, pediatric upper arm circumference <12.5 cm, with lower skinfold thickness.

   The main reasons that cause innutrition are lack of nutrients or excessive consumption. Innutrition is usually seen in patients with long-term and serious diseases. Innutrition may result from excessive consumption of protein and fat, which is observed in patients with active tuberculosis, tumors, metabolic diseases (such as diabetes) and some endocrine diseases (such as hyperthyroidism).
2. Overnutrition
   Also known as hypernutrition, refers to excessive accumulation and (or) abnormal distribution of fat, characterized by weight gain and obesity (BMI ≥ 30). According to the etiology, obesity is categorized as primary and secondary obesity.
   (a) Primary obesity: Also known as simple obesity. Primary obesity is common in clinic, and can be categorized as obesity with genetic predisposition and obesity due to excessive intake of calories.
   (b) Secondary obesity: Secondary obesity is often caused by some endocrine and metabolic diseases, such as hypothalamic pituitary diseases, Cushing syndrome, hypothyroidism, polycystic ovary syndrome, and insulinoma. Long-term use of chlorpromazine, insulin, glucocorticoids and other drugs promoting protein synthesis may result in obesity (drug induced obesity).

Patients with Cushing syndrome show fat redistribution due to significant increase of cortisol in plasma. Typical Cushing syndrome is characterized by excessive accumulation of fat in face and trunk, and limbs are relatively thin and small, which is called concentric obesity. Patient with Cushing syndrome is usually accompanied with full moon face, sanguineous appearance and skin stretch marks.

42.1.6 Consciousness

Consciousness refers to individual's cognition and awareness ability to the surroundings and their own state, which is a comprehensive performance of central nerve system functional activity. Conscious activities mainly comprise five aspects: cognition, thinking, emotion, memory and orientation. Diseases that affect brain functional activities may result in consciousness abnormality, called disturbance of consciousness, which may be manifested as excited and restless, thought disorders, weakened verbal ability, abnormal emotional activities and increased unconscious action. According to clarity or wakefulness, disturbance of consciousness is categorized as somnolence, lethargy and coma.

Inquiry, careful observation and examination are the main methods for evaluation of patients' consciousness. Pain stimulation test and pupil reflex test may be used to determine disturbance of consciousness in patients with serious diseases. In clinic, Glasgow coma scale (GCS) is used to determine the consciousness state (see Table 42.2).

According to the scale, eye opening, verbal and motor responses are scored respectively from 1 to 6, and the consciousness state is evaluated by the total score results. The lowest total score is 3, and the maximum is 15. Generally, score 9 or higher is considered as being conscious, the higher the score, the better the state of consciousness. Scoring under 8 is considered as coma, and fewer than 3 is called deep coma.

Table 42.2 Glasgow coma scale

Evaluation items	Indicators	Score
Eye opening response	Open eyes spontaneously	4
	Open eyes in response to calling	3
	Open eyes in response to painful stimuli	2
	No response to painful stimuli	1
Verbal response	Accurate orientation	5
	Confused occasionally	4
	Give an irrelevant answer	3
	Incomprehensible voice	2
	No verbal response	1
Motor response	Obey instructions	6
	Locate painful stimuli accurately	5
	Escape painful stimuli	4
	Flexion reaction to painful stimuli (Decorticated posture)	3
	Extension reaction to painful stimuli (Decerebrated posture)	2
	No response to painful stimuli	1
Total point		3–15

42.1.7 Mental State

Mental state refers to the functional status of brain in response to various stimuli of external environment. Mental disorders are abnormal phenomena of emotional, cognitive or behavioral alteration, accompanied with painful experience and (or) functional impairment.

42.1.7.1 Disorders of Sensation and Perception

1. Disorders of sensation
   Sensation is the direct reflection of brain to different stimuli, such as color, sound, temperature and odor. Common disorders of sensation include:
   (a) Hyperesthesia: Intolerable to general stimuli from surroundings. Hyperesthesia is usually seen in patients with neurosis, menopausal syndrome.
   (b) Hypoesthesia: Unable to perceive or with limited ability to perceive intense stimuli from surroundings. Hypoesthesia is usually seen in patients with depression, stupor and disturbance of consciousness. Loss of sensation refers to complete deficiency of perceiving ability, showing as blindness, deafness and aphonia, which may be observed in hysteria.
   (c) Senestopathia: A sense of discomfort or insufferable feeling within the body, such as the sense of throat blockage, abdominal airflow and gastrointestinal torsion. Senestopathia is usually seen in hypochondriasis, somatization disorder, schizophrenia and depressive episode.
2. Disorders of perception
   Perception is a complete image, which is formed in the brain with the aid of previous experience, after integrated with various attributes of objective things. Common disorders of perception include:
   (a) Illusion: A distorted perception of objective things. Illusion is usually seen in patients with delirium, and occasionally observed in normal person.
   (b) Hallucination: Perceptual experience without realistic stimulation action on sensory organs. A hallucination is often coexisting with delusion. Based on differently involved sensory organs, hallucination may manifest as auditory hallucination, visual hallucination, olfactory hallucination, tactile hallucination and visceral hallucination.
3. Psychosensory disturbance
   One can perceive objective things, but faulty perception is generated with some specific properties, such as size, shape, color, distance, position, etc. Psychosensory disturbance is usually seen in patients with epilepsy, which may appear visual distortion and space perception disorders.

42.1.7.2 Thinking Disorders

Thinking is the indirect and resumptive reflection of brain on objective things. As the highest form of human cognitive activities, thinking includes analysis, synthesis, comparison, generalization, judgment and reasoning. In clinic, thinking disorders are categorized as thinking form disorders and thinking content disorders. Thinking form disorders mainly present as hypermetamorphosis, slow thinking, poor thinking, slack thinking, cracked thinking and intermitted thinking. Thinking content disorders usually manifest as delusions, including delusions of persecution and delusion of reference.

42.1.7.3 Attention Disorders

Attention is the process of mental activity directing and concentrating on certain things. Disorders of attention may present as hyperprosexia, aprosexia, hypoprosexia, and transference of attention.

42.1.7.4 Memory Disorders

Memory is the recurrence of the past experience. Clinically common disorders of memory include hypermnesia, hypomnesia and amnesia.

42.1.7.5 Intelligence Disorders

Intelligence refers to the ability to understand objective things and to solve practical problems with knowledge. Clinically common disorders of intelligence include mental retardation, dementia, etc.

42.1.7.6 Disorientation

Orientation refers to the ability to judge the time, place, characters and personal identity. Disorientation refers to the wrong understanding or loss of cognition to one's surroundings and situation, which is observed in patients with symptomatic or organic mental disorders accompanied with disturbance of consciousness or severe dementia.

42.1.7.7 Affection Disorders

Affection refers to the attitude towards objective things and subsequent inner experience. Disorders of affection may manifest as elation, depression, anxiety, phobia, panic, labile, apathy, emotional vulnerability, emotional numbing, irritability, pathological passion, parathymia, emotional infantility and affective ambivalence.

42.1.7.8 Will Disorders

Will is the mental process that one consciously sets goals, and overcomes difficulties to achieve the goals. Disorders of will may display as hyperbulia, hypobulia, abulia, parabulia, and ambitendency.

42.1.7.9 Disorders of Action and Behavior

Disorders of action and behavior, also known as psychomotor disorders, are usually observed in patients with mental diseases. Common disorders of action and behavior include psychomotor inhibition, psychomotor excitement, stereotyped action, echopraxia, mannerism, and forced action.

42.1.7.10 Disturbance of Consciousness

Consciousness refers to one's capability to understand and respond to the surroundings or one's own state. Disorientation is an important symbol of disturbance of consciousness. Disturbance of consciousness may manifest as reduced consciousness clarity, narrowed consciousness span, and altered consciousness content.

42.1.7.11 Disturbance of Insight

Insight, also known as comprehension or introspection, refers to the ability to recognize and judge one's mental illness. Lack of insight is a typical manifestation of psychosis.

42.1.8 Tone and Voive

Tone refers to the pitch of one's speech. Tone is related nerve and vocal organs, for instance, hoarseness occurs in recurrent laryngeal nerve paralysis, laryngitis, vocal cord edema or polyp. Nasal voice is seen in patients with acute rhinitis or nasosinusitis.

Voice refers to the speed and rhythm of speech. Abnormal voice may manifest as slow or irregular language, which is seen in Parkinsonism, chorea, athetosis, and cerebrovascular diseases.

42.1.9 Facial Features and Expression

Facial features and expression are important indicators for emotion status evaluation. Some diseases show characteristic facial features and expression, which have great values for differential diagnosis. Common typical facial features are as follows:

1. Acute facies
   Reddening facies, restlessness, and pained expression, sometimes accompanied with flaring alae nasi, herpes labialis. Acute facies is usually seen in patients with acute febrile diseases such as lobar pneumonia, malaria, and epidemic cerebrospinal meningitis.
2. Chronic facies
   Haggard facies, with gloomy complexion, dim eyes, worried expression. Chronic facies is observed in patients with chronic wasting diseases, such as malignant tumor, cirrhosis, and severe tuberculosis.
3. Anemic facies
   Pale facies, pale lips and tongue, tired expression. Anemia facies is seen in patients with anemia caused by various diseases.
4. Hepatic facies
   Thin cheeks, gloomy facies, facial brown pigmentation, sometimes with spider angiomas. Hepatic facies is observed in patients with chronic liver diseases.
5. Nephrotic facies
   Pale facies, facial edema. Nephrotic facies is seen patients with chronic kidney diseases.
6. Hyperthyreosis facies
   Astonished expression, blepharodiastasis, exophthalmos, bright and shining eyes, excited and restless, agitated and irritable (Fig. 42.3). Hyperthyreosis facies is seen in patients with hyperthyroidism.
7. Myxedema facies
   Sallow complexion, with facial edema, thick and wide face, dull eyes, unresponsive, languid mood, thin hair, hypertrophic tongue with pale color. Myxedema facies is seen in patients with hypothyroidism.
8. Mitral facies
   Dim complexion, purplish red cheeks, and mild lips cyanosis. Mitral facies is seen in patients with rheumatic mitral stenosis.
9. Acromegaly facies
   Enlarged skull, longer face, enlarged and bulged jaw, thickened forehead skinfold, ridgy superciliary arch and cheekbones, enlarged nose and ears, hypertrophic lips and tongue, increased teeth space (Fig. 42.4).
10. Typhoid facies
    Indifferent expression, unresponsiveness showing no desire. Typhoid facies is seen in patients with high fever

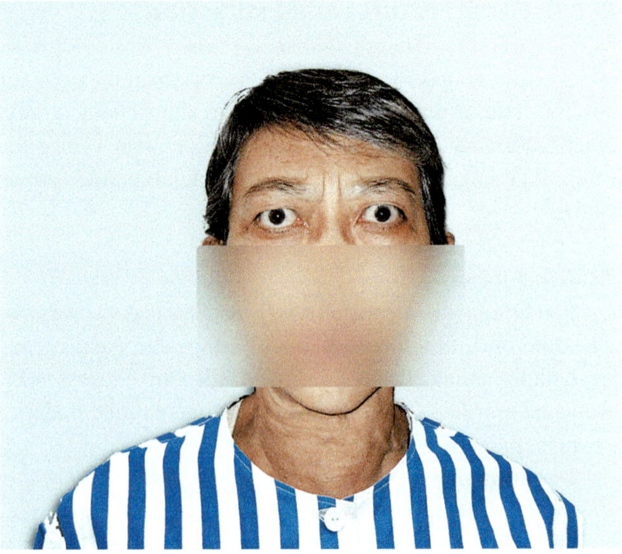

Fig. 42.3 Hyperthyreosis facies

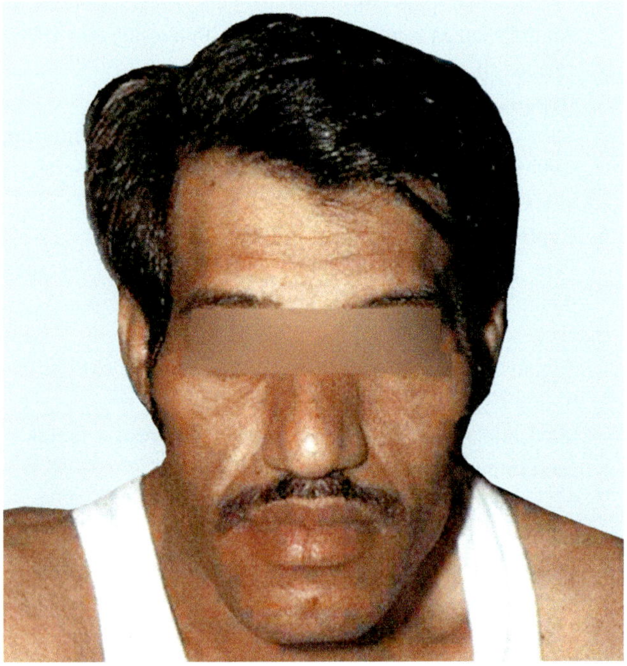

Fig. 42.4 Acromegaly facies

due to typhoid fever, cerebrospinal meningitis, and encephalitis.

11. Sardonic feature
    Lockjaw, facial spasm, showing a forced smile. Sardonic feature is seen in patients with tetanus.
12. Moon facies
    The face is round like a full moon, and the skin is red with sanguineous appearance, often accompanied with acne and whiskers. Moon facies is usually observed in patients with Cushing syndrome and long-term use of glucocorticoids.
13. Masked facies
    Stiff face without expression, like a mask. Masked facies is seen in patients with Parkinson's disease, encephalitis, cerebral vascular disease and brain atrophy.
14. Critical facies
    Also known as Hippocrates facies, with thin pale face, and sunken dull eyes. Critical facies is seen in patients with hemorrhoea, shock, dehydration, and acute peritonitis.

42.1.10 Position

Position refers to patient's body status. Some diseases show characteristic positions, which is useful for differential diagnosis. Common body positions are as follows:

42.1.10.1 Active Position

Active position refers to free movement of the body without restriction. Active position is seen in normal individuals, or patients in the early stage of diseases.

42.1.10.2 Passive Position

Patients with passive position are unable to adjust or change the position of the body by themselves. Passive position is observed in patients who are extremely weak or unconsciousness.

42.1.10.3 Compulsive Position

Compulsive position is a special position that patient is forced to take in order to relieve discomfort caused by disease. Common compulsive positions include:

1. Compulsive supine position
   Compulsive supine position is often accompanied with lower limbs flection, which helps to reduce abdominal muscle tension. Compulsive supine position is seen in patients with acute peritonitis.
2. Compulsive prone position
   Compulsive prone position can reduce back muscle tension, and is seen in patients with spinal diseases.
3. Compulsive lateral position
   Patients with pleural diseases often take lateral position with the affected side down, since this position can limit the moving of affected chest and reduce chest pain. In addition, lateral position is conducive to the compensatory breathing of the normal side. Compulsive lateral position is seen in patients with pleurisy or pleural effusion of one side.
4. Compulsive sitting position
   Also known as orthopnea. Patient sits on the edge of the bed, with hands extending against the knees or bed.

The position can lower the position of diaphragm, which facilitates chest and auxiliary respiratory muscles movement, increases pulmonary ventilation, and relieves burden of the heart. Compulsive sitting position is usually seen in patients with cardiopulmonary dysfunction.

5. Compulsive squatting
   During activities, patients are forced to stop due to dyspnea and palpitations, and take squatting position or knee-chest position in order to relieve discomfort. Compulsive squatting is seen in patients with cyanotic congenital heart disease.
6. Forced standing position
   Patient suffers a sudden precordial pain during walking, and is forced to stop immediately, pressing hand on the precordium. Patient can continue to walk only after the discomforts are relieved. Forced standing is seen in patients with angina pectoris.
7. Alternative position
   Patient shows restlessness, tossing and turning, due to abdominal pain attack. Alternative position is seen in patients with cholelithiasis, ascariasis of biliary tract, and renal colic.
8. Opisthotonos position
   The head is thrown backward, with thoracoabdominal convex, showing arched trunk, due to neck and back muscle rigidity. Opisthotonos position is seen in patients with tetanus, encephalitis and meningitis in children.

42.1.11 Posture

Posture is the state of behavior. Healthy individual has straight body, flexible limbs and coordinated action. Posture observation has clinical significances: (a) recognizing health status, for example, patients with congestive heart failure are more willing to take sitting position. (b) Posture can reflect spiritual state.

42.1.12 Gait

Gait refers to the walking manner. Some diseases have characteristic gait, and the followings are common typical abnormal gait:

1. Waddling gait
   Waddling gait is characterized by a duck-like walking. Waddling gait is seen in rickets, Kashin Beck disease, progressive muscular dystrophy, and congenital bilateral hip dislocation.
2. Drinking man gait
   Patients are unable to walk straightly, which is seen in cerebellar diseases, alcoholism and barbitals poisoning.
3. Ataxic gait
   Ataxic gait is characterized with unsteady gait, with wide foot space to prevent the body from tilting. Patient cannot keep balance when closing eyes, and has difficulty to walk in the dark. Ataxic gait is seen in patients with myeleterosis.
4. Festinating gait
   Difficult starting, walking with small, rapid steps. The walking is getting faster and faster, and seems unable to stop, lacking arm swing (Fig. 42.5). Festinating gait is seen in patients with Parkinsonism.
5. Steppage gait
   Due to weakened ankle muscles and affected foot ptosis, patient must lift the foot higher than in a normal stride while walking. Steppage gait is seen in patients with common peroneal nerve paralysis.
6. Scissors gait
   Due to hypermyotonia of lower limbs, especially extensor and adductor muscles, patient shows excessive adduction of lower extremities while walking, displaying crossed legs like scissors (Fig. 42.6). Scissors gait is seen in patients with cerebral palsy and paraplegia.
7. Intermittent claudication
   Patient was forced to stop walking due to sudden pain or weakness of lower limbs, and after taking a rest patient

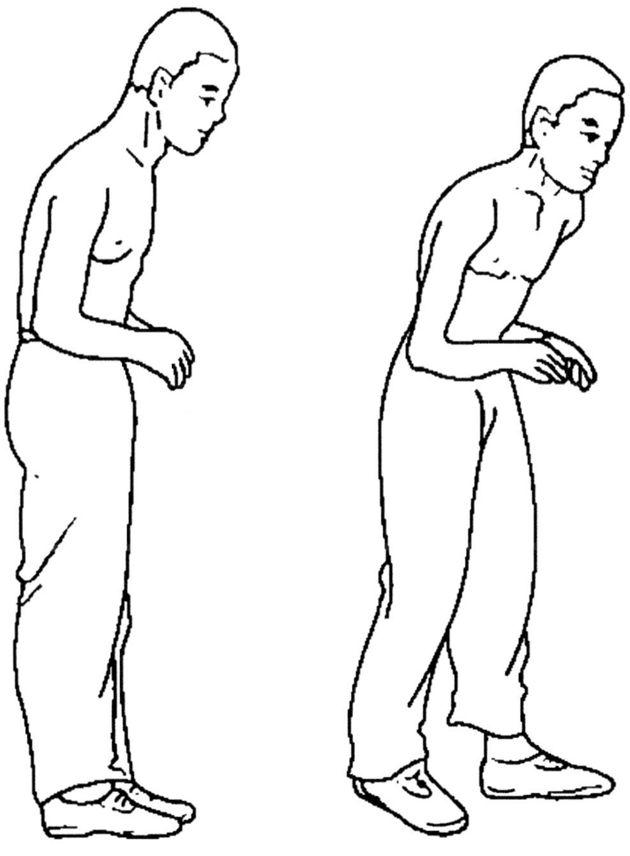

Fig. 42.5 Festinating gait

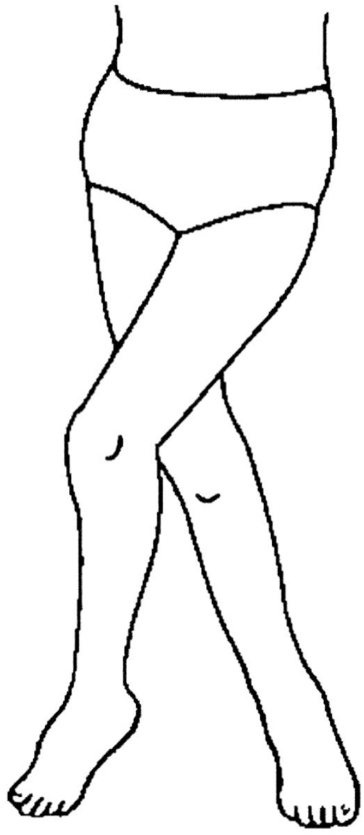

Fig. 42.6 Scissors gait

can walk again. Intermittent claudication is observed in patients with hypertension and arteriosclerosis.

42.2 Section 2: Skin

The skin is a barrier between the body and the external environment, which has important physiological functions. Skin lesions may be due to certain local reaction, or arise as manifestations of systemic diseases and responses. Therefore, a comprehensive check of the skin is an indispensable part of physical examination, which forms the basis of proper diagnosis of disease. In addition to color, humidity and elasticity alterations, skin lesions may be displayed as rash, desquamation, hemorrhage, edema, subcutaneous nodules or scar.

42.2.1 Color

Skin color may be different due to racial heredity. In the same race, it varies owing to capillaries distribution, pigmentation and subcutaneous fat thickness.

1. Pallor
   Pale skin and mucous membranes may be due to anemia, peripheral capillaries spasm or insufficient blood filling, which may result from cold, shock, collapse and aortic valve insufficiency. Nail bed, palm prints, conjunctiva, oral mucosa and tongue are proper sites for skin color examination. If pallor is only observed in extremities, this may related to arterial spasm or obstruction, such as Raynaud's disease and thromboangiitis obliterans.
2. Redness
   Redness is caused by skin capillary dilatation, increased blood flow or red blood cells. In physiological conditions, it can be the results of drinking and sports. In pathological conditions, redness may be the manifestation of febrile diseases such as lobar pneumonia and certain poisonings (such as atropine poisoning, carbon monoxide poisoning). Persistent skin redness is observed in Cushing's syndrome, long-term use of corticosteroids and polycythemia vera.
3. Cyanosis
   Skin and mucous membrane are purple, which is often observed in the tongue, lips, cheeks and extremities. Cyanosis is found in reductive hemoglobin increasing, or abnormal hemoglobinemia.
4. Stained yellow
   Stained yellow is usually observed in the following situations:
   (a) Jaundice: Increased serum bilirubin concentration makes the skin, mucous membranes and body fluids yellow. Visible jaundice can be observed when serum total bilirubin concentration exceeds 34.2 μmol/L. Jaundice of skin and mucous membranes are characterized by: (**A**) Jaundice first appeared in the sclera, on the rear of the hard palate and soft palate mucosa. Skin jaundice will emerge following continuing increase of serum bilirubin concentration. (**B**) Yellow sclera is non-uniform; jaundice is light near the limbal, while a relatively deeper yellow will be observed in sclera far from cornea.
   (b) Increased carotene: Excessive consumption of carrots, pumpkins, oranges and orange juice causes elevation of blood carotene, and when carotene in blood is above 2.5 g/L, the skin will turn yellow. (**A**) Yellowing first appeared in the skin of palm, foot, forehead and nose; (**B**) Yellowing generally does not occur in sclera and oral mucosa; (**C**) Serum bilirubin concentration is normal; (**D**) After stopping eating carotene-rich vegetables or fruits, yellowing will fade away.
   (c) Long-term use of medicines (such as mepacrine and furans, which contain yellow pigment), will cause skin yellow as well. (**A**) Yellowing first appeared in the skin, yellow sclera can be seen in severe cases. (**B**) Yellow sclera is non-uniform, heavy yellowing is observed near the limbal, which is different from jaundice.

5. Pigmentation
   Primary chronic adrenal hypofunction (Addison's disease) has systemic skin hyperpigmentation, with oral mucosa and gingival pigmentation, which results from weakened inhibition effect of adrenal cortical hormone on melanocyte stimulating hormone (MSH). Cirrhosis, advanced liver cancer, acromegaly, leishmaniasis, malaria and the use of certain drugs (such as arsenic agent, antineoplastic drug busulfan), can cause varying degrees of skin pigmentation as well. Massive transfusion-induced secondary hemochromatosis may appear brown or bronze skin pigmentation, which is due to the deposition of hemosiderin.
6. Achroma
   Achroma is found in patients with Vitiligo, leukoplakia and albinism.
   (a) Vitiligo: Depigmentation spots with different size, may expand gradually, without symptoms. Vitiligo is occasionally found in patients with hyperthyroidism, adrenal insufficiency and pernicious anemia.
   (b) Leukoplakia: Small depigmentation spots with round or oval shape, often occur in oral mucosa and female genital, and some of them may develop to cancer.
   (c) Albinismus: Achroma appears in the skin of total body and hair. Patient has photophobia due to eye uveal depigmentation. Albinismus is a hereditary disease, caused by congenital tyrosinase synthesis disorder.

42.2.2 Moisture and Sweating

Moisture is related to skin excretion function which is controlled by sweat and sebaceous glands. Heavy sweating, less sweating or no sweating may occur in pathological conditions, which may provide clues for diagnosis. Extreme dry skin are found in patients with vitamin A deficiency, mucinous edema, dehydration and scleroderma. Night sweating is a common symptom of tuberculosis. Cold sweating is seen in patients with shock or collapse who have heavy sweating with cold extremities. Autonomic nervous system dysfunction may cause paroxysmal sweating. Increased sweating is also seen in hyperthyroidism, rickets, lymphoma and sequela of encephalitis.

Body odor arises from skin glands excretion, especially from apocrine, which generates more odor substance. Urine sweat refers to sweat containing and smelling of urine, which is seen patients with uremia.

42.2.3 Skin Elasticity

Skin elasticity is related to age and nutritional status. Hand back or arm inside are the places used for skin elasticity examination. Skin is pinched with index finger and thumb, releasing after 1–2 s, and observe the speed of skin folds recovery. Skin elasticity is good or normal if the skin folds recovered quickly. Less elasticity refers to slow recovery of skin folds, which is observed in patients with long wasting disease, malnutrition and severe dehydration. Increased skin elasticity is observed in patients with fever, since fever accelerates blood circulation, accompanied by full filling of peripheral blood vessels.

42.2.4 Skin Eruption

Skin eruption is usually a manifestation of systemic diseases. There are different types of skin eruption, caused by infectious diseases, medicines or other substances leading to allergic reactions and skin diseases. Skin eruption may be specific regarding to its appearance and shape. Observation and recording of skin eruption should consist of: the time of appearance and disappearance, the order of development, distribution, morphological characteristics, size and arrangement, color and surface, with or without symptoms, etc. Common skin eruptions in clinical are as following:

1. Maculae: Maculae manifested as local skin redness, generally without depression and bulge. Maculae are seen in typhus, erysipelas and rheumatic erythema multiforme.
2. Roseola: Roseola is a kind of bright red circular maculae, 2–3 mm in diameter. The roseola subsided under pressure or after tightening the surrounding skin. Roseola usually appears on the chest and abdomen, and is a typical manifestation of typhoid and paratyphoid.
3. Papules: Eruption is red with bulge, which is seen in drug rash, hives, eczema, etc.
4. Maculopapule: Papule surrounded with skin redness, is found in scarlet fever, rubella and drug rash.
5. Urticaria: The skin slightly bulged, being pale or pink, with limited edema. Urticaria varies in size and shape, caused by rapid onset of skin allergies, and dissipated without leaving any traces,
6. Bleb: Limited cavity lesions with bulge, displayed variable color due to different liquid contained in the cavity. The liquid may be serum or lymph fluid, and the diameter is lee than 1 cm. This kind of bleb is called vesicle, and is seen in herpes simplex and chicken pox. Bleb, showing a diameter greater than 1 cm, is called bullous. Pustule contains pus, which may be primary or secondary to blisters infection. Bleb may be found in burns. Diabetes may have scalded blisters or bullae in their hand or foot, which is associated with glucose metabolism disorders.

42.2.5 Desquamation

Desquamation is the result of constant keratosis and shedding of normal stratum corneum. In pathological conditions, mass desquamation may be observed. For example, rice bran-like desquamation is seen in convalescence of measles and seborrheic dermatitis; Flaky desquamation is seen in scarlet fever and exfoliative dermatitis; Silvery white scaly desquamation is observed in psoriasis.

42.2.6 Subcutaneous Bleeding

Skin appears purple when patient has subcutaneous bleeding (with old hemorrhage, the skin is brown due to hemosiderin deposition). The color does not change under pressure, without bulge except hematoma. The size and distribution of bleeding spots varied depending on patient's condition: (**A**) petechia, <2 mm in diameter; (**B**) purpura, 3–5 mm in diameter; (**C**) ecchymosis, >5 mm in diameter; (**D**) hematoma, skin bulged with flaky hemorrhage. Bleeding spots sometimes occur in the mucosa, and the clinical significance is the same as subcutaneous hemorrhage.

42.2.7 Spider Angioma and Liver Palms

Spider angioma is formed by expansion of terminal branches of skin small artery, morphologically similar to spider (Fig. 42.7). Spider angioma varied in size, often seen in the area of the superior vena cava distribution, such as face, neck, hand back, upper arms, chest and shoulders. Pressed the center of spider angioma (i.e., the central arterioles main branch), the radial network of small blood vessels will disappear, and the spider angioma will appear again when the pressure is removed.

Liver palms are the skin redness of thenar and hypothenar, faded after pressure, which is seen in chronic liver diseases.

Generally, the formation of spider angioma and liver palms is due to weakened estrogen inactivation by liver, which is seen in acute and chronic hepatitis, liver cirrhosis; However, it is also observed in healthy pregnant women, which may result from increased level of estrogen during pregnancy.

42.2.8 Edema

Edema is the excessive accumulation of fluid in subcutaneous tissue and interstitial. Pitting edema refers to skin depression

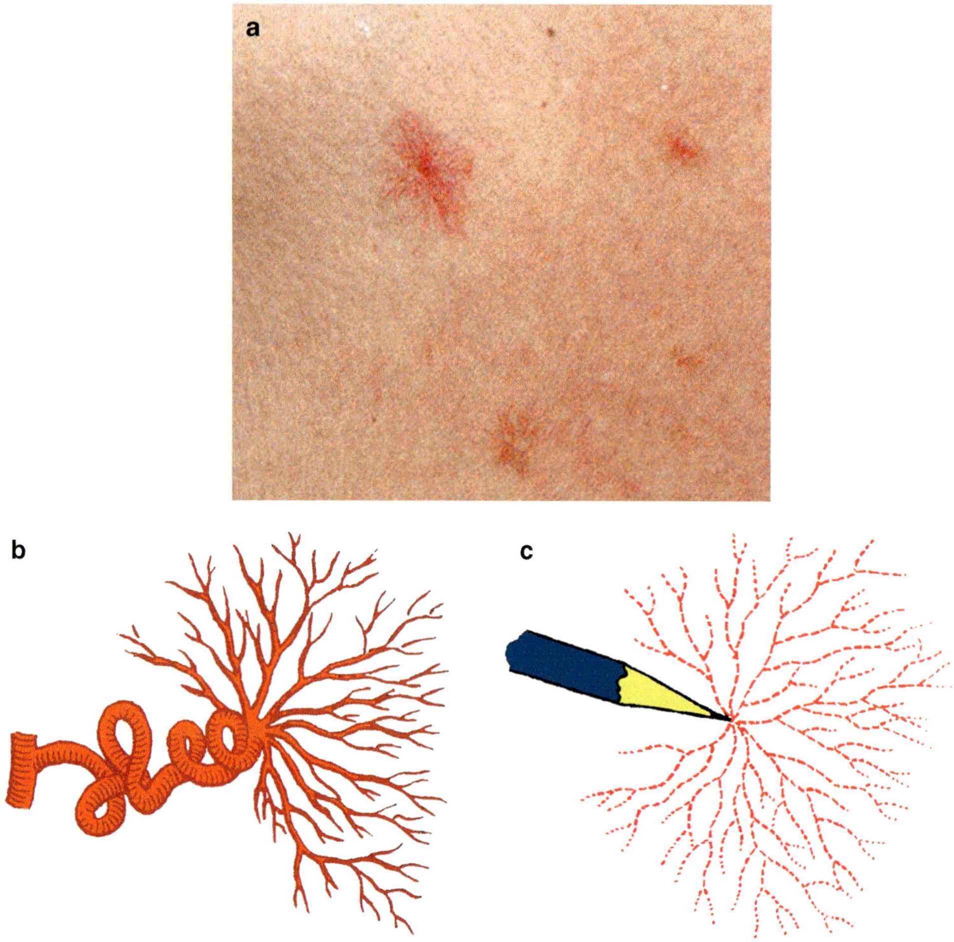

Fig. 42.7 Spider angioma

(usually medial skin of tibialis anterior), when pressed with finger for 3–5 s. Myxedema is the edema of face, supraclavicular, medial skin of tibialis anterior, hand back and instep, characterized by dry rough skin with pale or yellowish color, without depression after pressure. Myxedema is usually found in patients with hypothyroidism. Elephantiasis is characterized by rough, asymmetric skin thickening of lower limbs, with pores and skin fold, occasionally involving scrotum, labia majora and upper limbs. Elephantiasis is observed in filariasis, without depression after pressure.

In clinical, edema is classified as mild, moderate and severe edema.

- Mild edema: Edema is only appeared in the eyelids, infraorbital soft tissue, tibialis anterior, ankle subcutaneous tissue. Tissues displayed mild depression after finger pressing, and restored quickly. In early stage of edema, patient may only show rapid weight gain without sign of edema.
- Moderate edema: The whole body has visible edema, with obvious or deep tissue depression and restored slowly after finger pressing.
- Severe edema: Severe tissue edema in the whole body, skin of the lower part of the body is tight and shiny, even showing liquid exudation. Some patients sometimes are accompanied by pleural effusion or ascites, and genitals may show severe edema as well.

42.2.9 Subcutaneous Nodules

Large subcutaneous nodules can be found by inspection, and palpation is required to detect smaller nodules. After palpation, nodule size, location, hardness, mobility, with or without tenderness, should be noted. Common subcutaneous nodules are as follows:

1. Rheumatism nodules
   Rheumatism nodules are located at joint extensor side of subcutaneous tissue, especially at the elbow, wrist, knee, occiput, or spinous of thoracic and lumbar spine. The nodules are slightly hard and painless, without skin adhesion and swelling. Rheumatism nodule is often associated with heart inflammation, and is one the manifestations of active rheumatism.
2. Rheumatoid nodules
   Distributed symmetrically, is usually located at joint bulge areas, such as extensor side of forearm, near elbow olecranon, occiput and Achilles tendon. The size of Rheumatoid nodules may range from a few millimeters to several centimeters in diameter, hard as rubber with no tenderness.Rheumatoid nodule simplies the presence of active rheumatoid.
3. Metacercaria nodules
   Located in trunk, limbs, subcutaneous or intramuscular, occasionally occurred in the neck, breasts and genitals subcutaneous. The nodule is round or oval, with smooth surface, like soybean. The number of nodules varies in different patient, without tenderness, has no adhesion with the skin, and the texture is hard with flexibility. Metacercaria nodule is seen in cysticercosis.
4. Tophus
   Tophus is the deposition of needle-like crystals of urate in the subcutaneous connective tissue, causing chronic foreign-material-like reaction due to blood uric acid level exceeding the saturation concentration. Tophus, presented as yellow-white nodules, with varied sizes, is usually found in auricular, metatarsophalangeal and finger (toe) joints. Tophus is the characteristic lesion of gout.
5. Erythema nodosum
   Erythema nodosum is usually found in young women, occurs in the leg extensor side with symmetric distribution. Chronic erythema nodosum is seen in hemolytic streptococcus infection, autoimmune diseases, certain drugs (such as bromine, oral contraceptives, etc.) and leprosy.
6. Panniculitis nodules
   Panniculitis nodules are usually occurred in the thigh, with medium hardness, clear boundary and significant tenderness. The nodules have little mobility due to skin adhesion, subsided after lasting for several weeks. Although panniculitis nodule is self-limited, skin sag and pigmentation are common after its disappearance.
7. Arteritis nodules
   Arteritis nodules are commonly found in the lower and upper limbs, occasionally found in trunk, face and shoulders. Nodules, located along superficial artery, mostly 0.5–2.0 cm in diameter, had hard texture with tenderness. Arteritis nodules are self-limited after appearing for more than a week, and are usually observed in nodal polyarteritis.
8. Osler nodule
   Osler nodule appeared at fingertips, toes, thenar or hypothenar muscles, with blue or pink color and tenderness, is observed in infective endocarditis.

42.2.10 Ulcer and Erosion

Ulcer refers to skin defects or destruction reached to dermis or under dermis, with scar left after healing. (**A**) Ulcers occur above the malleolus of legs, and this kind of ulcer is often seen in inflammation around the vein, thrombophlebitis or recurrent cellulitis. (**B**) Small ulcers in the mouth, genitalia and anus, and this kind of ulcer are usually observed in active tuberculosis with decreased immune function. (**C**) Chancroid, occurred at genitalia, susceptible to bleeding, is a kind of painful, round or oval ulcer.

Erosion refers to skin lesions showing a wet surface, due to excoriation or skin damage. Erosion is seen in eczema, diaper dermatitis, contact dermatitis, and does not leave scars after healing.

42.2.11 Scar

Scar is defined as patch formed by connective tissue proliferation, due to tissue repair after dermal lesions. The surface of atrophic scar is lower than the surface of surrounding normal skin, while hypertrophic scar is higher than the surrounding skin. Scar provided evidence of certain diseases, for example, healed scar at the surgical incision site is a mark of surgery. Similar-sized scars in the face are frequently found in patients who suffered from smallpox.

42.2.12 Hair

The color and appearance (being curved or straight) of hair, are determined by human ethnicity. The amount, thickness and distribution of hair are not only associated with age and gender, but also influenced by genetic, nutritional and psychiatric status. The amount of hair may be different in normal people. Generally, males present more body hair, and the pubic hair has diamond-shaped distribution, while females have less body hair, and the pubic hair is distributed as inverted triangular.

The amount and distribution of hair may facilitate diagnosis of certain diseases. Hair diseases are generally classified as hair loss, hair increase, hair discolor and hair metamorphism.

42.3 Section 3: Lymph Nodes

The status of lymph nodes is closely related to the occurrence, development, diagnosis and treatment of many diseases, especially cancers. Lymph nodes distributed in the whole body, only superficial lymph nodes may be found by general examination.

42.3.1 Normal Lymph Nodes

Under normal circumstances, superficial lymph nodes are very small, with smooth surface, mostly 0.2–0.5 cm in diameter, soft by palpation, without tenderness. The lymph nodes are often in chain or group distribution, without adhesion with the adjacent tissue, and usually are not accessible.

Distribution of superficial lymph nodes

1. Head and neck (Fig. 42.8)
    (a) Preauricular lymph nodes: located in front of the tragus.
    (b) Postauricular lymph nodes: also known as the mastoid lymph nodes, located at the mastoid surface and sternocleidomastoid termination point.
    (c) Occipital lymph nodes: located in occipital subcutaneous, between trapezius starting point and sternocleidomastoid termination point.
    (d) Submandibular lymph nodes: near submandibular gland, in the middle of mandibular angle and chin.
    (e) Submental lymph nodes: located within the submental triangle, mylohyoid muscle surface.
    (f) Anterior cervical lymph nodes: located at the sternocleidomastoid surface and mandibular angle.

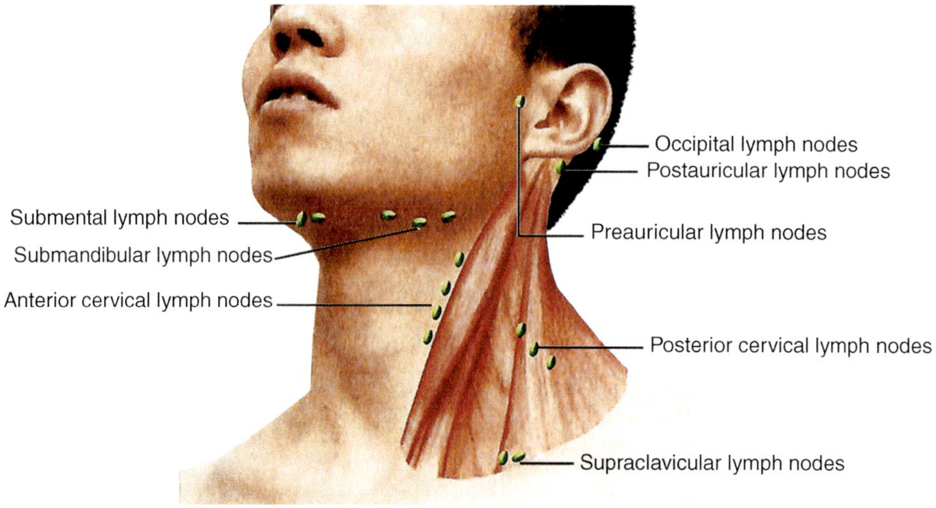

Fig. 42.8 Head and neck lymph nodes distribution

(g) Posterior cervical lymph nodes: located in the leading edge of the trapezius muscle.
(h) Supraclavicular lymph nodes: located at the angle area formed by clavicle and sternocleidomastoid.

2. Upper limb
   (a) Axillary lymph nodes (Fig. 42.9): Axillary lymph nodes form the largest group of upper limb lymph nodes, and are classified as five small groups: (A) Top axillary lymph nodes group: at the top of the axillary; (B) Central lymph nodes group: at the inner wall of axillary which is near to rib and serratus anterior muscle; (C) Chest muscle lymph nodes group: located in the deep and lower edge of pectoralis major; (D) Subscapular lymph nodes group: at the rear and deep folds of axillary; (E) Outer lymph nodes group: in the outer sidewall of axillary.
   (b) Upper trochlea lymph nodes: located in the intermuscular trench of biceps and triceps, 3–4 cm above the medial epicondyle, i.e., upper humeral trochlea.
3. Lower limb
   (a) Inguinal lymph nodes (Fig. 42.10): Located in femoral triangle, under inguinal ligament. Inguinal lymph node is classified as upper and lower groups: (**A**) Upper group: also known as inguinal ligament cross-group, located below the inguinal ligament, arranged in parallel with ligament; (**B**) Lower group: also known as inguinal lymph nodes vertical group, located at the upper end of saphenous vein, arranged along the vein.
   (b) Popliteal lymph nodes: in the confluence area of small saphenous vein and popliteal vein.

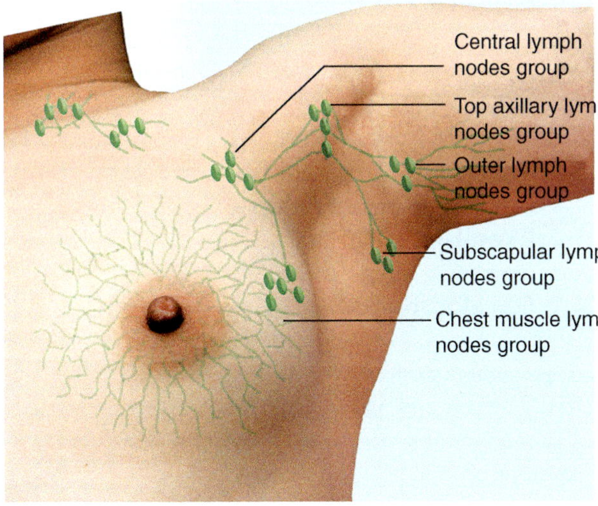

Fig. 42.9 Axillary lymph nodes distribution

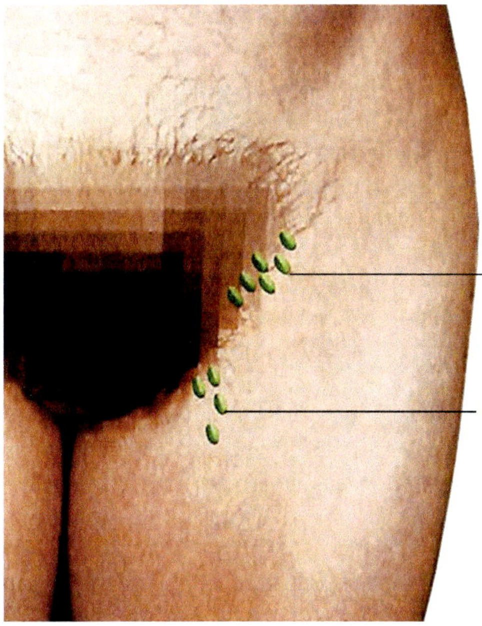

Fig. 42.10 Inguinal lymph nodes distribution

Table 42.3 Superficial lymph node groups and drainage areas

Lymph node groups	Drainage areas
Postauricular lymph nodes	Scalp
Deep cervical lymph nodes upper group (upper part of sternocleidomastoid)	Nasopharyngeal
Deep cervical lymph nodes lower group (lower part of sternocleidomastoid)	Throat, trachea, thyroid
Supraclavicular lymph nodes group	Left: esophagus, stomach Right: trachea, pleura, lung
Submandibular lymph nodes group	Mouth floor, buccal mucosa, gums
Submental lymph nodes group	Submandibular triangle, lips and tongue
Axillary lymph nodes group	Upper trunk, breast, chest wall
Inguinal lymph nodes group	Lower limb and perineum

42.3.1.1 Drainage Area of Superficial Lymph Nodes

Superficial lymph nodes are distributed as groups, and lymph fluid in certain area is collected by the corresponding lymph nodes groups (Table 42.3). Lymphadenopathy is usually caused by local inflammation or tumor.

42.3.2 Lymph Nodes Examination

42.3.2.1 Examination Order

The examination order for head and neck lymph nodes is as the following: preauricular lymph nodes, postauricular lymph nodes, occipital lymph nodes, submandibular lymph nodes, submental lymph nodes, anterior cervical lymph nodes, posterior cervical lymph nodes and supraclavicular lymph nodes. Upper limb lymph nodes: axillary lymph nodes, upper trochlea lymph nodes. The proper examination order for axillary lymph nodes is: top axillary lymph nodes group, central lymph nodes group, chest muscle lymph nodes group, subscapular lymph nodes group and outer lymph nodes group. For lower limb lymph nodes, the examination order is inguinal lymph nodes (upper and lower group) and popliteal lymph nodes.

42.3.2.2 Examination Methods

The examination of the lymph nodes consists of two steps: inspection and palpation.

1. Head and neck lymph nodes palpation
   Patient takes sitting or lying position, slightly bows the head. Examiner stands in front of or behind the patient, put the finger pulp closely on the skin surface, moving from the shallow to the deep site of local lymph nodes by slipping palpation (Fig. 42.11).

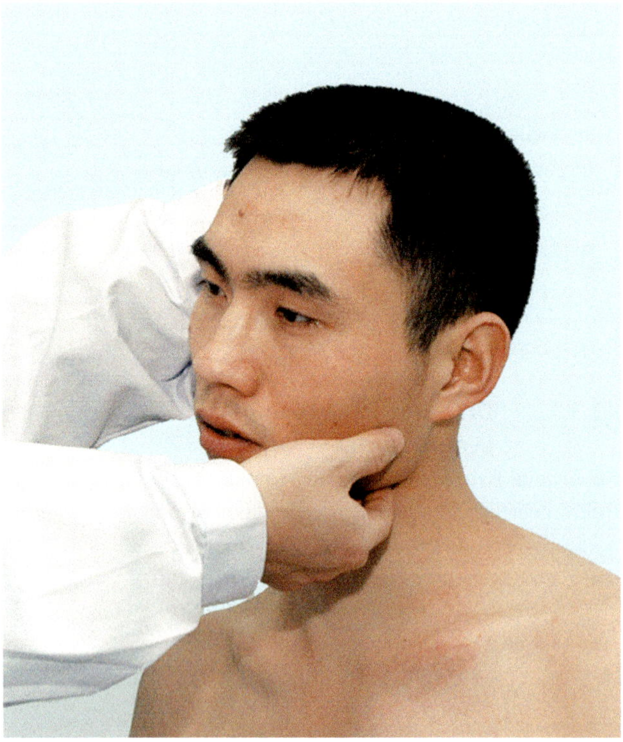

Fig. 42.11 Submandibular lymph nodes palpation

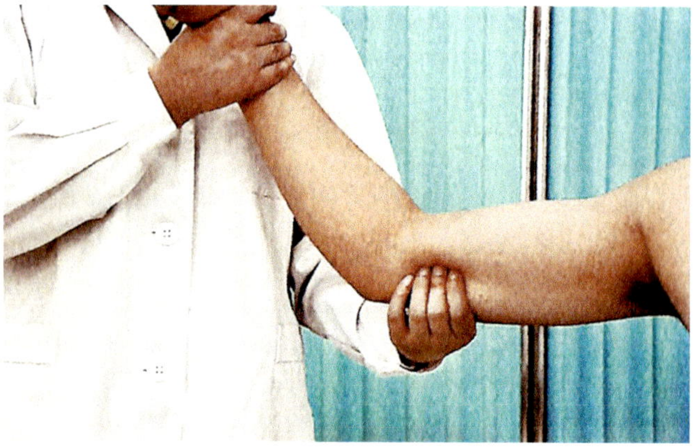

Fig. 42.12 Upper trochlea lymph nodes palpation

2. Axillary lymph nodes palpation
   Five groups of right and left axillary lymph nodes are checked by examiner's left and right hand respectively, usually from left to right.
3. Upper trochlea lymph nodes palpation
   Upper trochlea lymph nodes are generally unable to be found in normal persons (Fig. 42.12).
4. Inguinal lymph nodes palpation
5. Popliteal lymph nodes palpation

42.3.2.3 Examination Contents

If lymph nodes are found, the location, size, shape, number, arrangement, surface characteristics, texture and mobility of lymph nodes should be noticed. Whether the lymph nodes have tenderness, adhesions or clear boundaries should be mentioned as well. In addition, local skin with or without redness, swelling, scar or fistula may provide diagnostic evidence for certain diseases.

42.4 Section 4: Common Abnormities and Differential Diagnosis in General Examination

42.4.1 Developmental and Stature Disorders

Developmental disorders refer to incoordination and inconsistency between age and intelligence or physical growth. Short stature and tall stature are the common stature disorders in clinic.

42.4.1.1 Short Stature

The height is significantly lower than the normal standard, when compared with the normal individuals who have the same race, age and gender in the same region.

Etiology

1. Familial and Genetic Factors
   Familial and genetic factors are related to the physique of family. Some families have chromosomal abnormalities, such as Turner syndrome.
2. Delayed puberty
   Delayed puberty usually has family history. Bone growth and sexual development are generally delayed for about 4 years.
3. Malnutrition or metabolic disorders
   Certain chronic diseases may lead to malnutrition and metabolic disorders, and the growth and development may be affected if those chronic diseases occur before adulthood. Common chronic diseases which may cause malnutrition and metabolic disorders are as follows: tuberculosis, schistosomiasis, chronic enteritis or diarrhea, chronic malaria, leishmaniasis, syphilis, congenital or acquired heart disease, chronic lung disease, chronic pancreatitis, malabsorption syndrome, liver cirrhosis, chronic kidney disease, diabetes and neurological diseases, etc.
4. Endocrine diseases
   Such as stay ailment, youth mucous edema, pituitary function abate dwarfism, precocious puberty, etc.
5. Bone diseases
   Such as achondroplasia, congenital osteogenesis imperfecta, kaschin-beck disease, rickets, etc.

Clinical Characteristics and Differential Diagnosis

The clinical characteristics of short stature may vary due to different diseases.

1. Familial short stature
   The development of bone and tooth, and sexual maturation are normal, although the stature is short. The endocrine function is normal and no any other diseases are found.
2. Turner syndrome
   Turner syndrome is the congenital abnormal sexual differentiation caused by sex chromosome abnormality, which is characterized by female appearance, short stature, webbed neck (the shape of the connection between neck and shoulder is similar to a wing), elbow valgus, ovary and genitalia agenesis, primary amenorrhea and secondary sexual characteristics agenesis. The intelligence may be normal, and some patients may have internal organs deformity.
3. Progeria
   Progeria is a rare disease, characterized by early stop of growth and development with extreme short stature, although the patient is normal at birth. Progeria phenomenon refers to senescence of youth, characterized by facial wrinkles, physical decline, loss of hair and skin relaxation, which behaves like an elder person. Patients with progeria phenomenon may have systemic atherosclerosis, and the lifespan is short.
4. Delayed puberty
   Delayed puberty is characterized by growth retardation in childhood with short stature. Patients have normal intelligence and endocrine function, and without any other diseases. The adolescence may be delayed to over 18 years old, and the final height may be normal.
5. Short stature due to hypothyroidism
   (a) Cretinism: Hypothyroidism, occurred in fetal or neonatal period, can lead to cretinism. Symptoms such as drowsiness, slow response, feeding difficulty, hoarse crying, constipation, umbilical hernia, etc., may appear shortly after the birth. With age increasing, more abnormalities may appear, such as short stature, stubby limbs. Other clinical manifestations of cretinism may present: Cretinism face (large head, low forehead, flat and saddle nose, wide eye span, small eye fissure, eyelid edema, thick lips); Intelligence development disorders; Late teething, delayed fontanel closing; Dry, cold, coarse and thick skin; Goiter or atrophy, etc.
   (b) Juvenile myxedema: Juvenile myxedema occurs in children who have hypothyroidism, characterized by short stature, bone development retardation, varied degrees of mental retardation and low metabolism. Patients with juvenile myxedema do not have cretinism face.
6. Hypopituitarism dwarfism
   The development is normal during the first 2–3 years period after birth, then growth retardation and short stature will appear gradually. Patient has proportional bone growth and normal mental development, although without gonads and secondary sexual development.
7. Sexual precocity
   Sexual precocity refers to sexual development before the age of 8 for girls, or before 9 for boys.

42.4.1.2 Tall stature

The height is significantly higher than the normal standard, when compared with the normal individuals who have the same race, age and gender in the same region.

Etiology

1. Genetic factors It is the most common cause for tall stature.
2. Endocrine dysfunction Such as, excessive growth hormone secreted by adenohypophysis, hypogonadism, lack of pituitary gonadotropins, testicular seminiferous tubules hypoplasia, testicular dysgenesis.
3. Others Hypothalamic lesions, such as craniopharyngioma, glioma, inflammation, etc.

Clinical Characteristics and Differential Diagnosis

1. Constitutional tall stature
   Constitutional tall stature is usually related to genetic background, not a morbid state. The well-proportioned tall stature is accompanied by good physical strength and normal fertility, without any endocrine dysfunction and other diseases.
2. Advanced puberty
   Generally, advanced puberty refers to sexual development occurs before the age of 9 in female, and before 10 for male. The body stature is in the normal range after growing up, which is different from constitutional tall stature.
3. Gigantism
   Gigantism is caused by hypersecretion of pituitary growth hormone before epiphyseal fusion, characterized by rapid body growth and development, which is more apparent in adolescence.
4. Tall stature due to hypogonadism
   Hypothalamic lesions, pituitary gonadotropin deficiency and gonadal dysgenesis may lead to lack of androgen or estrogen, which in turn results in bone overgrowth, delayed epiphyseal fusion and tall stature.

42.4.2 Coma

Coma is the most severe disturbance of consciousness, caused by extreme inhibition of the cerebral cortex and subcortical network structure. Patients have continued disruption, or complete loss of consciousness, characterized by disappearance of pain reaction and voluntary movement. Patients with coma can't be awakened by strong stimulation, without independent activities due to extreme inhibition of higher nervous activity. Coma usually occurs in severe brain diseases or dying period of somatic diseases. Clinically, coma can be classified as mild, moderate and deep coma.

42.4.2.1 Etiology

1. Extracranial disease
   Extracranial diseases, such as metabolic disorders, poisoning and systemic infection, can directly affect the metabolism of brain cells, or cause brain ischemia and hypoxia, which in turn leads to coma.
   (a) Metabolic encephalopathy: Different kinds of metabolic abnormalities, abnormal osmotic pressure, acid-base imbalance, lack of nutrients, temperature imbalances, ischemia, hypoxia, poisoning, drug overdose or trauma, may cause brain cells dysfunction or damage.
   (b) Toxic encephalopathy: Different kinds of poisoning, such as infections, medicines, pesticides, harmful gas, harmful solvents, metal, plant (bitter almond, mildew sugar cane, toadstool, gingko nuts), animals (fugu, snake bites, bee sting), physical factors (such as high fever, drowning, electric shock, radiation).
   (c) Systemic diseases: Such as systemic lupus erythematosus (SLE), leukemia, diffuse intravascular coagulation (DIC), etc.
2. Intracranial disease
   Coma is caused by oppression of brainstem reticular formation and thalamus dispersion system, resulting from intracranial structural lesions, increased intracranial pressure or brain displacement due to occupying effect.
   (a) Space-occupying or destructive lesions: Such as hematoma, bleeding, infarction, tumors, focal infection (abscess, cerebral parasitic disease), granuloma, etc.
   (b) Diffuse lesions: Inflammation, degeneration, tumor, poisoning, trauma, vascular disease, epilepsy, parasitic infections, etc.

42.4.2.2 Clinical Characteristics and Differential Diagnosis

The differential diagnosis of coma includes differentiation of the coma state and coma etiology. First, try to determine whether it is coma or not; then, try to find out the causes of coma, which is critical for further proper treatment and prognosis assessment.

1. Differentiation of coma state
   (a) Special types of unconsciousness: Catochus is a special type of unconsciousness, in which patient is in waking state but without awareness. Catochus may be observed in decorticated syndrome, akinetic mutism and vegetative state. The clinical manifestation of catochus is severe loss of language and motor response, although spontaneous eye opening and awakening-sleep cycle are preserved.
   - Decorticated syndrome: Decorticated syndrome refers to loss of cortical function (although subcortical structure function remains) due to extensive cerebral cortex damage. Clinical manifestations of decorticated syndrome are as follows: Awakening-sleep cycle disturbance; Subcortical unconscious activities (e.g., staring, looks like awaking without language response, etc.) remain, accompanied by active reflections (e.g., eye blinking, swallowing, chewing, pupillary light reflex, corneal reflection, etc.). Decorticated syndrome is usually found in extensive ischemia anoxic encephalopathy, severe brain trauma, encephalitis, poisoning and cortex-striatum spinal cord degeneration.
   - Akinetic mutism: Akinetic mutism, also known as coma vigil, is another type of catochus due to the

damage of upper part of brainstem and thalamus reticular activating system. Patients with akinetic mutism have intact cerebral hemisphere and efferent pathways, and the awakening-sleep cycle is normal. Akinetic mutism is usually found in patients with brainstem infarction.

- Vegetative state: Vegetative state is a state of catochus resulting from serious damage of brain hemisphere, in which the brainstem function remains, and the awakening-sleep cycle is preserved. Persistent vegetative state (PVS) refers to such a catochus state continues for at least 1 month.

(b) Similar coma state: A state or symptom, which is similar to coma or looks like coma, including pseudocoma and other diseases.

- Pseudocoma: Pseudocoma is a mental condition in which patients can't express or react, different from real loss of consciousness. Pseudocoma may presents as locked-in syndrome, hysterical unreacted state, stuporous state and abulia.
  - Locked-in syndrome: Locked-in syndrome, also known as efferent losing state, is due to the lesion of pontine base portion, resulting in bilateral blocking of corticobulbar tract and corticospinal tract. The efferent functions of motor nerves under abducens nerve nucleus are lost, while oculomotor nerve and trochlear nerve functions are intact. Locked-in syndrome is usually seen in cerebrovascular diseases, demyelinating disease (central pontine myelinolysis), craniocerebral trauma and tumors.
  - Hysterical unreacted state: Patient often has eyelid blinking, with blinking reflex or even eyes opening after strong stimulation.
  - Stuporous state: Eye opening reaction is exist, may accompanied with ceroid flexibility or negativism. Stuporous state is usually observed in patients with depressive stupor of severe depression, catatonic stupor of the schizophrenia, and reactive catatonia of the reactive psychosis.
  - Abulia: Patients are awake and aware of their situation, being silent due to lack of initiation, without locomotor activity. Abulia is usually seen in patients with bilateral frontal lesions.
- Others
  - Syncope: Syncope is a transient loss of consciousness caused by a sudden transient extensive cerebral hypoperfusion or hypoxia.
  - Hypnolepsy: Hypnolepsy is characterized by irresistible short sleeping attacks, accompanied with abnormal sleeping. Most patients with hypnolepsy are accompanied with cataplexy disorder, sleeping paralysis, sleeping hallucination, which is called "Tetralogy of Hypnolepsy".
  - Aphasia: Patients with complete aphasia, especially when accompanied with quadriplegia, cannot response to external stimuli.

2. Differential diagnosis of coma

Characteristics of disease initiation and course of illness are particularly important for differential diagnosis of coma. Generally, coma characterized by sudden onset, reaching peak rapidly, is seen in patients with vascular lesions, acute inflammation, trauma, or poisoning. Coma caused by tumors is usually demonstrated as chronic onset and gradual disease progression. Intermittent episodes of coma are usually seen in patients with epilepsy, migraine or periodic paralysis.

(a) Coma accompanied with focal neurological signs: Etiology of coma may be defined by comprehensive analysis of neurological locating signs with other clinical features such as age, gender, history characteristics, physical examination and auxiliary examination.

- Traumatic coma: For patients with a history of trauma, intracranial hematoma should be taken into consideration, which includes brain contusion, epidural hematoma and subdural hematoma. CT or MRI shows intracranial hemorrhage or skull fracture, which is helpful for differential diagnosis.
- Non traumatic coma: Non traumatic coma is mainly observed in patients with destructive or space-occupying brain lesions, such as cerebral hemorrhage, cerebral infarction, encephalitis, brain abscess and brain tumors.
  - Sudden onset: Cerebrovascular disease should be considered if patient has a history of hypertension, diabetes, atherosclerosis or rheumatic heart disease.
  - Gradual onset: Intracranial space-occupying lesions should be considered if patient has signs of increased intracranial pressure, such as headache, vomiting and papilloedema. It is usually seen in patients with brain tumors, subdural hematoma, brain abscesses or cerebral granuloma.
  - Fever as the prodromal symptom: It is usually seen in patients with intracranial infections, such as brain abscess, encephalomyelitis, viral encephalitis, sporadic encephalitis, or cerebral venous thrombosis.

(b) Coma accompanied with meningeal irritation sign:

- Sudden onset: It is usually observed in subarachnoid hemorrhage, which is characterized by severe headache and vomiting induced by stress.

Table 42.4 Differential diagnosis of coma due to cerebrovascular diseases

	Hemorrhagic cerebrovascular diseases		Ischemic cerebrovascular diseases	
	Cerebral hemorrhage	Subarachnoid hemorrhage	Cerebral infarction	Cerebral embolism
Age	Usually over 50	Around 40	Mainly middle-aged and old patients	Mainly young adults
Etiology	Hypertension, cerebral arteriosclerosis	Congenital aneurysms, vascular malformations	Atherosclerosis	Rheumatic heart disease
Predisposition	Agitated with elevated blood pressure	Agitated with elevated blood pressure	Relaxed with low blood pressure	Atrial fibrillation onset
Onset	Acute (minutes, hours)	Sudden (seconds, minutes)	Chronic (hours, days)	Sudden (seconds, minutes)
Transient ischemic attack history	No	No	Usually yes	Maybe yes
Headache, vomiting	Yes	Fiercely	No	No
Hemiplegia	Usually	No	Yes	Yes
Disturbance of consciousness	Usually	Maybe yes, mainly with elder patients	Yes	Usually no
Cerebrospinal fluid	Maybe blood red with high pressure	Homogenous blood red with high pressure	Normal	Normal
CT or MRI	High density image in early stage	Localized image of blood	Low density image 24–48 h after onset	Local lesion displayed 24–48 h after onset

Differential diagnosis of coma caused by cerebrovascular diseases is shown in Table 42.4.

- Onset with fever: Coma with fever is usually seen in patients with various meningitis and encephalitis, such as suppurative meningitis, tuberculous meningitis, cryptococcal meningitis, encephalitis B, forest encephalitis, herpes simplex virus encephalitis, acute disseminated encephalomyelitis, etc.
- Coma without focal neurological sign or meningeal irritation sign: This kind of coma is usually seen in patients with systemic diseases, including metabolic encephalopathy and toxic encephalopathy.

Common causes of coma are summarized in Table 42.5.

Table 42.5 Common causes of coma accompanied with different signs

Accompanied signs	Common causes
Fever	Coma after fever is seen in patients with severe infection, heat stroke; Fever after coma is seen in patients with cerebral hemorrhage, barbiturate poisoning.
Hypothermia	Shock, mucous edema, glycopenia, hepatic encephalopathy, sedative drug poisoning and frostbite.
Hypertension	Cerebral infarction, cerebral hemorrhage, subarachnoid hemorrhage, hypertensive encephalopathy
Hypotension	Shock, critical period of severe diseases
Papilledema	Hypertensive encephalopathy, intracranial space-occupying lesions
Miosis	Morphine, barbitone and organophosphate poisoning
Dilated pupils	Cerebral hernia, traumatic brain injuries, severe hypoxia, alcohol poisoning, atropine poisoning, cyanide poisoning, botulism
Meningeal irritation sign	Encephalitis, meningitis and subarachnoid hemorrhage
Abnormal breath odor	Rotten apple smell, ammonia smell, alcohol smell, and pungent garlic smell are seen in patients with diabetic ketoacidosis, uremia, alcoholism and organophosphorus pesticide poisoning respectively
Bradycardia	Increased intracranial pressure, cardiac conduction block, hypothyroidism
Mucocutaneous hemorrhage	Severe sepsis and hemorrhagic diseases
Epileptic seizure	Encephalitis, cerebral hemorrhage, cerebral trauma, intracranial space-occupying lesions, hypoglycemia
Myotonia	Hypocalcemia, tetanus, diffuse encephalopathy
Amyostasia	Ethanol or sedatives poisoning, sympathomimetic drug poisoning
Paralysis	Cerebral infarction, cerebral hemorrhage, cerebral trauma and intracranial space-occupying lesions

42.4.3 Pigmentation

Pigmentation refers to deepened skin color due to abnormally increased skin pigment.

42.4.3.1 Etiology

1. Genetic background
   Such as lentigo, juvenile acanthosis nigricans, acra pigmentation, Peutz-Jeghers syndrome, familial progressive pigmentation, neurofibromatosis.
2. Endocrine and metabolic diseases
   Such as Addison's disease, ectopic adrenocorticotropic hormone syndrome (ectopic ACTH syndrome), ectopic adrenocorticotropic hormone releasing hormone syndrome (ectopic pregnancy syndrome), chloasma, pregnancy, renal insufficiency, biliary cirrhosis, hepatolenticular degeneration, idiopathic pulmonary hemosiderosis, amyloidosis skin amyloidosis, etc.
3. Physical, chemical factors and medicine
   Such as sunburn, ultraviolet light or radiation exposure, contamination of gold, silver, bismuth, mercury, or arsenic.

Drugs, such as chlorpromazine, anti-leprosy drugs, anti-malarial drugs, amiodarone, contraceptives, busulfan, etc.

4. Nutritional factor
   Such as deficiency of Vitamin B12 and Vitamin A.
5. Post-infection or cutaneous inflammatory lesions
   Pigmentation appears after systemic infections, such as malaria, leishmaniasis, schistosomiasis, tuberculosis, secondary syphilis. Cutaneous inflammatory lesions, such as compressed moss, chronic eczema and neurodermatitis, may present pigmentation as well.
6. Tumor
   Pigmentation may be observed in patients with lymphoma, malignant melanoma, pigment basal cell carcinoma, ependymoma, etc.
7. Others
   Such as systemic lupus erythematosus (SLE), scleroderma, dermatomyositis, tattoo, explosive dust particle deposition, etc.

42.4.3.2 Pathogenesis

Pigmentation is caused by multiple factors mainly through the following pathways: (a) Increase tyrosinase activity: more melanin is synthesized due to increased tyrosinase activity, which is seen in inflammation or skin leisions; (b) Increased melanocyte stimulating hormone (MSH) secretion, or decreased MSH inhibitor: resulting in increased melanocyte activity and melanin synthesis, which is seen in nervous system diseases, endocrine and metabolic factors (such as pregnancy, adrenocortical hypofunction); (c) Increased melanocyte populations: resulting in increased melanin synthesis due to genetic background.

Clinical Manifestations

1. Localized or extensive hyperpigmentation of skin and mucous membrane
   Systemic pigmentation is usually seen in patients with familial progressive pigmentation, drug rash, Addison's disease, and malignant tumor with acanthosis nigricans.
2. Accompanied symptoms
   Skin lesions of nodules, plaques and thickened skin may be observed in patients with malignant melanoma and acanthosis nigricans.
3. Manifestations of primary disease
   In addition to hyperpigmentation, characteristic manifestations may be observed in certain systemic diseases, such as chronic liver disease, cirrhosis, renal insufficiency, connective tissue disease.

Differential Diagnosis

As a characteristic manifestation, pigmentation is observed in a variety of diseases, and here are two major disease categories.

1. Common dermatosis with pigmentation
   (a) Chloasma, or Melasma: Chloasma is brown, or light black spots often appeared in Zygomaticum, forehead, upper lip, or around eyes. Patient with chloasma has no symptoms, and chloasma mainly appears in pregnancy.
   (b) Freckles, or lentigo: Freckles is brown, or light black spots, mainly observed in females without symptoms.
   (c) Lentigo simplex: Pigmentation shows as brown, or dark brown spots, 1–3 mm in diameter, without symptoms, and has no relationship to sunlight.
   (d) Familial progressive hyperpigmentation: Familial progressive hyperpigmentation is an autosomal dominant genetic disease, characterized by systemic diffuse brown or dark brown, patch or speckled pigmentation after born.
   (e) Pigmentation macularis multiplex idiopathica: Pigmentation with dark brown or light black patches usually appears in the trunk, occasionally occurs in the limbs.
   (f) Hyperkeratosis of the nipple and areola: Unilateral or bilateral hyperkeratosis of the nipple and areola is accompanied with pigmentation and infiltration hypertrophy.
   (g) Acanthosis nigricans: Acanthosis nigricans is light brown or dark brown papilloma pigmentation or verrucous hypertrophy of skin.
   (h) Mongolian spot: Mongolian spot is congenital dermal melanocytosis, and may appear in any part of the body, especially lumbosacral region and hips.
   (i) Acropigmentation: Acropigmentation is genetic pigmentation of fingers or toes in babies or children, occasionally occurred in the knee and elbow.
   (j) Peutz-Jeghers syndrome: Peutz-Jeghers syndrome, also known as dark spots polyp syndrome, is an autosomal dominant genetic disease, characterized by round or oval, brown or black spots in lips, oral buccal mucosa, gums, hard palate, tongue, or around the mouth. Polyps usually appear at the age of 10–30, and may be found in any part of the gastrointestinal tract, especially in the small intestine.
   (k) Malignant melanoma: Malignant melanoma derives from melanocyte or nevus cells of skin, and should be distinguished in the early stage of disease. Malignant melanoma should be taken into consideration if the following alterations happened: the color of pigmentation becomes deeper; the black spot appears from normal skin; the skin lesion gets enlarged with pain and burning, or ulcer appears on the surface with scabby or bleeding, or around which satellite nevus appears.

2. Pigmentation due to systemic diseases
   Pigmentation is sometimes one manifestations of systemic disease.
   (a) Hemachromatosis: Hemachromatosis is derived from metabolic disorders, usually accompanied with diabetes, hepatomegaly or cirrhosis, myocardial diseases, and cardiac dysfunction.
   (b) Addison's disease: Addison's disease is the primary adrenocortical hypofunction caused by tumors or autoimmune diseases, which is characterized by fatigue, weight loss, dizziness, nausea, vomiting, hypotension, irregular menstruation, or even coma in severe cases. Pigmentation spot may appear in mouth, gums, lips, or tongue.
   (c) Hyperthyroidism: Patient with hyperthyroidism may present anterior tibial myxedema, diffuse patchy pigmentation, and skin angiotelectasis.
   (d) Hepatolenticular degeneration: Hepatolenticular degeneration is a systemic disease caused by copper metabolism disorder. Light green pigment spots appear in lower limbs, occasionally display on the face, neck and genitals. Characteristic feature of hepatolenticular degeneration is greenish brown Kayser-Fleischer pigment ring around the cornea.

42.4.4 Lymphadenopathy

Normal superficial lymph nodes are small, soft, smooth, movable, without tenderness, and usually are not palpable. Lymphadenopathy refers that the lymph node is more than 0.5 cm in diameter, with tenderness, or palpable. Lymphadenopathy may be caused by local disease, or is a clinical manifestation of certain systemic diseases.

42.4.4.1 Etiology

1. Infection Lymphadenopathy may be caused by various pathogens, such as virus, chlamydia, helix, protozoa, bacteria, parasites, etc.
2. Allergy or anaphylaxis Such as drug fever, etc.
3. Connective tissues diseases Such as Sjogren's syndrome, systemic lupus erythematosus (SLE), Still disease, etc.
4. Hematological diseases Such as lymphoma, leukemia, plasma cells diseases, malignant histiocytosis, etc.
5. Metastasis of malignant tumors
6. Others Such as snakebite, hypogammaglobulinemia, necrotizing hyperplastic lymphadenopathy, etc.

42.4.4.2 Clinical Characteristics and Differential Diagnosis

Clinical characteristics of lymphadenopathy, such as onset, position, accompanied symptoms and pathogens, are helpful for differential diagnosis. According to the distribution, lymphadenopathy is classified as localized or generalized lymphadenopathy.

1. Localized lymphadenopathy
   (a) Infectious lymphadenopathy
      - Non-specific infectious lymphadenitis: Non-specific infectious lymphadenitis is caused by acute or chronic inflammation in lymph node drainage region. Lymph nodes caused by acute inflammation are often soft, tender, smooth without adhesion, with limited enlargement, and the enlarged lymph nodes will shrink or subside quickly after inflammation disappears.
      - Specific infectious lymphadenitis: (a) Lymph node tuberculosis: Enlarged lymph nodes often appear around the neck blood vessels, with multiple occurrence, hard in early stage, painless, and may adhere to each other or adjacent tissues. (b) Gonorrhea: Gonorrhea is the purulent infection of genitourinary system due to Neisseria gonorrhoeae, leading to bilateral tender groin lymphadenopathy. (c) Chancroid: Chancroid refers to multiple painful genitals ulcers due to haemophilus ducreyi infection. (d) Syphilis: Syphilis is the infection of genitourinary system due to cadaverous helicoid.
      - Simple lymphadenitis: Simple lymphadenitis is the acute inflammation of lymph node, medium hardness with tenderness, and usually occurs in cervical lymph nodes.
   (b) Lymph node metastasis of malignant tumor: Lymphadenopathy due to malignant tumor metastasis has characteristic enlarged lymph node: hard, smooth or protuberant surface, without tenderness, very limited mobility, and the boundary is not clear when it adheres to adjacent tissues. (a) Thoracic tumors, such as lung cancer, may metastasize to right supraclavicular fossa, or axillary lymph node groups. (b) Gastric cancer, esophageal cancers are more often to metastasize to the left supraclavicular fossa lymph node groups. Such an enlarged lymph node is called Virchow lymph node, which is often a sign of metastasis from gastric, or esophageal cancer. (c) Groin lymphadenopathy may result from advanced tumor metastasis from perineum, crissum and lower abdomen.
2. Systemic lymphadenopathy
   (a) Infectious lymphadenopathy: (a) Virus infections, such as infectious mononucleosis syndrome, acquired immunodeficiency syndrome (AIDS), etc. (b) Bacterial infections, such as brucellosis, hematogenous disseminated pulmonary tuberculosis, leprosy, etc. (c) Treponemal infections, such as syphilis,

leptospirosis, etc. (d) Protozoa and parasitic infections, such as kala-azar, filariasis, toxoplasmosis, etc.

(b) Connective tissues diseases: Such as Sjogren's syndrome and systemic lupus erythematosus (SLE).

(c) *Hematological Diseases: Such As Leukemia, Lymphoma, Etc.*

Key Terms

1	Vital sign	生命体征
2	Blood pressure	血压
3	Systolic blood pressure, SBP	收缩压
4	Diastolic blood pressure, DBP	舒张压
5	Body mass index, BMI	体重指数
6	Moon facies	满月脸
7	Coma	昏迷
8	Lymphadenopathy	淋巴结病

Study Questions

1. What is the normal axillary temperature?
2. What are the reference values of blood pressure?
3. Try to describe subcutaneous bleeding according to the size and distribution of bleeding spots?
4. What are the common causes of lymphadenopathy?

Suggested Websites

http://cc.scu.edu.cn/G2S/Template/View.aspx?action=view&courseType=0&courseId=1887

http://cc.scu.edu.cn/G2S/Template/View.aspx?action=view&courseType=0&courseId=6 (Fei Chen).

43 Physical Examination of Head

Gang Chen and Rui Zeng

Head, Eyes, Ears, Nose and *Throat* (HEENT) exam is the initial portion of general physical examination, after the vital signs. A thoughtful examination, including inspection and palpation, could provide useful clues of systemic illness. In order to examine the special structures and sensory function of eyes, ears and nose, several instruments and techniques are usually required.

43.1 Section 1: Hair and Scalp

For hair examination, observe the color, distribution, texture and pattern of any loss of the hair. The color and texture of the hair vary by race and age. Hair turns grey and white with aging. In addition to age, a variety of conditions can cause hair loss, such as typhoid fever, hypothyroidism, alopecia areata, chemotherapy and radiotherapy. To examine the scalp, part the hair to expose the area for viewing, observe the color and look for scaliness,, boil, carbuncle, scar, erythema, or other lesions.

43.2 Section 2: Skull

Inspect the skull for the general size, contour and any deformities. Palpate the skull with finger pads. Note any tenderness, lumps and deformities. The head circumference was measured above the supraorbital ridges and around most prominent part of the back of the head using a non-stretchable, flexible tape. A newborn's head circumference is usually 34 cm. It increases by 12 cm during the first year of life, and almost ends up with an average of over 53 cm at 18 years old. Premature closure of the sagittal suture and coronal suture may cause a misshaped head.

G. Chen
Department of Endocrine, Fujian Medical University, Fuzhou Shi, China

R. Zeng (✉)
Department of Cardiology, Sichuan University, Chengdu, China

1. Microcephaly is defined as head circumference more than 2 standard deviations below the mean for age and sex. The closure of the fontanelles occurs between 12–18 months, and premature closure of fontanelles can cause poor development of brain resulting in small head size and intellectual disability.
2. Oxycephaly**,** also known as tower skull, is a condition in which the skull becomes pointed due to premature closure of the sagittal suture and coronal suture. It is a common presentation of rare genetic disorder such as acro-cephalosyndactylia (Apert syndrome) (Fig. 43.1).
3. Macrocephaly is a condition in which the head circumference must be above at least 2.5 standard deviations from the mean for age and sex. The "setting sun sign" is an early indicator of hydrocephalus, in which there is a forced downward deviation of both eyes resulting in disappearance of a part of the iris below the lower eyelid (Fig. 43.2).
4. Dolichocrany is a relatively long skull with large cranial length, and moderate breadth. Dolichocrany is presented in Marfan syndrome and acromegaly.
5. Deforming skull is characterized by adult bone destruction and regrowth leading to the deformity of skull. It is often caused by Paget disease.

In addition, note any movement disorders of the head. Cervical spondylosis causes a limitation of head movement. Parkinson's disease is characterized by neurological disorders including involuntary head movement. De Musset's sign is an indicator of aortic regurgitation, in which rhythmical nodding of the head coincides with the pulse.

43.3 Section 3: Face

Face is the central organ of sense and expressing emotion, and it is also crucial for human identity. Face examination may detect HEENT disorders as well as systemic illnesses. Note the facial expression and contour. Observe for skin color, asymmetry, scars, edema, and masses.

X.-H. Wan, R. Zeng (eds.), *Handbook of Clinical Diagnostics*, https://doi.org/10.1007/978-981-13-7677-1_43

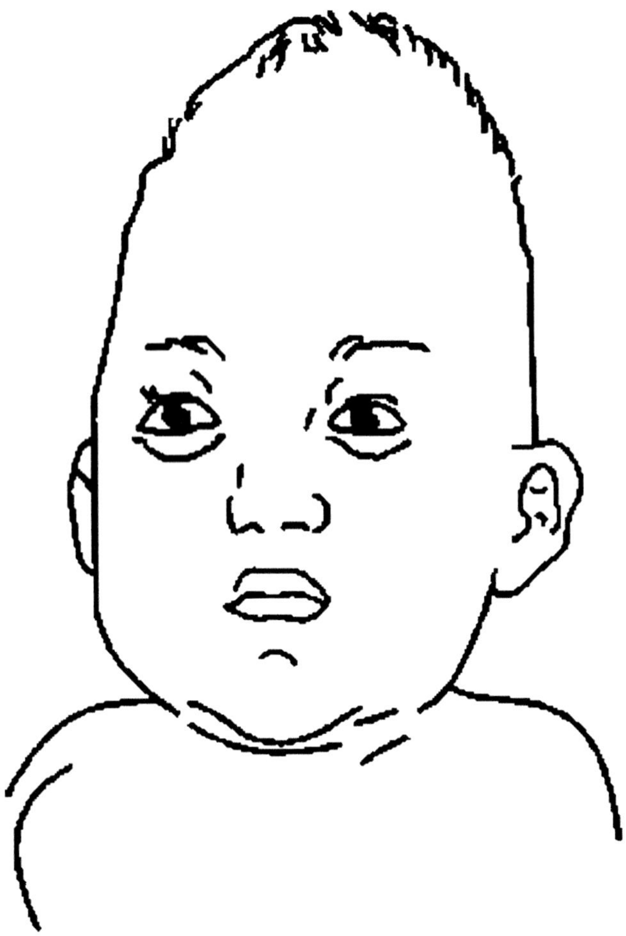

Fig. 43.1 Oxycephaly

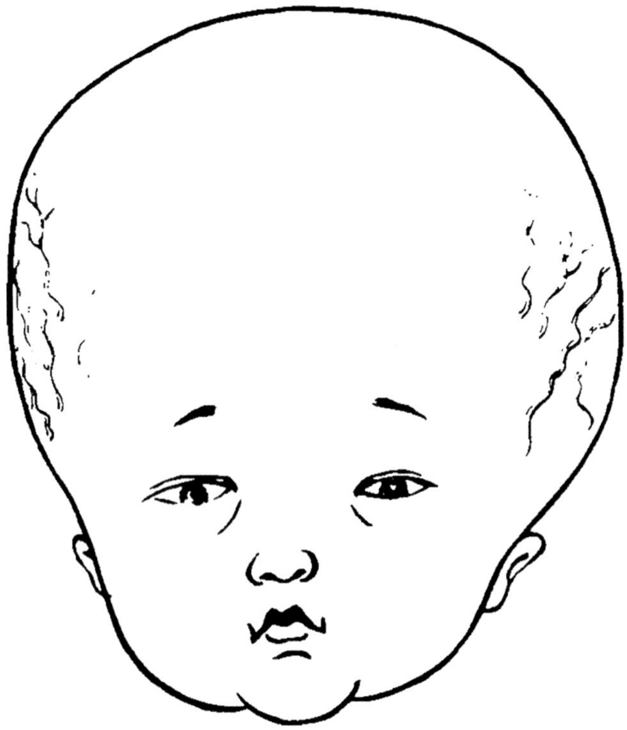

Fig. 43.2 Macrocephaly

43.3.1 Eyes

An basic eye examination usually consists of a series of tests and inspections of: visual function, external eye, anterior segment, and internal eye. The assessment of visual function includes tests of visual acuity, visual field, color vision and stereopsis. The external eye examination consists of the inspection of eyelid, lacrimal gland and duct, palpebral fissures, medial and lateral angles. Anterior segment is the front structures of eyes including the cornea, iris, ciliary body, and lens. Lastly, ophthalmoscopic exam is required to examine the internal eye structures, such as optic disc, arteries, veins, and retina.

43.3.1.1 Vision Testing

1. Visual acuity: There are two types of visual acuity: near visual acuity and far visual acuity. Near visual acuity refers to the ability to see the close subjects, such as reading and sewing. Visual acuity was measured by standardized vision charts.

   Far vision was tested at 5 m. with vision charts. Ask the patient to cover one eye with a card, and to prevent pressing on the eye. Instruct the patient to read the smallest line of print possible. Record the reading of visual acuity at the side of this line. Repeat the test for the other eye. For logMAR chart, normal visual acuity is defined as 1.00 decimal. For those who have already worn glasses, a refraction test is usually required to check the visual acuity corrected by glasses. Position the patient who cannot read the largest letter of chart closer to the chart until the patient can see the smallest line, then record the value of actual distance minus 50 m (the distance in which normal people can read the largest line) as the reading of visual acuity. If the patient cannot read the largest line at 1 m. from the chart, record the distance that the patient can correctly count the number of fingers as Count Fingers/distance (CF/cm). If the distance is less than 5 cm, visual acuity can be recorded as Hand move/distance (HM/cm), Light Perception (LP), or No Light Perception (NLP).

   Near vision was tested at 33 cm with a pocket chart. The normal reading is defined as 1.0. The patient can choose their own distance to access the best visual acuity and refraction function. Near visual test estimates the central vision and the accommodation ability. This test helps to identify prebyopia, cataract and other retina and vitreous diseases in patients aged over 45.
2. Visual field: The visual field is the entire area seen when the eyes are fixed in one direction. The confrontation visual field test estimates peripheral vision. To perform the test, the examiner faces the patient at eye level, about 1 m apart. Instruct the patient to occlude one eye while the other eye is fixated on the examiner's eye. Use the examiner's own visual fields as a reference. The examiner

slowly moves the fingers from outside the patient's peripheral field towards the center of the vision to see whether the patient can recognize the fingers in each of the four quadrants. When abnormality is detected, further tests with an automated diopsimeter are usually required.

Common defects of the visual field include concentric contraction of the visual field, scotoma (area of blind spots), hemianopia (half loss of visual field) and bitemporalheianopia. Visual field test is needed when the patient has glaucoma, retinitis pigmentosa, age-related macular degeneration and stroke, etc.

3. Color sensation: Color sensation abnormalities include color blindness (color vision deficiency) and color amblyopia (reduced color vision). Color vision deficiency can be either inherited or acquired. Sex-linked congenital red-green color vision defect is the most common form. About 4.7% of males and 0.7% of females are colorblind. The reasons for acquired color vision deficiencies may be ocular pathology, retinal disorders and intracranial injury. Color vision test is a mandatory screening test for occupations where color vision is essential, such as the military, medical care, arts or electronics.

   Color sensation is tested with an Ishihara chart at a distance of 50 cm. If the patient fails to recognize the numbers or figures after 5–10 s, color blindness or amblyopia should be considered.

43.3.1.2 External Eye Examination (Fig. 43.3)

1. Eyelids
   (a) Entropion is defined as inward turning of a portion (usually the lower lid) of the eyelids. Congenital disorders, aging, scarring and repeated trachoma infection could be the causes of entropion.
   (b) Ptosis refers to a drooping upper eyelid. Bilateral ptosis can be caused by congenital ptosis and myasthenia gravis. Unilateral ptosis is seen in oculomotor nerve palsy induced by subarachnoid hemorrhage, diphtheria, cerebral aneurysm, trauma and inflammation.
   (c) Lagophthalmos is a condition in which the eyelids are unable to close completely. Hyperthyroidism may cause bilateral lagophthalmos. Unilateral lagophthalmos is common in unilateral facial nerve palsy (Bell's palsy).
   (d) Palpebral edema is an early manifestation of mild edema because of the abnormal accumulation of liquid in the loose tissue under eyelids. The common causes of palpebral edema include nephritis, chronic liver disease, malnutrition, anemia, and angioneurotic edema.

   Xanthelasma is sharply demarcated, slightly raised yellowish plaques on or around the eyelids. It is caused by deposits of fat underneath the skin, and is seen in patients with dyslipidemia. In addition, note any masses, tenderness and trichiasis (inversion of eyelashes).
2. Lacrimal sac: Instruct the patient to observe the upper outer portion of upper lid. Note any swelling, asymmetry and tearing. Gently evert the upper lid, have the patient gaze to the opposite side, and observe the gland. Palpate over the medial canthal area for any enlargement and masses. Palpation over Lacrimal sac area may cause reflux of tears in patients with lower lacrimal drainage channel obstruction. In chronic dacryocystisis, pressure may cause purulent reflux. Avoid performing this exam in patient with acute dacryocystisis.
3. Conjunctiva: The conjunctiva consists of three parts: palpebral conjunctiva, ocular conjunctiva and fornix conjunctiva. To perform the exam, instruct the patient to look upwards, and gently pull the lower 1/3 portion of the low eyelid. Observe the color of the sclera and the vascular pattern of the scleral and palpebral conjunctivae. Usually the examiner uses the right hand to exam the patient's left eye and vice versa (Fig. 43.4).

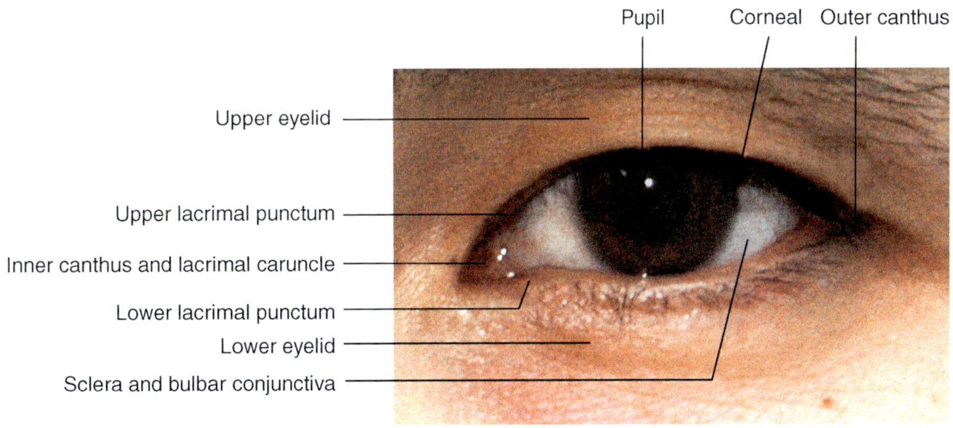

Fig. 43.3 The structure of external eye

Conjunctivitis and keratitis may cause conjunctival hyperemia (pink eye).Follicular conjunctivitis is seen in active trachoma. Pale conjunctiva indicates anemia, and jaundice causes conjunctiva to turn yellowish. Conjunctival petechiae may be one of the cutaneous manifestations of infective endocarditis. Patient with hypertension may present with subconjunctival hemorrhage (red eyes). In general, all of the signs of conjunctivitis are more severe in the lower conjunctiva than in the upper one except for trachoma.

4. Eyeball: Note the contour and movement of eyeball (Fig. 43.5).
   (a) Exophthalmos is defined as abnormal protrusion of the eyeball. Bilateral exophthalmos is commonly seen in hyperthyroidism. In addition, the other eye signs include: (A) Stellwag's sign is infrequent blinking of the eye. (B) Graefe's sign is a laggingof upper eyelid following the downward movement of the eyeball. (C) Möbius sign refers to the impairment of ocular convergence. (D) Joffery's sign is a lack of wrinkling of the forehead when the patient gazes upwards. Unilateral exophthalmos is commonly caused by orbital cellulitis, and by retro-orbital tumor under some circumstances (Fig. 43.6).
   (b) Enophthalmos is the opposite of exophthalmos, in which the eyeball sinks backward into the orbit. Bilateral exophthalmos is seen in dehydration, and orbital adipose atrophy. Unilateral exophthalmos is seen in Horner syndrome and orbital fracture.
   (c) Extraocular muscles (EOMs) and eye movements: To examine the extraocular muscles movements, instruct the patient to fix gaze straight ahead. The examiner holds up a finger about 30–40 cm in front of the patient. Ask the patient to follow the finger through six cardinal positions of gaze without head movement. The sequence is usually left-up/left-down/left-right-up/right/−down/left. Note the speed, smoothness and symmetry of movements. Lack of coordinated movement suggests problems with corresponding extraocular muscle or cranial nerve that innervates the muscle. Ptosis refers to failure of lid opening. Lid lag is found in hyperthyroidism with exposure of sclera over iris as the patient moves eyes downwards. Paralytic squint is defined as the eyes are unable to focus together because of weakness of

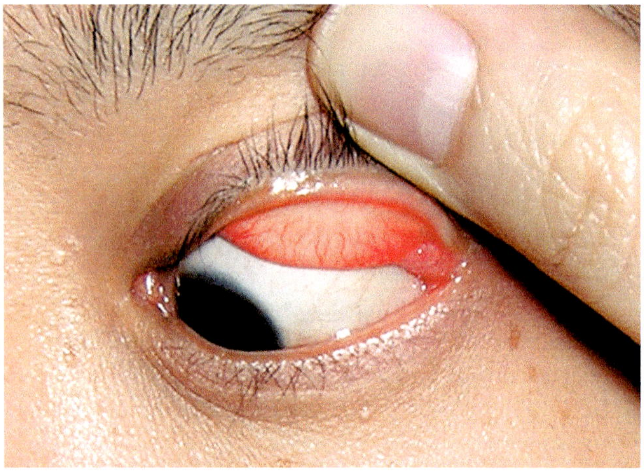

Fig. 43.4 Evert the eyelid to exam the upper eyelid

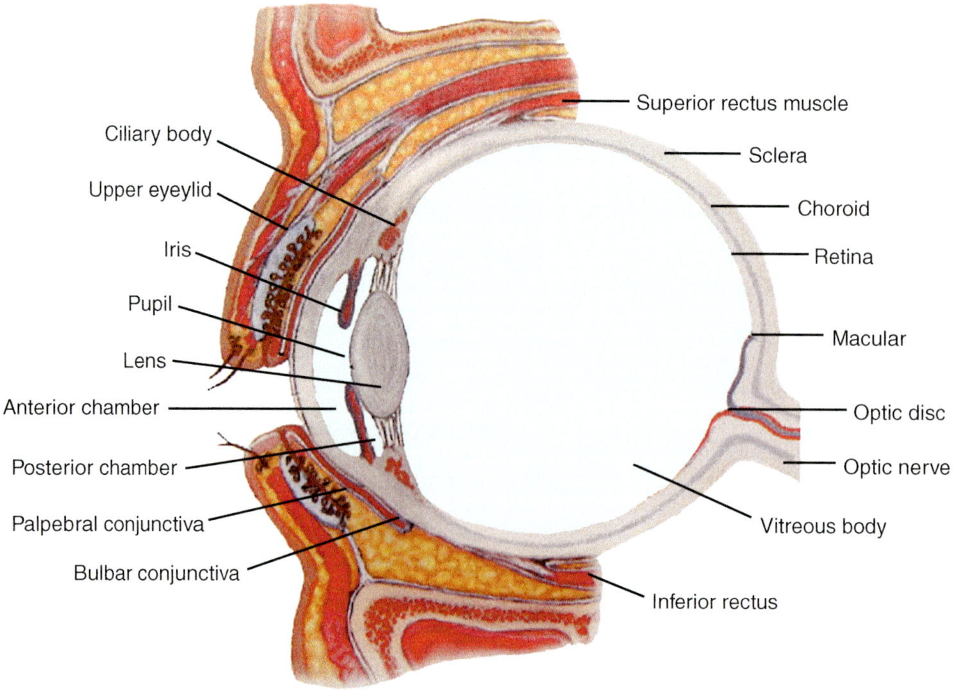

Fig. 43.5 Sagittal section of the eyeball

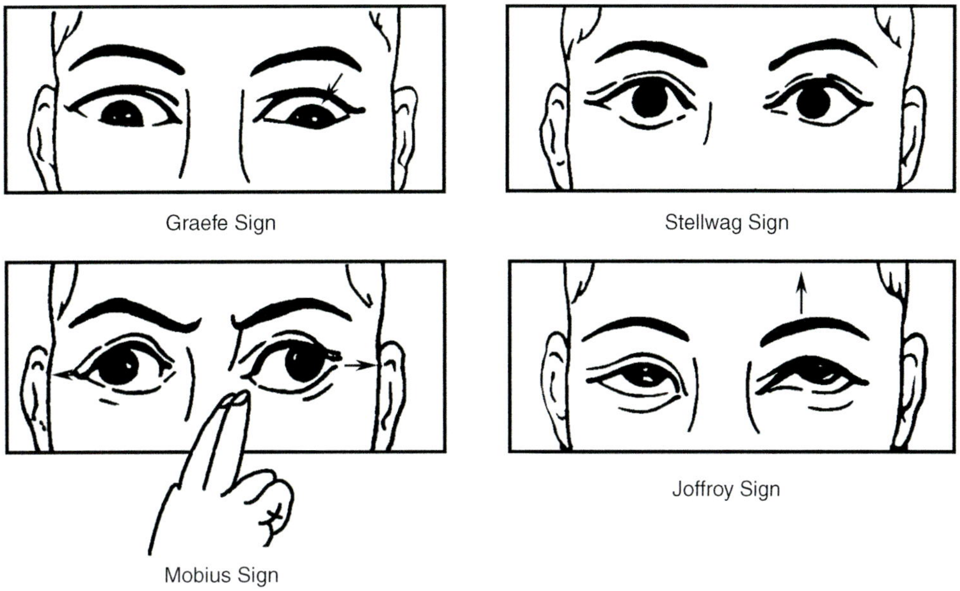

Fig. 43.6 Eye sign of hyperthyroidism

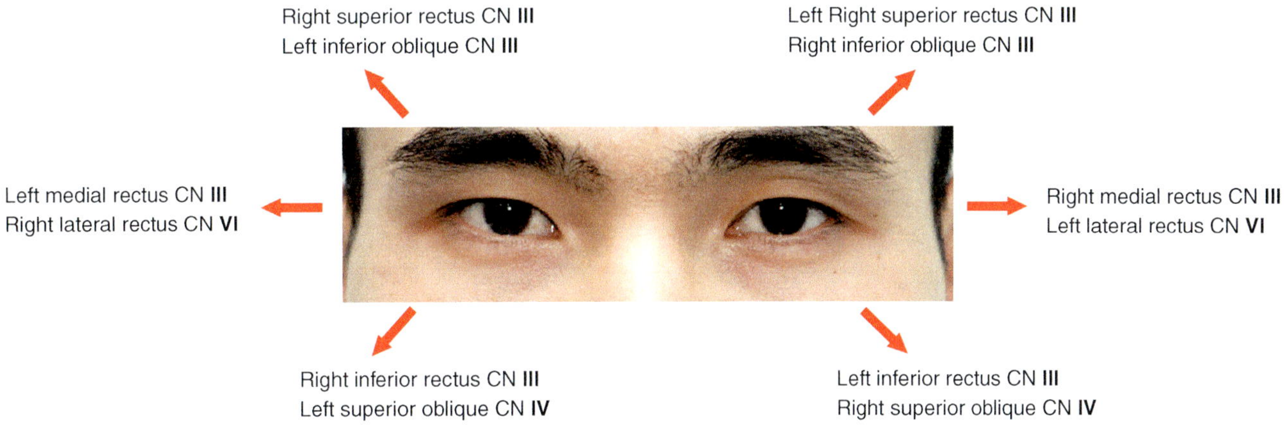

Fig. 43.7 Eye movement and corresponding extraocular muscle or cranial nerve innervation

extraocular muscle or cranial nerve as a result of cerebral diseases such as craniocerebral trauma, nasopharyngeal darcinoma, encephalitis, cephalomeningitis, encephalopyosis and cerebrovascular disease (Fig. 43.7).

(d) Nystagmus is involuntary rhythmic eye movement, characterized by a slow initiating phase and a fast corrective phase. In general, horizontal nystagmus is more common than vertical or rotary nystagmus. Give the eye straight or rotary movement and observe nystagmus or "jerkiness" of eyes. Common causes of acquired nystagmus include certain drugs (alcohol and phenytoin), head injury, Meniere's disease and stroke.

(e) Intraocular pressure(IOP) is the fluid pressure within the eye. Intraocular pressure is measured by Tonometry or palpation. The patient looks downward and the examiner gently applies pressure with index fingers to the superior portion of lids alternatively, and then estimates the force required indenting the orbital wall. Hypotony is defined as low intraocular pressure less than 5 mmHg which is usually caused by dehydration or ocular atrophy. Ocular hypertension is commonly seen in glaucoma.

43.3.1.3 Anterior Segment

1. Cornea
   Cornea is rich in sensory nerve and sensitive to stimulation (such as touching and foreign body). Observe the transparency of cornea with penlight, and note any nebula, corneal leucoma, keratomalacia, corneal ulcer corneal neovascularization. Central corneal nebula and leucoma may affect the central vision. Corneal neovascu-

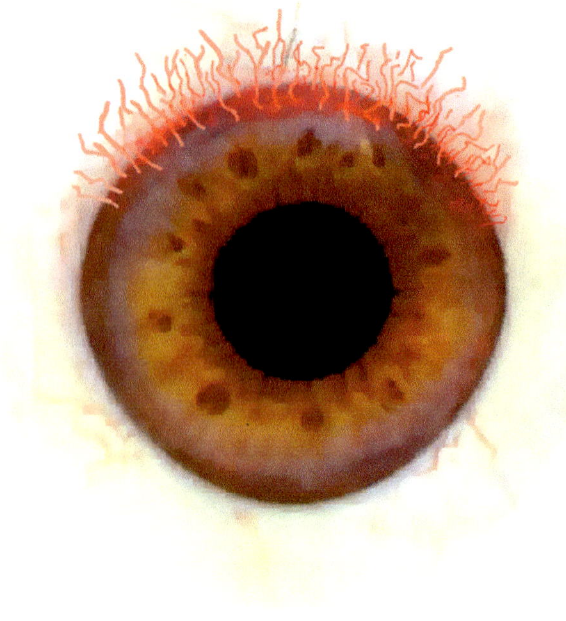

Fig. 43.8 Corneal neovascularization

larization and scarring are usually caused by advanced stage of trachoma (Fig. 43.8).

Keratomalacia occurs in general malnutrition in infants and young children due to vitamin A deficiency. Arcus senilis is the grey or white opaque around the margin of cornea in elderly. It may be related to dyslipidemia. Kayser–fleischer ring is golden-brown or brownish pigmented rings in peripheral corneal opacity caused by copper deposition in Wilson disease.

2. Sclera is the white outer layer of the eyeball. Yellowish sclera is a symptom of jaundice, and it should be differentiated from irregular fatty deposits on the sclera in old patients. Excessive consumption of carrots or drugs such as atebrine may also cause yellowing of sclera around the margin of cornea.
3. Iris is the colored ring-shaped membrane of anterior part of uvea with the pupil in its center. The pupil size is controlled by the iris sphincter and dilator muscles. Observe the shape, color, vascularity and any nodules. Loss of radial pattern within the iris is seen in iritis, iris swelling and atrophy. Abnormal shape and iris dehiscence are usually caused by iris adhesion to lens, injury and congenital coloboma of iris.
4. Pupil is the hole in the center of iris. The normal size is 3–5 mm in diameter. Pupillary constriction is controlled by iris sphincter muscle innervated by parasympathetic fibers from oculomotor nerves. The dilator muscle, which is innervated by sympathetic nerves from the superior cervical ganglion, controls pupillary dilatation. Inspect the size, shape, symmetry, reaction to light and accommodation of pupils
   (a) The size and shape of pupil Normal pupils are round and equal. Oval pupils can be associated with glaucoma and intracranial tumor. Irregular pupils can be seen in iris adhesion. Normally, the size of pupil is small in infants and old people, and large in adolescent. The pupil gets wider in the dark but narrower in light or upon stimulation. Pupillary constriction(also called miosis) is seen in iritis, organophosphate poisoning, and certain drugs such as pilocarpine, morphine and chlorpromazine. Pupillary enlargement, or mydriasis, is caused by injury, superior cervical sympathetic nerve stimulation, absolute glaucoma, optic atrophy and the application of certain drugs such as atropine and cocaine. Pupil dilation and loss of light reflex usually suggest brain death. Horner's syndrome is caused by sympathetic paralysis of the cervical sympathetic chain. It is characterized by miosis, ptosis, and anhidrosis (inabilitytosweatnormally), with or without enophthalmos.
   (b) Anisocoria refers to unequal pupils, and is usually seen in cerebral diseases, such as injury, tumor, syphilis of the central nervous system, and cerebral hernia. Pathologic anisocoria reflects an abnormality in the muscles of the iris or in the parasympathetic or sympathetic pathways that innervate the pupil. Anisocoria associated with loss of pupillary reaction usually suggests midbrain disorders.
   (c) Reaction to light Have the patient to look into the distance, shine a light into pupil, and observe the papillary constriction in the same eye (direct reaction). Then shine again into the same pupil, and observe the papillary constriction in the contralateral eye (consensual reaction). Repeat this procedure on the opposite eye. Patients in coma usually present with abnormal direct and consensual reactions.
   (d) Accommodation Instruct the patient to look at the examiner's finger about 1 m. away, and then follow the finger brought just beyond the end of the patient's nose (around 5–10 cm from the eyeballs). Normal convergence reflex consists of constriction of pupils, and convergence of eyes. The process of adjusting lens curvature is called accommodation. Alternatively, papillary constriction, convergence of eyes and lens adjustment can also be called near reflex. Loss of convergence reflex and accommodation is seen in ciliary muscle and in ocular medial rectus paralysis induced by oculomotor injury.

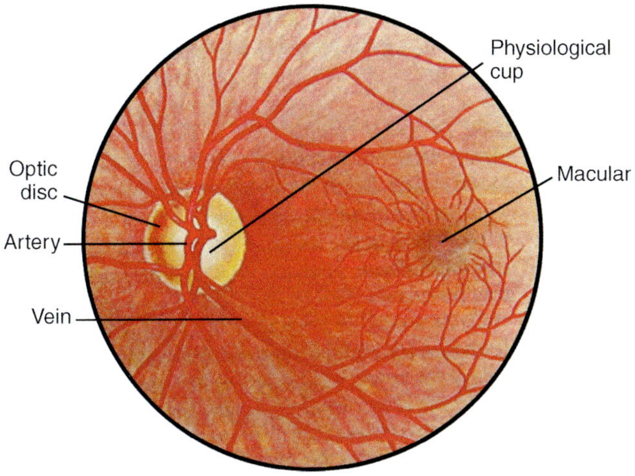

Fig. 43.9 Fundus exam of the left eye

43.3.1.4 Fundus Exam (Fig. 43.9)

Ophthalmoscopy is required for fundus examination. This test can be performed without pupil dilatation. Normal optic disc is round or oval-shaped with a pink and sharp edge and a central cup. The retinal arteriovenous ratio (A/V ratio) is 2:3. Inspect optic disc, vessels, macula and every area of retina. Note the color, margins, shape, size of the disc, any exudates or hemorrhages, and any arteriosclerosis.

Papilledema is seen in cranial tumor, cerebral abscess, traumatic brain hemorrhage, meningitis and cerebritis. The mechanism is central retinal venous occlusion caused by elevated intracranial pressure. As shown in Table 43.1, abnormalities of the optic disc can be seen in some systemic illnesses.

Table 43.1 Abnormalities of the optic disc

	Fundus changes
Hypertensive atherosclerosis	Early stage: arteriospasm Advance stage, irregular and tighter constrictions of the retinal artery, called "AV nipping". Late stage, arteriolar necrosis, retinal edema, cotton-wool spots, flame-shaped hemorrhage, and disc edema
Chronic kidney disease	Optic disc swelling, retinal edema, cotton-wool spots, and flame-shaped hemorrhage
Pregnancy toxemia	Retinal arteriospasm, edema and exudative retinal detachment
Diabetes	Retinal vein tortuosity and dilation with splinter or dotted hemorrhage
Leukemia	The edges of optic disc become obscure; retinal veins develop dilation, tortuosity, and beading of the retinal veins; vascular sheathing; cotton-wool spots; flame-shaped hemorrhages; Roth spots

43.3.2 Ear

Ear is the organ of hearing and balance. There are three compartments: external ear, middle ear and inner ear.

1. The external ear
   (a) Auricle Inspect the contour, size, position of ear lobes, and symmetry. Note any deformity, injury, scaring, redness, swelling, lumps, fistulous tract. Tophi are deposits of uric acid crystals found in patients with gout. Gently pull and palpate the auricle for texture and tenderness. Red and swollen auricle associated with tenderness suggests inflammation.
   (b) External auditory canal Inspect the skin and drainage. Yellow exudates with itching suggest otitis externa. Lumps on the ear can cause auditory canal redness and swelling. Movement of the auricle is painful in otitis externa but not in otitis media. Blood and cerebral spinal fluid which is caused by fracture of skull base may drain from the ear. Tinnitus (ringing) can be seen in narrowness of external ear canal, foreign bodies in ear and cerumen.
2. Middle ear
   Gently pull the auricle upward and backward and observe the tympanic membrane using an otoscope. Inspect the color, transparency, and position of the tympanic membrane. Note any perforation. Foul-smelling discharge from the middle ear may suggest cholesteatoma.
3. Mastoid
   The mastoid process is filled with cavities called "air cells" (sinuses) that connect to the middle ear. Inflammation of middle ear can cause mastoiditis, which is red and swollen behind ear. Complications of mastoiditis include intracranial extension and cranial abscess formation.
4. Auditory acuity
   Auditory acuity can be estimated by several screening tests. In a quiet room, ask the patient to occlude one ear. Move the fingers/watch from 1 m. towards the patient's ear. Instruct the patient to acknowledge the rubbing of the examiner's fingers/watch sounds. Use the examiner's own hearing as a reference. Repeat this procedure on the opposite ear. Record the distance and compare the results of the two ears. People with normal auditory acuity can hear fingers rubbing or watch sounds approximately 1 m away from the ear.

   Hearing loss can be caused by cerumen, foreign bodies in ear, auditory nerve injury, vascular sclerosis, otitis media and otosclerosis. For patient with abnormal auditory acuity in screening test, further tests for hearing evaluation, including tuning fork tests and electroaudiometry, are usually performed to make a diagnosis.

43.3.3 Nose

1. The shape of a nose: Inspect the skin color and contour of external surface of nose. Hyperpigmentation on the bridge of nose may be caused by sun damage or pigmentation disorders such as visceral leishmaniasis and chronic liver disease. Patients with SLE may develop a characteristic red, flat facial rash over the bridge of the nose, which is called butterfly rash. Rosacea is characterized by facial redness on the central face including tips and wings of nose. (Fig. 43.10) The mechanism is small and superficial blood vessel dilating and tissue thickening. Since nasal fracture is one of the most common bone injuries, patient with nosebleeds should be examined for nasal fracture or transposition. Saddle-nose is nasal dorsal depression caused by nasal fracture, nasal dysplasia, congenital syphilis and leprosy.
2. Nasal flaring: It is the nostrils widen while breathing. The common cause is dyspnea induced by lobar pneumonia, asthma, and cardiac asthma.
3. Nasal septum: Nasal septal displacement is a common physical disorder. Only severe cases associated with difficulty breathing can be called nasal septal deviation. Symptoms of nasal septal deviation include headache due to nasal obstruction, or nose bleeding caused by mucous membrane irritation. Nasal septal perforation is the hole in nasal septum. The patient can hear a whistling noise when breathing. A white light shined in one nasal cavity and seen in the other suggests septal perforation. The common causes can be chronic inflammation and injury.

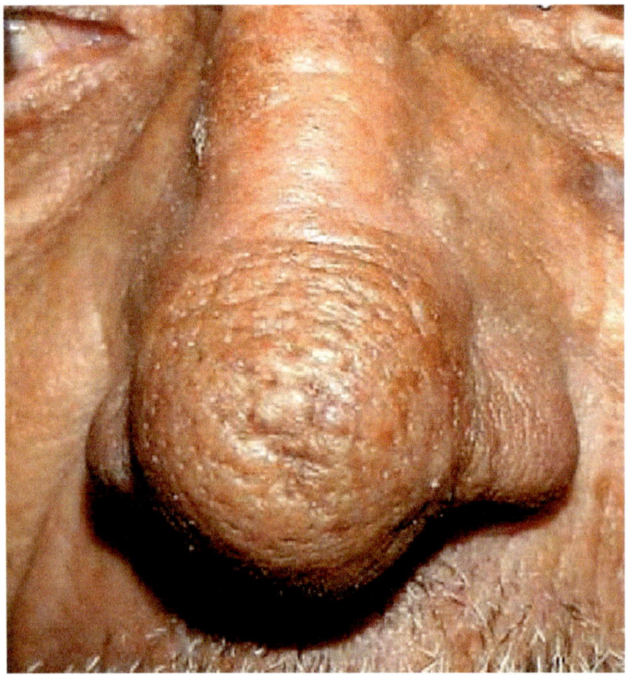

Fig. 43.10 Rosacea

4. Epistaxis: It is also called nosebleed. Unilateral nosebleed can be caused by nasal diseases, such as trauma, inflammation, blood vessel injury, nasopharyngeal carcinoma, nasal septal deviation. Bilateral nosebleeds can be seen in systemic illnesses, such as infectious diseases (viral hemorrhagic fevers, typhoid fever), hematological diseases (thrombocytopenic purpura, aplastic anemia, leukemia, hemophilia), hypertension, liver diseases, vitamin C or D deficiency. Endometriosis should be considered if a woman presents with periodic nosebleeds.
5. Nasal mucosa: Acute nasal mucosa swelling, caused by nasal cavity obstruction and discharges, is usually seen in acute rhinitis. Thickening of the nasal mucosa is more commonly found in chronic rhinitis. Nasal mucous atrophy, nasal crusting, foul-smelling discharge, roomy nasal cavities and bad smell are common symptoms of chronic atrophic rhinitis. Tilting the tip of nose with pen light, and inspect the nasal vestibule, nasal floor and inferior nasal concha. Examination of the concha nasalis media, middle meatus, olfactory cleft and upper nasal septum requires an otoscope.
6. Rhinorrhea is also known as a running nose. It is a condition where the nasal cavity is filled with mucus or discharge. Thick phlegm and mucus is seen in catarrh inflammation. Green or yellow mucus suggests purulent inflammation in nasal cavities or sinus.
7. Nasal sinuses are the four paired air-filled spaces that surround the nasal cavity and connect to nasal cavities. Sinusitis will occur when the drainage of mucus within the sinuses is blocked. Symptoms of sinusitis may include nasal obstruction, rhinorrhoea, headache and tenderness over sinus (Fig. 43.11).

The procedures for the examination of the sinuses are as follows.

- Maxillary sinuses: The patient's head is fixated by the hands of the examiner. The examiner places the thumbs upward just below the cheekbone. Percuss the cheekbone with middle finger tip of the examiner's right hand. Note any tenderness and compare on either side.
- Frontal sinuses: The examiner uses thumbs to press up on the frontal sinuses from under the bony brows, avoiding pressure on the eyes. Alternatively, the examiner can percuss the frontal sinuses by tapping with the middle finger on this area. Patients are asked whether they feel painful during this examination.
- Ethmoidal sinuses: The patient's head is fixated by the hands of the examiner. The examiner places the thumbs in the medial angle of the eye against the roof of the eye socket, and applies pressure. Note any tenderness and make a comparison on either side.
- Sphenoid sinuses: Sphenoid sinuses lay hidden within the skull, and cannot be examined by palpation.

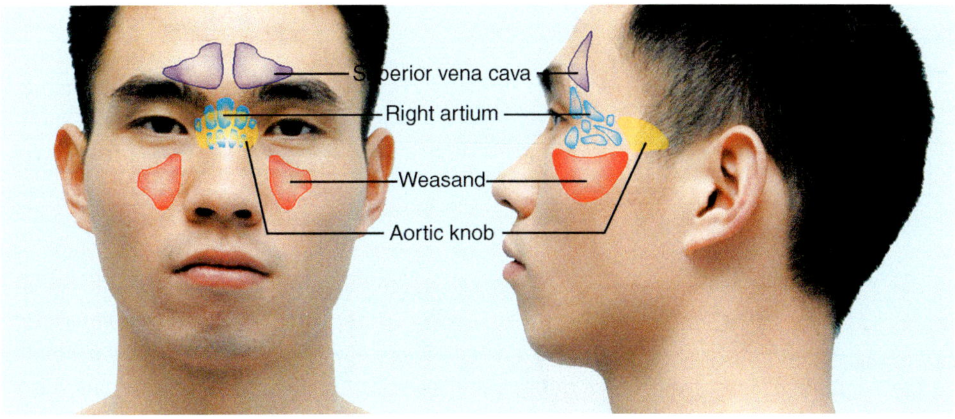

Fig. 43.11 The position of nasal sinuses

43.3.4 Mouth

Oral examination includes examination of lips, organs and tissues in oral cavity and breath odor.

1. Lips
   Inspect the color and moisture of the lips. Note any scarring and cracking. Normal Lips are red due to rich capillaries distribution and thin epidermis in this area. Pale lips are a symptom of inadequate oxygenation due to the low hemoglobin level or poor blood supply. The common causes are anemia, fainting, and aortic insufficiency. Cyanosis is blue discoloration of lips due to an increase in desaturated hemoglobin, which is seen in heart failure and respiratory failure. Cracked lips can be caused by dehydration. Herpes labialis is a group of blisters occurring between the lips and skin caused by herpes simplex virus infection. The symptoms typically begin with itching, and then heal with crusting within 7 days. It is usually associated with lobar pneumonia, common cold, meningococcal meningitis and malaria. Cleft lips are congenital malformation. Red spots in lips and mouth can be seen in hereditary hemorrhagic telangiectasia, which turn white when pressure is applied. Unpainful lips swelling can be caused by angioedema, which progresses rapidly.

   Chapping and fissuring of the lips can be caused by riboflavin deficiency. Large mouth with puffy lips can be seen in myxedema, acromegaly and cretinism.
2. Oral mucosa
   Inspect the oral mucosa for color, ulcers, consistency and nodules with a tongue blade in a good light condition. Normal oral mucosa is pink and smooth. Generalized dark blue pigmentation is presented in adrenal insufficiency (Addison disease). Bruising and petechiae are manifestations of bleeding disorders or vitamin C deficiency. Koplik spots occur in early phase of measles. They are small white spots found in the oral mucosa opposite the upper first and second molars. An enanthem is a widespread symmetrical rash with small spots, which occurs in German measles, scarlet fever and certain drug poisoning.

   Painful ulcers can be caused by recurrent aphthous stomatitis. Oral thrush is a condition that fungus Candida albicans accumulates on the oral mucosa. It is a common infection in infants and the elderly due to long-term use of broad spectrum antibiotics and antitumor drugs.

   Ask the patient to cling the tongue to the roof of the mouth, inspect the mucous membrane underneath. Palpation may be needed to assess a lesion in the soft tissues of the floor of mouth.
3. Teeth
   Inspect the number and condition of teeth. Note any dental caries, missing teeth, dentures and residual root. Record the abnormities of teeth in the format shown below.

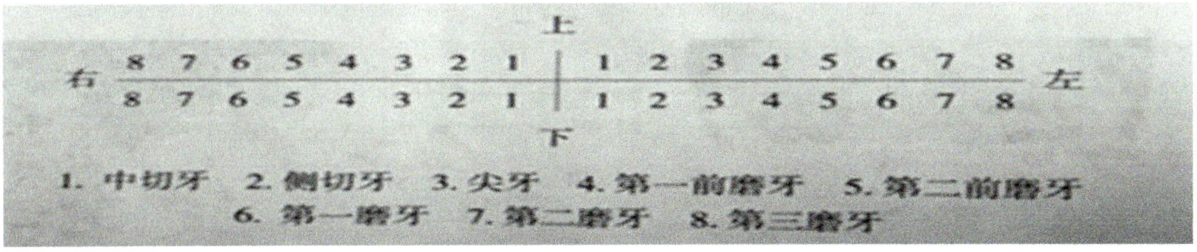

上	Upper	4. 第一前磨牙	First premolar
下	Lower	5. 第二前磨牙	Second premolar
左	Left	6. 第一磨牙	First molar
右	Right	7.第二磨牙	Second molar
1. 中切牙	Central incisor	8. 第三磨牙	Third molar
2. 侧切牙	Lateral incisor;		
3. 尖牙	Left ventricle		

For example 1| represents upper right central incisor, 4| represents right lower first premolar, 5|5 / |7 represents upper left and right second premolars, and lower left second molar.

The shapes and colors of the teeth are useful for clinical diagnosis. Hutchinson's teeth are a sign of congenital syphilis, in which the teeth are more widely spaced and smaller than normal, and central incisors have notches on the biting surfaces. Dental fluorosis (mottled enamel) refers to brown discoloration on the enamel due to high level of fluoride in drinking water. Widely spaced teeth are seen in acromegaly.

4. Gum
Inspect the gum for color and swelling. Retract the lips and cheeks, check the gums with gloves for bleeding and pus. Normal gum is pink, firm, moisture with tight margins. Swollen gum can be caused by chronic periodontitis. Bleeding gums can be caused by gum problems such as dental tartar, as well as systemic disease such as liver diseases, Vitamin C deficiency, and hematological disease. If pus is seen between the teeth and gums upon applying pressure on the gums, chronic periodontitis should be considered. Burton's line is the blue-purplish line on the gums caused by lead poisoning. The history of lead exposure could be useful for the clinical diagnosis.
5. Tongue
Ask the patient to stick out the tongue, inspect the tongue for color, texture, moisture, symmetry and size. Palpate any lesions of hardness with gloves. Tough abnormities can be useful clues for systemic illnesses.
(a) Dry Tongue Persistent dryness of tongue may be due to local disorders of the salivary glands, as well as systemic illnesses, such as Sjogren's syndrome, diabetes, nerve injury and atropine. In addition, other conditions, including mouth breathing, heavy smoking and alcohol consumption, may also cause dry tongue. Deep lateral furrows on dry tongue can be seen in severe dehydration.
(b) Swollen tongue Temporary tongue swelling can be seen in glossitis, stomatitis, cellulitis, abscess, hematoma and angioedema. Persistent swollen tongue can be caused by myxedema, cretinism, Down syndrome, and tongue tumor.
(c) Geographic tongue is a benign condition in which patches on the surface of the tongue are characterized by loss of lingual papillae with irregular, smooth, red, map-like appearance and slightly raised borders. The reasons for geographic tongue are still unknown. Riboflavin deficiency may be related to this condition.
(d) Fissured tongue is characterized by deep grooves in the dorsum of the tongue. It can be caused by Down syndrome and riboflavin deficiency, in association with geographic tongue. Some patients may complaint about soreness.
(e) Strawberry tongue is characterized by bumpy appearance of tongue papilla and its distinct red color. It is commonly associated with scarlet fever, and prolonged fever.
(f) Beefy tongue refers to "beefy" or "fiery red and sore" glossitis caused by vitamin B12 deficiency.
(g) Smooth tongue refers to the absence of papillae on the dorsum of the tongue due to anemia and malnutrition.
(h) Hairy tongue is a dark, furry appearance of tongue due to dead skin cells on the tiny papillae. It's usually seen in old patients, smokers and those patients with long term use of broad spectrum antibiotics.
(i) Abnormal movement of tongue Hyperthyroidism can cause a trembling tongue. Asymmetric protrusion of tongue indicates a lesion of CN XII.
6. Pharynx and tonsil
Pharynx is divided into three compartments (Fig. 43.12).
(a) Nasal pharynx is above the soft palate and posterior to the nasal cavities. The adenoids are a mass of lymphoid tissue in this area, which present at birth and in childhood, but shrink by adulthood. Enlarged adenoids may cause nasal obstruction, mouth breathing and nasal voice. Unilateral nosebleeds, ringing in the ears and hearing loss may be early symptoms of nasopharyngeal cancer.
(b) Oral pharynx is below the soft palate, behind the mouth, and superior to the hyoid bone. It is in front of the superior constrictor muscle and the cervical vertebrae. The tonsil lies in the front of the pharyngopalatine and behind the palatoglossal arch. To examine the oral pharynx, instruct the patient to open the mouth and ask the patient to say "ah" or place a tongue blade in outer 2/3 of the arched tongue. Inspect the soft palate, anterior and posterior pillars, uvula, tonsils, and posterior pharynx wall with a penlight. Note the color, symmetry, any exudates or swelling, and the degree of tonsil enlargement (Fig. 43.13).

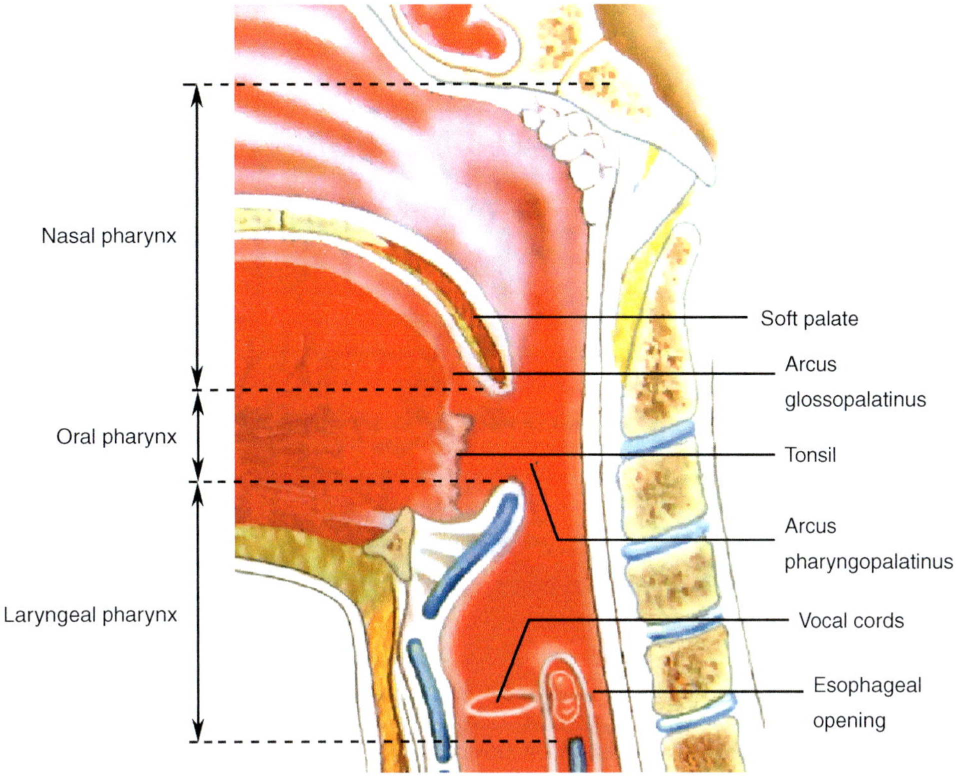

Fig. 43.12 The three compartments of pharynx

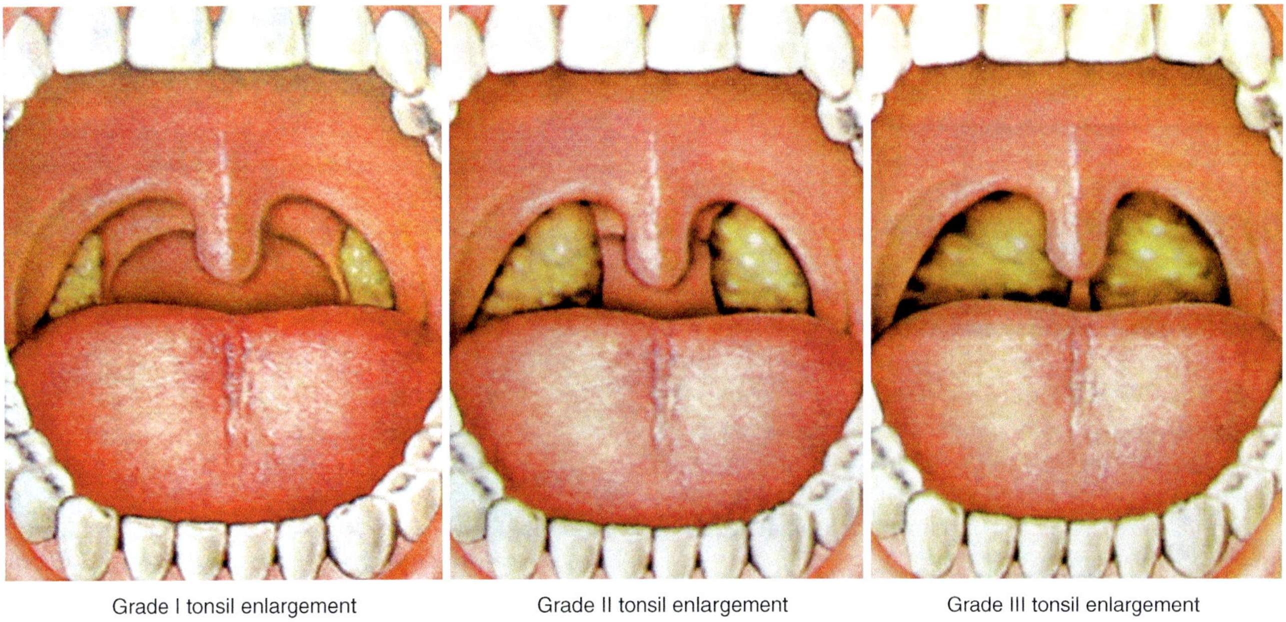

Fig. 43.13 The position of tonsil and enlarged tonsil grading

Pharyngitis can cause hyperemia and swelling of the pharynx covered with exudates. Chronic pharyngitis may present with swollen, hypertrophic and red pharynx membranes and enlarged follicles in the posterior pharynx wall. In acute tonsillitis, enlarged tonsils are covered with white exudates or gray scum which can be removed without bleeding. This condition should be differentiated from pseudomembrane found in diphtheria which causes bleeding after being removed. The three scales of tonsils enlargement are as follows: I, Tonsil enlargement does not exceed the pharyngeal arch palate; II, tonsil enlargement exceeds the pharyngeal arch palate, but not the

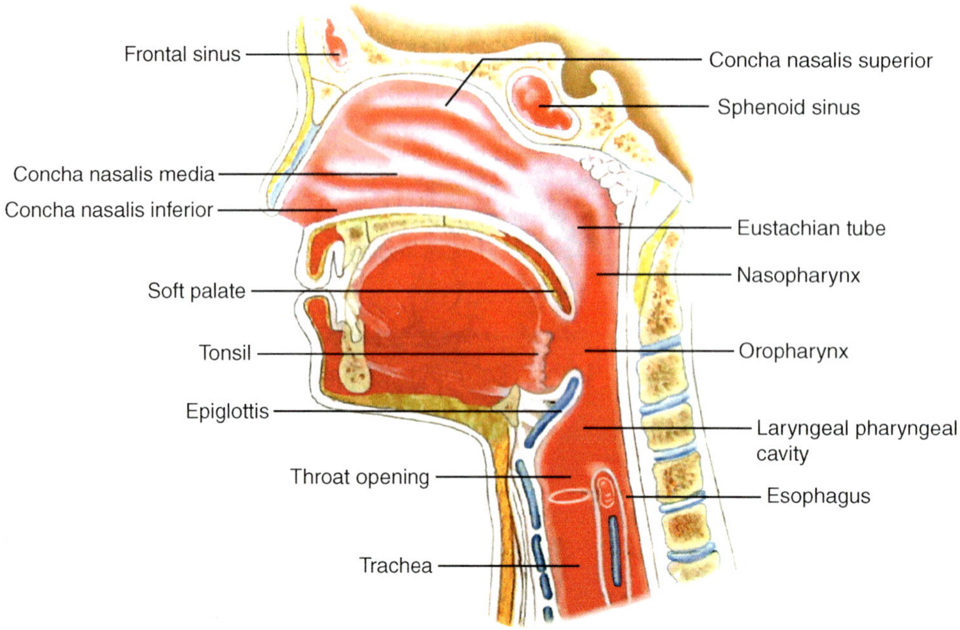

Fig. 43.14 Sagittal section of nasal pharynx

midline of the posterior pharyngeal wall; and III, tonsil enlargement exceeds the midline of the posterior pharyngeal wall.

(c) Laryngeal pharynx, also known as hypopharynx, is the area below the oral pharynx. It communicates with larynx anteriorly, and opens into the esophagus inferiorly. Examination of laryngopharynx requires direct or indirect laryngoscopy.

7. Larynx

The Larynx is a tube-shaped organ that connects the lower portion of pharynx with the trachea. It is the organ that is responsible for voice production, and consists of cartilage, ligaments, muscles, and mucous membrane. Normal voice production relies on the harmony work of three subsystems: a power source (lungs), the vibrator (vocal folds, or larynx) and the resonator (throat, nose, mouth, and sinuses and teeth).Any abnormalities or changes in those subsystems may cause voice disorders. Common symptoms of laryngitis are hoarseness, loss of voice, and score throat. Persistent loss of voice may indicate larynx cancer (Fig. 43.14).

Halitosis, also known as bad breath, is the unpleasant odor presenting in the exhaled breath. The source of bad breath can be the oral cavity, nasal passages, lungs or systemic diseases.

Local disorders in the mouth, such as gingivitis and periodontitis, can cause bad breath. Fetid odor is caused by alveolar abscess. Gum bleeding can cause blood smell. Bad breath can be present in systemic diseases. For example, a fruity odor of the breath is a sign of diabetic ketoacidosis. An ammonia odor may indicate liver failure. A pungent garlic-like odor suggests organophosphorus poisoning.

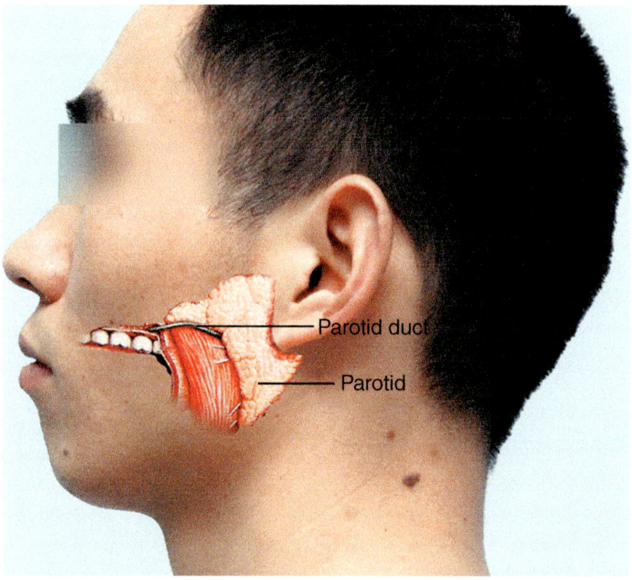

Fig. 43.15 The position of parotid gland and parotid duct

43.3.5 Parotid Gland

The parotid gland is localized in the parotid space, wrapping around the angle of mandible up to the tragus of ear with an extension on the cheekbone. On examination, inspect the region of parotid gland for swelling, asymmetry, opening of a fistula and scarring. Palpate from behind the patient, ask the patient to clench teeth, and then check for tenderness, enlargement or texture for any lumps. In addition, look inside the mouth at the opening of parotid duct (Stensen's duct), which is opposite to upper second molars. Normal parotid gland is soft and impalpable. Parotid gland swelling can be caused by the following conditions (Fig. 43.15).

1. Epidemic parotitis, also called mumps, is a generalised infection caused by a paramyxovirus, resulting in acute onset of unilateral or bilateral tender swelling of paroid gland. It can be associated with acute pancreatitis, orchitis and oophoritis. Mikulicz syndrome is characterized by the painless enlargement of parotids, lacrimal gland and salivary gland.
2. Acute suppurative parotitis is acute unilateral infection of the parotid gland. It occurs in patients with poor oral hygiene and debilitation, particularly among elderly postoperative patients. On examination, a pus discharge from Stensen duct can be seen after massaging the parotid gland.
3. Parotid tumor Benign mixed tumor is a firm and movable nodular mass with an obvious border. A painful and rock-hard mass with fixation to adjacent structures usually suggests malignant parotid tumor, which may be associated with facial nerve paralysis.

Key Terms		
1	Head	头
2	Eyes	眼
3	Ears	耳
4	Nose	鼻
5	Throat	喉
6	Scalp	头皮
7	Skull	头颅
8	Face	颜面
9	Vision Testing	视力测试
10	Extraocular Muscles	眼外肌
11	Pupil	瞳孔
12	Auditory Acuity	听力
13	Sinuses	鼻窦
14	Tonsil	扁桃体
15	Parotid Gland	腮腺

Study Questions

1. How to perform the examination of the eyes &vision?
2. How to perform the examination of nasal sinuses?
3. Describe normal findings of the head, ear, nose and throat exam.
4. Identify anatomic landmarks of the head, ear, nose mouth, throat.

Suggested Readings and Websites

1. www.med-ed.virginia.edu/courses/pom1/pexams/HEENT
2. Bickley LS. Bates'Guide to physical examination and history taking. tenth ed: Lippincott Williams & Wilkins; 2009. (Gang Chen)

44 Physical Examination of Neck

Gang Chen and Rui Zeng

Neck exam is performed in a quiet and well-lit room. The patient should be seated in a comfortable position. Expose the neck down to the shoulders. Remove any jewelry. Gently perform the exam, particularly for those with suspected cervical diseases.

44.1 Contour and Cervical Triangles

Normal neck is upright and symmetrical. Ask the patient to look up a little bit, inspect the neck for contour, scarring, masses and symmetry. Laryngeal prominence is larger in men than in women. The vessels are invisible as the patient is seated.

For the purpose of description, each side of the neck was divided into two triangles bounded by the sternomastoid muscle. For the anterior triangle, the borders are the clavicle inferiorly, and the midline anteriorly. For the posterior triangle, the borders are the clavicle anteriorly, and the trapezius anteriorly.

44.2 Posture and Movement

Normal neck makes basically six movements: flexion, extension, lateral rotation (left and right), lateral flexion (left and right). On examination, fix the head with one hand, inspect the concavity of cervical spine, and observe trapezius and sternomastoid muscles. Check the range of active and passive motion. Dropped head deformity can be caused by cachexia, myasthenia gravis, acute anterior poliomyelitis, and progressive muscular atrophy. Torticollis (wry neck) is an abnormal, asymmetrical neck posture as a result of cervical muscle injury, scarring and congenital muscular torticollis or contracture. Congenital muscular torticollis is characterized by a shortening or excessive contraction of the sternocleidomastoid muscle. Limited range of motion with pain can be caused by inflammation of soft tissues, neck sprain, hypertrophic spondylitis, cervical tuberculosis and tumor. Neck stiffness is a sign of meningeal irritation caused by meningitis and subarachnoid hemorrhage.

G. Chen
Department of Endocrine, Fujian Medical University, Fuzhou, China

R. Zeng (✉)
Department of Cardiology, Sichuan University, Chengdu, China

44.3 Skin and Mass

1. Skin Note any spider angioma, signs of inflammation (boils, carbuncle) and other conditions such as scarring, fistula, neurodermatitis and psoriasis.
2. Masses Note the location, size, number, shape, delimitation (discrete or matted together), mobility, consistency, and any tenderness. Enlarged, soft and tender lymph nodes may suggest acute nonspecific lymphadenitis. Metastatic nodes are hard and usually associated with mediastinal, thorax and abdominal disorders. Generalized, non-tender lymph nodes enlargement can be seen in hematological diseases. A painless, smooth, round, rubbery mass can be cystic tumor. Neck masses of variable size without systemic symptoms can be cysts. Enlarged thyroid or thyroid nodules can be differentiated from neck masses by the upward movement induced by swallowing water.

44.4 Vessels

Jugular vein is visible in a supine position, but invisible at 45° inclination or seated. Jugular venous distension or pulsation at 45° inclination indicates abnormal conditions. Central venous pressure (CVP) can be estimated by measuring the jugular venous pressure (JVP). On examination, the patient's trunk is at 45° inclination. Turn the head slightly towards left shoulder to relax the muscles. Internal jugular vein is located

X.-H. Wan, R. Zeng (eds.), *Handbook of Clinical Diagnostics*, https://doi.org/10.1007/978-981-13-7677-1_44

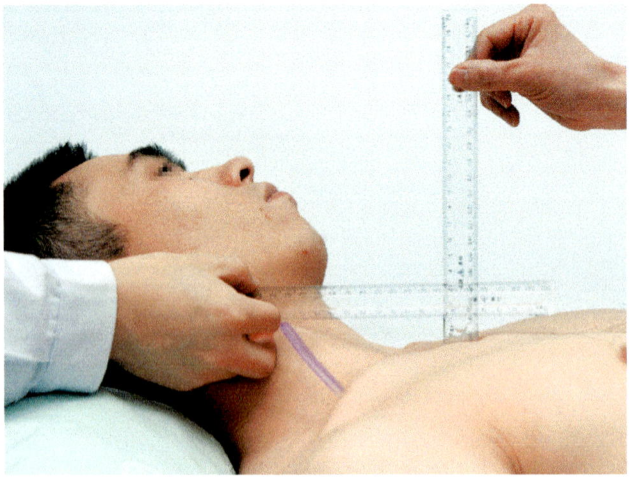

Fig. 44.1 Measurement of jugular venous pressure

at the root of the neck between clavicular and the heads of sternoclidomastoid. Apply light tangentially and inspect for upper level of venous pulsations, waveform and respiratory variation. Measure the elevation of venous pulsations above the sternal angle (Lewis angle). For estimating CVP, add 5 cm to the measurement of JVP since right atrium lies 5 cm below the sternal angle. If the measurement of JVP is more than 4cm, the estimated CVP will be more than 9 cm, which suggests elevation of CVP. Common causes of CVP elevation include right ventricular failure, pericardial effusion, constrictive pericarditis, superior venacava (SVC) obstruction and other diseases which induce high intrapleural and Intra-abdominal pressure (Fig. 44.1).

Hepatojugular reflux refers to a distension of the jugular vein that occurs when applying pressure over the abdomen. This sign can be seen in congestive heart failure because the dilated sinusoids in the liver. Jugular venous pulsation is visible in tricuspid regurgitation. Collapse of Jugular vein in supine position usually suggests volume depletion. The internal jugular vein is the preferred site to assess CVP because it is in direct line with the right atrium. If the internal jugular vein is not detectable, the external jugular vein can be an alternative site to perform the test.

Normal carotid pulse is weak and invisible under resting conditions, and becomes detectable after vigorous physical exercises. Carotid pulse amplitude can be detected in several conditions such as aortic valve regurgitation, hypertension, hyperthyroidism, and severe anemia. A prominent carotid pulse should be differentiated from JVP. Carotid pulse is vigorous, single and palpable. JVP is un-palpable, multiphasic and variable with respiration or pressure.

For auscultation of vessels, ask the patient to be seated, and place the bell of the stethoscope over each carotid artery. If bruits are present, note location, radiation, intensity, pitch, quality, timing, and relationship to respiration or body position. Bruits can be caused by atherosclerotic stenosis in carotid artery and vertebral artery. A Bruit of carotid artery stenosis can be auscultated over the bifurcation of the carotid artery. It is high-pitched blowing radiated to mandibular area during mid- systole. The cervical venous hum is heard over the internal jugular veins. It is a continuous high-pitched sound varied with respiration or position. In addition, supraclavicular bruits during systole can be heard in subclavian or vertebral artery stenosis. A continuous venous hum is auscultated in the right supraclavicular fossa as the right internal jugular vein and brachiocephalic vein have straight access to the superior vena cava. This venous hum can be obliterated upon pressure.

44.5 Thyroid

Thyroid is a butterfly-shaped organ located below the thyroid cartilage and anterior to the trachea, extending to either side. A thyroid gland usually weights 15–25 g. It is soft, smooth, and impalpable (Fig. 44.2).

1. Inspection Inspect the thyroid in a neutral position. Observe its size and symmetry. Normal thyroid is not visible. Mild enlargement can be seen in some adolescent girls. Instruct the patient to swallow a sip of water, and watch the upward movement of the thyroid. Extending the neck can improve the visualization of thyroid.
2. Palpation Palpate the isthmus and lateral lobes. Note the contour and texture of thyroid.
   - Thyroid isthmus lies below cricoid cartilage, overlying the 2–4th tracheal rings. Locate the isthmus by palpating upward from the suprasternal notch to the cricoid cartilage. Ask the patient to swallow a sip of water, feeling for the upward movement of the isthmus. Note any thickening, enlargement and masses.
   - Lateral lobes There are two approaches for palpating the thyroid gland. Use one hand for each lobe. Ask the patient to swallow a sip of water as feeling for the movement of the thyroid gland.

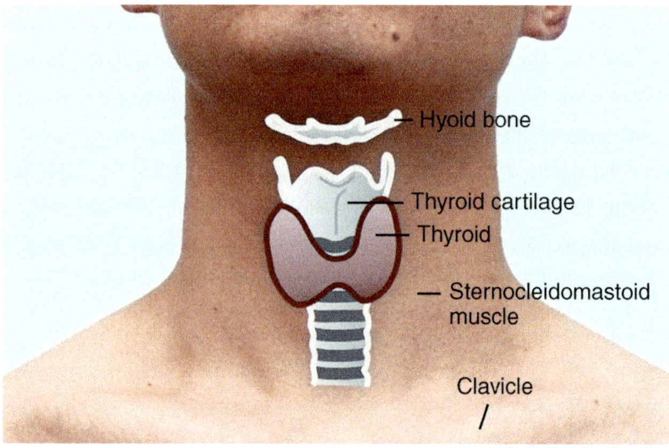

Fig. 44.2 The position of thyroid

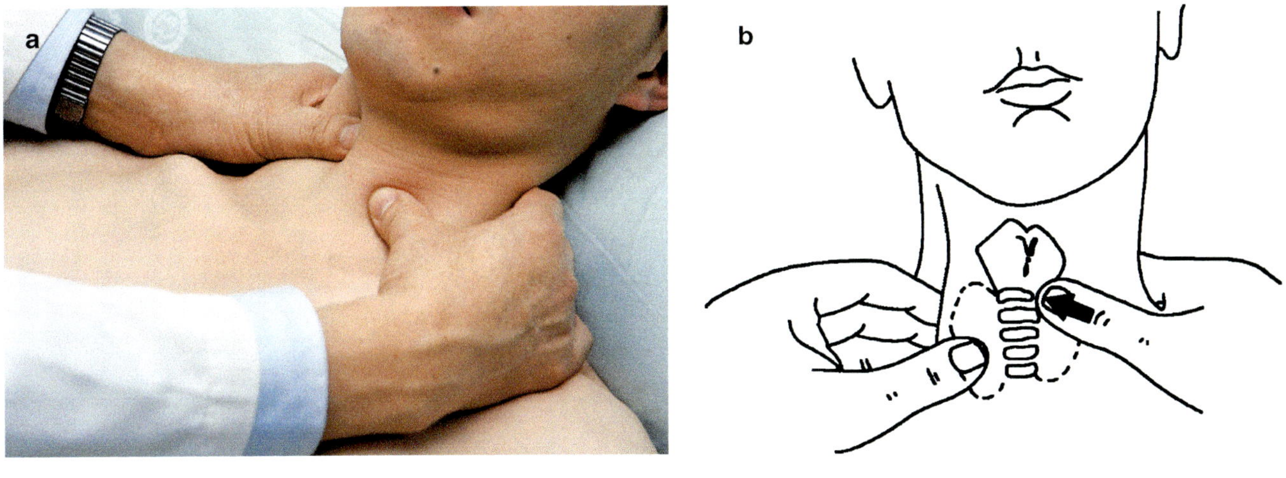

Fig. 44.3 Anterior approach

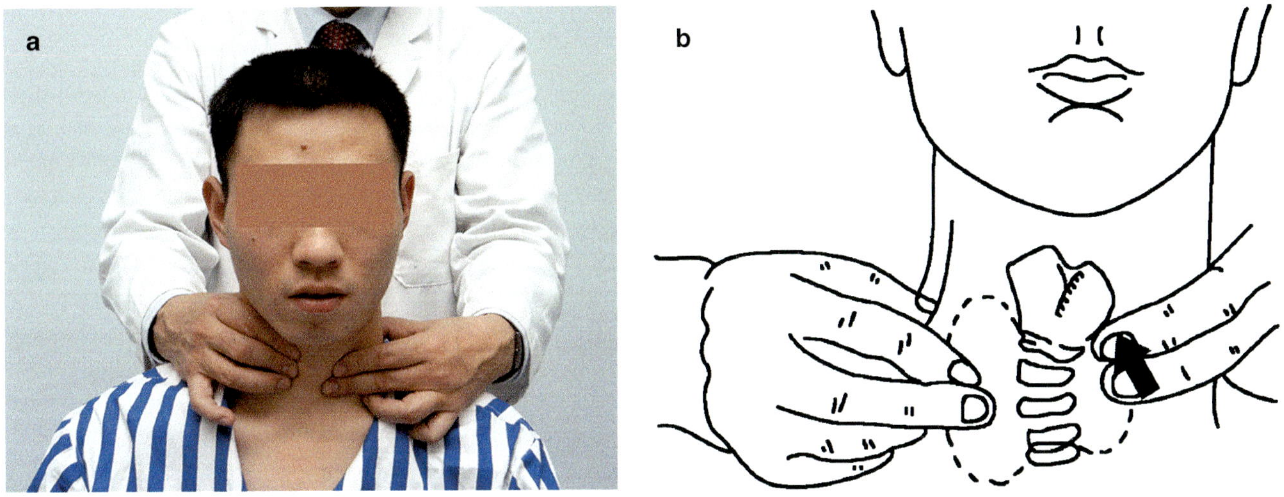

Fig. 44.4 Posterior approach

For the anterior approach, the examiner is in front of the patient. Displace the larynx with one thumb. Use the other thumb to palpate the lateral lobe with the sternocleidomastoid muscle retracted by the index and middle fingers of the same hand. Repeat the procedure for the other lobe by reversing the hand (Fig. 44.3). For the posterior approach, the examiner stands behind the patient. Push the trachea with the index and middle fingers of one hand. Use the index and middle fingers of the other hand to feel the lateral lobe with the thumb of the same hand pushed forward sternocleidomastoid. Repeat the procedure for the other lobe by reversing the hand (Fig. 44.4).

3. Auscultation The enlarged thyroid should be auscultated for bruits using the diaphragm of stethoscope. Bruits and venous hum are characteristic signs for Grave's disease. Systolic bruits have been reported in thyrotoxicosis. The enlarged thyroid can be divided into three classifications (Fig. 44.5). Class I The thyroid is palpable, however, not visible in normal position of the neck; Class II The thyroid is palpable and easily visible within the medial edge of sternocleidomastoid. Class III The thyroid extends beyond lateral edge of the sternocleidomastoid. Common causes of enlarged thyroid are as follows.

- Hyperthyroidism The enlarged thyroid is soft and a thrill may be felt by palpation. In addition, a bruit may be heard on the thyroid gland.
- Simple goiter, also called diffuse nontoxic goiter, can become extremely large with or without nodules. No signs of hyperthyroidism will be shown.
- Thyroid cancer can be hard and irregular nodules on palpation. Due to the slow growth rate, it should be differentiated from thyroid adenoma or enlarged anterior cervical lymph nodes.
- Chronic lymphocytic thyroiditis (Hashimoto's thyroiditis) can cause diffuse or nodular enlargement of the thyroid gland. It should be differentiated from thy-

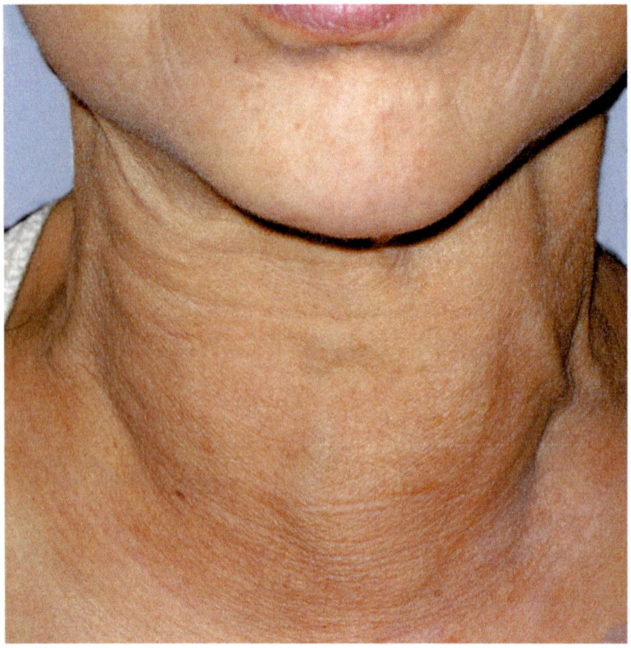

Fig. 44.5 Thyroid enlargement

roid cancer by carotid arterial pulsation. The carotid arterial pulsation can be felt on the edge of lateral lobes in Hashimoto's thyroiditis but not in thyroid cancer due to its infiltration into the tissues around the arteries.

- Parathyroid adenoma Parathyroids are located on the posterior side of the thyroid. Parathyroid adenoma may cause the protrusion of thyroid, which will move upward while swallowing. Symptoms and signs are important for the differential diagnosis.

44.6 Trachea

Trachea is located in the middle of the neck. Trachea exam is performed with the patient in a seated or supine position (Fig. 44.6). Gently bend the head to relax the sternomastoid muscle, place the examiner's index and ring fingers on suprasternal notch and use the middle finger to feel the trachea. Note the spaces between trachea and the sternomastoid, which should be equal on either side. The directions of tracheal deviation may indicate the underlying causes. Disorders causing tracheal deviation away from affected side include:

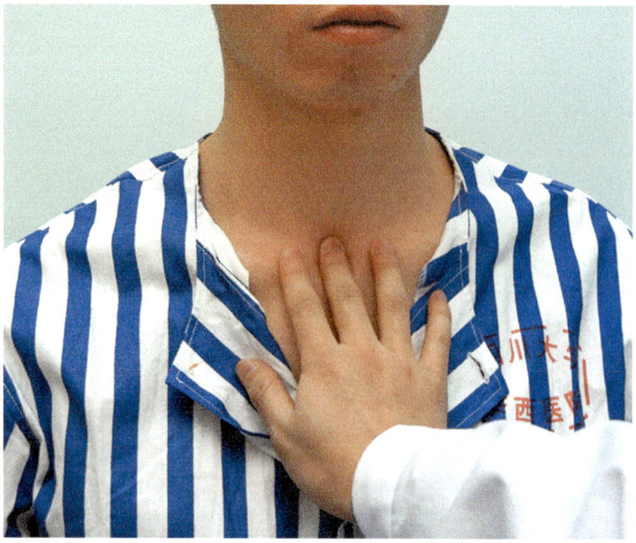

Fig. 44.6 Trachea examination

tension pneumothorax, large pleural effusion, mediastinal mass, and neck tumors. On the other hand, lung disorders causing tracheal deviation towards the affected side can be atelectasis pneumonectomy, fibrosis and atelectasis. Oliver's sign refers to the downward movement of trachea during systole in aortic aneurysm.

Key Terms		
1	Neck	颈部
2	Central venous pressure	中心静脉压
3	Jugular venous pressure	颈静脉压
4	Thyroid	甲状腺
5	Trachea	气管

Study Questions

1. How to examine and access neck masses?
2. How to measure JVP and CVP by inspection and palpation?
3. How to perform the palpation of the thyroid?
4. Please describe normal findings of the neck.
5. Identify anatomic landmarks of the neck.

Suggested Reading and Website

https://meded.ucsd.edu/clinicalmed/abbreviation.htm

Swartz MH. Textbook of physical diagnosis. 7th ed: Elsevier; 2014.

Physical Examination of Chest

45

Jianping Zhao, Weihong Jiang, and Rui Zeng

The chest is the upper part of the trunk between the neck and abdomen. The bony framework of chest is composed of the sternum, ribs and vertebral column. The skin, muscles, pleurae and the bony framework constitute the thorax. The diaphragm and thorax form the thoracic cavity, which is divided into two lateral compartments and one central compartment. The lateral compartments contain the left and right lungs and pleural cavities. The central compartment, occupied by the mediastinum, contains the pericardium, heart, great vessels, trachea, esophagus, thoracic duct, thymus, nerves, lymphatic vessels and lymph nodes. The purpose of chest examination is to determine whether the thoracic organs are in physiological or pathological state. The examination of chest wall, thorax and breast is mainly performed by inspection and palpation, while the heart and lungs should be examined in the sequence of inspection, palpation, percussion and auscultation.

45.1 Landmarks of the Chest Wall

Landmarks of the chest wall include bony landmarks, natural fossae and imaginary lines, which can be used to mark the position and contour of the thoracic organs, describe the location and range of the signs, and instruct the site of puncture or surgery.

45.1.1 Bony Landmarks

1. **Suprasternal notch** It is located at the top of the sternum and can be felt as a depression at the base of the neck.
2. **Manubrium sterni** It is the upper portion of the sternum with a hexagonal shape. Its upper part connects bilaterally to the sternal end of each clavicle, and its lower part connects to the body of the sternum.
3. **Sternal angle** The junction of the manubrium and the body of the sternum produces a slight angle protruding anteriorly, the angle of Louis. It connects bilaterally to the second costal cartilage and indicates the tracheal bifurcation, the upper level of the atria, the demarcation of upper and lower parts of mediastinum and the inferior border of the fourth thoracic vertebra.
4. **Xiphoid process** It is the most inferior portion of the sternum. Its bottom connects to the body of sternum. The length of xiphoid process varies widely in normal population.
5. **Suprabdominal angle** The angle between the right and left costal margins formed by the medial borders of the seventh to tenth costal cartilages, also termed infrasternal angle, is approximately 70°–110° in normal condition. It can be narrower in slender and wider in dumpy persons, and widens slightly during deep inspiration. The underlying region contains the left lobe of liver, stomach and pancreas.
6. **Rib** There are 12 pairs of ribs. They are curved and flat bones. The first seven sets of ribs, known as true ribs, are directly attached to the sternum through their own costal cartilages. The following five sets are known as false ribs, three of these sharing a common cartilaginous connection to the sternum, while the last two (ribs 11 and 12) are termed free ribs. They are attached to the vertebrae only, and not to the sternum or cartilage coming off of the sternum.
7. **Intercostal space** Ribs and their cartilages are separated by intercostal spaces that are occupied by intercostal muscles, vessels and nerves. The intercostal space between two ribs is numbered by the rib above it (Fig. 45.1).
8. **Scapula** It is a flat triangular bone that lies on the posterolateral aspect of the thorax, overlying the ribs 2–8.

J. Zhao
Department of Respiratory, Huazhong University of Science and Technology, Wuhan, China

W. Jiang
Department of Cardiology, Central South University, Changsha, China

R. Zeng (✉)
Department of Cardiology, Sichuan University, Chengdu, China

X.-H. Wan, R. Zeng (eds.), *Handbook of Clinical Diagnostics*, https://doi.org/10.1007/978-981-13-7677-1_45

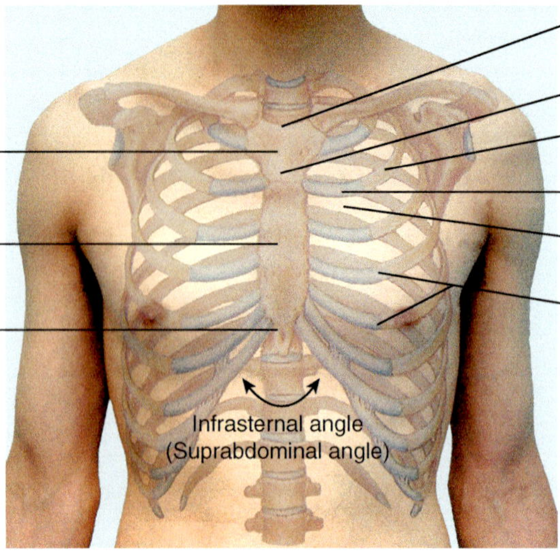

Fig. 45.1 The bony landmarks of the anterior chest wall

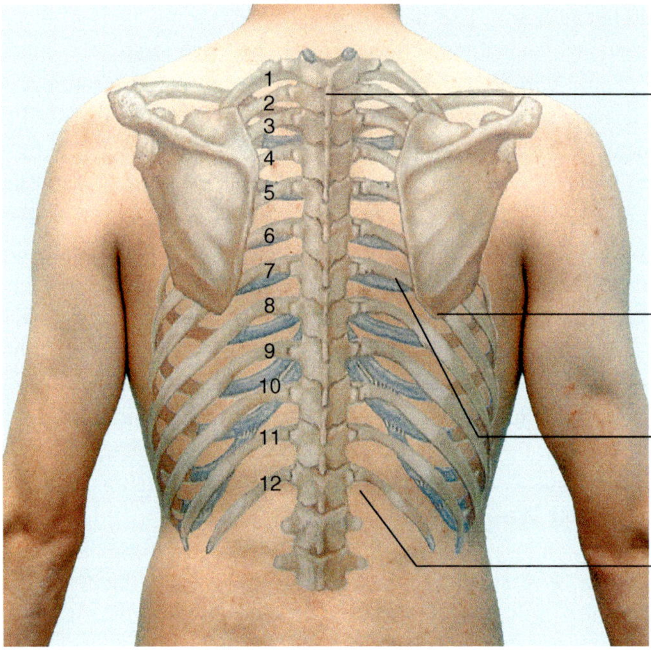

Fig. 45.2 The bony landmarks of the posterior chest wall

The spine of scapula and the acromion are palpated easily. When the upper limb is in the anatomical position, the inferior angle of the scapula lies at the level of the eighth thoracic vertebra, near the inferior border of the seventh rib or the seventh intercostal space.

9. **Spinous process** It marks the posterior midline. The seventh cervical spinous processis the most prominent one, which usually serves as the landmark for counting the thoracic vertebrae (Fig. 45.2).

45.1.2 Imaginary Lines

1. **Anterior midline** Namely midsternal line, a vertical line drawn through the middle of the sternum.
2. **Sternal line** **(L, R)** Vertical lines running along the vertical edges of the sternum and parallel to the anterior midline.
3. **Parasternal line** **(L, R)** Vertical lines at the middle of sternal line and midclavicular line.
4. **Midclavicular line** **(L, R)** Vertical lines drawn through the middle points of the clavicles and parallel to the anterior midline (Fig. 45.3).
5. **Anterior axillary line** **(L, R)** Vertical lines drawn along the anterior axillary folds and parallel to the anterior midline.
6. **Posterior axillary line** **(L, R)** Vertical lines parallel to the anterior midline and extending vertically along the posterior axillary folds.

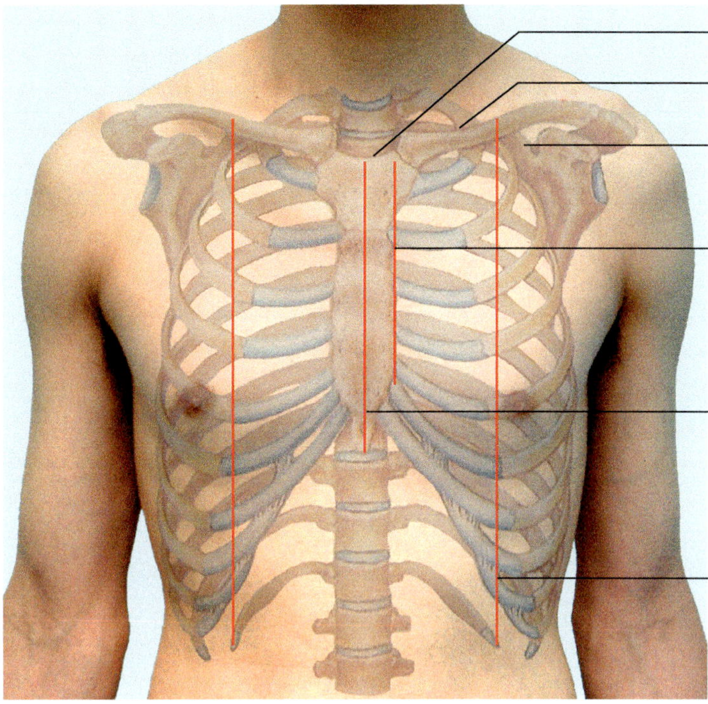

Fig. 45.3 The natural fossae and imaginary lines of the anterior chest wall

7. **Midaxillary line** (**L**, **R**) Vertical lines drawn from the vertex of the axilla and parallel to the anterior midline.
8. **Posterior midline** Namely midspinal line, a vertical line passing through the posterior spinous processes of the vertebrae.
9. **Scapular line** (**L**, **R**) Vertical lines parallel to the posterior midline and passing through the inferior angle of the scapula (Fig. 45.4).

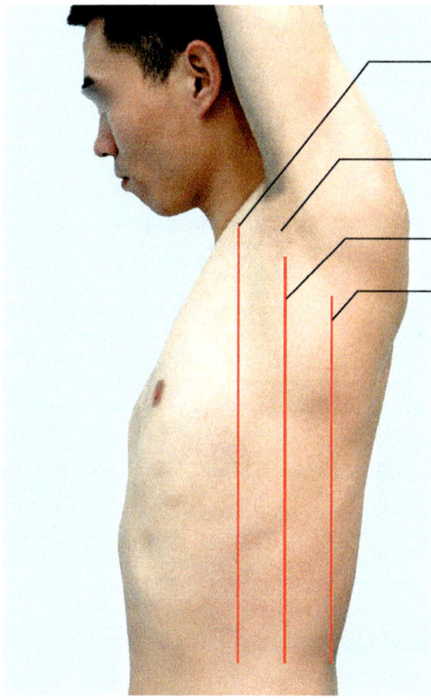

Fig. 45.4 The natural fossae and imaginary lines of the lateral chest wall

45.1.3 Natural Fossa and Anatomic Region

1. **Axillary fossa** (**L**, **R**) The pyramidal space inferior to the glenohumeral joint and superior to the skin and axillary fascia at the junction of the arm and thorax.
2. **Suprasternal fossa** The depressed region above the manubrium sterni, the trachea lies behind it in normal condition.
3. **Supraclavicular fossa** (**L**, **R**) The indentation immediately above the clavicle corresponding to the upper part of the lung apex.
4. **Infraclavicular fossa** (**L**, **R**) The indentation immediately below the clavicle with its lower border at the third rib, corresponding to the lower part of the lung apex.
5. **Suprascapular region** (**L**, **R**) The region above the spine of scapula with its upper lateral margin at the upper edge of the trapezius, corresponding to the lower part of the lung apex.
6. **Infrascapular region** (**L**, **R**) The region between the line through the inferior angles of scapula and the horizontal line through the twelfth thoracic vertebra.
7. **Scapular region** (**L**, **R**) The region inferior to the spine of scapula, superior to the inferior angle of scapula, and outside the medial border of scapula.
8. **Interscapular region** (**L**, **R**) The region between the medial borders of the two scapulae (Fig. 45.5).

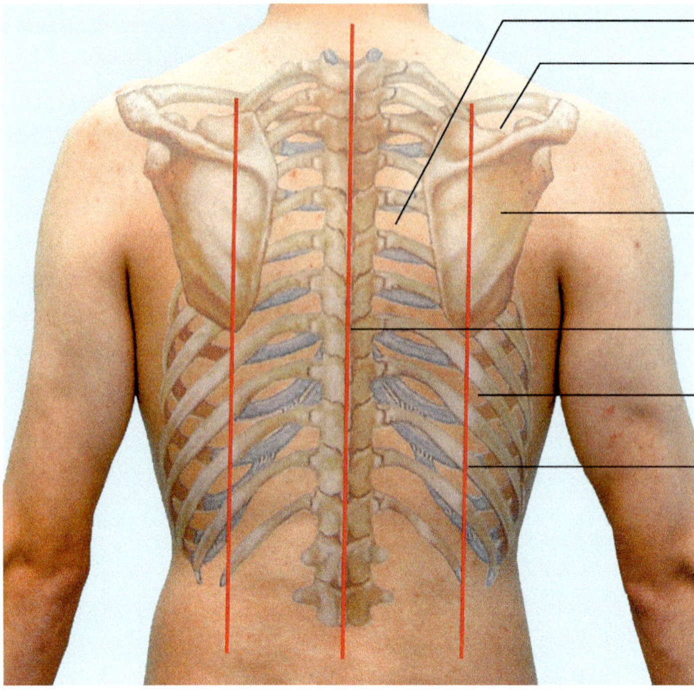

Fig. 45.5 The anatomic regions and imaginary lines of the posterior chest wall

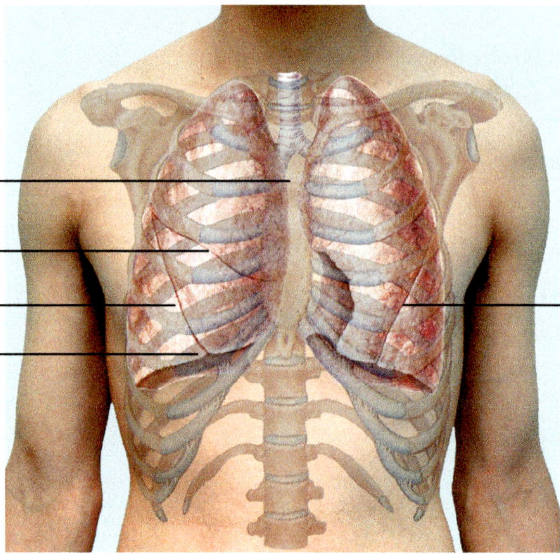

Fig. 45.6 Topography of lungs (anterior view)

45.1.4 Topography of Lungs and Pleura

The trachea descends anterior to the esophagus, enters the superior mediastinum and divides into right and left main bronchi at the level of the sternal angle. The right main bronchus is wider, shorter and steeper, while the left one is slender and oblique. The topography of lungs is shown in Figs. 45.6, 45.7, 45.8 and 45.9.

1. **Lung apex** It is blunt superior end of the lung ascending 2–4 cm above the inner third of the clavicle.
2. **Superior boundary of the lung** Its projection on the anterior chest wall forms an upward arc. It begins from the sternoclavicular joint, runs upward and outward to the level of the first thoracic vertebra, and then downwardly and outwardly ends at the border point of middle and inner third of the clavicle.
3. **Lateral boundary of the lung** It extends from the superior boundary of the lung, and approaches the inner surface of the lateral chest wall.
4. **Medial boundary of the lung** It descends from the sternoclavicular joint, the two sides nearly meet each other at the sternal angle, then runs down along the anterior midline and separates at the fourth costal cartilage level. The right boundary continues almost vertically downward, turns rightward at the sixth costal cartilage, and runs down to meet the inferior boundary. The left boundary turns leftward to the anterior end of the fourth rib, along

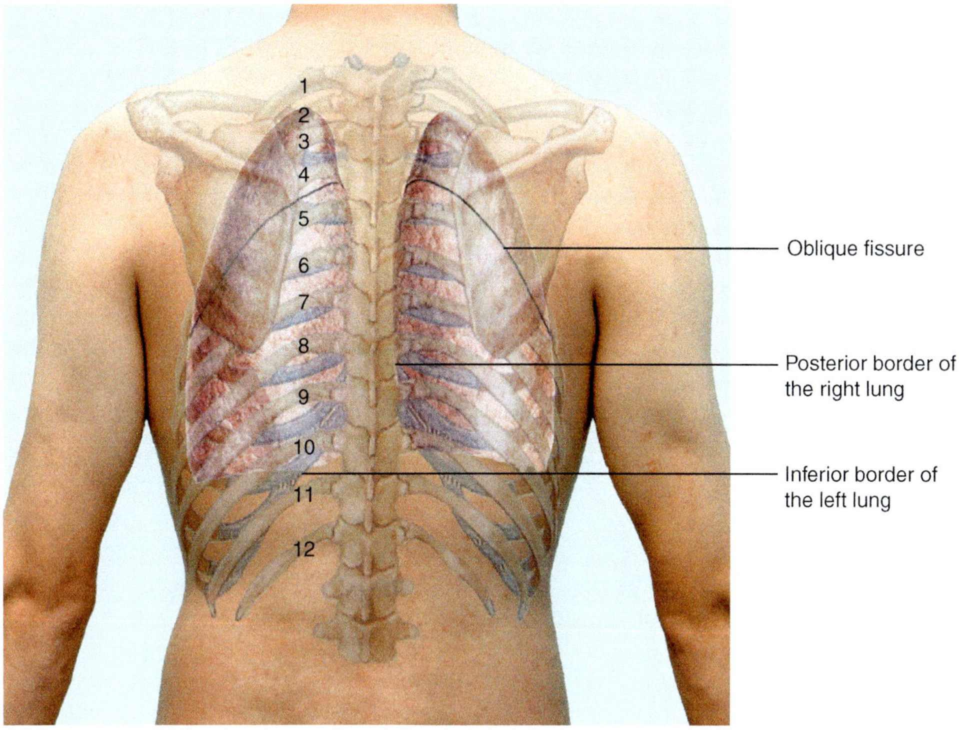

Fig. 45.7 Topography of lungs (posterior view)

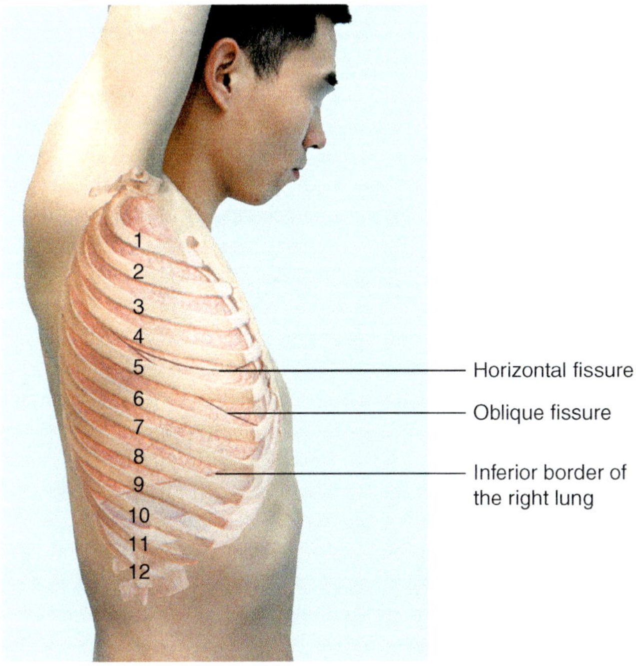

Fig. 45.8 Topography of the right lung (lateral view)

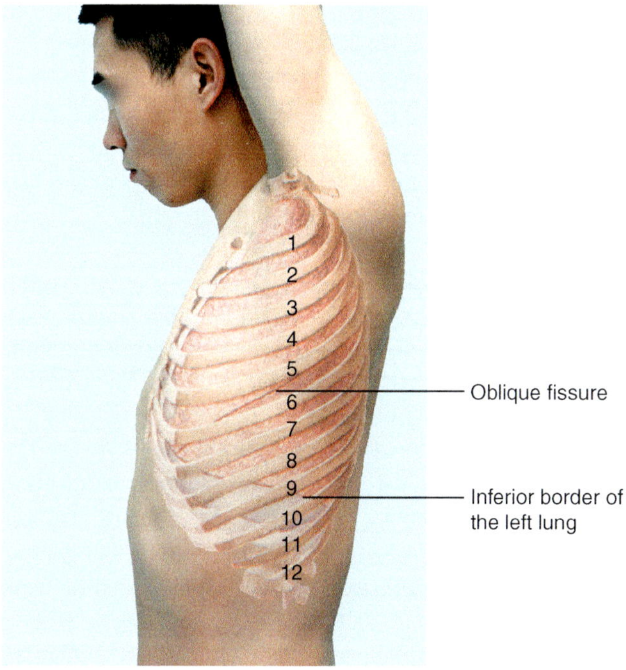

Fig. 45.9 Topography of the left lung (lateral view)

the anterior ends of ribs 4–6 downward, then turns left again at the level of the sixth costal cartilage to meet the inferior boundary.

5. **Inferior boundary of the lung** The inferior margins of the lungs extend to the sixth interspace at the midclavicular line, to the eighth interspace at the midaxillary line, and to the tenth interspace at the scapular line.

6. **Pleura** Each lung is enclosed in a serous pleural sac that consists of two continuous membranes, visceral pleura and parietal pleura. The visceral pleura covers the surface of the lungs and the parietal pleura lines the pulmonary cavities, adhering to the thoracic wall, the mediastinum and the diaphragm.

The interlobar fissures are situated between the lobes of the lungs. Both lungs have an oblique fissure, which begins from the anterior chest at the level of the sixth rib at the midclavicular line, extends laterally upward to the fourth rib at the posterior axillary line, and ends at the posterior chest at the spinous process of the third thoracic vertebra. The horizontal fissure is present only on the right and divides the right upper lobe from the right middle lobe. It begins from the fourth rib at the posterior axillary line, and ends at the right edge of sternum at the level of the fourth interspace.

45.2 Chest Wall, Thorax and Breast

45.2.1 Chest Wall

The physical examination of the chest wall includes inspection and palpation. The examiner should pay attention to the following aspects in addition to the nutrition, skin color and swelling, and lymph nodes.

45.2.1.1 Vein

Normally the venous pattern of the chest wall is barely perceptible. Superficial veins are sometimes visible in the subjects with little subcutaneous fat or the surface of breastfeeding women's breasts. The direction of blood flow should be determined if the superficial veins are distended or varicose. The common causes are portal hypertension, obstruction of the inferior or superior vena cava or the brachiocephalic vein, and substernal goiter.

Subcutaneous Emphysema

Subcutaneous emphysema is a condition that occurs when air or gas gets into tissues under the skin. Swelling of the chest wall can be inspected. In palpation, a characteristic crepitus or sensation of grasping snow can be detected for the movement of stored air in the subcutaneous tissue. The common causes for the subcutaneous emphysema of chest wall are thoracic trauma, ribs fracture, lung diseases such as tuberculosis, thoracic close drainage and thoracentesis, and artificial pneumothorax.

Chest Wall Tenderness

Normally there is no tenderness on chest wall. In intercostal neuritis, costal chondritis, soft tissue inflammation of chest wall and rib fractures, there may be tenderness in the involved portion. Tenderness and percussion pain of the sternum are common in the patients with leukemia.

45.2.1.2 Intercostal Space

It must be mentioned whether the intercostal space is narrow or bulging. Retraction of the intercostal space during inspiration indicates the obstruction of the respiratory tract. The so-called "three depression sign" includes the depressions of intercostal space, suprasternal fossa and supraclavicular fossa during inspiration. Bulging of the intercostal space can be seen in patients with massive pleural effusion, tension pneumothorax or severe emphysema.

45.2.2 Thorax

Normally, the thorax is bilaterally symmetrical and elliptical. In normal adults, the anterioposterior diameter of the thorax is shorter than the transverse diameter, and the ratio is approximately1:1.5. In the elderly and children, the anterioposterior diameter is a little shorter than or equal to the transverse diameter. Common changes of the thorax are shown in Fig. 45.10.

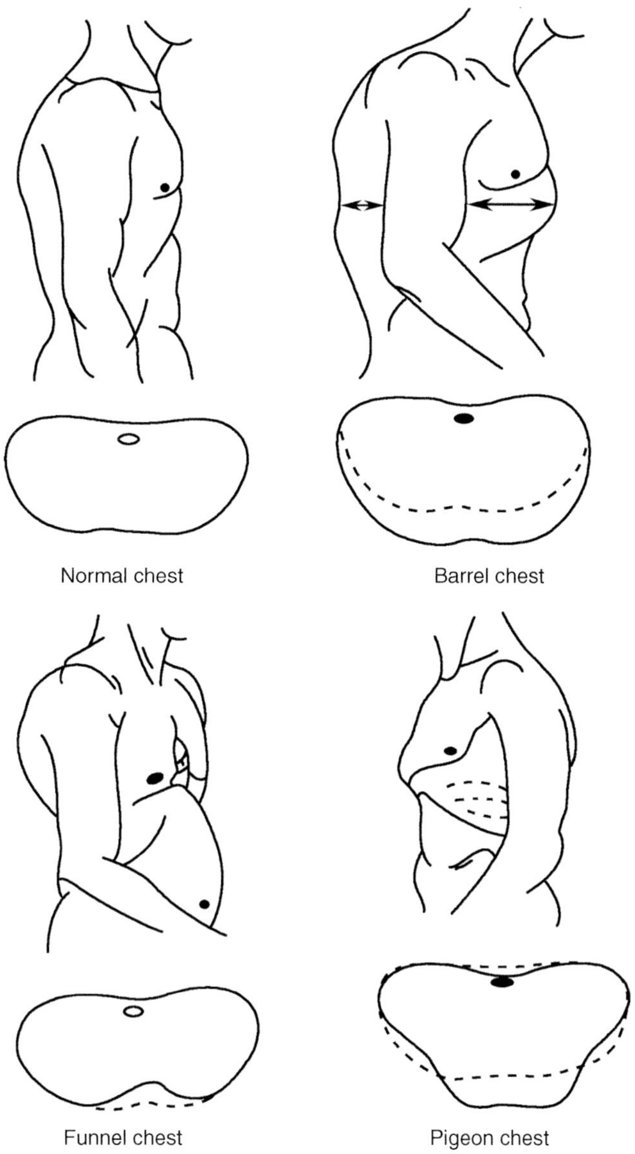

Fig. 45.10 Common changes of the thorax

45.2.2.1 Flat Chest

The thorax is flat and the anterioposterior diameter is less than half of the transverse diameter. This can be seen in the slender adults or patients with chronic consumptive diseases such as tuberculosis.

45.2.2.2 Barrel Chest

Barrel chest is a condition characterized by a significant increase in the anteroposterior diameter. This diameter is sometimes approximately equal to or even greater than the transverse diameter, resulting in the cylindric thorax. The angle between the ribs and spine is usually more than 45°. The interspaces become wider and full, and the infrasternal angle becomes greater. This can be seen in infants, the elderly or obese subjects, also seen in patients with asthma exacerbation or emphysema.

45.2.2.3 Rachitic Chest

Rachitic chest is a deformed thorax caused by rachitis, seen mostly in childhood. The sternal ends of rachitic ribs bulge at their costochondral junctions like rosary, termed rachitic rosary. The lower anterior part of ribs turns outward, where the rib cage along the attachment of the diaphragm is compressed to form a sulcus on the chest wall, called Harrison groove. The anteroposterior diameter is a little longer than the transverse diameter, the sternum is bulging and the adjacent ribs are depressed. This kind of thoracic deformity is called pigeon chest.

45.2.2.4 Funnel Chest

Funnel chest is the reverse of the pigeon chest. The lower costal cartilages, inferior sternum and xiphoid process are retracted toward the spine. Most cases are congenital.

45.2.2.5 Unilateral Deformation of the Thorax

Unilateral bulging of the thorax can be seen in massive effusion, pneumothorax, unilateral severe compensatory emphysema, giant pulmonary cyst, tumors, diaphragmatocele, etc. Unilateral retraction of the thorax is usually seen in atelectasis, pulmonary fibrosis, extensive pleural thickening and adhesion, etc.

Local Bulge of Chest Wall

Local bulge of chest wall may be caused by chest wall masses or intrathoracic lesions including skin nodules of chest wall, costal cartilage apophysis, rib lumps, manubrium sterni or suprasternal fossa apophysis, and precordial prominence.

Spine Malformations

The lordosis, kyphosis or scoliosis (Fig. 45.11) can result in asymmetric thorax, seen in congenital malformations, spine trauma, tuberculosis, etc.

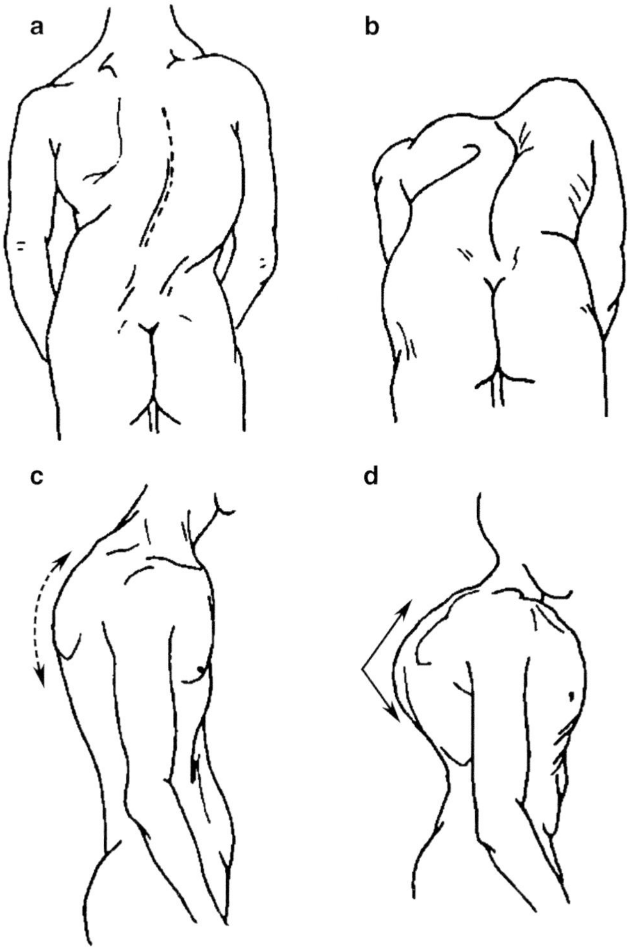

Fig. 45.11 Spine malformations

45.2.3 Breast

The breasts lie against the pectoral fascia of the anterior chest wall. In normal children and males, they are rudimentary. Female breasts become larger during adolescence, they are hemispheric, and the nipples also develop to cylindrical shape. The adult female breasts extend from the second rib to the sixth rib and from the sternal line to the midaxillary line. The upper outer part of breast may extend to the apex of the axilla. The nipple is usually at the level of the fourth intercostal space or the fifth rib. The breast is divided into four quadrants by imaginary vertical and horizontal lines intersecting at the nipple. The quadrants are named upper lateral, lower lateral, lower medial and upper medial (Fig. 45.12).

45.2.3.1 Inspection

1. **Symmetry and size** The two breasts are generally symmetrical in healthy females in the sitting position. Obvious enlargement of one breast can be seen in congenital

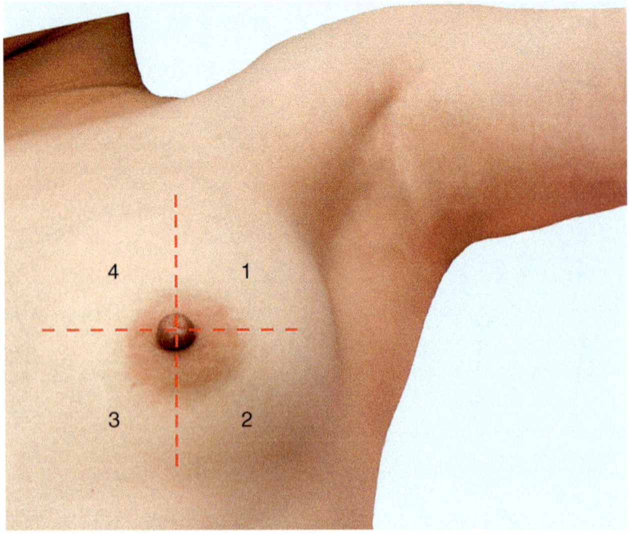

Fig. 45.12 Quadrants of the breast

malformation, cystogenesis, inflammation or tumors. Shrinkage of one breast often results from the maldevelopment.

2. **Skin of breast** Skin erythema of the breast is often associated with inflammation or cancer. Inflammation is always accompanied by local swelling, fever and pain. The skin color in breast cancer is usually dark red without fever or pain. Edema of the breast is seen in inflammation. However subcutaneous lymphatic obstruction by tumors can also lead to the lymphedema, which is always accompanied with depressed hair follicle and thickened skin, the involved skin looks like orange peel or pig skin. Local skin retraction of the breast may be caused by trauma or inflammation, which could also be an early sign of breast cancer.
3. **Nipple** Normal nipples are cylinder shaped. The size and color of the two nipples are similar. Nipple retraction since childhood indicates maldevelopment, while recent retraction suggests cancer or inflammation. The bloody discharge from the nipples is most often seen in breast cancer, while the clear and yellow secretion is usually seen in chronic cystic mastitis.
4. **Areola** The nipple is surrounded by pigmented circular skin called the areola. The color of areolae can range from pink to brown. The size and shape of areolae are also highly variable. The inspection of areolae includes the size, shape, symmetry, color and surface characteristics. Pregnancy or use of contraceptive pills can darken the areolae.

The axillary fossae and supraclavicular fossae should be observed to find whether there are masses, erythema, ulcerations, fistula or scars after inspection of the breasts.

45.2.3.2 Palpation

Breast palpation is performed in the sitting or supine position. When the patient lies supine, put a small pillow under the scapula and have the patient place her hands behind the head, so the breasts rest symmetrically on the chest wall. In the sitting position, have the patient sit in a chair with the arm down, or have the patient raise her arms over the head or press her hands downward on the hips if necessary.

Palpation should be performed from the upper outer quadrant clockwisely for the left breast and anticlockwisely for the right one. Every quadrant should be palpated superficially and then deeply. It should be noted whether there are nodules or discharge when palpating the nipples and areolae. In addition, the axillary fossae and supraclavicular fossae should be checked for lymphadenectasis. The following signs should be noted when palpating the breasts:

1. **Consistency and elasticity** Increase in consistency and loss in elasticity suggest the infiltration of subcutaneous tissue by inflammation or cancers. In addition, the consistency and elasticity of the nipples should also be checked.
2. **Tenderness** Local tenderness of the breast suggests inflammation, while tenderness is rare in breast cancer.
3. **Masses** Masses in the breast, the following items must be accurately described:
   - Location: use the nipple as the center of a clock face, state the o'clock position and the radial distance from the nipple.
   - Size: describe the length, transverse diameter and thickness of the mass in centimeters, e.g. 2 cm × 1 cm × 1 cm.
   - Number: single mass is common in breast cancer, while multiple masses are often seen in galactoma and mastofibroma.
   - Contour: note whether the shape is regular or not, the margin is smooth or not, the mass is fixed to the breast tissue or not. Benign masses usually have a smooth and regular contour, while malignant ones are often irregular and fixed.
   - Consistency: it can be described generally as soft, fluctuant, firm or hard. Benign tumors are usually soft or fluctuant, while malignant ones are often firm or hard.
   - Tenderness: Moderate to severe tenderness often results from inflammatory lesions, while tenderness is not common in malignant lesions.
   - Mobility: it should be determined whether the mass is movable or not. If the mass is movable only in a certain direction or fixed, it should also be determined whether the mass is fixed to the skin, the surrounding tissue or the deep structures. Most benign tumors are freely mobile, and inflammatory lesions

are less movable. Malignant masses are movable in the early stage. However, they become fixed with the disease progression due to the invasion of cancer into the surrounding tissues.

45.3 Lungs and Pleura

The physical examination of the lungs and pleura is the key of chest examination. The patient is examined in sitting or supine position. The lungs and pleura examination usually includes inspection, palpation, percussion and auscultation.

45.3.1 Inspection

45.3.1.1 Breathing Movement

Breathing movement is accomplished through the contraction and relaxation of the diaphragm and intercostal muscles. Normally, the inspiration is an active movement, leading to the expansion of the thorax, increasing the intrathoracic negative pressure and expansion of the lungs, resulting in the air flowing into the lungs from the upper respiratory tract. The expiration is a passive movement depending on the elastical recoil of the lungs and thorax, the air in the lungs is exhaled with the increased alveolar pressure.

1. **Thoracic respiration** and **diaphragmatic respiration** In healthy male adults and children, respiration is mainly driven by the diaphragm, so the lower part of thorax and the upper abdomen move up and down substantially, forming the diaphragmatic respiration. While the respiration in females is mainly dependent on intercostal muscles, this is called thoracic respiration. Actually, the two types of respiration exist simultaneously with different degrees. Diminished thoracic respiration and increased diaphragmatic respiration can be seen in extensive pneumonia, pulmonary edema, severe pulmonary tuberculosis, massive pleural effusion or pneumothorax. Diminished diaphragmatic respiration and increased thoracic respiration can be seen in peritonitis, massive ascites, extreme hepatosplenomegaly, giant abdominal tumor or advanced pregnancy.
2. **Paradoxical breathing** Normally, the expansion of thorax during inspiration is accompanied with the bulging of abdomen. The paradoxical inward motion of the abdomen as the rib cage expands during inspiration is termed paradoxical breathing, which can be seen in diaphragmatic paralysis or fatigue.
3. **Dyspnea** Namely difficulty in breathing, the manifestations may include mouth breathing, shrugging, orthopnea and sweating. Dyspnea is divided into inspiratory dyspnea, expiratory dyspnea and mixed dyspnea based on the phases when dyspnea appears.

45.3.1.2 Respiratory Frequency

The respiratory rate in the newborn is about 44 cycles per minute, and the rate diminishes gradually until maturity. At rest, the normal rate in adults is between 12 and 20, and the ratio of respiration to pulse is 1:4.

1. **Tachypnea** It is defined as increased respiratory rate over 24 cycles per minute, mainly seen in fever, pain, hypoxia, anemia, hyperthyroidism and heart failure. In general, the body temperature rises 1 °C, the respiratory rate increases 4 cycles per minute.
2. **Bradypnea** It is defined as decreased respiratory rate less than 12 cycles per minute, often seen in narcotic or sedative overdose or increased intracranial pressure (Fig. 45.13).

45.3.1.3 Respiratory Depth

1. **Shallow breathing** It can be seen in respiratory center inhibition or respiratory muscle weakness such as narcotic or sedative overdose or Guillain-Barre Syndrome, also seen in severe intestinal tympanites, ascites, obesity

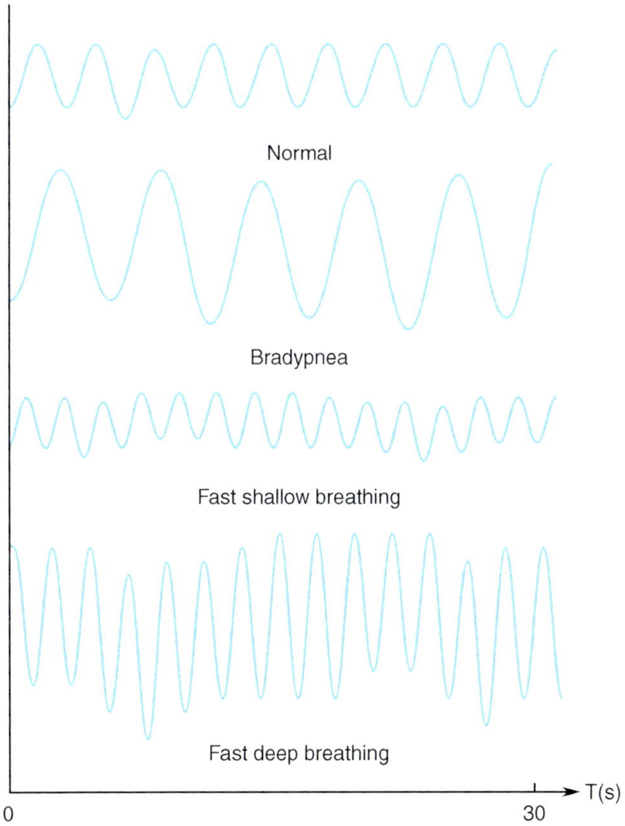

Fig. 45.13 The changes of respiratory frequency

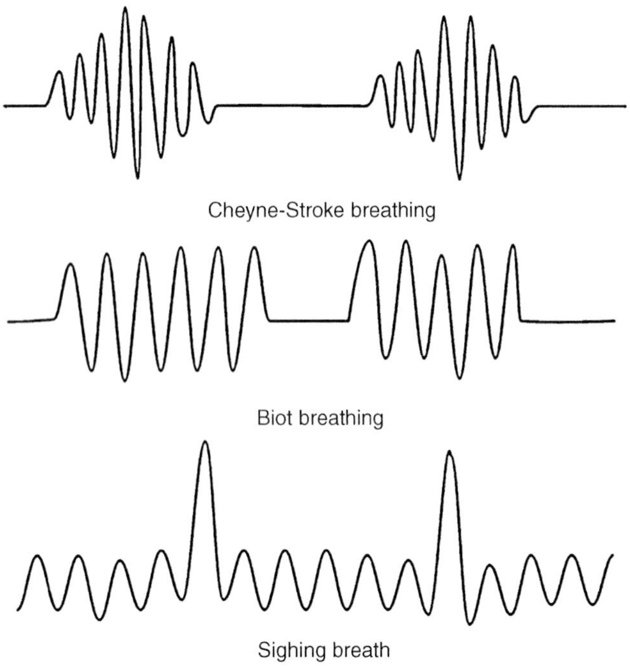

Fig. 45.14 The changes of respiratory rhythm and range

or lung disease such as extensive pneumonia, pulmonary edema, massive pleural effusion or pneumothorax.

2. **Deep breathing** It is often seen in strenuous exercise, excessive emotion or overstress. The deep breathing in diabetic ketoacidosis or uremic acidosis is termed Kussmaul breathing. The decreased pH of body fluids stimulates the respiratory center, which causes hyperventilation.

Respiratory Rhythm and Range

At rest, normal respirations are regular and smooth. The rhythm and range may change in many disease states (Fig. 45.14).

1. **Tidal breathing** It is also known as Cheyne-Stroke breathing. Both respiratory rhythm and range change in this breathing pattern. Respirations are interrupted by periods of apnea. In each cycle, the rate and amplitude of successive breaths increase to a maximum, then progressively diminish into the next apneic period. Each cycle of tidal breathing lasts 30 s to 2 min, and the apneic period lasts 5–30 s. Mild tidal breathing can be seen in the sleep of the elderly. However, in most cases, it implies a critical illness with poor prognosis, seen in central nervous system diseases, uremia, diabetic ketoacidosis and barbitalism.
2. **Biot breathing** It is an uncommon variant of tidal breathing, periods of apnea alternate irregularly with series of breaths of equal depth that terminate abruptly. The pathogenesis of Biot breathing is almost the same as tidal breathing, however the inhibition of respiratory center is more serious, the patient's condition and prognosis is much worse. The diseases that cause Biot breathing are similar to those causing the tidal breathing.
3. **Sighing breath** The normal respiratory rhythm at rest is occasionally interrupted by a long, deep sigh. It is commonly seen in panasthenia, psychentonia or depression.

45.3.2 Palpation

In addition to the skin temperature, humidity, tenderness and masses, the thoracic expansion, vocal fremitus and pleural friction fremitus are the key items for palpation.

45.3.2.1 Thoracic Expansion

It is the movement range of the thorax during respiration and is usually examined on the anterior or posterior lower thorax. When testing the expansion of the anterior lower chest, place your hands on the chest with the extended thumbs lying along the inferior edges of the costal margins, and their tips nearly touching (about 2 cm). When testing the expansion of the posterior lower chest, place your thumbs at the level of the tenth rib. To provide slack, press the soft tissues and pull your hands medially until your thumbs meet over the vertebral spines. Have the patient inspire deeply, watch the divergence of your thumbs as the thorax expands, and feel the range and symmetry of respiratory movement (Fig. 45.15).

1. **Unilateral increase in thoracic expansion** It occurs when the contralateral lung expansion is restricted, such as contralateral diaphragmatic paralysis, pulmonary atelectasis and rib fractures.
2. **Unilateral decrease in thoracic expansion** It results from the unilateral decrease of lung elasticity or air content, or restricted lung or thoracic expansion caused by the unilateral pleural thickening or rib and soft tissue lesions.
3. **Bilateral increase in thoracic expansion** It can be seen in diseases that cause the diminished diaphragmatic respiration, such as ascites, hepatosplenomegaly, giant abdominal tumor, acute peritonitis and subdiaphragmatic abscess.
4. **Bilateral decrease in thoracic expansion** It can be seen in central nervous system diseases, peripheral neuropathy, respiratory muscle weakness or extensive lung lesions.
5. **Paradoxical respiration of the bilateral thorax** It usually results from traumatic injury to the thorax in which multiple adjacent ribs are broken in multiple places. The healthy side of thorax expands during inspiration, while the injured side retracts. On the contrary, the health side retracts during expiration, and the injured side expands.

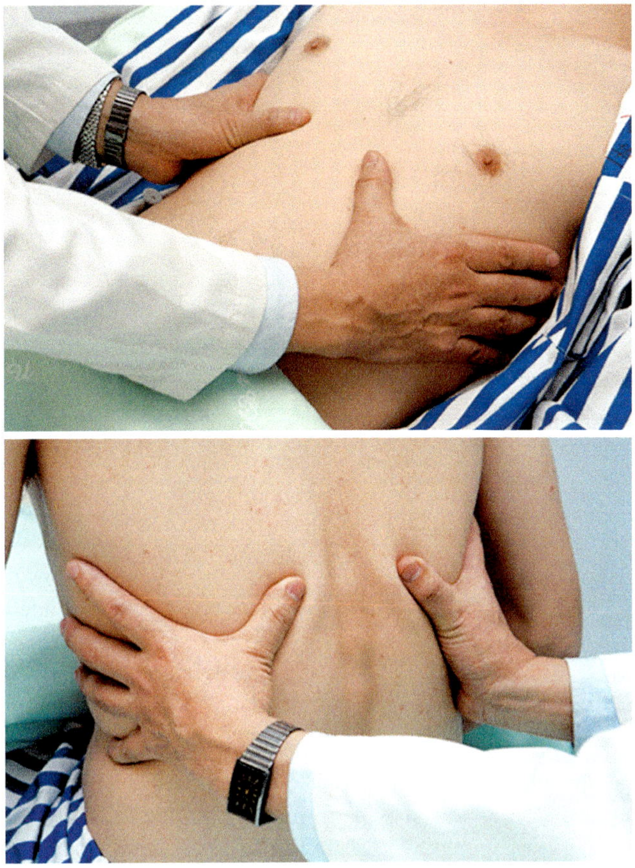

Fig. 45.15 Thoracic expansion

45.3.2.2 Vocal Fremitus

During speech, the patient's vocal cords set up vibrations in the bronchial air column that are conducted to the thoracic wall through the lung septae, where they may be perceived by vibratory palpation, as vocal fremitus. The intensity of vocal fremitus is associated with the conductivity of the lungs and chest wall, so it can reflect the characteristics of intrathoracic lesions. Place your palms or the ulnar sides of your hands on the patient's chest wall symmetrically and ask the patient to repeat the test words "yi", using the same pitch and intensity of voice each time. Feel the vibrations and compare symmetrical parts of the chest sequentially. The techniques for palpating the vocal fremitus are shown in Fig. 45.16. The locations and sequence are shown in Fig. 45.17.

Vocal fremitus is decreased or absent in the following situations: (1) alveoli contain too much gas such as emphysema; (2) bronchial obstruction caused by bronchial carcinoma, bronchial tuberculosis or increased bronchial secretions; (3) massive pleural effusion or pneumothorax; (4) severe pleural thickening and adhesion; (5) subcutaneous emphysema or edema of the chest wall.

Vocal fremitus is increased in the following situations: (1) lung consolidation such as lobar pneumonia; (2) large cavity in the lung, especially when the cavity is close to the chest wall and the surrounding tissue is infiltrated by inflammation, such as cavitary pulmonary tuberculosis and pulmonary abscess; (3) compression atelectasis.

Fig. 45.16 The detection of vocal fremitus

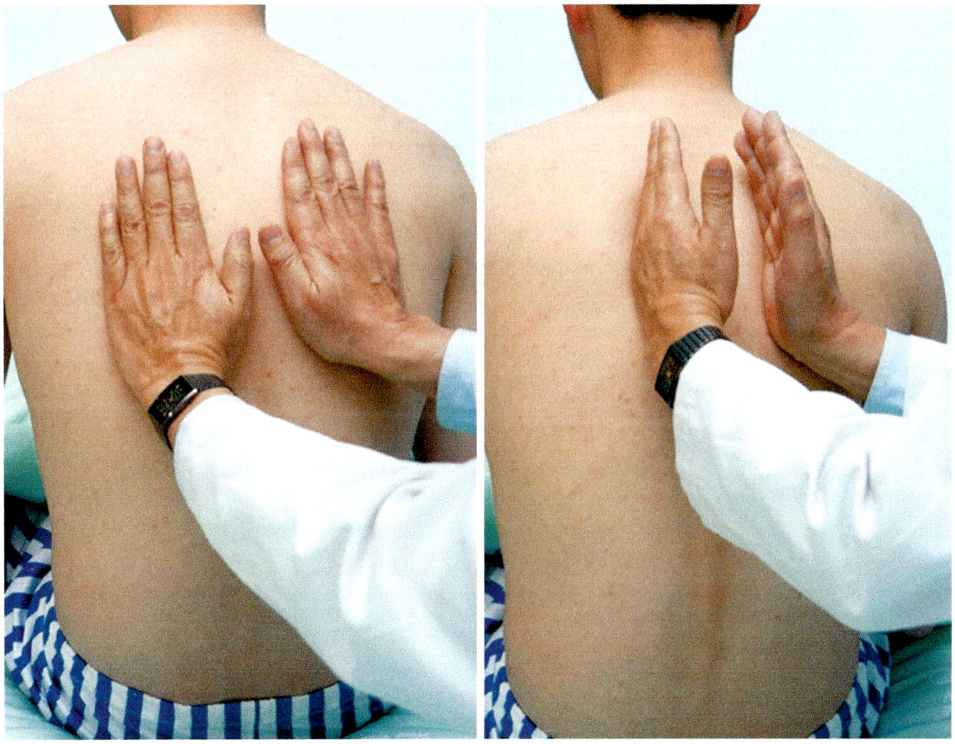

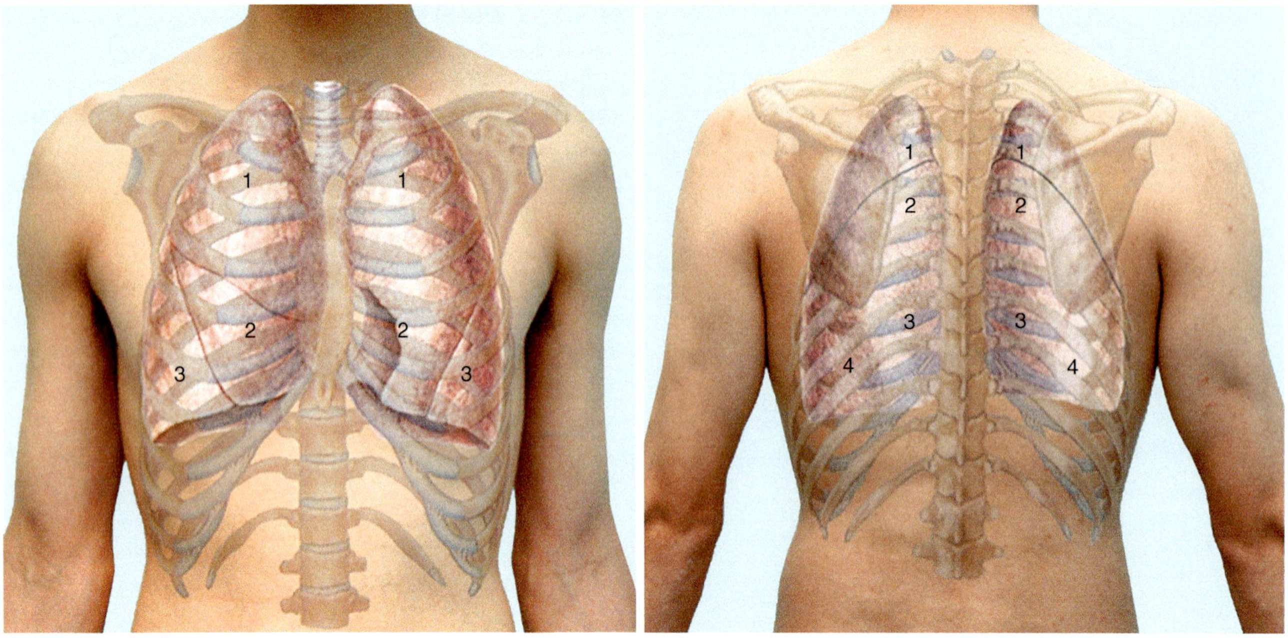

Fig. 45.17 The locations and sequence for palpating the vocal fremitus

45.3.2.3 Pleural Friction Fremitus

Normally, there is no pleural friction fremitus during breathing movement. It may be felt when the pleural layers are inflamed and lose their lubrication. The tactile sensation is like two pieces of leather being rubbed together. This sign is most obvious in the lower part of the thorax. It can be palpated during both phases of respiration and is more obvious at the end of inspiration and the beginning of expiration. The friction fremitus disappears when the patient holds the breath. Have the patient take deep and slow breaths in the supine position and place your palms on the patient's chest to feel for friction fremitus. It may be felt in the following diseases: (1) pleuritis; (2) primary or secondary pleural tumors; (3) severe pleural dryness such as severe dehydration; (4) lung diseases involving the pleura such as pneumonia; (5) others such as diabetes mellitus and uremia.

45.3.3 Percussion

45.3.3.1 Techniques of Percussion

Have the patient relax and breathe evenly in the sitting or supine position, percuss the chest symmetrically from the top down and from anterior to posterior part. Hyperextend the middle finger of your left hand as the pleximeter finger and place its distal interphalangeal joint firmly against the patient's chest wall. The pleximeter finger is usually placed in the intercostal space with its direction parallel to the ribs. However the direction should be parallel to the spine when percussing the interscapular region. With the end of your right middle finger (plexor finger), use a quick flick of the wrist to strike the pleximeter finger 2–3 times, and then withdraw your striking finger quickly. This is called mediate percussion. Sometimes, the immediate percussion is performed by striking the thoracic wall directly with the fingers or hand.

45.3.3.2 Normal Percussion Notes of the Thorax

The normal percussion note of the lungs is resonance, but there is a little difference among various parts. The percussion note is relatively dullin the upper part of the anterior thorax than the lower part, relatively dull in the upper right part of the thorax than the upper left part, relatively dull in the posterior chest than the anterior chest. It is relatively dull in the lower right lung due to the influence of the liver. The percussion note is tympany in the area near the stomach bubble (Fig. 45.18).

45.3.3.3 Percussion of the Lung Boundary

1. **Superior boundary of the lung**
   It is the width of the apices. Its inner side is the cervical muscle, and its outer side is the shoulder girdle. Have the patient sit and stand behind him, percuss from the central part of the anterior edge of the trapezius muscle to inner side and outer side respectively until dullness replaces resonance. The width of the resonant boundary is the width of apices, normally 4–6 cm. The right one is slightly narrower than the left one. Narrowed boundary is often seen in pulmonary tuberculosis, pneumonia, lung tumors, pleural thickening or encapsulated pleural effusion at the apices. Widened boundary is often seen in pulmonary emphysema, pneumothorax or pulmonary bulla at the apices.

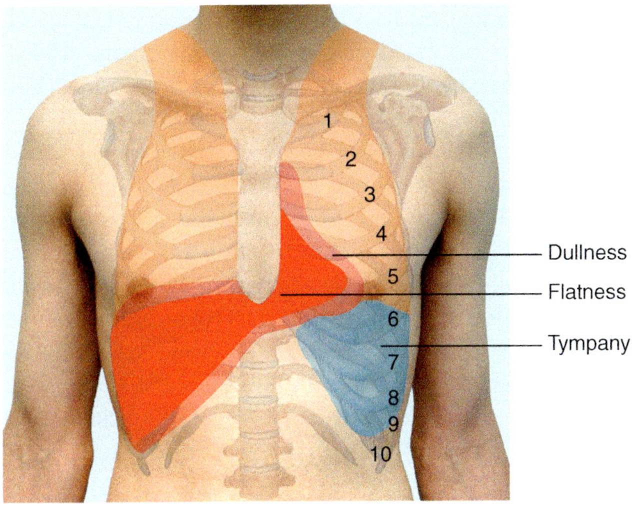

Fig. 45.18 Normal percussion notes of the anterior chest

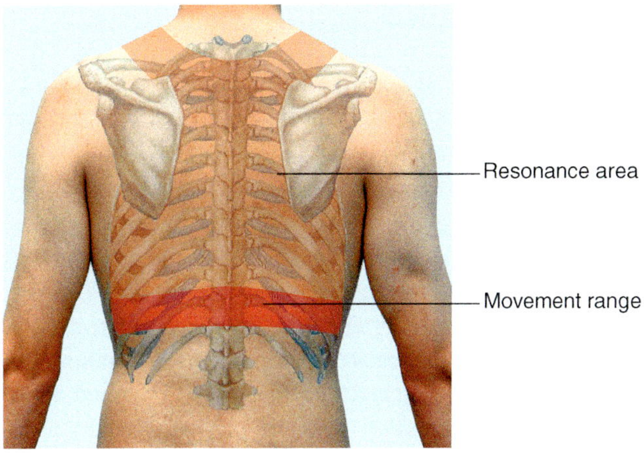

Fig. 45.19 Normal movement range of the inferior lung boundary

2. **Anterior boundary of the lung**
   Normally, the anterior boundary of the lung is equivalent to the cardiac dullness. The right boundary is at the sternal line and the left one is at the parasternal line from the fourth to sixth interspace. The dullness area between the two boundaries enlarges in patients with cardiomegaly, pericardial effusion, aortic aneurysm or hilar lymph node enlargement, while it narrows in patients with pulmonary emphysema.
3. **Inferior boundary of the lung**
   Percuss the inferior boundary of the lung at the midclavicular, midaxillary and scapular lines. Have the patient breathe calmly and percuss from the top down until dullness replaces resonance to determine the level of inferior lung boundary. At rest, it is located at the sixth interspace at the midclavicular line, the eighth interspace at the midaxillary line and the tenth interspace at the scapular line. However it varies slightly in different somatotypes and development situations. In pathological conditions such as pulmonary emphysema, pulmonary bulla and abdominal viscera prolapse, the inferior lung boundary descends. It ascends in pulmonary atelectasis, pleural effusion, meteorism, ascites, giant intraabdominal tumors, phrenoparalysis, etc.
4. **Movement range of the inferior lung boundary**
   It is equivalent to the diaphragmatic movement range during deep breathing. Firstly, determine the level of the inferior lung boundary during quiet respiration. Secondly, ask the patient to take a deep breath and hold it, percuss downward until dullness replaces resonance and mark the level. Thirdly, ask the patient to exhale deeply and hold breath, percuss the inferior lung boundary again and mark the level. The distance between the two marks is the movement range of the inferior lung boundary. It is usually examined at the scapular line, normally 6–8 cm (Fig. 45.19). It is decreased in patients with pulmonary emphysema, atelectasis, pulmonary fibrosis, pulmonary inflammation or edema, etc.

45.3.3.4 Abnormal Percussion Notes of the Thorax

When lung resonance is replaced by dullness, flatness, hyperresonance or tympany, pathological changes of lung, pleura, diaphragm or chest wall are suggested. The type of abnormal percussion note depends on the nature, extent and location of the lesions. Deep lesions, lesions with diameter less than 3 cm or a small amount of pleural effusion cannot be detected by percussion.

1. **Abnormal dullness or flatness** It results from the reduction of air content in lung tissue, non air containing lesions, pleural lesions or localized swelling of the chest wall tissue.
2. **Hyperresonance** It results from the decrease in pulmonary elasticity and increase in air content in lung tissue, such as pulmonary emphysema.
3. **Tympany** It results from the marked increase in air content in lung tissue such as pulmonary bulla, huge cavity and pneumothorax. In huge cavity with superficial location and smooth wall, or tension pneumothorax, the percussion note is tympany with metal-like echoes, called amphorophony.
4. **Dullness-tympany** When the alveolar wall is relaxed and the air content is reduced, such as pulmonary atelectasis, congestive or dispersed phase of pneumonia and pulmonary edema, the percussion note is a mixed sound which has the characters of both dullness and tympany, called dullness-tympany.

45.3.4 Auscultation

Auscultate the lungs with the patient in the sitting, semi-reclining or recumbent position. Preferably, have the patient sit with the chest fully exposed. Demonstrate how you wish the patient to breathe through the mouth, deeper and slightly more forcefully than usual. Start auscultating with the stethoscope diaphragm anteriorly at the apices and work downward, then listen to the back, comparing symmetrical points sequentially. The sites of auscultation of the anterior chest include the supraclavicular fossae, the upper, middle and lower parts at the midclavicular lines, the upper and lower parts at the anterior axillary lines and at the midaxillary lines, totally 16 sites. The sites of auscultation of the back include the upper and lower parts at the posterior axillary lines and in the interscapular region, and the inner and outer parts in the infrascapular region, totally 12 sites. Auscultate each point at least 1–2 respiratory cycles. During auscultation, note the location, loudness, pitch and quality of the breath sounds and adventitious sounds, and their relationships to the respiratory phases.

45.3.4.1 Normal Breath Sounds

1. **Bronchial breath sound** It is the sound of turbulence produced by the respiratory air flow through the glottis, trachea or main bronchi. Bronchial breath sound is loud and high pitched. The expiratory sound is louder and higher pitched and lasts longer than the inspiratory sound. Normally, it is heard in the suprasternal notch and over the sixth and seventh cervical spines and the first and second thoracic spines.
2. **Vesicular breath sound** It is produced by the respiratory air flowing through the bronchioli and alveoli. It is soft and low pitched. The inspiratory sound is louder and higher pitched and lasts longer than the expiratory sound. Normally, it is heard almost over the entire lung surface, except the sites where bronchial and bronchovesicular breath sound can be heard.
3. **Bronchovesicular breath sound** It is a mixed sound which has the characters of both bronchial and vesicular breath sound. The inspiratory sound is similar to vesicular breath sound, but louder and higher pitched. The expiratory sound is similar to bronchial breath sound, but softer, lower pitched and shorter in duration. Normally, it is heard over the first and second interspace near the sternum and the interscapular region at the level of the third and fourth thoracic spines (Fig. 45.20).

45.3.4.2 Abnormal Breath Sounds

Abnormal Vesicular Breath Sound

1. **Diminished or absent vesicular breath sound** This is usually caused by the decreased transmission of vesicular breath sound, the restriction of the thorax or lung expansion, or the decreased alveolar ventilation or airflow volume and velocity due to the insufficient respiratory drive or increased resistance. It can be unilateral, bilateral or localized.
   - Decreased transmission of vesicular breath sound: pneumothorax, pleural effusion or pleural thickening.
   - Restriction of the thorax or lung expansion: unilateral diminished vesicular breath sound can be seen in complete atelectasis, malpositioned endotracheal tube with tip in one main bronchus or rib fractures. Bilateral decrease can be seen in advanced pregnancy, massive ascites or giant abdominal tumor. Localized decrease can be seen in lobar atelectasis.

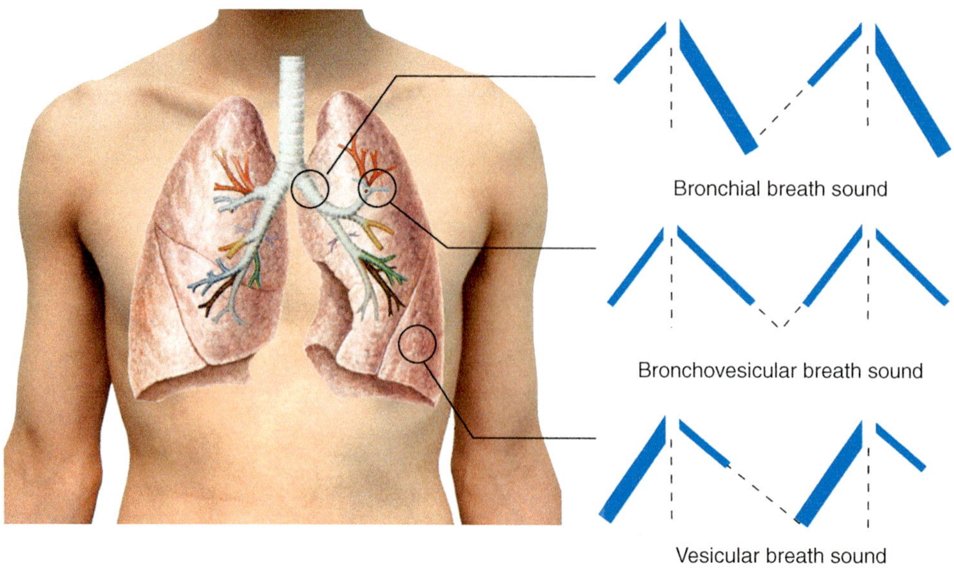

Fig. 45.20 The three types of normal breath sounds

- Insufficient respiratory drive: unilateral decrease can be seen in diaphragm paralysis. Bilateral decrease can be seen in respiratory center inhibition, narcotic or sedative overdose, hypokalemia or respiratory muscle fatigue.
- Increased airway resistance: unilateral decrease can be seen in central lung cancer or lymphoma. Bilateral decrease can be seen in chronic bronchitis, asthma or obstructive pulmonary emphysema. Localized decrease can be seen in bronchial tuberculosis, foreign body or tumor.

2. **Increased vesicular breath sound** This is mainly caused by the increased alveolar ventilation or airflow volume and velocity due to the enhanced breathing movement or the increased transmission due to the thin chest wall. It can be unilateral or bilateral. The common causes are as follows:
   - Physiological enhancement: infants or adults with thin chest wall or in physical activity.
   - Pathological enhancement: fever, hypermetabolism, anemia or acidosis. Unilateral lung or pleural lesions result in contralateral increase in vesicular breath sound as compensation, such as pneumonia, pneumothorax, etc.
3. **Extension of expiratory sound** This is mainly caused by the increased lower airway resistance, common in chronic bronchitis or asthma attack. In addition, reduced lung tissue elasticity also results in the extension of expiratory sound such as emphysema.
4. **Discontinuous breath sound** Due to the local pulmonary inflammation or bronchial stenosis, the air cannot enter the alveoli smoothly, which results in discontinuous breath sound. It is also termed cogwheel breath sound, common in patients with pneumonia.
5. **Coarse breath sound** It is caused by the mild edema or inflammatory infiltration of the bronchial mucosa, seen in the early stage of bronchitis or pneumonia.

Abnormal Bronchial Breath Sound

Bronchial breath sound heard at the locations where vesicular breath sound should be heard is abnormal bronchial breath sound, also termed tubular breath sound.

1. **Lung consolidation** It facilitates transmission of breath sound. The location, range and intensity of bronchial breath sound are associated with the location, size and depth of lesions, the larger and the shallower the lesion, the louder the sound, and vice versa. Abnormal bronchial breath sound is often heard in the consolidation stage of lobar pneumonia, pulmonary embolism or cheesy pneumonia.
2. **Large cavity in the lung** When there is a cavity in the lung surrounded by consolidated lung tissue and communicating with the bronchi, the breath sound resonates in the cavity and is transmitted well. So the bronchial breath sound can be heard clearly, often seen in pulmonary abscess or cavitary pulmonary tuberculosis.
3. **Compression atelectasis** In pleural effusion or massive pericardial effusion, compression at electasis facilitates transmission of breath sound. So the bronchial breath sound may be heard over the area above pleural effusion or the compressed part of the lower left lung. The sound is weak and distant.

Abnormal Bronchovesicular Breath Sound

When the consolidated part is small and mixed with normal lung tissue or the consolidated part is deep and covered by normal lung tissue, abnormal bronchovesicular breath sound can be heard. This is common in bronchopneumonia, pulmonary tuberculosis, early stage of lobar pneumonia or over the area of atelectasis above pleural effusion.

45.3.4.3 Rales

Rales are adventitious sounds that are absent in the normal lung, including moist rales and rhonchi.

Moist Rales

Moist rales are produced by the air bubbling through thin secretions in the respiratory tract such as exudate, sputum, blood, mucus and pus during inspiration, also called bubble sounds. They may also result from the opening and closing of alveoli and small airways during respiration.

1. **Characteristics of moist rales** They are intermittent and transient, and apparent during inspiration, especially at the end of inspiration, sometimes in the early phase of expiration. The location is fixed and the quality is invariable. Medium and fine rales can exist simultaneously. Coarse and medium rales may disappear after coughing, while rales caused by bronchiectasis and fine rales do not disappear after coughing.
2. **Classification of moist rales**
   - Moist rales are classified into loud rales and non-loud rales according to the loudness. Loud rales are produced because there is good conductive medium around the lesions, which are common in pneumonia, pulmonary abscess or cavitary pulmonary tuberculosis. Non-loud rales result from the decreased transmission when the lesions are surrounded by lots of normal lung tissue. The sounds are distant.
   - Moist rales are classified into coarse, medium, fine rales and crepitus according to the quality. Coarse rales, also named as large bubble sound, occur in the trachea, main bronchi or cavity in the early phase of inspiration. They are common in bronchiectasis, severe pulmonary edema, or pulmonary tuberculosis

or abscess with cavities. Medium rales, also named as medium bubble sound, occur in the medium sized bronchi in the middle phase of inspiration. They are common in bronchitis or bronchopneumonia. Fine rales, also named as fine bubble sound, occur in the small bronchi in the late phase of inspiration. They are common in bronchiolitis, bronchopneumonia, pulmonary congestion or pulmonary infarction. Velcro rales, the high pitched fine rales, can be heard at the base of the lungs of patients with diffuse interstitial pulmonary fibrosis at the end of deep inspiration. Crepitus, very fine and uniform rales, can often be heard in the terminal phase of inspiration. Crepitus is very similar to the sound produced by rubbing hair next to the ear. It is common in the inflammation or congestion of bronchioles and alveoli such as pulmonary congestion, early stage of pneumonia and pulmonary alveolitis.

- Moist rales are classified into localized and bilateral diffuse rales according to the location. Localized and fixed rales indicate local lesions such as pneumonia, pulmonary tuberculosis, bronchiectasis, pulmonary abscess and pneumonia secondary to lung cancer. Moist rales at the base of both lungs are heard in pulmonary congestion due to heart failure. Bilateral diffuse moist rales are heard in acute pulmonary edema, bronchopneumonia or chronic bronchitis.
- Moist rales are classified into early and late inspiratory rales according to the time of their occurrence. Late inspiratory rales can be heard in pneumonia or diffuse interstitial pulmonary fibrosis. Early inspiratory rales are often heard in chronic obstructive pulmonary disease. Both early and late inspiratory rales can be heard in congestive heart failure (Fig. 45.21).

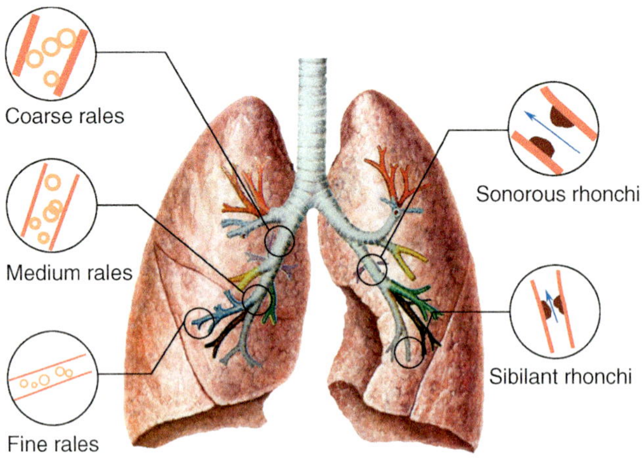

Fig. 45.21 Mechanism and sites of rales generation

Dry Rales/Rhonchi

Dry rales/rhonchi are produced by the turbulent air flow due to the stenosis or partial obstruction of the trachea, bronchi or bronchioles, which may be caused by bronchospasm, edema, secretions, intraluminal neoplasm or foreign body, or the compression by extraluminal enlarged lymph nodes or mediastinal tumors.

1. **Characteristics of rhonchi** They are continuous, relatively long, musical and high pitched adventitious sounds, and can be heard in both phases of respiration, especially during expiration. Rhonchi are variable in intensity, quality and location. Rhonchi that occur in the trachea or main bronchus may be heard without a stethoscope.
2. **Classification of rhonchi**
    - Rhonchi are classified into sibilant and sonorous rhonchi according to the pitch. Sibilant rhonchi are high pitched with a basic frequency over 500 Hz. They usually occur in the small bronchi or bronchioles. Sonorous rhonchi are low pitched with a basic frequency about 100–200 Hz, which often occur in the trachea or main bronchi.
    - Rhonchi are classified into diffuse rhonchi and localized rhonchi according to the location. Diffuse rhonchi are heard in chronic bronchitis, bronchial asthma, obstructive pulmonary emphysema or cardiac asthma. Localized rhonchi are heard in endobronchial tuberculosis, lung cancer or bronchial foreign body.

45.3.4.4 Vocal Resonance

The techniques for vocal resonance are basically the same as for vocal fremitus. Ask the patient to repeat the word "yi" and auscultate the voice sounds on the chest wall with a stethoscope. Normally, voice sounds are faint and indistinct. An increase or decrease in vocal resonance can be found by comparing the two sides. Vocal resonance has the same clinical significance as vocal fremitus, but is more sensitive.

1. **Bronchophony** Both the intensity and clarity of vocal resonance are increased. Bronchophony is often accompanied by increased vocal fremitus, dullness on percussion and abnormal bronchial breath sound, and heard in patients with lung consolidation.
2. **Pectoriloquy** It is a kind of bronchophony that is more intense and louder. Syllables are heard distinctly. Pectoriloquy is often heard in a large area of lung consolidation.
3. **Egophony** Not only the intensity is increased but the quality is also changed. There is a nasal or bleating quality. The spoken "yi" is changed to "A". It is often heard in the area of compressed lung above a moderate amount of pleural effusion, or in the area of lung consolidation with a small amount of pleural effusion.

4. **Whispered pectoriloquy** To improve the sensitivity of vocal resonance, ask the patient to whisper the word "yi". Normally, only a very faint and indistinct voice is heard, however whispered pectoriloquy can be heard distinctly in lung consolidation. This sign is particularly valuable in the diagnosis of lung consolidation.

45.3.4.5 Pleural Friction Rub

Pleural friction rubs occur when inflamed, unlubricated surfaces of pleurae rub together during respiration. Have the patient in the sitting or supine position and auscultate the chest with a stethoscope, rubs can be heard in both phases of respiration, especially at the end of inspiration and the beginning of expiration. They may be ephemeral and disappear after several respiratory cycles, also may last for several days or even longer. Rubs disappear when the patient holds the breath, which can be used to differentiate them from the pericardial friction rub. The most common site for a friction rub to be heard is the lower anterolateral chest wall. Rubs can disappear or reappear with the change of body position. Rubs disappear when the pleurae are separated due to the increasing of pleural effusion and reappear when the pleurae contact again due to the decreasing of pleural effusion. The common causes are the same as pleural friction fremitus. Schematic diagrams of rhonchi, moist rales and pleural friction rub are shown in Fig. 45.22.

45.4 Heart Examination

Cardiac physical examination is a basic skill for physicians to diagnose cardiovascular disease. Physicians can get preliminary diagnostic indications from patient's history and physical examination, meanwhile, those information can provide a reference for physicians to choose further supportive examination. Although there are increasing advanced medical technological methods, cardiac physical examination can be amongst the most diagnostic if done correctly and carefully. Knowledge of cardiac physiology and auscultation techniques can often determine a diagnosis, or help to form a strong differential diagnosis.

Physicians need a quiet and comfortable environment with adequate light to perform the physical examination. Inspection, palpation, percussion, and auscultation are performed in a sequential order. On special occasions, patients should alter body positions when it is necessary, we should evaluate those signs throughout the body for evidence of hemodynamic sufficiency or insufficiency.

45.4.1 Inspection

Cardiac inspection begins with the patient in supine position. Sitting position is also acceptable for an outpatient's inspection. Physician stands on the right side of the patient with his

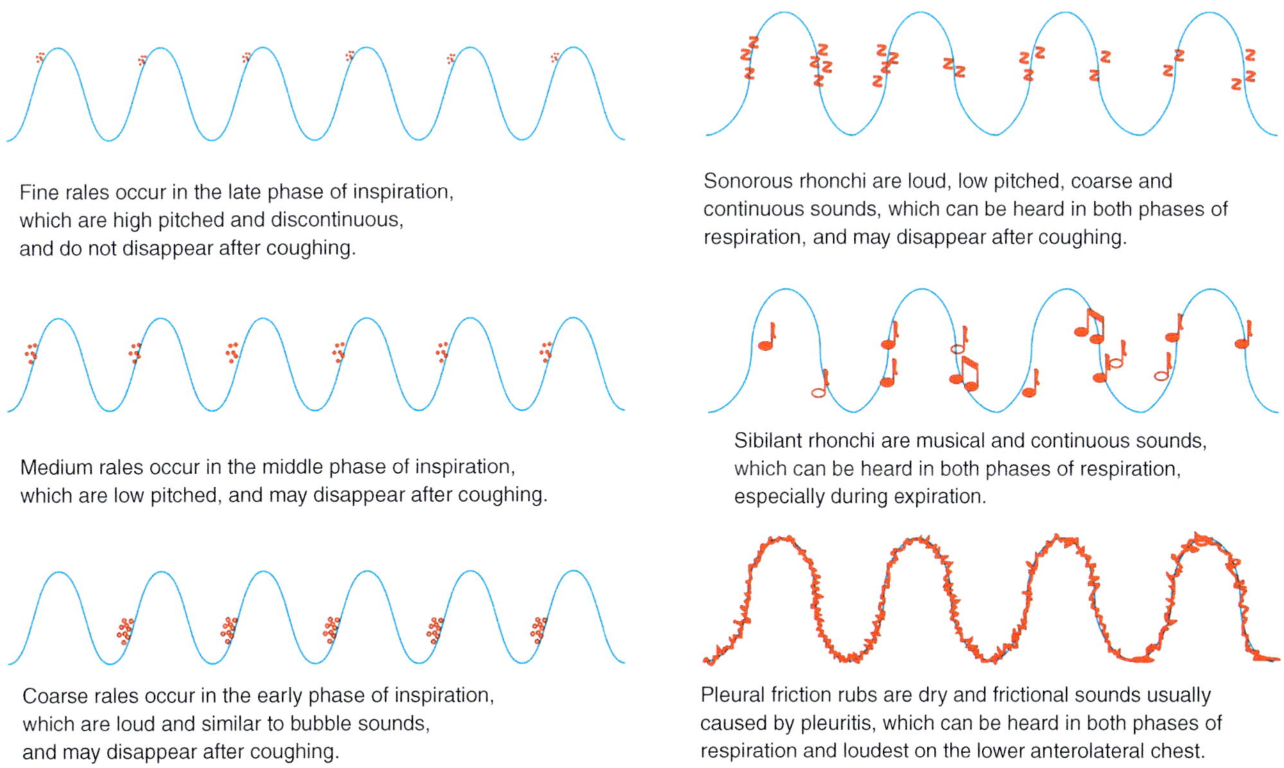

Fig. 45.22 Schematic diagrams of rhonchi, moist rales and pleural friction rub

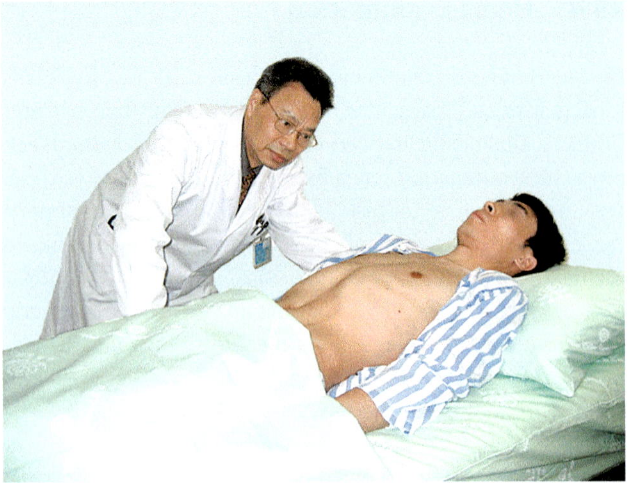

Fig. 45.23 Cardiac inspection

chest fully exposed, to inspect the chest of breathing pattern and respiratory motions by vertical or horizontal observation (Fig. 45.23).

45.4.1.1 Thoracic Deformity

Normal thorax is symmetrical. Physicians should pay more attention on any thoracic deformity which is associated with cardiac abnormality during cardiac inspection.

1. Protrusion of precordium:
   Protrusion of precordium is usually observed at the inferior segment of sternum over 3rd, 4th, and 5th intercostal space. This is mostly due to congenital heart disease, results in right ventricular hypertrophy. In those patients with tetralogy of Fallot, pulmonary valve stenosis and rheumatic valvular disease, their growth of chest wall was interferenced by ventricular hypertrophy during childhood. Chronic pericarditis with massive pericardial effusion may also lead to protrusion.
2. Pectus carinatum, pectus excavatum and spinal deformity:
   If anyone above in a severe situation may change the location of the heart to indicate heart abnormality, like spinal deformity with kyphoscoliosis could cause pulmonary heart disease, and pectus carinatum often accompany with Marfan syndrome.

45.4.1.2 Apical Impulse

The apical impulse is formed by the apex regional vibration with the left ventricular systole. The normal apex beat can be palpated in the 5th left intercostal space, inside the midclavicular line about 0.5–1.0 cm, with impulse range around 2.0–2.5 cm. In some special conditions, apical impulse is impalpable when the patient is obesity, woman with mastoptosis and so on.

1. Apical impulse displacement
   (a) Physiologic conditions:
   - Body shape: Thoracic diaphragm will be elevated in obese people compared to normal people, and then their heart will be horizontal while their apical impulse present in the 4th left intercostal space, at the point of intersection with the outside of left midclavicular line. On the contrary, for lean people (especially in a standing position), their heart will be upright, and their apical impulse occur inside-downward displaced to the 6th left intercostal space.
   - Age: In infants and children, their heart lie horizontal with their apical impulse occur in the fourth left intercostal space medial to the nipple.
   - Posture and position: The apical impulse occurs upward in decubitus position compared to sitting position due to the elevation of the diaphragm. The apical impulse presents on right side and displacement is around 1.0–2.5 cm in the **right lateral decubitus position**. On the contrary, left displacement is 2.0–3.0 cm in the left decubitus position. In case of adhesive pericarditis and pleurisy, there is no change of the apical impulse in lateral decubitus position.
   - Pregnancy: The diaphragm lies gradually upward and the heart is horizonal, the apical impulse is displaced outside and upward.

   (b) Pathophysiologicconditions:
   See attached Table 45.1.

Table 45.1 Pathological factors of apical impulse displacement

Factors	Displacement	Common diseases
Cardiac factors		
Left ventricular enlargement	Left-downward	Aortic regurgitation
Right ventricular enlargement	Leftward	Mitral stenosis
Whole ventricular enlargement	Left-downward, cardiac dullness increased on both sides	Dilated cardiomyopathy
Dextrocardia	In the right side of chest wall	Congenital dextrocardia
Non-cardiac factors		
Mediastinum displacement	Ill side	One side pleural adhesion, thickening or atelectasis
	Ill side contralateral	One side pleural effusion or pneumothorax
Diaphragm displacement	Left-outside	Massive ascites, the heart is horizontal due to diaphragm elevation
	Inside-downward and the 6th intercostal space	Severe emphysema, the heart is upright due to diaphragm depression.

2. The change of strength and range of apical impulse
   (a) Physiological factors: The strength of apical impulse is associated with the thickness of the chest wall. The apical impulse will be weaker and the range will be smaller in case of obesity or people with narrow intercostal space, whereas the apical impulse will be stronger and has a wider range caused by a severe physical activity or excited emotions.
   (b) Pathological factors
      - Cardiac diseases: (a) There will be a stronger apical impulse and a wider range in a patient with the left ventricular hypertrophy. (b) The apical impulse becomes weaker in case of myocardial injury (such as acute myocardium infraction, dilated cardiomyopathy). (c) When there is pericardial effusion, the apical impulse becomes weaker or even vanished.
      - Non-cardiac factors: (a) Hyperthyroidism, fever, or severe anemia could result in the apical impulse getting stronger with a wider range. (b) The apical impulse will be weaker or even vanished when there occur with massive aerothorax, effusion or emphysema on the left side.
3. Inward Impulse: Normal Apical Impulse is Towards the chest wall, however, inward impulse has the contrary direction on cardiac contraction. It always occurs in constrictive pericarditis because of the pericardial adherence with the circumambient tissues; or due to severe right ventricular hypertrophy, in addition, the clockwise rotation of the heart also leads to inward impulse due to the left ventricular moving backward.

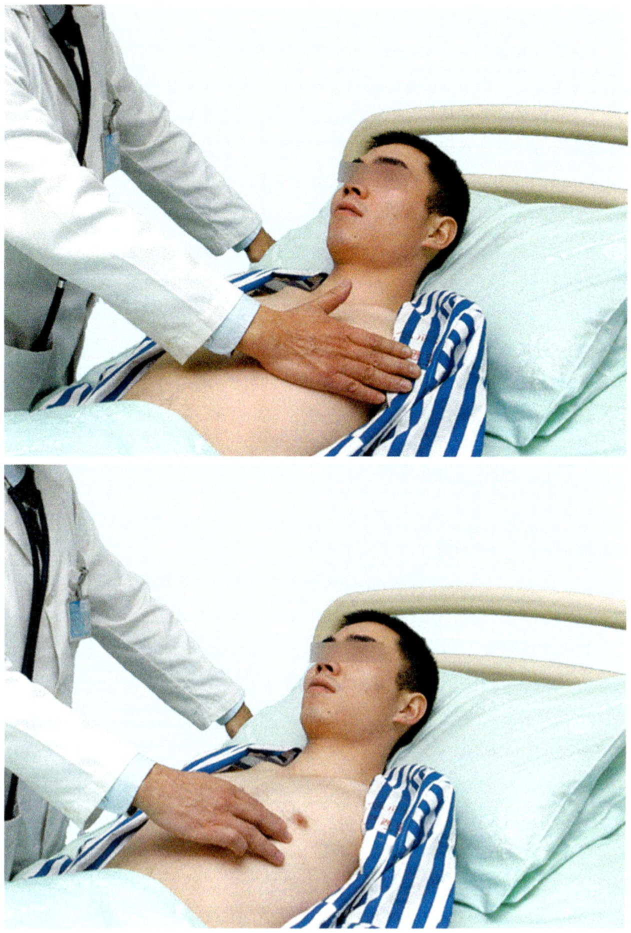

Fig. 45.24 Palpation of apical impulse

45.4.1.3 Abnormal Precordial Pulsation

The abnormal precordial pulsation in different position means different clinical significance (Table 45.2).

45.4.2 Palpation

Cardiac palpation could further confirm the findings observed on inspection. Inspection and palpation are inseparably interrelated. Functions of palpation are to discriminate textures, dimensions, consistencies and temperature. The examiner could apply his whole palm, ulnar side of palm (hypothenar), index or middle finger to perform cardiac palpation (Fig. 45.24), and adjust the pressure against the chest wall to maximize the sensitivity and result during the palpation.

Table 45.2 Abnormal precordial pulsation

Position	Peroid	Clinical significance
2nd intercostal space at the left sternal border	Systole	1. Pulmonary hypertension or pulmonary artery expansion 2. Physical activity or emotional excitement in some normal young people
2nd intercostal space at the right sternal border	Systole	1. Aortic aneurysm, aortic arch aneurysm or ascending aorta and aortic arch expansion 2. Aortic regurgitation, severe anemia, hyperthyroidism
3rd and 4th intercostal space at the left sternal border	Systole	Right ventricular hypertrophy
Subxiphoid	Systole	Right ventricular beat or aortaventralis beat

45.4.2.1 Apical Impulse and Abnormal Precordial Pulsations

Palpation can not only further determine the location, intensity and size of the apical impulse and abnormal precordial pulsations, but also reveal cardiac rate and rhythm. As the apical impulse gently lifts the palpating fingers with each systole, it can provide vital information to determine systole, S1 and thrill duration.

Heave or lift impulse is a forceful and sustained outward motion throughout systole and has great amplitude. In patient with left ventricular hypertrophy (LVH), lift impulse can be palpated at apex, and a sustained left parasternal lift impulse is the reliable indication of a large right ventricle.

The xiphoideusal pulsation may be found in cardiac inspection incase of right ventricular hypertrophy or abdominal aortic pulsation caused by abdominal aortic aneurysm. There are two kinds of identification methods as following: Firstly, to instruct patients inhale deeply, pulsation is enhanced for right ventricular beats whereas is weakened for abdominal aorta. Secondly, placing the finger flat on xiphoid, under upward pressure of the anterior chest wall, beating is enhanced in patients on deep breathing and impacts fingers to end for right ventricular beats whereas pulse is weakened and impacts fingers to palm for abdominal aortic pulsation. In addition, xiphoideusal pulsation also occurs in some lean people due to the normal abdominal aorta beating or right ventricular beats when the heart is in dropping position.

45.4.2.2 Thrill

Thrill is a superficial vibratory sensations felt on the skin overlying an area of turbulence. It is also called purring thrill as it is similar to respiratory tremor palpated at the throat of a resting cat. It is a distinctive physical sign in organic heart disease.

The mechanism of thrill is similar to heart murmur (Fig. 45.35). Thrill is most commonly produced by the flow of blood from one chamber to another through a restricted or narrowed orifice. The intensity of the thrill varies depend on the velocity of the blood flow, the degree of narrowing of the orifice and the difference in pressure between the two chambers of the heart. It is also associated with chest wall thickness, the thinner for chest wall (such as in children and lean people), the easier to be palpated. Thrill may occur in systole, diastole, presystole or continuous. It is usually common in some patients with congenital heart disease or valves stenosis whereas it's seldom found in valve insufficiency unless serious mitral valve or tricuspid valve insufficiency.

Any thrill should be described by its location, time in cardiac cycle, and its mode of extension or transmission. The examiner can determine its time by palpating apical impulse or carotids impulse, auscultation can also be applied to determine the relationship between thrill and heart sound (Table 45.3).

Table 45.3 Clinical significance of precordial thrill

Peroid	Location	Common disease
Systole	Second intercostal space, right sternal border (2ICS-RSB)	Aortic stenosis
	Second intercostal space, left sternal border (2ICS-LSB)	Pulmonary valvular stenosis
	Third and fourth intercostal space, left sternal border	Ventricular septal defect
Diastole	Cardiac apex	Mitral stenosis
Continuous	Second intercostal space, next to left sternal border	Patent ductus arteriosus

45.4.2.3 Pericardial Friction Rub

Pericardial friction rub is a to-and-fro grating sensation. The rub is caused by fibrinous pericarditis, in which visceral and parietal pericardium become coarse. It is easily palpated at the 3rd and 4th left intercostal space and left sternal border, also called as Bare Area, wherein no lung tissue cover the heart surface. Pericardial friction rubs are present during both phases of cardiac cycle, and often are more readily palpated with the patient sitting erect and leaning forward during the end period of deep inspiration. Pericardial friction rub is similar to pleural friction, but the palpation location is different, and pericardium friction rub won't disappear while holding breath. However, in the presence of pericardial effusion the rub will usually disappear because of the separation of visceral and parietal layers by the accumulated fluid.

45.4.3 Percussion

Cardiac percussion can confirm the heart borders, size of the contour and position in the thoracic cavity. The percussion on the bare area with no lung tissue covered at the surface of the heart is flat, called as absolute cardiac dullness. The percussion on area covered by lung tissue is dull, called as relative cardiac dullness. The real heart border is refer to relative cardiac dullness, which reflect the full size of heart (Fig. 45.25).

45.4.3.1 Percussion Method

Usuallywe employ indirect percussion for relative cardiac dullness. The examiner hyperextends the left middle finger as the pleximeter finger, parallel to intercostal space when a

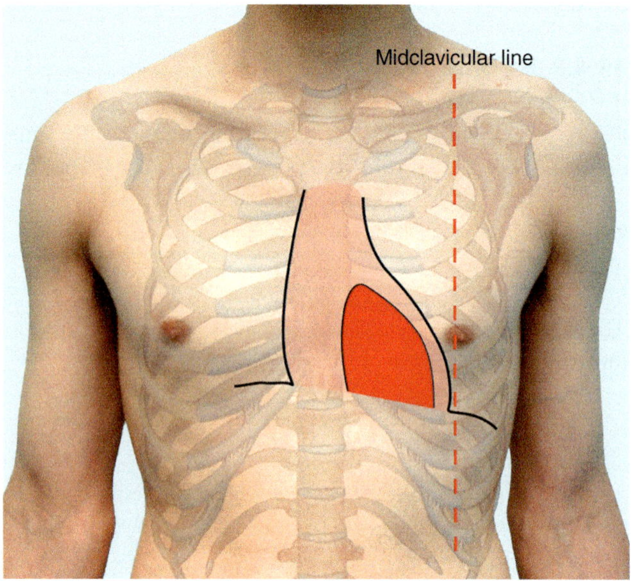

Fig. 45.25 Absolute cardiac dullness and relative cardiac dullness

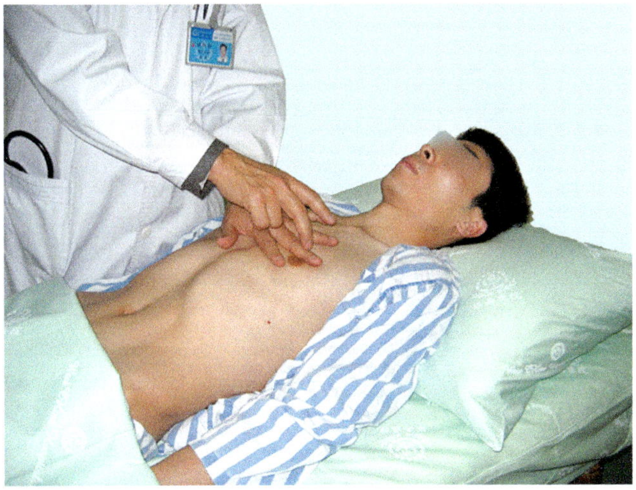

Fig. 45.26 Heart border percussion

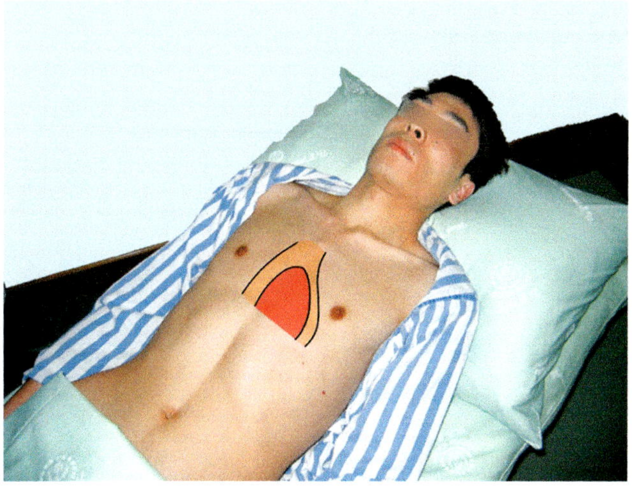

Fig. 45.27 Cardiac dullness border

patient lies supine on an examining table, and perpendicular when patient sits (Fig. 45.26). During percussion, the examiner should press pleximeter finger firmly on the surface that is to be percussed, and put the right forearm quite close to the surface with the hand cocked upward, then move medially until cardiac dullness is noticed. The border is perceived better by repetitive thumping the point at which the percussion note becomes dull. Light percussion will mostly produce a clear cardiac border, but a heavier percussion may be neccessary for people with a thick chest wall.

45.4.3.2 Percussion Sequence

Cardiac percussion starts from left to right, from outside to inside, and from the bottom up. It usually starts from 2 to 3 cm lateral to the point of maximal impulse, which is outlined by percussing in the 5th, 4th, 3rd and 2nd left intercostal space sequentially, starting from the anterior axillary line towards the sternum. The point at which percussion note becomes dull represents the left heart border, and the beginner should mark with a skin pencil where the note changes (Fig. 45.27).

To get the right heart border, percussion of upper margin of liver should be performed first along the right midclavicular line, starting from the 2nd right intercostal space sequentially and moving downward until liver dullness is noticed. The right heart border is outlined by percussing from one intercostal space above the upper margin of liver (usually from the 4th intercostal space) to the 2nd right intercostal space sequentially, moving medially until cardiac dullness is noticed (Fig. 45.27).

At the end, the distance from left mid-sternal line to the left and right border should be measured and recorded, measure the distance from mid-sternal line to left mid-clavicular line, all the data should be recorded as shown in Table 45.4. The normal range of relative cardiac dullness border in healthy adults is listed in Table 45.4.

Table 45.4 Normal cardiac dullness

Right heart border (cm)	Intercostal space	Left heart border (cm)
2–3	2	2–3
2–3	3	3.5–4.5
3–4	4	5–6
	5	7–9

The distance from mid-sternal line to left mid-clavicular line is about (8–10 cm)

45.4.3.3 The Heart Borders

Left heart border in the 2nd, 3rd, 4th and 5th left intercostal space are formed by pulmonary trunk, left auricular appendix and LV, respectively. At the junction of the blood vessel and the left heart, the inward depression is called heart waist. Right heart border in the 2nd right intercostal space is formed by ascending aorta and superior vena cava, and the borders below the 3rd right intercostal space is R2 (Fig. 45.28).

45.4.3.4 Variation and Clinical Significance

Many factors, either cardiac or non-cardiac factors, can affect cardiac dullness range, contour and position in the thoracic cavity.

1. Heart disease:
   Cardiac dullness will be enlarged in case of atrial and ventricular enlargement, pericardial effusion and so on. The most common variations with changes in area of cardiac dullness are listed in Table 45.5.
2. Non-cardiac factors
   (a) Emphysema: The cardiac dullness decreases and is even difficult to hear.
   (b) In patients with pleural effusion, pulmonary Infiltration or consolidation, lung tumor and enlargement of mediastinal lymph node, the cardiac dullness will be overlapped or covered.

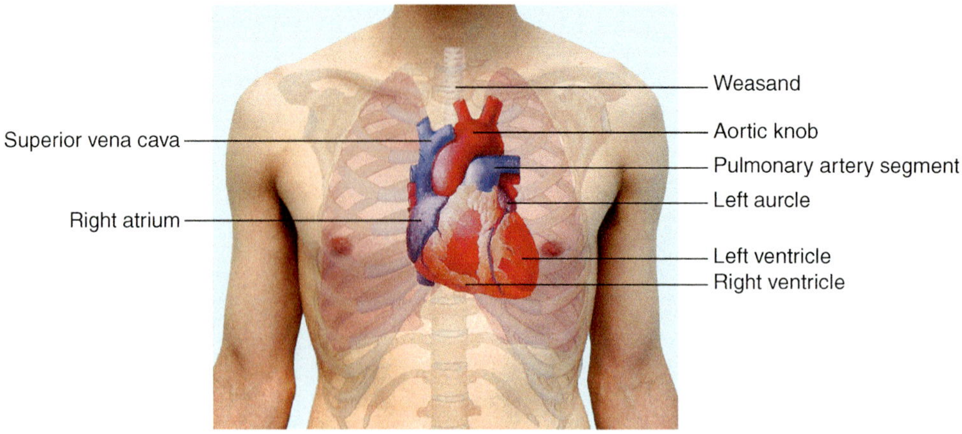

Fig. 45.28 Projection of heart and large blood vessel on the chest

Table 45.5 The changes of cardiac dullness and related common heart disease

Factors	Cardiac dullness	Common disease
LV enlargement	Leftward and downward displacement, cardiac waist becomes deeper and the heart silhouette looks likes a shoe. It is also called aortic heart (Fig. 45.29)	Aortic insufficiency
RV enlargement	Mildly enlarged: Cardiac dullness extends towards left and upward, the absolute heart border is enlarged, but relative heart border is normal. severely enlarged: Cardiac dullness extend both to right and left.	Cor pulmonale or atrial septal defect
LV and RV enlargement	Cardiac dullness extends on both sides. Left heart border extends to left and downward.	Dilated cardiomyopathy
LA enlargement or combined with pulmonary trunk enlargement	left atrium enlargement: heart border extends in 3rd left intercostal space, and cardiac waist disappear. left atrium and pulmonary artery enlarged: The pulmonary artery exaggerates to left, cardiac waist fills out. The cardiac silhouette looks likes a pear, and it is also called mitral heart (Fig. 45.30).	Mitral Stenosis
Dilatation of aorta	The base border of the heart will be widened usually accompanied by systolic pulsation.	Ascending aortic aneurysm
Pericardial effusion	Cardiac dullness extends to both right and left, the relative heart border is almost same with absolute heart border. The cardiac silhouette changes following the change of patient's position, the cardiac silhouette looks likes triangular flask when patients sits, and the base border of the heart will be widened in supine position.	Pericardial effusion

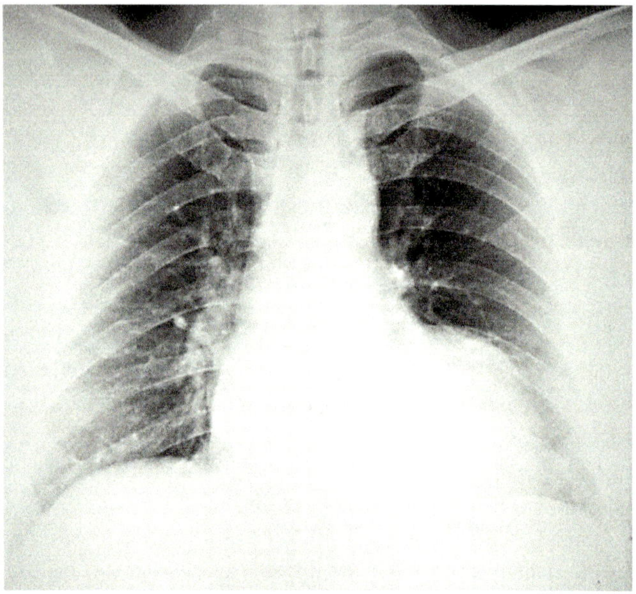

Fig. 45.29 "Aortic heart"

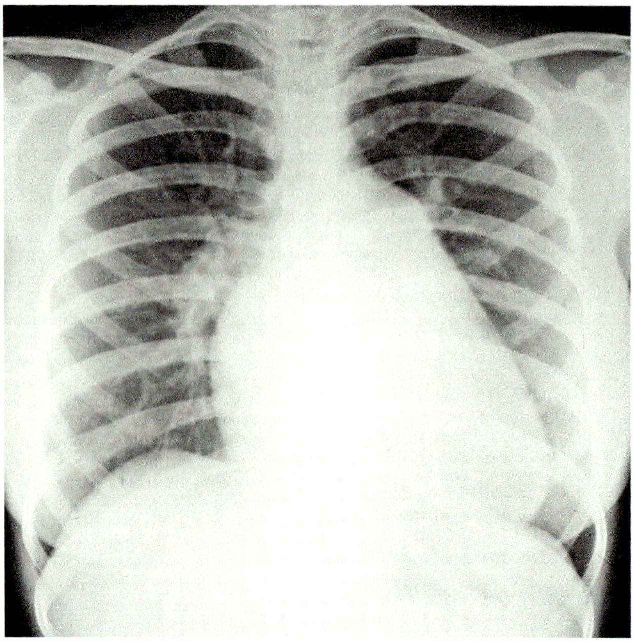

Fig. 45.30 "Mitral heart"

(c) Unilateral pleural effusion or pneumothorax: The cardiac border will extend to the healthy side.
(d) Unilateral pleural adhesion, pleural thickening and atelectasis: The cardiac border will extend to the diseased side.
(e) Massive peritoneal effusion or giant intraperitoneal tumor: The diaphragm elevates and heart position becomes transverse resulting in cardiac dullness extending to the left.
(f) Increased gastric gas content: The Traube tympany area enlarges affecting the accuracy of left heart border on percussion.

45.4.4 Auscultation

Cardiac auscultation is one of the most important and difficult part of cardiac physical examination. There are heart rate, cardiac rhythm, heart sound, extra heart sounds, heart murmur and pericardial friction sound. Skilled cardiac auscultation is not only the basis for clinical diagnosis but also could provide us lots of informations.

A patient could take a sitting or lying position with fully chest exposed during auscultation. If necessary, the patient could change his position, hold the breath or implement appropriate physical activities to make some sounds or murmurs clearer. There are two types of stethoscope microphones for cardiac auscultation: bell microphone and diaphragm microphone. Bell microphone is for low-pitched sounds, such as diastolic rumbling murmurs of mitral valve and fetal heart sounds from maternal intrauterine whereas diaphragm microphone is for all the high-pitched sounds, such as respiratory sounds, bowel sounds and diastolic sighing murmurs of aortic valve, etc.

45.4.4.1 Auscultatory Valve Area and Sequence

Sounds produced by valve opening and closing may propagate to different areas. The clearest sound area is called "auscultatory valve area", which is not equal to the valve anatomic location, which means that the auscultatory areas do not correspond with the surface markings of the heart valves. There are five auscultatory areas in cardiac auscultation, and their locations are described in Fig. 45.31: (a) Mitral area: the apex point of maximal impulse; (b) Pulmonary area: the left second intercostal, space just parasternal line; (c) Aortic area: the right second intercostal, space just parasternal line; (d) The second aortic area: the left third intercostal, space just parasternal line, also known as Erb area. (e) Tricuspid area: the left lower sternal border (4th, 5th left intercostal space). Auscultatory valve area should be appropriately adjusted according to the cardiac structure and position.

Cardiac auscultation should be started in a systematic way, usually in counter clockwise sequence: starting from

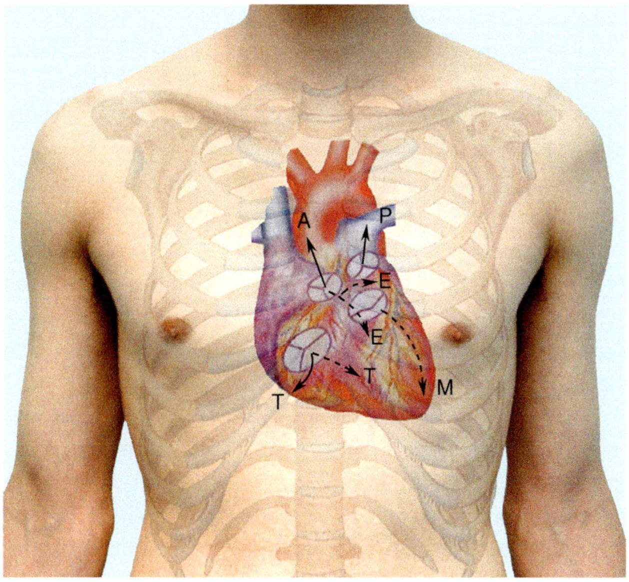

Fig. 45.31 Anatomy of heart valves and auscultatory valve area. *M* Mitral valve (MV) area, *A* Aortic valve (AV) area, *E* The second aortic valve area (Erb area), *P* Pulmonary valve (PV) area, *T* Tricuspid valve (TV) area

MV area, then PV area, to AV area, to second AV area, and TV area respectively.

45.4.4.2 The Contents of Auscultation

Cardiac auscultation refer to heart rate, rhythm, heart sound, extra sounds, murmur and pericardial friction sound.

Heart Rate

It means the number of heart beats per minute (bpm), usually heard at the apex. In normal adults heart rate is 60–100 bpm which may be a little bit faster in women and children (more than 100 bpm in children under the 3 years) and slower in elderly. More than 100 bpm in adults or more than 150 bpm in infants is called tachycardia whereas less than 60 bpm in adults is called bradycardia.

Tachycardia and bradycardia may be transient or persistent, which can be caused by physiological factors, pathological factors or by drugs. For example, heart rate increases under some physiological conditions, such as during physical activity and excitement. It also increases under some pathological conditions with increased sympathetic activity, such as fever, anemia, hyperthyroidism, etc. Physiological or sinus bradycardia is a common condition found in healthy person and in an athletes. Pathological bradycardia can be caused by intracranial hypertension, obstructive jaundice, thyroid hypofunction, sick sinus syndrome, etc.

Cardiac Rhythm

It means the rhythm of the heart beat, which is regular in normal adults. Some young adults and children may have sinus arrhythmia, whose speed is changed along with breath, which behaves as faster during inspiration and slower during exhalation. It's usually of no clinical significance. The most common arrhythmias are premature beats and atrial fibrillation (AF).

Premature beat is a sudden heart extra systole in the period of regular heart beats and then followed by a longer compensatory pause. If premature beat appears regularly, they could be named bigeminal beats or trigeminal beats, and so on. Bigeminal beats: every sinus beat is followed by a premature beat continuously. Trigeminal beats: every two sinus beats are followed by a premature beat continuously. According to the sources, premature beats are divided into three types as atrial, junctional and ventricular premature beats. Only by auscultation cannot distinguish the type of premature beats, so that all types must be diagnosed by ECG. Especially, frequent premature beats could be mostly caused by a variety of organic heart diseases, it also could be induced by mental stimulation, fatigue, excessive drinking, tea, drugs, and so on.

There are threecharacteristics to auscultate the atrial fibrillation like followings: (a) Irregularly irregular rhythm; (b) Variable intensity of first heart sound; (c) Heart rate is greater than pulse rate (Pulse deficit). It is caused by absolute irregularity of ventricular rhythm. Premature ventricular contraction can not transport enough blood to the peripheral blood vessels, resulting in the weakening of the pulse. Atrial fibrillation is usually caused by mitral stenosis, hypertension, coronary atherosclerotic heart disease, hyperthyroidism, etc. The unexplained atrial fibrillation is idiopathic.

Heart Sound

The first heart sound (S1), the second heart sound (S2), the third heart sound (S3) and the fourth heart sound (S4) are successively named according to the occurrence in sequence during the cardiac cycle (Fig. 45.32). Their mechanisms and

Fig. 45.32 Cardiac cycle

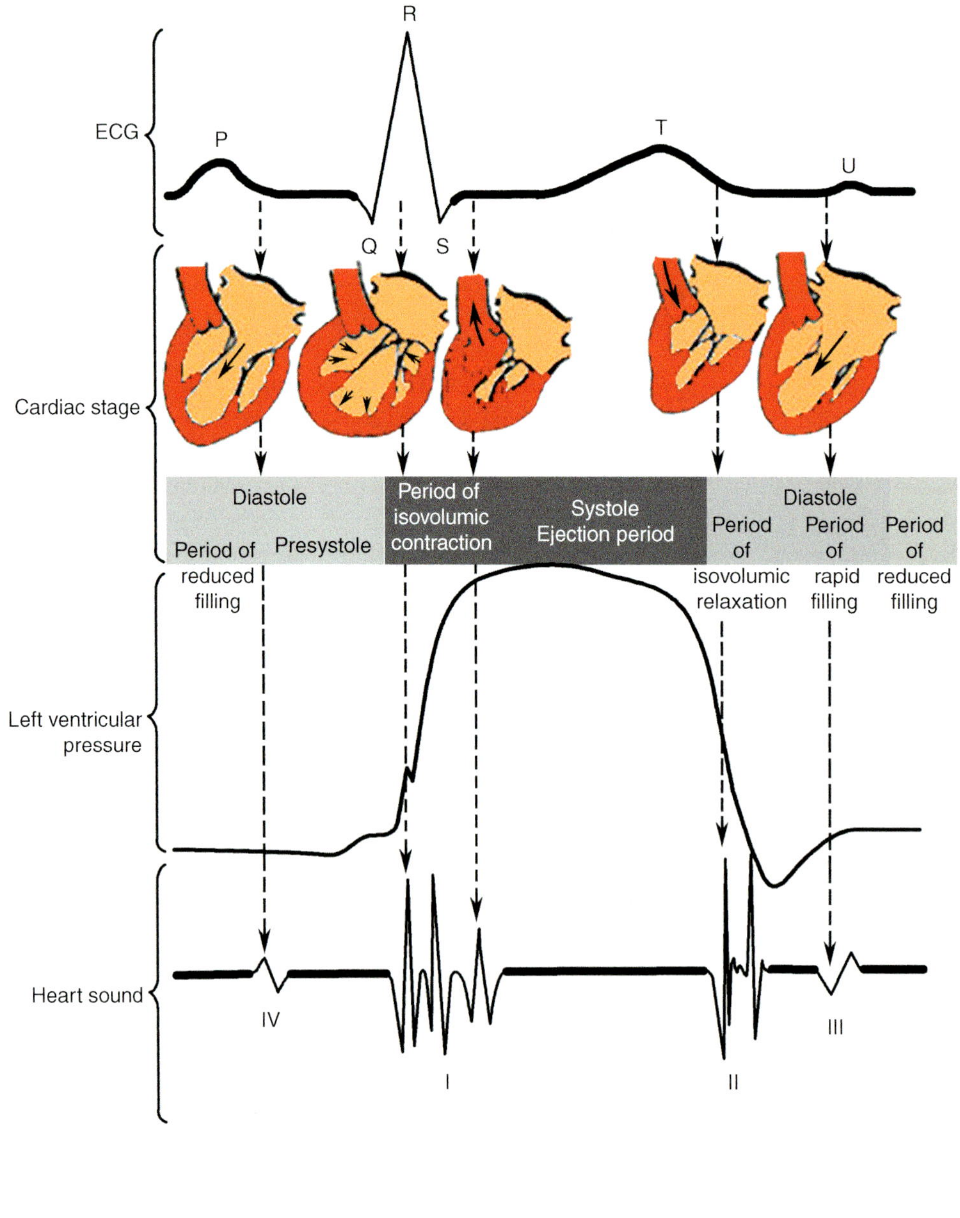

Table 45.6 Mechanisms and characteristics of heart sound

Heart sound	Mechanisms	Characteristics
S1	It is mainly produced by vibration generated by closure of the mitral and tricuspid valves. In addition, vibrations generated by opening of the semilunar valve, ventricular contraction and shocks of large vessel walls caused by rush of blood flow are also involved in the generation of S1. At the beginning of ventricular contraction, closure of the mitral valve is slightly earlier than the tricuspid valves. Usually this distinguish is hard to be heard, so we can only hear one sound by auscultation. S1 marks the beginning of systole.	It is low-pitched, loud intensity and long-lasting (≈0.1 s). It occurs simultaneously with the apex beat and is heard best at the apex.
S2	It is mainly produced by vibration generated by closure of aortic and pulmonary valves. In addition, vibrations generated by opening of atrioventricular valve and shock of ventricular wall caused by rush of blood flow are also involved in the generation of S2. S2 is composed of A2 and P2. A2 is produced by the closure of the aortic valve, and P2 is produced by the closure of the pulmonary valve. A2 is earlier than P2. Similarly, this distinguish is hard to be heard, so we can only hear one sound by auscultation. S2 marks the beginning of diastole.	The S2 is higher and sharper in pitch as well as lower in intensity and shorter in time than S1 (≈0.08 s). It doesn't occur simultaneously with the apex beat. And it is heard best at the bottom of the heart.
S3	It occurs at the beginning of diastole and the end of rapid filling period. S3 is produced by the sudden vibrations of ventricular wall, chordae and papillary muscles after the blood flow rapidly rushes the ventricular walls from the atria.	It is low-pitched, low intensity and short-last (≈0.04 s). It is limited at the apex or the inner of the apex. And it can be best heard if the patient is in left lateral decubitus position with breath held at end expiration.
S4	It occurs late in diastole and just before systole. Generally, it is produced by the distensions and vibrations of atrioventricular valve and its associated structures such as valves, annulus, chordae and papillary muscles during atrial contraction.	It is a low-pitched and low-intensity sound, which is heard best at the apex and its inner side. It is a sign of a pathologic state.

Table 45.7 Differences between S1 and S2

	S1	S2
Mechanism	Closure of atrioventricular valve	Closure of semilunar valve
Symbol	Ventricular systole	Ventricular diastole
Pitch	Low	High
Quality	Blunt	Brittle
Intensity	Loud	Weak
Duration	Long (about 0.1 S)	Short (about 0.08 S)
Best heard	At the apex	At the base
Apex beat	Synchronism	After apex beat

characteristics are shown in Table 45.6. In normal condition only S1 and S2 sounds could be heard, and S4 usually cannot be heard. The rare extra sound S3 can be heard in both normal and abnormal situations whereas if S4 sound could be heard, which it indicates a sign of a pathological situations.

It is essential to identify the first sound (S1) and the second sound (S2), which is very important for further determining the cardiac cycle phase of murmurs and extra heart sounds. Generally, the key points to identify S1 and S2 area are in following Table 45.7:

In case of complex arrhythmias, the key point to identify S1 and S2 are:

(a) Apex or carotid pulse is synchronous with S1. It is more convenient to discern S1 by carotid pulse.
(b) When it is difficult to identify S1 and S2 on auscultation at the apex, the stethoscope microphone is kept at the bottom of the heart including pulmonary valve area or aortic valve area would be a better choice, S1 is become easier to be found once S2 is identified.

Changes of Heart Sound

1. Change of sound intensity: The loudness of heart sound can be affected by many factors, such as lung, chest wall, thoracic cavity, pericardium, etc. However, myocardial contraction, valves' position, valves' structure and valves' elasticity play a most important role in all factors.
   (a) Changes of S1:
   - S1 increase: It occurs mostly in mitral stenosis during its early peroid. As the narrowed valve orifice limits ventricular filling, the left ventricular pressure accelerates and the systolic phase shortens. Because of all the above, the vibration amplitude of mitral valve during the closed period is increased, then S1 increases. However, S1 decreases with the stiffening and thickening of mitral valve cusps.
   - S1 decrease: It occurs in mitral insufficiency, aortic insufficiency and prolonged P-R intervals. Over-filling left ventricular in diastolic and the mitral valve in a higher position at the beginning of systolic, results in the decrease of the vibration amplitude of mitral valve during its closed period. In addition, S1 decreases in myocarditis, myocardiopathy, myocardial infarction and heart failure due to decrease of myocardial contractility.
   - S1 inconsistency: The intensity of S1 is inconsistent in atrial fibrillation and complete atrioventricular

block. The cannon sound which usually occurs in complete atrioventricular block is a loud S1 i.e. produced by the contraction of atria and ventricle at the same time.

(b) Changes of S2: S2 is composed of A2 and P2. P2 is louder than A2 in young people and children. As the sound volume changes with the age, in adults P2 will gradually decrease to become the same as A2, whereas till elderly, A2 will gradually increase and the P2 will be lower.

- S2 increase: mainly depends on the pressure within the aorta and pulmonary artery and the situation of semilunar valve. Increased S2 at aortic valve area is due to the increased pressure within the aorta (such as hypertension, aorta atherosclerosis). Increased S2 at pulmonary valve area is a symbol of pulmonary hypertension (such as pulmonary heart disease, left to right shunt congenital heart diseases, and mitral stenosis with pulmonary hypertension).
- S2 decrease: It occurs in case of decreased systemic and pulmonary circulating resistance, decreased circulating blood volume and stiff semilunar valve, for example, hypotension and aortic valve stenosis. S1 and S2 are often increased by exercise, anemia, hyperthyroidism due to increased myocardial contraction. Heart sound is also clearer in those people with thinner chest wall, but not louder. S1 and S2 are often decreased by shock, serious myocardial damage and etc. Conduction of heart sound decreases in case of obesity, pericardial effusion, left pleural effusion and emphysema.

2. Change of quality: If the original low blunt properties of S1 disappear and become similar with S2 when the heart rate is fast, thus we call it "pendular rhythm", which means the patient must be with a severe damaged myocardial situation, such as extensive AMI and severe myocarditis. If accompanied with tachycardia, it sounds like the heart sound of an embryo, called embryocardia.
3. Splitting of heart sounds:
   In normal physiology, the closure of atrioventricular valve (mitral valve and tricuspid valve) or semilunar valve (aortic valve and pulmonary valve) is asynchronous. The closure of tricuspid is about 0.02–0.03 s delay than the mitral valve, and the closure of pulmonary valve is about 0.03 s delay than aotic valve, and these differences cannot be found by auscultation. However, if the closure interval of valves prolongs for some pathological reasons, S1 or S2 can be divided into two sounds, and then it could be detected by auscultation, thus defined as splitting of heart sounds.
   (a) Splitting of S1: The mitral sound occurs slightly earlier than tricuspid sound as mitral valve closes significantly before the tricuspid valve allowing both valve to make a separate sound. Split S1 is common in RBBB as in RBBB electrical impulse reach the left ventricle earlier than the right ventricle resulting in increase of left ventricle pressure before that of right ventricle. The delay in closure of tricuspid valve results in split of S1 sound on auscultation.
   (b) Splitting of S2: It is due to the unsynchronized closure of the aortic and pulmonary valve. It usually occurs during inspiration and in mitral stenosis associated with pulmonary hypertension or pulmonary stenosis. During deep inspiration the returned blood volume of right heart usually increases, which can cause the delay of the right ventricular constriction and the pulmonary valve closure. Split S2 can also be heard in mitral insufficiency and ventricular septal defect. It is because the left ventricular ejection time is shortened in these cases, resulting in early closure of aortic valve. Fixed splitting of S2 indicates the presence of Atrial septal defect which remains unchanged through inspiration and expiration. Paradoxical splitting or reversed splitting of S2 occurs in the case of delay of aortic valve closure relative to pulmonary valve. It occurs due to the delay of the left ventricular emptying as in LBBB, aortic stenosis and severe hypertension (Fig. 45.33).

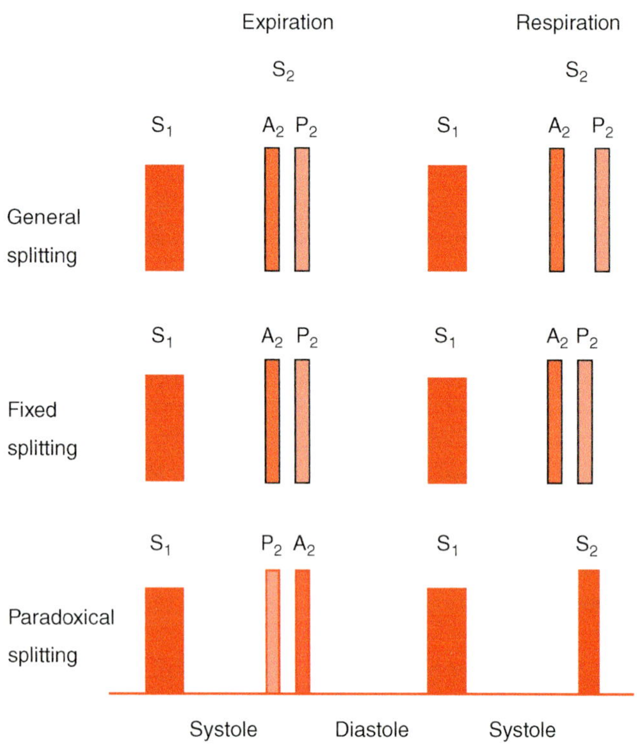

Fig. 45.33 Splitting of S2 diagram. S1: the first heart sound; S2: the second heart sound; A2: aortic valve component of S2; P2: pulmonary valve component of S2

Extra Cardiac Sound

It means additional heart sounds other than the normal heart sounds. It is pathologic and mostly occurs after S2, called diastolic extra cardiac sound. If it occurs after S1, it is called systolic extra cardiac sound.

1. The extra sounds in diastole period
   (a) Gallop rhythm: It is the extra heart sound in diastolic phase. It refers to abnormal rhythm of the heart on auscultation. The gallop rhythm contains another sounds, S3 and S4, depending upon from where the added sound comes. Gallop is a sign of serious myocardial damage. According to the starting of the extra sound, it can be classified into three types: (a) protodiastolic gallop: It is also called as ventricular gallop or pathological S3. It is commonly found in heart failure, acute myocardial infarction, severe myocarditis and dilated cardiomyopathy. The appearance of it is caused by the overload of ventricle which results in the vibration of ventricular wall. It is low-pitched and often accompanied with fast heart rate. Left ventricular gallop is detected at the apex on auscultation, and right ventricular gallop is usually heard under the xiphoid or at the fifth left intercostal space. Physiologic S3 can be heard in normal children and teenagers in left lateral decubitus position at the end of expiration, but without fast heart rate. (b) late diastolic gallop: It is termed as S4 or atrial gallop. It occurs in late diastole, just before S1 when the atrium contracts to force the blood flowing into the left ventricle. S4 is an important sign of diastolic heart failure and ischemia. It is a low-pitched sound, heard best at the apex with the patient in the left lateral decubitus position. c. Summation gallop: The rhythm in which the gallop sound is due to the superimposition of S3 and S4. It usually occurs in middle diastolic gallop and is comprised by the overlapping of early and late diastolic gallop. In normal conditions, Gallop rhythm may be heard in young person or athletes but at the same time it can be a sign of serious cardiac problems like heart failure and other cardiomyopathies. When the gallop rhythm contain both S1 and S2 it forms a quadruple gallop.
   (b) Opening snap: It is also called the mitral valve slapping sound which is common for mitral stenosis and soft superior valve. At the early diastolic period, the blood flow of left atrium quickly passes through the narrow mitral valve into the left ventricle under high pressure. It causes the mitral valve leaflets to quickly open and close producing the slapping sound. It sounds high-pitched, briefness, and sonorousness and is clearly detected in the apex. The opening snap indicates a flexible valve, and it is a significant evidence that the valve is suitable for mitral commissurotomy.
   (c) Pericardial knock: It is found in constrictive pericarditis. On rapid ventricular filling at early diastolic phase, the ventricular diastolic enlargement gets blocked by thicken pericardium which leads to ventricular vibration and the extra sound. It can be clearly detected at the left sternum.
   (d) Tumor plop: Left atrial myxoma produces a diastolic sound called tumor plop. This sound is produced from ventricular obstruction in flow that occurs as the tumor comes to rest over mitral annulus. It's a low frequency diastolic murmur that's heard in apex and 3/4th left intercostal space. The tumor plop is caused by the sudden tension of collision avoidance rooms, walls and valves because myxoma flow into the left chamber during diastolic blood phase.
2. The extra sounds in systolic period: The extra sounds appears in the systolic period which is divided into early phase, metaphase and later phase.
   (a) Early systolic ejection click: It is also called ejection sound, i.e., heard at early systolic period. It is a high pitched sounds that occur at the moment of the maximum opening of the aortic or the pulmonary valves. The mechanism is that the arterial wall of pulmonary artery or aorta vibrates as both of them expand at the period of ventricular contraction. In addition, the strong open of semilunar valve or sudden restriction during stenotic valve opening can produce the sound in the case of high resistance of aortic or pulmonary artery. According to the location of heart sounds, it can be divided into pulmonary ejection click and aortic ejection click: (1) Pulmonary ejection click: It can be heard best in the pulmonary valve area and usually occurs in patients with pulmonary hypertension, idiopathic pulmonary artery expansion, mild to moderate pulmonary stenosis and atrial or ventricular septal defect. (2) Aortic ejection click: It is usually heard best at the aortic valve area. It occurs in hypertension, aortic aneurysm, aortic stenosis, aortic insufficiency and the coarctation of aorta, etc. But the murmurs will disappear when the valve calcifies or the activity of the valve decreases.
   (b) Mid and late systolic click: It is a high-frequency sound in mid-systole that results from the halting of prolapsed mitral valve leaflets. It sounds like a padlock voice "ka-ta". The clearest sound is best heard at the apex. The click always indicates mitral valve prolapse. The mechanism is that when atrioventricular valve falls into left atrium at mid and late systolic phase, the valve leafs suddenly tense or the chordae tendineae suddenly tightens resulting in vibration. Mitral valve prolapse is also accompanied with late

Table 45.8 The characteristics of the rhythm and splitting of cardiac auscultation

	Location	Quality	Duration	Impact of respiration	Clinical manifestation
Physiological S_3	Apex or inside-upside	Weak and low	Early diastolic, S_2–S_3 <S_1–S_2	Obvious in the end of expiration	Normal teenagers
Splitting of S_2	Pulmonary valve area	Short and fast	The interval of the two parts of S_2 > 0.03 s	Obvious in the end of inspiration	Normal teenagers, pulmonary artery stenosis
Splitting of S_1	Apex	Short and fast	The interval of the two parts of S_1 > 0.03 s		Pulmonary hypertension
VG	Apex (left ventricle) or blow of xiphoid (right ventricle)	Weak and low	In early diastolic, with fast heart rate which makes S2 and S3 sound the same, as well as S1 and S2.	Obvious in the end of expiration (left ventricle) or inspiration (right ventricle)	Myocardium damage
AG	Inside apex	Weak and low	In late diastolic, about 0.1 s earlier than S_1	Obvious in the end of expiration	Myocardium hypertrophy with damage
OS	Inside apex	High tone, short, and sharp: slapping sound	In early diastolic, about 0.05–0.06 s later than S2		Mitral stenosis
PK	Left sternum	middle frequency, loud, short and fast	In early diastolic, about 0.09–0.12 s later than S2		Constrictive pericarditis
tumor plop	Inside apex	low tone, change with position	About 0.08–0.12 s later than S2		Atrial myxoma
EC	Aortic valve area or pulmonary valve area	High tone, sharp and short burst sound	About 0.05–0.07 s later than S1		Aortic stenosis or pulmonary hypertension
MLC	Apex or inside apex	High tone, sharp and short sound with late systolic murmur	At least 0.08 s later than S_1		Mitral valve prolapse

S1: the first sound; S2: the second sound; S3: the third sound; S4: the fourth sound; VG: ventricular gallop; AG: atrial gallop; SG: summation gallop; OS: opening snap; PK: pericardial knock; EC: early systolic ejection sound; MLC: middle to late systolic click

systolic murmur and this phenomenon is called as mitral valve prolapse syndrome.

3. Iatrogenic extra heart sounds: they include artificial valve sound and artificial pacemaker sound.

The characteristics of some triple rhythm and splitting of heart sound can be seen in Table 45.8 and Fig. 45.34.

Cardiac Murmurs

The abnormal heart sound heard in systole or diastole besides the normal heart sound and the extra heart sound is called cardiac murmurs. It is of great significance to determine the murmurs for correct diagnosis.

1. Mechanism of production of murmurs: Normal blood flow presents a laminar flow that can not produce the sounds. However, when blood flow accelerates or get through narrow valves, laminar flow turned to be turbulent flow or vortices. Turbulent flow or vortices vibrate the heart wall, vascular wall, valve and chordae tendineae, and then therelative murmurs are generated at the corresponding location. Specific mechanisms are as follows (Fig. 45.35).
2. Characteristics of murmurs:
   (a) Location and conducting direction: Murmurs are usually best heard over the diseased area. For example, if the murmurs are best heard at the apex, it always represents that the diseased region is mitral valve. The conducting direction of murmurs is determined by the direction of blood flow. The murmurs produced from mitral valve insufficiency usually conduct to left subaxillary region, and the murmurs produced from aortic stenosis conduct towards the neck. However, the murmurs produced from mitral stenosis are restricted to the apex. If we hear a murmur in any auscultatory area of heart, we must consider whether the murmur is from the relative valve area or is conducted from other diseased area.
   (b) Timing: There are three basic types of murmurs: systolic, diastolic and the murmurs occur in both systole and diastole. Murmurs can be further classified as early, mid, late and whole phase murmurs according to the phase of the cardiac cycle when they occur.
   (c) Quality: It means the pitch and the tone of the murmurs. Depending on the different pitches, the murmurs can be divided into soft or rough murmurs. The

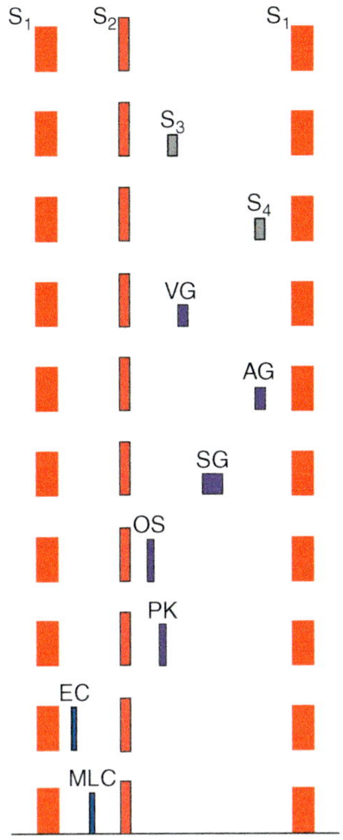

Fig. 45.34 Several significant triple rhythm diagram

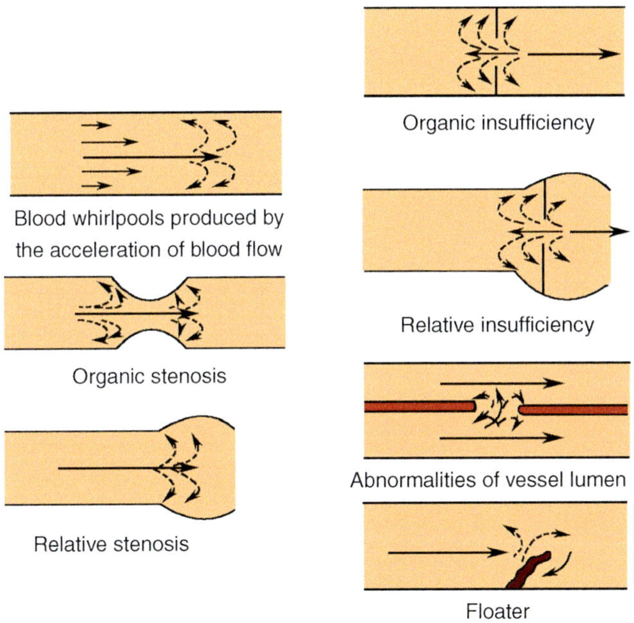

Fig. 45.35 Mechanisms of generation of murmurs

tones of the murmurs can be described as blowing, rumbling, jet-like, sigh-like, machine-like, musical, birdsong-like, etc. Different pitches and tones of murmurs can reflect different pathological condition. It is helpful to diagnose the heart disease by the quality of the murmurs. A diastolic roughly rumbling murmur at the apex is a feature of mitral stenosis. A systolic blowing murmur at the apex usually reflects mitral insufficiency. A soft blowing murmur at the apex is a functional murmur. The diastolic sigh-like murmur at second aortic valve area reflects aortic insufficiency.

(d) Intensity and form: Intensity is the loudness level of murmurs, and form means the changes of the loudness level in different phases of cardiac cycle. The intensity of the murmurs depends on the following factors: (a) The severity of the lesion vessel: in general, the narrower the lesion vessel is, the louder the murmur becomes. However, the murmurs will be weakened or even disappear if the lesion vessel is so narrow that the blood flow significantly decreases. (b) The velocity of blood flow: When the blood flow accelerates, the murmurs become louder. (c) The pressure gradient of crossing valve: The higher the pressure gradient between the two sides of valve orifice or abnormal channel is, the louder the murmur becomes. If the area of ventricular septal defect increases, the pressure gradient between left and right ventricle will decrease, resulting in weakening or even disappearance of the murmur. (d) Myocardial contractility: The stronger the myocardial contractility is, the louder the murmur becomes. The decreased myocardial contractility in heart failure causes the blood stagnation, resulting in weak intensity murmur. After improvement of the heart function, the myocardial contractility increases, the blood flow accelerates, resulting in louder murmurs. In addition to the above factors, some factors other than heart can weaken the murmurs, such as chest wall thickening, pulmonary emphysema, pericardial effusion, etc. Usually Levine 6 classification is used to grade the intensity of systolic murmur(Table 45.9), whereas the

Table 45.9 Levine 6 classification for systolic murmurs

Grade	Intensity	Auscultation characteristics	Thrill
1	Very faint	Barely audible	No
2	Quiet	Audible but soft	No
3	Moderately loud	Easily audible	No/Yes
4	Loud	Easily audible and associated with a thrill	Yes
5	Very loud	Easily audible, associated with a thrill, and still heard with the stethoscope only lightly on the chest	Obvious
6	Very loud	Easily audible, associated with a thrill, and still heard with the stethoscope off of the chest	Intense

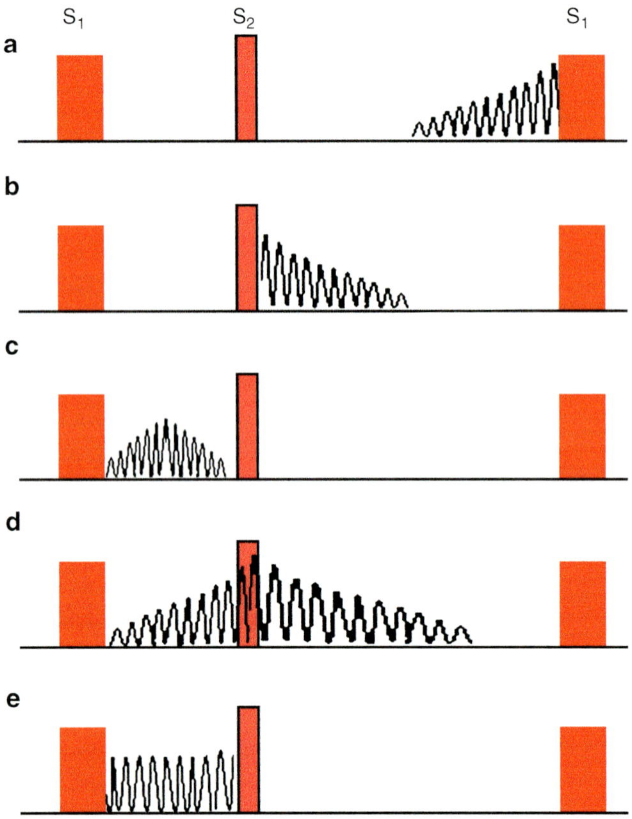

Fig. 45.36 Schematic of various types of heart Murmurs. (a) Crescendo murmur; (b) Decrescendo murmur; (c) Crescendo-decrescendo murmur; (d) Continuous murmur; (e) Plateau murmur

diastolic murmurs are described as mild, moderate and severe.

The intensity of murmurs is recorded in numerator. The denominator is six. For example, grade 2 murmur can be recorded as 2/6.

Murmurs' form refers to the changes of murmurs during a heartbeat. It is classified into five types (Fig. 45.36): (a) Crescendo murmur: found in mitral stenosis; (b) Decrescendo murmur: found in aortic insufficiency; (c) Crescendo-decrescendo murmur: found in aortic stenosis; (d) Continuous murmur: distributed in both phases, gradually increased in systolic phase whereas decreased in diastolic phase. It can be found in patients with ductus arteriosus. (e) Plateau murmur: found in mitral regurgitation.

(e) The impacts of body position, respiration and exercise: murmurs can be increased or decreased by different positions, exercise, deep inspiration, breath-hold, etc. (a) Body position: The murmur of mitral stenosis isheard better in left recumbent position. The murmur of aortic insufficiency is more clear when patient is sitting upright and leaning forward. In supine position, the murmurs of mitral, tricuspid and pulmonary valve regurgitation are more obvious. Changing the position from lying or squatting to standing may decrease the intensity of murmurs of Mitral insufficiency, Tricuspid insufficiency, Aortic insufficiency, Pulmonary Stenosis and Pulmonary insufficiency, whereas increase the murmurs of hypertrophic obstructive cardiomyopathy. (b) Respiration: During deep inspiration, the pressure within the thorax decreases, the venous return and the output volume of right ventricle increase, therefore the murmurs related to right heart increase. When performing valsalva maneuver, the pressure within the thorax increases, the venous return decreases, therefore the murmurs generated by the valves decrease normally, whereas the murmur of hypertrophic obstructive cardiomyopathy increases. (c) Exercise: exercise increases the heart rate and blood volume so the murmur increases in a certain heart rate range.

3. Clinical significance of heart murmurs: The murmur plays an important role in the treatment and diagnosis of heart diseases. Some patients with heart murmurs may not have heart disease but some patients with heart disease may not have murmurs. Murmurs can be classified as organic murmurs and functional murmurs according to the presence or absence of heart disease. Organic murmurs are produced from the place accompanied with an organic lesion. Functional murmurs include the following types: (a) Physiological murmur. (b) The murmurs arising from the systemic diseases that cause the hemodynamic changes such as hyperthyroidism. (c) The murmurs generated by the relative valve insufficiency or stenosis are always related to pathological significance. Although there is no pathological change of valve in the relative valve insufficiency and stenosis, the murmurs are still pathological. Contrary to pathological murmurs, functional murmurs are usually harmless. It is systolic, soft, blowing, without a thrill. The differences between the physiological and pathological murmurs are described in Table 45.10.

Table 45.10 The differences between the physiological and pathological murmurs

Different points	Physiological murmurs	Pathological murmurs
Age	Young person and children	Indeterminable
Location	Cardiac apex and/or pulmonary valve area.	Indeterminable
Quality	Soft and blowing	harsh, blowing and high-pitched
Duration	Short	Long, usually in the whole systole.
Intensity	≤Level 2/6	≥Level 3/6
Thrill	No	≥Level 3/6, ususlly with thrill.
Conduction	Limited	Wide

The feature and clinical significance of the organic murmurs are described according to the different phase and location as follows:

1. Systolic murmurs
   (a) **Mitral valve area:** It mainly occurs in rheumatic mitral insufficiency. It is harsh, blowing, and high-pitched. Its intensity is usually equal or greater than grade 3/6. It can persist throughout the systole, even cover S1 and conduct towards the left subaxillary region.
   (b) **Aortic valve area:** It occurs in aortic stenosis with various causes. It is mid-systolic, jet-like, loud, harsh, and crescendo-decrescendo. It conducts towards the neck, and always presents with thrill and decreased A2.
   (c) **Pulmonary valve area:** It occurs in pulmonary stenosis. It is mid-systolic, jet-like, and harsh. Its intensity is usually equal or greater than grade 3/6. It is always with thrill and decreased P2.
   (d) **Tricuspid valve area:** It is rare and usually occurs in tricuspid insufficiency. Its auscultation feature is similar to murmurs produced by mitral insufficiency but not the same. It can be accompanied with jugular vein and liver pulse in systole.
   (e) **Other areas:** In the patients with ventricular septal defect, loud and rough systolic murmur over the third or fourth left intercostal space just lateral to the sternum. In Atrial septal defect, a jet-like systolic murmur with increased P2 and intensity of 2/6–3/6 can be heard at the second and third intercostal space, left to the sternal border.
2. Diastolic murmurs
   Mitral valve area: It mainly occurs in rheumatic mitral stenosis. It is a mid or late diastolic, low-pitched, rumbling, and crescendo murmur with loud S1 and thrill. It is limited at the apex of heart and can be heard more clearly if the patients lie in the supine or lateral position. In moderate or severe aortic valve insufficiency the increase of left ventricular diastolic filling makes the mitral valve in a half-closed state, which generates a murmur called Austin Flint murmur. It must be distinguished from organic mitral stenosis murmur (Table 45.11).

Table 45.11 Distinguish for diastolic murmurs in mitral area

	Organic mitral stenosis	Austin Flint
Feature	Harsh, crescendo, in mid or late diastole, usually with thrill.	Soft, decrescendo, in mid or late diastole, without thrill.
S1 increase	Yes	No
Opening snap	Maybe	No
Atrial fibrillation	Usually with	Without
Heart shadow in X-ray	Pear-shaped heart with enlarged left atrium and right ventricle.	Boot-shaped heart, with enlarged left ventricular.

   Aortic valve area: It occurs in aortic insufficiency with various causes. The murmur is sigh-like and decrescendo. It radiates to the left lower part of sternum and apex of the heart. It is best heard at the second aortic area, in the sitting position leaning forward and on holding breath after a deep inspiration. It is usually heard in rheumatic aortic insufficiency. It also occurs in aortic insufficiency due to congenital heart disease, idiopathic aortic valve prolapse, syphilitic aortitis and Marfan syndrome.

   Pulmonary valve area: It is rarely caused by the organic heart disease. In general, it is a functional murmur produced by relative pulmonary insufficiency which is caused by dilatation of pulmonary artery. The murmur is soft, limited, decrescendo, diastolic, blowing and usually accompanied with increased P2. It is called Graham Steel murmur which is louder at the end of inspiration and usually occurs in mitral stenosis with pulmonary arterial hypertension.

   Tricuspid valve area: It is restricted to the fourth and fifth left intercostal space in the sternal border. The murmur is low-pitched, rumbling and louder at the end of deep inspiration. It occurs in tricuspid stenosis and is rarely heard.
3. Continuous murmurs: It usually occurs in patents with ductus arteriosus. This murmur which persists from systole to diastole even covering S2, is harsh and machine-like. It is best heard at second intercostal space, left to the sternal border and usually with thrill. The continuous murmur also occurs in aortopulmonary septal defect, and is best heard at third intercostal space, left to the sternal border. In addition, continuous murmur can also be heard in coronary arteriovenous fistula and coronary aneurysms rupture.

Pericardial Friction Sound

It is produced due to the rubbing of the parietal and visceral surfaces of the pericardium. The murmur is harsh, high-pitched and superficial, like paper rubbed against each other. It is heard best at the apex of the heart and the third/fourth intercostal space left to the sternal border in the sitting position leaning forward at the end of expiration. Typical pericardial friction sound shows three phases: atrial systole, ventricular systole and ventricular diastole. Sometimes, pericardial friction sound only occurs in ventricular systole or both ventricular systole and diastole. Pericardial friction sound begins at the same time as heart beat. It even exists when holding breath, which is different from pleural friction sound. The common causes of pericardial friction rub are infectious pericarditis (TB, purulent pericarditis, etc) and non-infectious pericarditis (acute myocardial infarction, uremia, post-cardiac injury syndrome and SLE). Pericardial friction sound disappears when pericardial effusion increases.

45.5 Vascular Examination

Vascular examination is an integral part for physical examination. This section focuses on the peripheral vascular examination including pulse, pressure, blood vessels and peripheral vessel signs.

45.5.1 Pulse

Pulse examination is mainly the palpation of the superficial artery, generally the radial artery and specifically the carotid artery, the femoral artery and the dorsal artery of foot. Palpate the artery wall with the tip of the index, middle and ring fingers. Compare and palpate both sides artery pulse, usually the difference is minimal for normal person. In certain condition as Takayasu arteritis, the difference is obvious or noticeable. To exclude Takayasu arteritis or Aortic coarctation, the pulse is compared and the pressure of upper and lower limbs are measured simultaneously to observe rate, rhythm, tone, strength, waveform and arterial wall elasticity during the palpation.

45.5.1.1 Pulse Rate

The clinical significances of the pulse rate and the heart rate are basically the same. Under normal circumstances, the heart rate and the pulse rate are consistent. But they would differ in some arrhythmias such as atrial fibrillation, or ventricular premature contraction. With the significant reduction of ectopic stroke volume, unable to perceive that makes the pulse rate less than the heart rate i.e. called pulse deficit.

45.5.1.2 Pulse Rhythm

The pulse rhythm reflects the rhythm of the heart. Pulse rhythm of normal individuals is the same as heart rhythm. Arrhythmias can influence the pulse rhythm. For example, with atrial fibrillation, the pulse rhythm of patients is absolutely irregular; pulse intensity ranges; pulse rate is less than the heart rate. Premature beat as bigeminy and trigeminy can cause bigeminal pulse and trigeminal pulse. The second-degree atrioventricular block can result in missed pulse rhythm called dropped pulse caused by cardiac arrest.

45.5.1.3 Tensity and Arterial Wall State

The pulse tension is related to the degree of arterial stiffness. To judge the pulse tension, two fingers are placed on the radial artery or temporal artery and the pressure is applied. For example, compress the radial artery and feel the existence of strip artery, like a cord, tortuous or nodular, suggestive of arteriosclerosis.

45.5.1.4 Strength

The strength of pulse is related to the cardiac output, pulse pressure and peripheral vascular resistance. Enhanced pulse with large amplitude is due to hyperkinemia, high pulse pressures and decent peripheral resistance, found in fever, hyperthyroidism, and aortic valve insufficiency. Whereas weakened pulse with small amplitude is due to hypokinemia, low pulse pressures and increased peripheral, found in resistance cardiac failure, aortic valve stenosis and shock i.e.

45.5.1.5 Pulse Wave

On palpation of the peripheral arteries, multiple abnormal pulse waves can be found which contribute in diagnosing the clinical diseases.

1. Normal pulse wave
   The normal pulse wave consists of ascending limb, wave crest and descending limb. The ascending branch occurs in the early phase of left ventricular contraction caused by left ventricular ejection on the aortic wall. Wave crest occurs in the middle and the late phase of the contraction during the metaphase to the final phase of systole i.e. caused by the aorta wall shocked during the blood far-end moving. The descending limb occurs in ventricular diastole when aortic valve close and aortic wall recoil, so that blood continues to flow to peripheral arteries. In obvious aortic sclerosis, the dicrotic wave tends to be less.
2. Water-hammer pulse
   The water-hammer pulse works like the tide water rising and falling down suddenly. It's caused by vasorelaxation, shunt or regurgitation existed in peripheral vessels. Shunt is common in hyperthyroidism, severe anemia and dermatophytosis. Regurgitation is often caused by aortic insufficiency, congenital patent ductus arteriosus and arterio-venous fistula. The examiner grasps patient's wrist in the radial artery and raises it above head, to feel the hasty and strong impulse like water-washed.
3. Pulsus alternans
   The pulsus alternans is a waveform of arterial pulse showing alternating strong and weak beats due to alternate strong and weak ventricular contractions. To exclude the respiratory effects, the patients are asked to hold the breath during examination. It is an indication of left ventricular systolic impairment.
4. Paradoxical Pulsus
   The paradoxical pulse is a kind of significantly weakened or disappeared pulse during a patient's inspiration. Normal pulse strength is not affected by respiratory cycle. But with cardiac tamponade and pericardial constriction, right ventricular diastole is limited and pulmonary vascular expand, blood flow from the pulmonary vein to the atrium becomes less, so the left ventricular ejection fraction decreases during the inspiration.
5. Pulsus Tardus
   It's a slow-rising pulse. On palpation the pulse is weak and delayed relative to its usually expected character. It is mainly found in severe aortic stenosis.

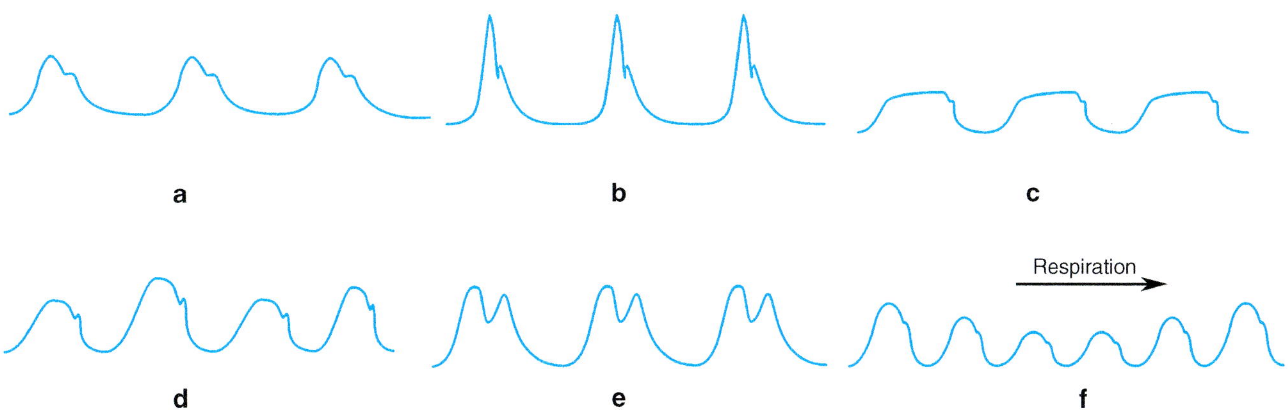

Fig. 45.37 The waveform of pulse waves. (a) Normal pulse. (b) Water-hammer pulse. (c) Pulsus tardus. (d) Pulsus alternans. (e) Dicrotic pulse. (f) Pulseless

6. Dicrotic pulse
   The dicrotic pulse is a pulse i.e. characterized by two peaks, the second peak occurring in diastole and being an exaggeration of the dicrotic wave, which exists when the stroke volume is weak, such as in severe heart failure. Bisferiens pulse which is characterized by the second peak occurring in late systole exists in severe aortic valve insufficiency with stenosis and occasionally in hypertrophic obstructive cardiomyopathy.
7. Pulseless
   Absence of pulse i.e. commonly found in following situations: (a) Severe shock, with unmeasurable blood pressure and impalpable pulse of peripheral arteries. (b) Polyarteritis, because of main artery occlusion, the pulse of the following parts of the blocked vascular can't be palpated. (c) Limb artery embolism, the pulse of the following parts of the vascular embolism can't be touched. (d) Electro-Mechanical Dissociation

   The pulse waves mentioned above are shown in Fig. 45.37:

45.5.2 Blood Pressure (BP)

Blood pressure, a vital sign, refers to systemic artery pressure in general. To measure BP is a important part in clinical physical examination.

45.5.2.1 Blood Pressure Measurement

There are two ways of blood pressure measurement, including direct measurement and indirect measurement.

1. Direct measurement
   Blood pressure is measured by a catheter-transducer system in direct measurement. The catheter serves to provide access to the artery (usually radial, brachial, or femoral artery) and also detects the pressure by connecting to pressure monitor via analog-to-digital converter. The blood pressure value collected by direct measurement is accurate and real-time. As it is an invasive examination method, and requires special equipment and advanced technology, this measurement is only applied to critical and surgical patients.
2. Indirect measurement
   Indirect measurement are obtained with a sphygmomanometer. The method and precautions of indirect measurement have been detailed in Sect. 3.1, Chap. 3, Part III.

45.5.2.2 Blood Pressure Standard

Epidemiological data show that blood pressure is somewhat variable depending on different sexes, races, jobs, physiological and environmental conditions. Systolic blood pressure (SBP) differs linearly with age increasing, and pulse pressure also increases gradually. In normal person, the blood pressure of one arm may differ by 5–10 mmHg from the other, and the blood pressure of the legs may be 20–40 mmHg higher than that of the arms. BP, especially SBP, can be affected by many factors. Exercise, tea, smoking, drinking, emotional excitement and stress can increase BP, so that it cannot be determined by only once BP measurement, and repeated BP measurements must be necessary. There are different criteria for hypertension in different countries. The definition and classification of Chinese adults' blood pressure can refer to general station examination in Sect. 2.1, Chap. 2, Part III.

45.5.2.3 Abnormal Blood Pressure

Abnormal blood pressure includes hypertension, hypotension, asymmetrical blood pressure between arms, decreased difference between arms and legs, and increased or decreased pulse pressure.

1. Hypertension
   Hypertension is defined as blood pressure higher than normal level [SBp ≥ 140 mmHg and (or) DBp ≥ 90 mmHg]. The results of blood pressure measurement should be recorded at least three times in different days without any anti-hypertensive agent. Hypertension for which no recognizable cause can be found is called essential or idiopathic hypertension, and the interaction of polygenic abnormality and environmental factors may be the causes. Hypertension caused by some diseases is called secondary hypertension (5%–10%), secondary causes include renal artery stenosis, renal disease, pheochromocytoma, primary aldosteronism, hypercortisolism, toxemia of pregnancy, large artery diseases, intracranial hypertension, etc.
2. Hypotension
   The blood pressure lower than 90/60 mmHg is called hypotension. Some serious causes of hypotension include shock, acute myocardial infarction, hemorrhage and languisher.
3. Asymmetrical blood pressure between arms
   In general, there is little or no significant difference in the blood pressure of the two upper extremities. Asymmetrical blood pressure between arms means that the SBP variation between arms is more than 10 mmHg. This condition is found mainly in polyarteritis, congenital arterial malformation and thromboangiitis obliterans.
4. Decreased difference between arms and legs
   If the blood pressure of the legs is equal or lower than that of the arms, it suggests that there must be arteriostenosis or arterial occlusion in the corresponding site. It usually occurs in coarctation of aorta, thoracoabdominal aorto-arteritis, iliac artery or femoral artery occlusion, etc.
5. Increased or decreased pulse pressure
   Increased pulse pressure means the pulse pressure is more than 60 mmHg. It is often caused by aortic insufficiency, patent ductus arteriosus, hyperthyroidism, severe anaemia and arteriosclerosis in the elderly. The decreased pulse pressure means the pulse pressure is less than 30 mmHg. It is mainly caused by aortic stenosis, heart failure, pericardial effusion, constrictive pericarditis, etc.
6. Pseudohypertension and Pseudohypotension
   (a) Due to the severe arteriosclerosis of brachial artery, the brachial artery is hard to be blocked by the sphygmomanometry. In this case, the measured BP must be higher than the actual BP, which is called pseudohypertension. In addition, some patients, whose BP is normal at home, exhibit a blood pressure level above the normal range in hospital, it is white-coat hypertension. In this condition, ambulatory blood pressure monitoring is helpful for to differentiate it (see the next chapter).
   (b) Pseudohypotension is a syndrome in which indirect blood pressure measurement by sphygmomanometer underestimates true intraarterial blood pressure, due to arterial medial sclerosis and calcification or operational problems.
      - There may be a long silent auscultatory gap between Korotkoff I and II in the elder, which leads to an underestimation of the actual SBP if the examiners mistake Korotkoff II for SBP. Therefore, we must continue inflating the cuff until the pressure increases to 30 mmHg after the brachial pulse disappears, and then deflating the cuff slowly until Korotkoff I sound is heard. Using this method can avoid the error in measurement.
      - Decreased arterial compliance in the elderly or in patients with severe arteriosclerosis can cause a delayed duration from Korotkoff IV sound to Korotkoff V sound, which can cause DBP underestimated. So if the pressure difference from Korotkoff IV to Korotkoff V is more than 20 mmHg, Korotkoff IV is a more accurate indication and should be taken as DBP, and the pressure at Korotkoff V should be recorded at the same time, for example 160/80–50 mmHg.

45.5.2.4 Ambulatory Blood Pressure Monitoring (ABPM)

Non-invasive ambulatory blood pressure monitoring is a newly-developed technique for diagnosis in recent years. It provides the mean value and dispersion of blood pressure over a 24-h period, and represents a true reflection of blood pressure sensitively and objectively, and obtains the blood pressure variability and the pattern of circadian BP changes, which are useful for further evaluating target organ damage and prognosis. Many studies have confirmed that the clinical value of blood pressure measured by ABPM is superior to office blood pressure.

China Hypertension Guidelines recommend that ABPM measuring device must be rigorously validated by hypertension societies and organization, such as BHS and AAMI. In clinical practice, measurements are often made every 15 or 20 min during daytime (6 am–10 pm) and every 30 min during nighttime (10 pm–6 am next day). According to 2013 ESC Guidelines for the management of arterial hypertension, the normal reference value of ambulatory blood pressure should be as follows: average 24-h BP <130/80 mmHg, average daytime (or awake) BP <135/85 mmHg and nighttime (or asleep) <120/70 mmHg. Daytime BP is normally 10–20% lower than that of nighttime. For Patients who are suspected of white-coat hypertension, masked hypertension (clinical blood pressure is normal while home-measurement of BP increases), refractory hypertension, paroxysmal hypertension, hypotension, and poor antihypertensive effect,

ABPM should be completed as a supplementary evaluation of BP besides conventional blood pressure measurements.

45.5.3 Vascular Murmur and Peripherial Vascular Sign

45.5.3.1 Venous Murmur

Venous murmur is usually not obvious. It could be heard most significantly under the clavicle, at the base of the neck. It is low-pitched, soft, continuous and best heard in sitting or standing position. It may disappear if the jugular vein is compressed. It is usually harmless and produced by venous flow rapidly flowing into superior vena cava. In addition, a venous murmur is heard surrounding the navel and upper abdomen in the cases of liver cirrhosis with portal hypertension, which leads to dilatation of collateral circulation and increase of flow velocities.

45.5.3.2 Arterial Bruit

Abnormal sound heard over the arteries is called arterial bruit. Arterial bruits are commonly heard at peripheral, pulmonary and coronary arteries. These sounds are low-pitched and may be more easily heard with the bell of the stethoscope. Common bruits that can be heard easily have been listed as follows:

(a) In patients with hyperthyroidism, continuous bruits at upper pole and lower pole of thyroid may be heard.
(b) In arterial stenosis caused by Takayasu's arteritis, a systolic bruit may be heard at supraclavicular region, posterior cervical triangle or back.
(c) A systolic bruit may be heard in superior abdomen and lower back in patients with renal artery stenosis.
(d) In patients with pulmonary arterio-venous fistula, a continuous bruit may be heard at the corresponding site of the chest.
(e) The continuous bruit also can be heard in patients with peripheral arterio-venous fistula.
(f) In patients with coronary arterio-venous fistula, a continuous or double phase bruits can be heard in the middle and distal segment of sternum. The bruit is soft and superficial, and sometimes is more obvious in diastole.
(g) A crescendo-decrescendo systolic bruit, which is heard at supraclavicular region, occurs in some healthy children and youth. The mechanism is still not clear. It is supposed that the bruit is from brachiocephalic branches of aortic arch.

45.5.3.3 Peripheral Vascular Signs

Besides increasing of pulse pressure and water-hammer pulse, there are some other peripheral vascular signs like pistol shot sound, Duroziez's sign, capillary pulsation sign and visible pulsation of carotid artery. If those signs above are found during physical examination means positive for the peripheral vascular signs, which is usually happened in those patients with severe aortic regurgitation, hyperthyroidism or severe anemia.

1. Pistol-shot sound
   The pistol-shot sounds, heard over the peripheral artery, such as femoral arteries (Traube's sign), is synchronous with heart beat.
2. Duroziez's sign
   A double phase and blowing murmur can be heard over the femoral artery by compressing it using the bell of stethoscope.
3. Capillary pulsation sign
   The alternate rhythmic blanching and reddening can be seen in the nails or lip compressed by fingers, when heart relaxes and contracts.
4. Visible pulsation of carotid artery
   Visible pulsation of carotid artery (Corrigan's sign) or deMusset's sign can be found when pulse pressure increases.

Key Terms

1	Thoracic respiration	胸式呼吸
2	Diaphragmatic respiration	腹式呼吸
3	Thoracic expansion	胸廓扩张度
4	Vocal fremitus	语音震颤
5	Bronchial breath sound	支气管呼吸音
6	Vesicular breath sound	肺泡呼吸音
7	Rale	啰音
8	Inward impulse	负性心尖搏动
9	Apical impulse	心尖搏动
10	Cardiac dullness border	正常心浊音界
11	Splitting of heart sounds	心音分裂
12	Gallop rhythm	奔马律
13	Pericardial friction sound	心包摩擦音
14	Capillary pulsation sign	毛细血管搏动征
15	Peripheral vascular signs	周围血管征

Study Questions

1. What are abnormal percussion notes of the chest and their common causes?
2. What are the definition, classification, characteristics and clinical significance of rales?
3. How to distinguish the normal S1 and S2?
4. How to identify functional and organic systolic murmurs?
5. What are the peripheral vascular signs? And in which situation it could be found?

Suggested Readings

Bettencourt PE, Del Bono EA, Spiegelman D, Hertzmark E, Murphy RL Jr. Clinical utility of chest auscultation in common pulmonary diseases. Am J Respir Crit Care Med. 1994;150:1291.

http://cc.scu.edu.cn/G2S/Template/View.aspx?action=view&courseType=0&courseId=1887.

46 Physical Examination of Abdomen

Fei Dai and Rui Zeng

Abdominal examination includes inspection, palpation, percussion and auscultation. The examination is performed following this sequence: inspection, auscultation, percussion and palpation. However, for a uniform format when recording the examination, we still conform to the basic steps of inspection, palpation, percussion and auscultation. There are two reasons to explain the change of the examination sequence: firstly, it's convenient to perform the auscultation of the abdomen after that of the heart; at the same time, it can also avoid negative impacts of a series of palpations on the auscultation of bowel sounds due to the alteration of gastrointestinal peristalsis. Palpation is the most important step in abdominal examination.

46.1 Section 1: Landmarks of the Abdominal Wall and Abdominal Areas

46.1.1 Abdominal Landmarks

Commonly used anatomic landmarks are illustrated as follows (Fig. 46.1):

1. Costal margin: The costal arch is composed of the eighth to tenth costal cartilage and the eleventh and twelfth floating ribs. The abdomen is bounded superiorly by its inferior margin, which is usually used in abdominal divisions and measurement of the liver and spleen.
2. Xiphoid process: It attaches to the cartilage at the inferior end of the sternum, serving as the upper bound of abdominal surface.
3. Upper abdominal angle: It is also called the infrasternal angle. As the crossing angle of bilateral costal arches to the root of xiphoid process, it is used for the judgement of somatotypes and measurement of the liver.
4. Umbilicus: The umbilicus, located at the center of the abdomen and between the third and fourth lumbar vertebrae, is the landmark of abdominal divisions and lumbar puncture.
5. Anterior superior iliac spine: It is the projecting point of the anterior iliac crest, functioning as the landmark of nine abdominal areas and the usual site of bone marrow puncture.
6. Lateral border of rectus muscles: It is equivalent to the continuation of the midclavicular line and usually serves as the position of surgical incisions. The gallbladder point is located at the junction of the right lateral border of rectus muscles and costal margin.
7. Midabdominal line: It is equivalent to the linea alba and is the continuation of the anterior median line, where hernias of linea alba are more likely to occur.
8. Inguinal ligament: Bilateral inguinal ligaments and the superior margin of pubic symphysis together form the lower bound of the abdominal surface, where it is the marker of the femoral artery and femoral vein and provides the site for inguinal hernia to pass through.
9. Costovertebral angle: It is the crossing angle of the twelfth rib on both sides of the back and the vertebral column, where the kidney percussion pain can be examined.
10. Pubic symphysis: It serves as the fibrous and cartilaginous connection between the two pubic bones and together forms the lower bound of the abdominal surface with pubic bones.

F. Dai
Department of Gastroenterology, Xi'an Jiaotong University, Xi'an, China

R. Zeng (✉)
Department of Cardiology, Sichuan University, Chengdu, China

X.-H. Wan, R. Zeng (eds.), *Handbook of Clinical Diagnostics*, https://doi.org/10.1007/978-981-13-7677-1_46

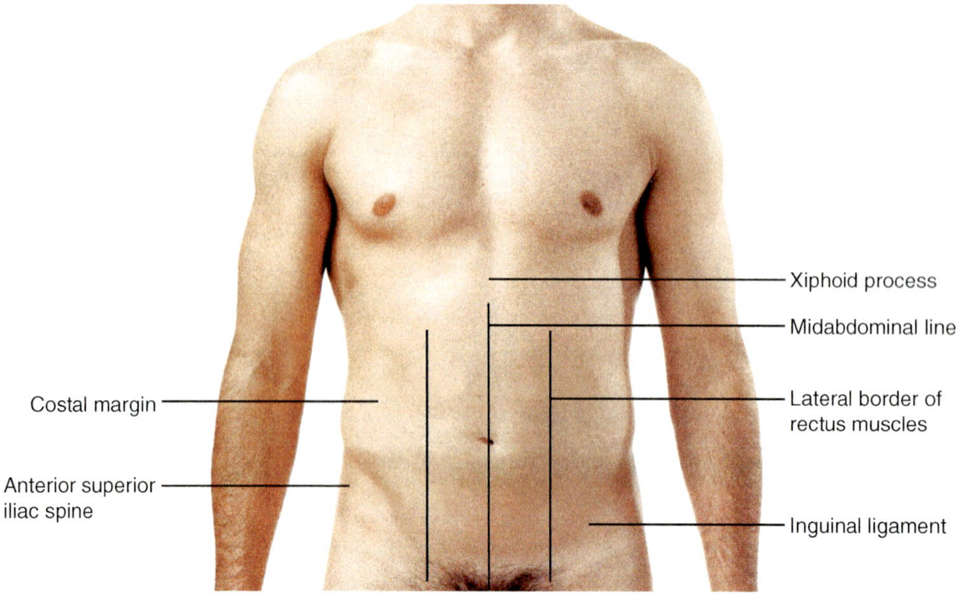

Fig. 46.1 Abdominal landmarks

46.1.2 Abdominal Areas

The abdomen can be divided into several areas with the aid of abdominal landmarks and some imaginary lines.

46.1.2.1 The Four Abdominal Quadrants

The abdomen is divided into four quadrants by two imaginary perpendicular lines crossing at the umbilicus. These four quadrants are the right upper quadrant, right lower quadrant, left upper quadrant and left lower quadrant (Fig. 46.2). Major organs underlying each of four quadrants are known as follows:

Right Upper Quadrant (RUQ)

Liver, gallbladder, pylorus, duodenum, small intestine, head of the pancreas, right adrenal gland, right kidney, hepatic flexure of colon, portion of the transverse colon, abdominal aorta.

Right Lower Quadrant (RLQ)

Cecum, appendix, portion of the ascending colon, small intestine, right ureter, distended bladder, right ovary, right fallopian tube, enlarged uterus, right spermatic cord.

Left Upper Quadrant (LUQ)

Left lobe of the liver, spleen, stomach, small intestine, body of the pancreas, tail of the pancreas, left adrenal gland, left kidney, splenic flexure of colon, portion of the transverse colon, abdominal aorta.

Left Lower Quadrant (LLQ)

Sigmoid colon, portion of the descending colon, small intestine, left ureter, distended bladder, left ovary, left fallopian tube, enlarged uterus, left spermatic cord.

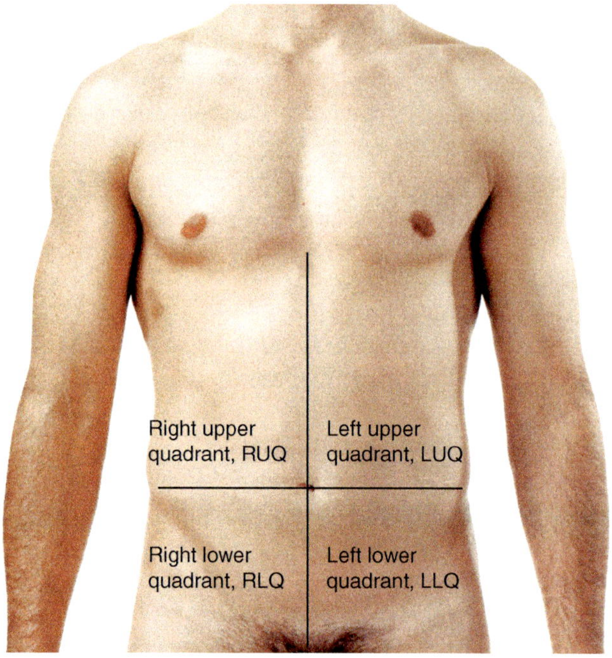

Fig. 46.2 The four abdominal quadrants

46.1.2.2 The Nine Abdominal Areas

The abdomen is divided into nine sections by two imaginary horizontal lines and two vertical lines. The upper horizontal line is drawn by joining bilateral costal margins, and the lower joining bilateral anterosuperior iliac spines. At right angles to these lines, another two lines are drawn across the middle of linking line formed by right and left anterosuperior iliac spine and the anterior median line. These four lines divide the abdomen into nine areas: right and left hypochondrium, right and left lumbar, right and left iliac region,

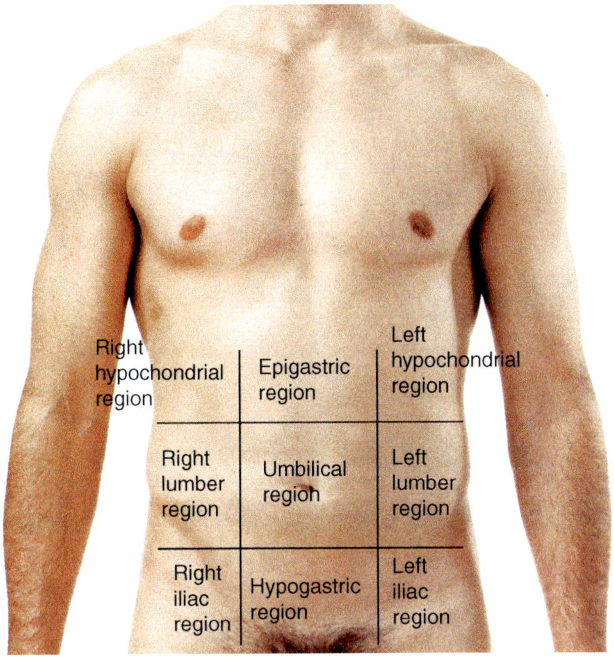

Fig. 46.3 The nine abdominal areas

epigastric, umbilical and hypogastric region (Fig. 46.3). Organs underlying each of nine areas are shown as follows:

1. Right hypochondrial region: Right lobe of the liver, gallbladder, hepatic flexure of colon, right kidney, right adrenal gland.
2. Right lumbar region: Ascending colon, jejunum, right kidney.
3. Right iliac region: Cecum, appendix, terminal ileum, lymph node, right ovary, right fallopian tube, right spermatic cord.
4. Left hypochondrial region: Spleen, stomach, splenic flexure of colon, tail of the pancreas, left kidney, left adrenal gland.
5. Left lumber region: Descending colon, jejunum or ileum, left kidney.
6. Left iliac region: Sigmoid colon, left ovary, left fallopian tube, left spermatic cord.
7. Epigastric region: Stomach, left lobe of the liver, duodenum, head and body of the pancreas, transverse colon, abdominal aorta, greater omentum.
8. Umbilical region: Descendant duodenum, jejunum and ileum, prolapsing stomach or transverse colon, ureter, abdominal aorta, mesentery and its lymph node, greater omentum.
9. Hypogastric region: Ileum, sigmoid colon, ureter, distended bladder or enlarged uterus.

In clinical practice, the four-quadrant method is frequently used with nine-section method as its supplement, for example, combined with epigastric, umbilical, hypogastric and lumber region. The location of major organs is illustrated in Fig. 46.4.

46.2 Section 2: Inspection

During abdominal inspection, the patient should keep warm, empty the bladder and take a supine position, as well as place the arm naturally on either side of the trunk. The abdomen should be exposed completely from the xiphoid process to pubic symphysis. The doctor should stand at the right side of the patient and inspect the abdomen from top to bottom in a certain order.

46.2.1 Abdominal Contour

46.2.1.1 Abdominal Protuberance

Abdominal protuberance refers to a condition that the anterior abdominal wall is significantly higher than the surface between the costal margin and pubic symphysis when the patient is in the supine position, presenting as a convex shape. It can be caused by physiological conditions such as obesity and pregnancy, or pathological factors such as ascites, peritoneal air and giant tumors. Different manifestations due to different situations are shown as follows.

Overall Abdominal Protuberance

Peritoneal Fluid

Ascites is an abnormal accumulation of fluid in the abdomen. The abdominal wall is lax in the supine position and fluid deposits at the flanks, making the abdomen flat and wide, which is called *frog belly*. If the patient lies on one side or sits up, the lower abdomen will be bulged because of downward movement of free fluid. When a large amount of ascites causes the increase of abdominal pressure, the abdomen will bulge like a globular belly and the umbilicus will also protrude. Ascites is commonly found in portal hypertension of liver cirrhosis, heart failure, constrictive pericarditis, peritoneal carcinomatosis, nephrotic syndrome, pancreatic ascites or tuberculous peritonitis etc. *Apical belly* results from peritonitis or infiltration of cancers, with the abdomen presenting as the apical shape.

Peritoneal Air

Peritoneal air is caused by a large amount of air accumulating within the gastrointestinal tract. Under this circumstance, the general shape of abdomen is globular, which is commonly seen in intestinal obstruction or enteroparalysis resulting from various reasons. The accumulation of air in the abdominal cavity known as *pneumoperitoneum*, occurs in

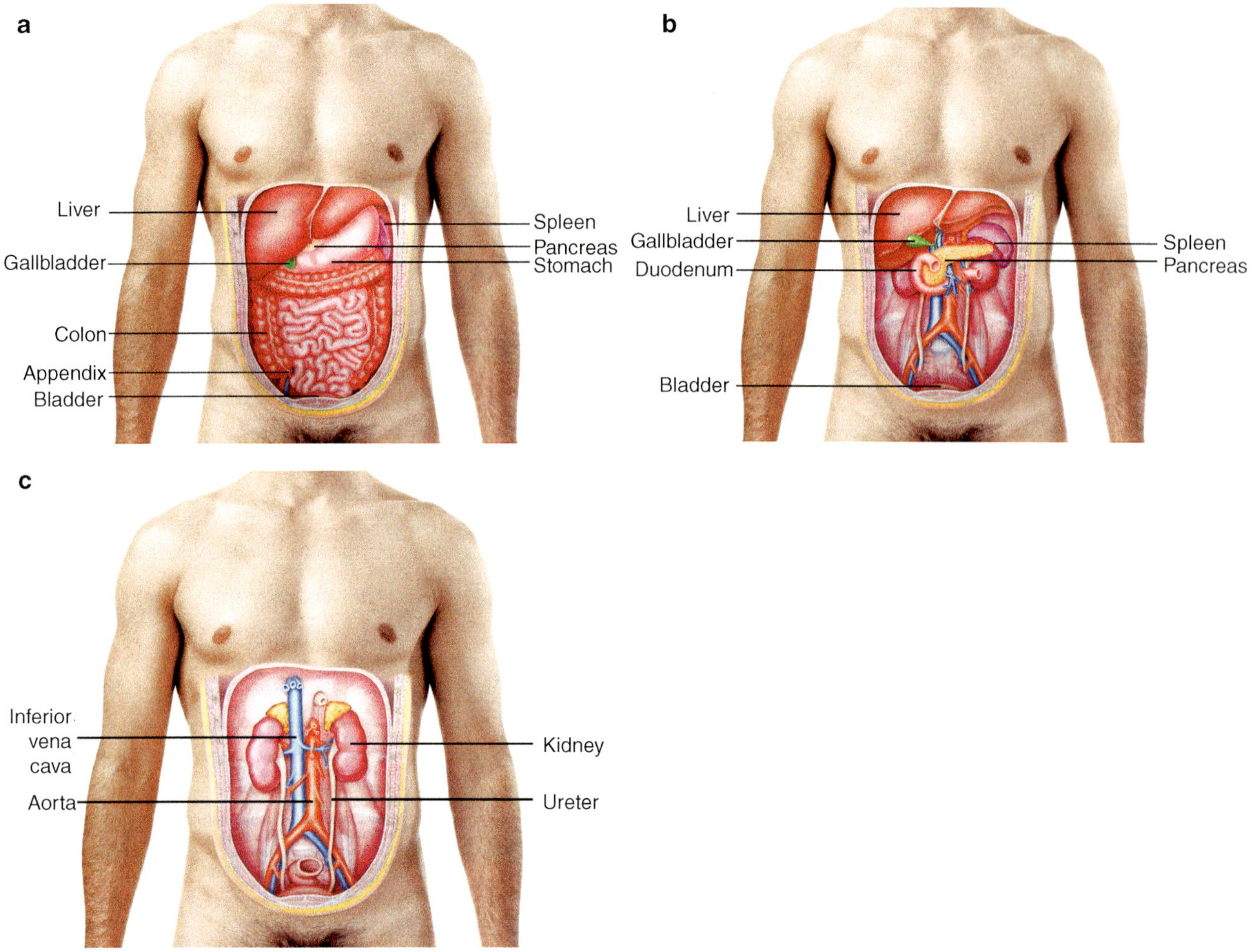

Fig. 46.4 Abdominal organs

the perforation of gastrointestinal tract or therapeutic artificial pneumoperitoneum, with the former accompanied by varying degrees of peritonitis.

Huge Abdominal Mass

Huge abdominal masses, such as full-term pregnancy, huge ovarian cysts and teratoma etc., can also result in overall abdominal protuberance.

Local Abdominal Protuberance

Local abdominal protuberance usually results from an enlarged viscera, intra-abdominal tumor or inflammatory mass, gastrointestinal flatulence, mass in the abdominal wall, and hernia etc. During inspection, it should be noted that whether protuberant sites and contours displace with respiration or change with postures, and whether pulsations exist or not. Organomegaly generally occurs in the site where the organ is located in and maintains its characteristics.

Local abdominal protuberance is sometimes attributed to masses in the abdominal wall (such as subcutaneous lipoma and tuberculous abscess etc.), rather than intra-abdominal lesions. What makes them identifiable is to raise the patient's head or legs for the purpose of tensing abdominal muscles, indicating that masses are located in the wall if they are more protrudent. Conversely, if they are not apparent or even disappear, it suggests that masses are within the abdominal cavity and obscured by hardened abdominal muscles due to contraction. However, abdominal conditions in the deep layer of abdominal muscles can also become blurred.

46.2.1.2 Abdominal Concavity

Abdominal concavity refers to a condition that the anterior abdominal wall is significantly lower than the surface between the xiphoid process and pubic symphysis when the patient is in the supine position. There are two kinds of concavity, that is, overall abdominal concavity and local abdominal concavity, with the former of greater significance.

Overall Abdominal Concavity

Overall abdominal concavity is observed in patients with emaciation and dehydration. *Scaphoid abdomen* is so called because the contour of the abdomen is shaped like a boat, with the anterior abdominal wall almost approximating to the spinal column, and costal arch, iliac crest as well as pubic symphysis appearing. This sign is commonly seen in cachexia, for instance, some chronic wasting diseases like tuberculosis and malignant tumors etc. Abdominal concavity occurring in inspiration often results from diaphragmatic paralysis and the upper airway obstruction.

Local Abdominal Concavity

Local abdominal concavity is less common and is frequently induced by contraction of an abdominal scar following surgery. When the patient stands erect or abdominal pressure is increased, concavity will be more marked.

46.2.2 States of Abdominal Wall

46.2.2.1 Skin Rash

Different kinds of rash suggest different diseases. Congestive or hemorrhagic rash commonly appears in exanthematous fever disorders or certain infectious diseases (such as measles, scarlet fever, typhoid fever as well as typhus), and drug allergies etc. Purpura or urticaria may be part of some systemic diseases, for example, anaphylactoid purpura and systemic urticaria. Herpes in one side of the abdomen or lumbar (distributing along spinal nerves) reveal herpes zoster.

46.2.2.2 Pigmentation

Normally, abdominal skin color is slightly lighter than the exposed area. Brown pigmentation in skin folds (such as inguen and the belt line) can be found in hypoadrenocorticism (Addison disease). A bluish discoloration of the left waist, resulting from extravasation of blood from retroperitoneal space into the skin beneath lateral abdominal wall (*Grey-Turner sign*), occurs in acute hemorrhagic pancreatitis or strangulated intestinal obstruction. A similar discoloration of the periumbilical region or lower abdominal wall is a sign following major intraperitoneal or retroperitoneal hemorrhage (*Cullen sign*), which is because of acute hemorrhagic pancreatitis or ectopic pregnancy rupture. For women in pregnancy, there is brown pigmentation in the midline between the umbilicus and pubis, gradually fading away after parturition.

46.2.2.3 Abdominal Striae

Abdominal striae are mainly distributed in hypogastric region and the area around the right and left lower abdomen, caused by fracture of dermal connective tissues due to the increased tension. White striae are common in obese or multiparous women; pink striae occur in the mid and third trimester of pregnancy, turning white after delivery and persisting for a long time; purple striae, common signs of hypercortisolism, can be encountered in vastus lateralis, shoulders and back, except for the lower abdomen and buttocks.

46.2.2.4 Scar

Abdominal scars mostly are remnants of injuries, operations or skin infections. Some surgical scars in specific areas usually suggest patient's operations.

46.2.2.5 Hernia

Abdominal hernia can be divided into two types: internal abdominal hernia and external abdominal hernia, with the former rare and the latter more common. It is formed by abdominal contents extruding from the body surface through the space or weak part of abdominal or pelvic wall. Umbilical hernia is frequently seen in infants and may be present in multipara or patients with massive ascites; incisional hernia may be present in the site where poor surgical scar healing happens.

46.2.2.6 Umbilicus

For patients undergoing abdominal protuberance, observing the umbilical position contributes to deduction of intra-abdominal lesions. For example, patients with umbilical downward displacement are mainly caused by hepatomegaly or ascites, and patients with upward displacement commonly caused by pelvic neoplasms or pregnancy.

46.2.2.7 Inguen

On inspection, it should be noted whether there are signs of abnormal masses, nodules in bilateral inguen and its symmetry, as well as signs of scars or swelling, and abnormal pulsation etc. If necessary, it also should be verified with the aid of palpation.

46.2.3 Veins of Abdominal Wall

Normally, subcutaneous veins of the abdominal wall do not appear unless the patient is emaciated or light-complexioned. They can also be seen in the aged whose skin is thinner and flabby, but they are usually straight rather than tortuous. In addition, epigastric veins also occur in various conditions that make abdominal inner pressure elevated, such as ascites, huge abdominal mass and pregnancy etc.

The abdominal veins being prominent and thick is referred to as abdominal wall varicosis, which is common in the impairment of circulation caused by portal hypertension or collateral formation due to the obstructed return of the superior or inferior vena cava.

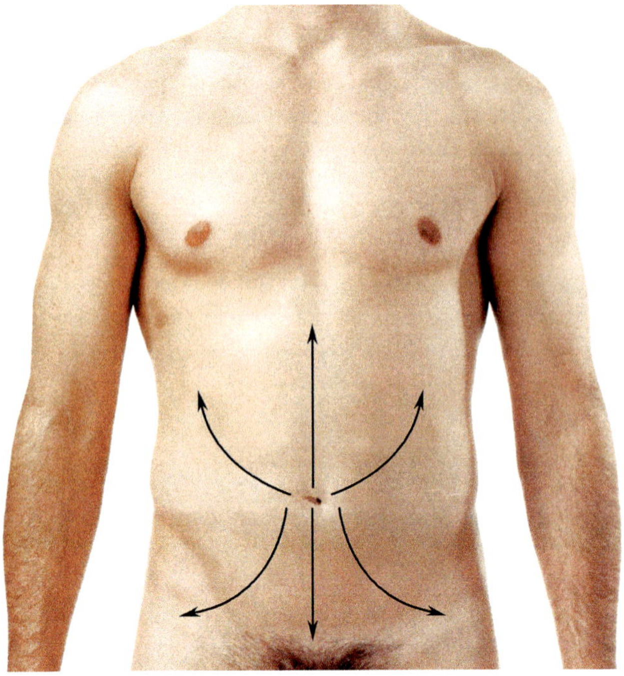

Fig. 46.5 Blood distribution and direction of superficial abdominal veins in portal vein obstruction

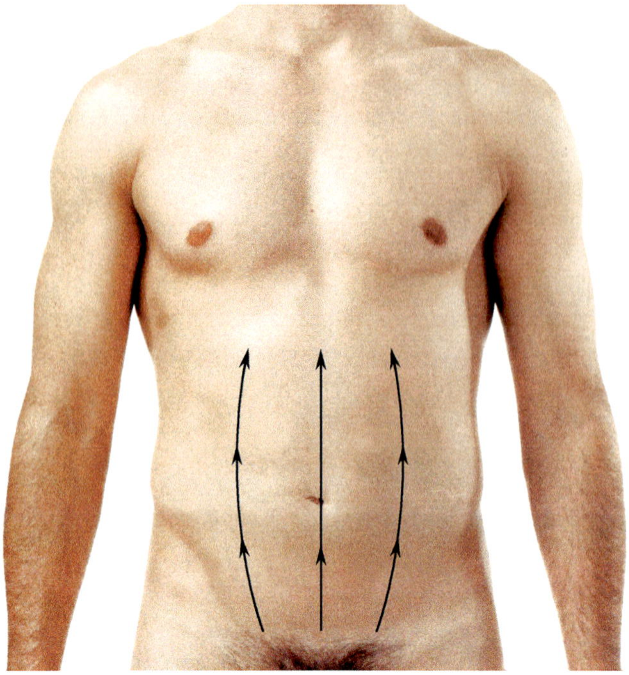

Fig. 46.6 Blood distribution and direction of superficial abdominal veins in obstruction of the inferior vena cava

It is known that normally, upper abdominal veins carry blood upward to the superior vena cava via thoracic and axillary veins, and lower veins drain blood downward to the inferior vena cava via great saphenous veins. As a result of significant portal hypertension, a cluster of varicose veins appear to radiate outward in all directions from the umbilicus, shaped like *caput medusae*, where venous blood murmur can often be heard (Fig. 46.5). In obstruction of the inferior vena cava, varicosities are mostly distributed in both sides of the abdominal wall, sometimes laterally in the buttocks as well as thighs, and the lower abdominal superficial veins also drain upward (Fig. 46.6). In an obstruction of the superior vena cava, the blood flow direction of superficial veins in the upper abdominal wall or chest wall is reversed, which can be demonstrated by a simple finger-pressing maneuver.

In order to identify the source of varicosity of the abdominal wall, it is necessary to examine blood flow direction. Choosing a segment of branch-free abdominal veins, the examiner places his right index finger and middle finger together on it, slides one compressing finger outward and empties blood between two fingers, then removes the finger to a certain distance and keeps the other tightly compressing, thus observing the venous rate of refilling. If the rate is fast, it suggests that the blood flow drains from the relaxing end towards the compressing, which can be verified by applying the same method to relax the other finger and observe venous refilling condition (Fig. 46.7).

46.2.4 Respiratory Movements

In normal people, the upward (with each inhalation) and downward (with each exhalation) movement of the abdominal wall at each breath is defined as an abdominal breathing exercise. Respiration in males and children is mainly abdominal, whereas that in females is commonly thoracic, with little movement of the abdominal wall.

Limitation of abdominal breathing may result from peritonitis, ascites, and acute abdominal pain, giant abdominal mass or pregnancy. In severe cases, such as acute peritonitis caused by gastrointestinal perforation or diaphragmatic paralysis, abdominal respiration will disappear. Enhancement of abdominal respiration is rare and frequently appears in hysterical breathing or thoracic diseases (pleural effusion etc.).

46.2.5 Gastral or Intestinal Pattern and Peristalsis

Normally, contours of the stomach and intestines and peristalsis do not appear unless the abdominal wall is very lax or thin as in the aged, multipara and lean individuals.

Once gastrointestinal obstruction occurs, gastral or intestinal segment in the proximal end will be protuberant due to dilatation, exhibiting contours of the stomach and intestines, which is known as *gastral or intestinal pattern*. Meanwhile, *peristalsis* will be observed due to the strengthened peristaltic motility in this site. Once intestinal paralysis

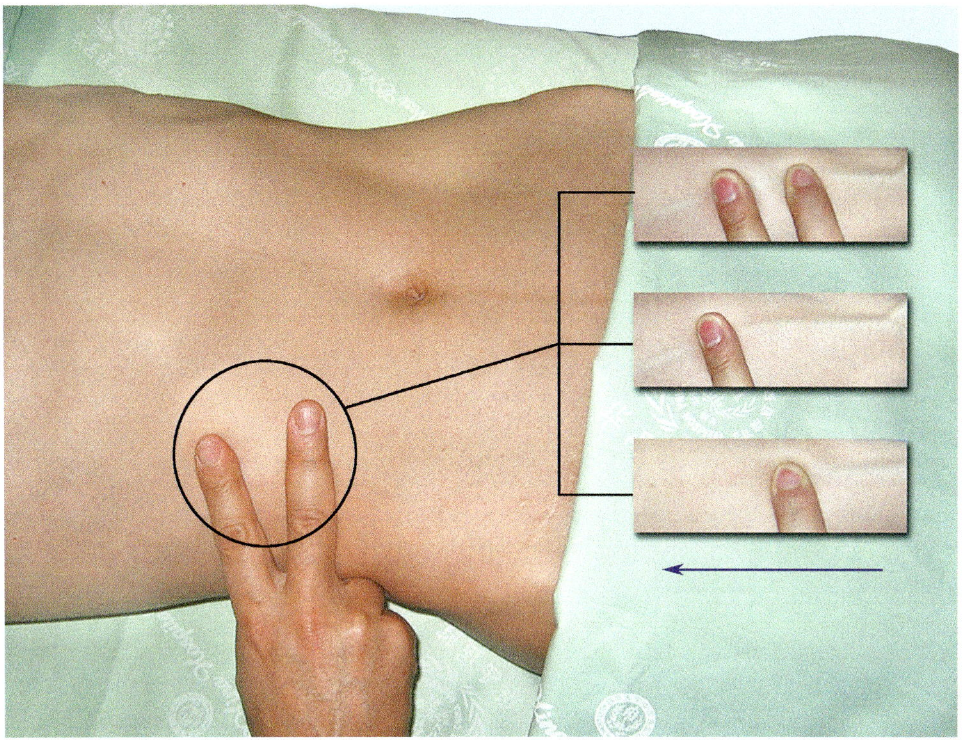

Fig. 46.7 Technique for examining venous blood flow direction

occurs, peristalsis will be absent. It is easier to observe peristalsis from the side and it can also be induced with hands slapping the abdominal wall.

46.2.6 Epigastric Pulsation

Epigastric pulsation, namely xiphoideusal pulsation, is mostly induced by abdominal aortic impulse and occurs in slender individuals. In cases such as abdominal aortic aneurysm and hepatic hemangioma, epigastric pulsation will be obvious, which can also be encountered in mitral stenosis or tricuspid insufficiency leading to right ventricular enlargement. The method to differentiate right ventricular beats with abdominal aortic pulsation, is illustrated in the eighth section of the sixth chapter about cardiac palpation.

46.3 Section 3: Auscultation

46.3.1 Bowel Sound

Gas and fluid in the intestinal canal flow with intestinal peristalsis, producing a kind of intermittent gurgling sound, which is referred to as a *bowel sound*.

Normal bowel sounds are produced approximately 4–5 times per minute with a large difference among frequency, intensity and pitch. Generally, since frequent and obvious bowel sounds appear after meals yet sparse and weak sounds occur at rest, normal bowel sounds can only be determined by the examiner's experience. Active bowel sounds, reaching up to over ten times per minute and showing a relatively low pitch as peristalsis increases, are noted in acute gastroenteritis and after the administration of laxatives or in massive hemorrhage of gastrointestinal tract. Increased bowel sounds with a characteristic loud, high-pitched tinkling quality, or even a metal tone, are regarded as hyperactivity and found in mechanical ileus. When there is a muscle strain of the intestinal wall due to various reasons, resulting in the weakened peristalsis, bowel sounds will also decrease or be heard over a period of minutes, which is called hypoactivity and is common in senile constipation, peritonitis and electrolyte disturbance (hypokalemia), as well as poor gastrointestinal motility etc. Absence of bowel sound after 3–5 min of continuous auscultation, known as disappearance of it, usually indicates acute peritonitis or paralytic ileus, which can be induced by fingers tapping or scratching the abdomen.

46.3.2 Blood Murmur

Blood murmurs include the arterial and venous, with the auscultation position being detailed in Fig. 46.8. Murmurs from arteries are often be heard in the middle or one side of the abdomen. Aortic systolic murmur (ejection murmur) in the middle of the abdomen usually suggests abdominal aneurysm or abdominal aortic constriction. In aneurysm, the pulsatory mass can be felt here; in constriction, pulsation

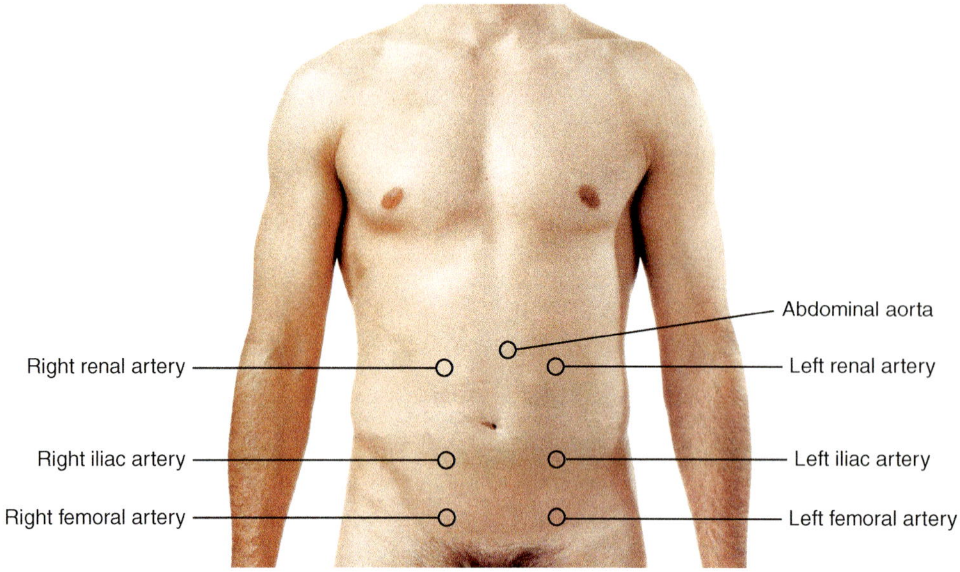

Fig. 46.8 Auscultation positions of abdominal vessels

will be weakened accompanied by blood pressure in lower limbs being lower than that in the upper, and pulse of dorsal arterial of the foot will not be palpated in severe cases. Systolic blood murmur in both sides of the upper abdomen, is a sign of renal artery stenosis and occurs in young patients undergoing hypertension, while the murmur in both sides of the lower abdomen indicates iliac artery stenosis. When hepatic artery or abdominal aorta is compressed by left liver cancer, a blowing murmur can also be heard in the site of the mass or a mild continuous murmur is heard in the tumor position. Murmurs from veins sound like a continuous hum, without systolic and diastolic properties, frequently appearing in the peripheral umbilicus or the upper abdomen. If there is severe varicosity of the abdominal wall, it commonly reveals portal hypertension associated with the formation of collateral circulation.

46.3.3 Friction Rubs

Under circumstances of splenic infarction, perisplenitis and perihepatitis or cholecystitis involving local peritoneum, friction rubs may be heard in corresponding parts as the patient takes deep breath, with sensation of friction being palpated in severe cases. Furthermore, friction rubs can also be heard in the abdominal wall in peritoneal fibrous exudative inflammation.

46.3.4 Scratch Test

The *scratch test* is used to assist in delimitation when palpation of liver inferior border is unclear. After the patient takes the supine position, the doctor holds the diaphragmatic head of stethoscope with his left hand and places it above the costal margin of the right midclavicular line, then gently scratches the right upper abdominal wall in "Z" shape from bottom to up with his right fingers on the right midclavicular line, or slightly scratches the abdominal wall from the distance to the diaphragm of stethoscope within the semicircular equidistant scope of the upper abdomen. Before it reaches the hepatic margin, the sound is remote and slight, but once it reaches liver surface, the sound is significantly enhanced and close-to-ear, which is because sound transmission by parenchymal organs is better than that by hollow organs. The test is usually applied to patients with thick abdominal wall or those who cannot cooperate with palpation satisfactorily, and sometimes it can also be used for differentiating whether the mass in the right upper abdomen is the enlarged liver or not. In addition, the method is also helpful in determining the stomach border.

46.4 Section 4: Percussion

Percussion of the abdomen is mainly to obtain the message of inflation of the gastrointestinal tract, presence of intraperitoneal pneumatosis, effusion and masses, as well as the size and percussion pain of some organs etc., usually cooperating with palpation to assist in judgement.

Both direct and indirect percussion can be applied to the abdomen, with the latter being preferable for its relative accurateness and reliability. Abdominal percussion is shown as follows.

46.4.1 Abdominal Percussion Sound

Normally, tympany is the most common percussion sound in the abdomen, except for dullness in the position of liver and spleen, in the site occupied by the enlarged bladder and

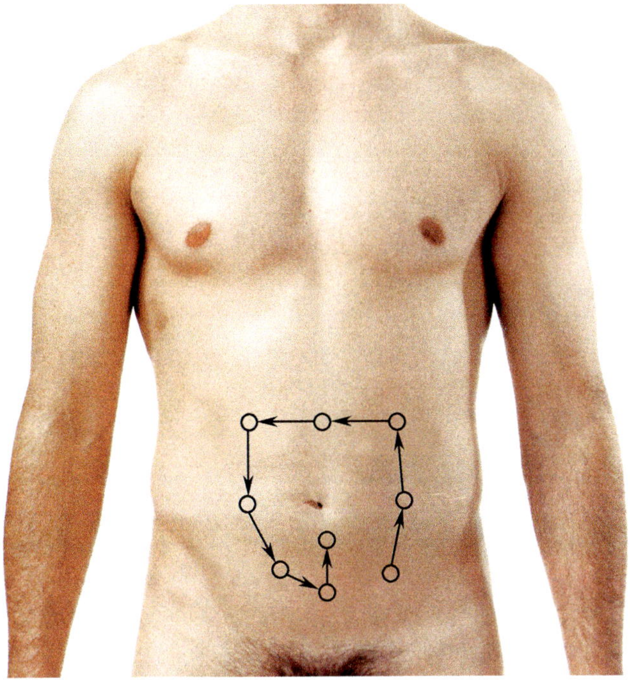

Fig. 46.9 Technique for abdominal percussion

uterus as well as in the abdominal flanks proximal to psoas. Presence of an extremely swollen liver and spleen or other organs, intraperitoneal tumors or massive ascites, shows that the scope of tympany is narrowed and dullness or flatness occurs in diseased areas. If there exist highly flatulent stomach and intestines, pneumoperitoneum caused by gastrointestinal perforation, the obvious tympany will expand or appear within the dullness border of the liver. General percussion, serving as the first step in abdominal percussion, can start from the left lower quadrant, and then reach to the right lower quadrant counterclockwise, and finally end in the umbilicus, by which the overall abdominal percussion sound can be acquired (Fig. 46.9).

46.4.2 Percussion of Liver and Gallbladder

Percussion of the upper border of the liver is operated from the pulmonary zone downward into the abdomen, along the right midclavicular line, right midaxillary line and right scapular line, with the percussion force being appropriate. The level of the shift from resonance to dullness is known as the upper border of the liver, where the border is also called the relative dullness border of the liver, since it is covered by the lung. Then percussing downward 1-2 intercostal space, the level of the shift from dullness into flatness is defined as the absolute dullness border of the liver, namely the lower border of the lung, where the liver is no longer shaded by the lung but is directly below the chest wall. Percussion of the lower border of the liver is preferably executed upward from abdominal tympanitic area along the right midclavicular line or median line. The level of the shift from tympany to dullness is the lower border of the liver, which is often determined with the help of palpation or auscultation because the border is overlapped with the stomach and colon and is difficult to be accurately percussed. Generally, the lower border of the liver felt by percussion is 1-2 cm higher than that by palpation. Attention should be paid to the body figure in determining the upper and lower border of liver. The normal liver of a healthy body is located along the right midclavicular line, with its upper border at the 5th intercostal space and the lower at the right subcostal margin, between which the distance is called liver span, and is about 9-11 cm; along the right midaxillary line, its upper border is located at the 7th intercostal space and the lower at the level of the 10th rib; along the right scapular line, its upper border is at the 10th intercostal space. Liver span of the pyknic shape is an intercostal space higher than the normal, while that of the slender shape is an intercostal space lower.

Expansion of the hepatic dullness border is encountered in hepatocarcinoma, liver abscess, hepatitis, hepatic congestion and polycystic liver etc. Narrowing of the hepatic dullness border appears in acute severe hepatitis, hepatic cirrhosis and gastrointestinal flatulence etc. Absence of liver dullness with replacement of tympany, mostly caused by coverage of free air on liver surface, is a significant sign of acute gastrointestinal perforation but it can also be seen in marked gastrointestinal inflation, interposition of the colon between liver and diaphragm, as well as in total situs inversus. The upward shift of the liver dullness border occurs in the right lung fibrosis, right lobe atelectasis, peumoperitoneum and meteorism etc., while the downward shift appears in emphysema and right tension pneumothorax, etc.

Percussion pain in hepatic region is common in hepatitis, hepatic abscess or hepatocarcinoma etc.

Clinically, the size of the gallbladder cannot be percussed since it is deeply located behind the liver. Only the presence of percussion pain in gallbladder region can be examined, which is also an important sign of cholecystitis.

46.4.3 Traube Semilunar Space

The *traube semilunar space*, located above the costal margin of the lower part of the left anterior chest and roughly presenting a semicircle, is formed by air-containing gastric fundal fornix. Its upper border is situated at the diaphragm and inferior lung margin, with the lower border at the costal arch, the left border at spleen and the right border at the left margin of the liver. The size of traube area is influenced by the amount of gastric air content and lesions of peripheral organs as well as tissues, with the long diameter being about 5–13 cm, and the transverse about 2.7–10 cm. Even in normal people, it still will enlarge on an empty stomach and narrow or disappear on a full stomach, which therefore can only be used as reference. Obvious narrowing or disappearance of traube semilunar space can be found in moderate and severe spleen enlargement, left pleural effusion, pericardial effusion and enlargement of left liver lobe, and also in acute gastric dilatation or drowning patients.

46.4.4 Percussion of Spleen

When palpation is not satisfactory or a tiny splenic margin is felt below the left rib, percussion of the spleen will be carried out to further examine the size of it, which preferably should be light and be operated along left midaxillary line. Normally splenic dullness can be percussed between 9 to 11 intercostal spaces along the left midaxillary line, with its scope being about 4–7 cm, and without passing over the anterior axillary line. Enlargement of the splenic dullness area occurs in splenomegaly due to various factors, while narrowing of it is seen in the left pneumothorax, gastric dilatation and meteorism etc.

46.4.5 Shifting Dullness

Influenced by gravity, much fluid in the intraperitoneal cavity will accumulate in the lower abdomen, where dullness can be percussed. On examination, when the patient lies on his back, tympany could be found because the middle part of the abdomen floats on fluid level due to intestinal gas, at the same time, dullness at bilateral flanks could be heard owing to accumulation of ascites. The examiner percusses the patient's abdomen at the umbilical level from the midabdomen toward the patient's left side. Once finding the dullness, the examiner should hold the pleximeter still, simultaneously, ask the patient to turn on his right side and then continue to percuss the same point again. If the sound changes from dullness to tympany, it implies that the dullness has been shifted to another position. Similarly, the examiner percusses the patient's abdomen toward the right side, then instructs him to roll onto the left side following the percussion of dullness, and keeps on percussing the same point again to confirm the shift of dullness. *Shifting dullness* because of changes of body positions functions as a vital method to confirm the presence of free fluid in abdominal cavity, through which a volume of free fluid greater than 1000 ml can be detected (Fig. 46.10).

If the amount is too little, shifting dullness would not be found by above-mentioned method. With condition permission, the examiner could ask the patient to take elbow-knee position so that the umbilicus is at the lowest level, and then percuss him from flanks toward the umbilicus. If percussion sound changes from tympany to dullness, it indicates ascites, which means the *puddle test* is positive (Fig. 46.11). Or asking the patient to stand up, the examiner will percuss dullness if fluid accumulates in the lower abdomen. The upper border of fluid is at a horizontal level, above which it is the floating intestinal flexure with percussion sound being tympany.

Attention should be paid to identify the following conditions that are easily mistaken for ascites:

1. Ileus, intestinal dilatation and retention of a large amount of fluid in the intestinal tract
   Shifting dullness will be percussed due to movement of the patient's body positions, frequently accompanied by the sign of ileus.
2. Huge ovarian cyst
   A huge ovarian cyst may also lead to a large area of dullness during percussion, but the sound would not shift. Differentiating points are as follows: a. Dullness resulting from ovarian cyst often occurs in midabdomen in the supine position with tympany in laterals, which is because bowels are pushed to bilateral flanks by the cyst (Fig. 46.12); b. Dullness of the ovarian cyst could not shift; c. *Ruler pressing test* can be used to differentiate huge ovarian cyst from real ascites. When the patient takes the supine position, the examiner puts a hard ruler on his abdominal wall horizontally and then presses the ruler downward with two hands. If the ovarian cyst exists, the pulsation of abdominal aorta will conduct to the hard ruler via the cyst, resulting in rhythmic pulsation of it. If ascites exists, the pulsation will not conduct, so that there will also be no such rhythmic pulsation of the hard ruler.

46.4.6 Percussion of Bladder

Bladder percussion is used to determine the degree of urinary bladder distention, which is generally carried out above the pubic symphysis, with tympany shifting into dullness from the top down. When the bladder is empty, tympany can be found but the outline of bladder cannot be percussed due to existence of bowels above the pubic bone. When the bladder is filled with urine, percussion sound above pubis shows circular dullness. If there is uterine enlargement during pregnancy, uterine myoma or the ovary cyst, dullness will also be percussed in this area, which should be given differentiation. The review result following micturition or catheterization, suggests bladder enlargement caused by urine retention if dullness changes into tympany. If ascites occurs, dullness can also be heard above the pubic bone, where the curve concaves to the umbilicus or is in a horizontal orientation. However, the curved upper border of the dullness area is convex to the umbilicus in bladder expansion.

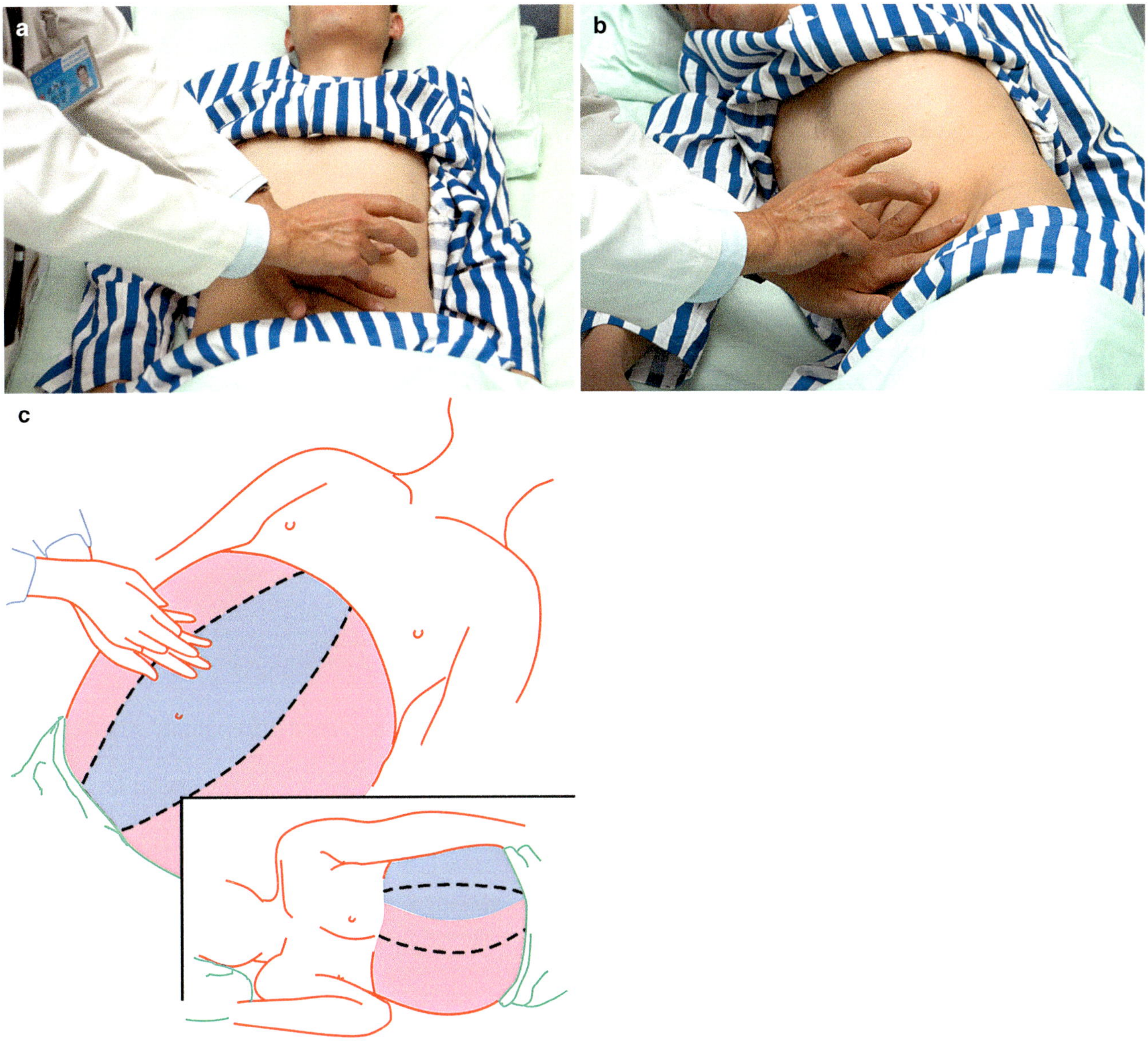

Fig. 46.10 Technique for testing for shifting dullness. (**a**) In the supine position (**b**) in the lateral position

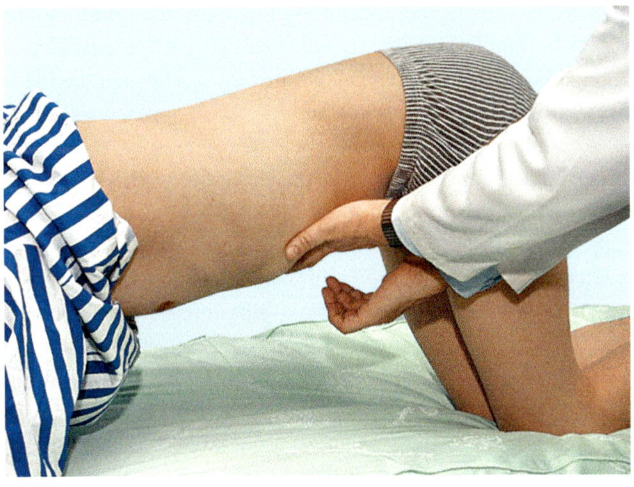

Fig. 46.11 Technique for puddle test

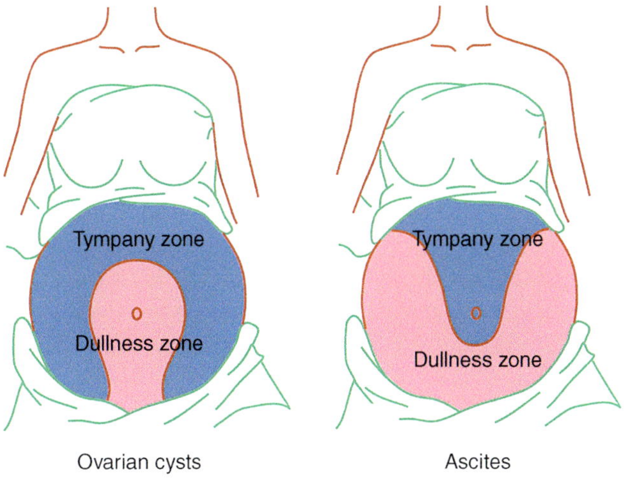

Fig. 46.12 Technique for differentiating between ovarian cysts and ascites percussion sound

46.4.7 Percussion Pain of Costovertebral Angle

Percussion of the costovertebral angle is mainly responsible for examining renal lesions. On examination, after the patient takes a sitting or lateral position, the doctor should put his left palm flat on the costovertebral angle (the renal region), and tap the left dorsum with the right-hand grip using light to medium force. Normally, there are no different degrees of percussion pain except for occurrence of nephritis, pyelonephritis, renal calculus, renal tuberculosis and perinephritis.

46.5 Section 5: Palpation

As a major method of abdominal examination, palpation plays a very significant role in recognition of abdominal signs and diagnosis of abdominal diseases. To achieve satisfactory abdominal palpation, the subject is required to take the supine position rather than sitting position on the bed. With the pillow under his head, the patient puts both hands on either side naturally and slightly separates both flexed legs, so that abdominal muscles can be relaxed to the greatest extent. The patient is asked to slightly open the mouth and calmly do abdominal breathing, with the diaphragm descending and abdomen elevating on inspiration as well as abdomen descending naturally on expiration, thus making subdiaphragmatic organs move up and down with breathing. On examination of the liver and spleen, the patient can also adopt the lateral position toward left and right respectively. The sitting or standing position can be assumed on the kidney examination, while elbow-knee position may be taken when examining abdominal tumors or ascites.

Standing at the right side of the subject and facing him, the examiner should try to keep the forearm at the same horizontal plane as the abdominal surface. During examination, firstly he places the whole palm flat on the abdominal wall to allow the patient to acclimate for a moment and feel the tenseness of abdominal muscles, and then the examiner gently palpates each part in order. The sequence of palpation generally starts from the left lower abdomen to all areas of the abdomen successively in a counter-clockwise direction, i.e. left lower abdomen→left upper abdomen→epigastric region→right upper abdomen→right lower abdomen→hypogastric region→ umbilicus (Fig. 46.9). The principle is that the examiner should palpate at the outset from the area not described as painful to the sickness site gradually, for the purpose of avoiding discomfort and conflict of the patient. On palpation, the examiner should also observe the patient's reaction and expression, as well as make simple conversation with him. If the patient remains tense or painful, comfort and explanation should be given to transfer his attention, thus reducing the tenseness of his abdominal muscles and ensuring the examination is completed successfully.

Light palpation is responsible for detecting the tenseness and resistance of the abdominal wall, superficial tenderness, lumps, pulsation and masses on the abdominal wall (subcutaneous lipoma and nodules, etc.); deep palpation can sense the conditions of abdominal organs such as liver, spleen, kidney and uterus etc.

46.5.1 Abdominal Tenseness

In normal individuals, the abdominal wall is somewhat tense. It is usually soft when palpated and easily depressed, which is defined as abdominal softness. Because some people (especially children) are not accustomed to being touched or tickled, this action may provoke an autonomic spasm of the abdominal muscles due to laughing, called strengthening of muscle resistance, which can disappear after appropriate induction or distraction and is not abnormal. Some pathological conditions can lead to an increase or decrease of whole or local abdominal tenseness.

46.5.1.1 The Increase of Abdominal Tenseness

This condition can be divided into several situations. The increase of tenseness, not accompanied by muscular spasm and dispensable tenderness, results from the increase of abdominal contents such as intestinal flatulence, pneumoperitoneum and massive ascites in the patient's abdominal cavity (usually transudate or hemorrhagic exudate). If the abdominal wall is palpated as obviously tense and even stiff, as hard as a board, it is called *board-like rigidity*, which is caused either by acute diffuse peritonitis due to acute gastrointestinal perforation or rupture of the viscera. In tuberculous inflammation or other chronic lesions, because of slow development of diseases leading to slow irritation to the peritoneum, and adhesion between the thickened peritoneum and bowels as well as the mesentery, the abdominal wall is palpated as pliable and tough, and is not easily depressed; it is referred to as a *dough kneading sensation*. This sign can also be seen in cancerous peritonitis.

Local abdominal tenseness frequently results from a visceral inflammation involving the peritoneum. For instance, tenseness of the upper or left upper abdominal muscles usually occurs in acute pancreatitis, of right upper muscles in acute cholecystitis and of right lower muscles often in acute appendicitis. Although peritoneal inflammation exists in the frail elderly, in patients with abdominal muscular dysplasia and massive ascites or in the obese, it does not result in an obviously-tense abdominal wall, as it does in the case of inflammation of pelvic organs.

46.5.1.2 The Decrease of Abdominal Tenseness

It is usually caused by the decrease or disappearance of abdominal muscular tension. On examination, flabby and inelastic abdominal wall and the decrease of whole abdominal tenseness are found in chronic wasting disease or drainage of a large amount of ascites, as well as in multiparous women or the frail elderly and dehydrated patients. Tension of the abdominal wall can disappear in paralysis of abdominal muscles due to spinal cord injury and myasthenia gravis. The decrease of local tenseness is rare and often results from local paralysis or a defect of abdominal muscles.

46.5.2 Tenderness and Rebound Tenderness

Normally, the patient does not respond in pain on general palpation, but only feels uncomfortable when deeply pressed. True tenderness is mostly derived from lesions in the abdominal wall or within the abdominal cavity. Unlike patients with tenderness caused by intra-abdominal lesions, when patients with superficial abdominal wall diseases are locally palpated, his tenderness will be marked as a result of tension of the abdominal muscles, and in the raising of the head and neck flexion. Lesions within the abdominal cavity, such as visceral inflammation, congestion, tumors, rupture and torsion, as well as peritoneal stimulation (inflammation and bleeding) etc., can elicit abdominal tenderness and related organs can also be discerned according to tenderness sites (Fig. 46.13). There is no local tenderness in early appendicitis, yet Mc Burney point tenderness occurs with the advancement of inflammation. Left lumbar tenderness is common in inflammation and tumor of the pancreatic body and tail, while right scapular tenderness frequently arises from gallbladder sickness. In addition, thoracic lesions, such as pneumonia of the lower lobe, pleurisy and myocardial infarction etc., also result in tenderness in epigastric region or hypochondrium. Pelvic diseases such as diseases of the urinary bladder, uterus and its adnexa, may give rise to tenderness in hypogastric region. Some tenderness-points in relatively fixed positions usually reflect specific diseases. For instance, gallbladder tenderness located at the junction of the midline of the right clavicle and costal margin is a sign of cholecystic illness; Mc Burney point tenderness, located at the junction of the lateral and middle thirds of the line joining umbilicus and the right anterosuperior iliac spine, marks lesion of appendix etc.

After occurrence of deep tenderness caused by palpation, the doctor should keep the index, middle and ring finger in place for a moment in order to make the tenderness stable, and then quickly release his hand. If the patient feels a sharp abdominal pain accompanied by an anguished expression or groan, it will be defined as rebound tenderness, which is a sign of parietal peritoneum resulting from inflammation. *Peritoneal irritation sign*, also called peritonitis triad, refers to the condition that the patient is palpated for abdominal tenseness, tenderness and rebound tenderness. When a parietal peritoneum has not been involved by visceral inflammation, only tenderness occurs without rebound tenderness.

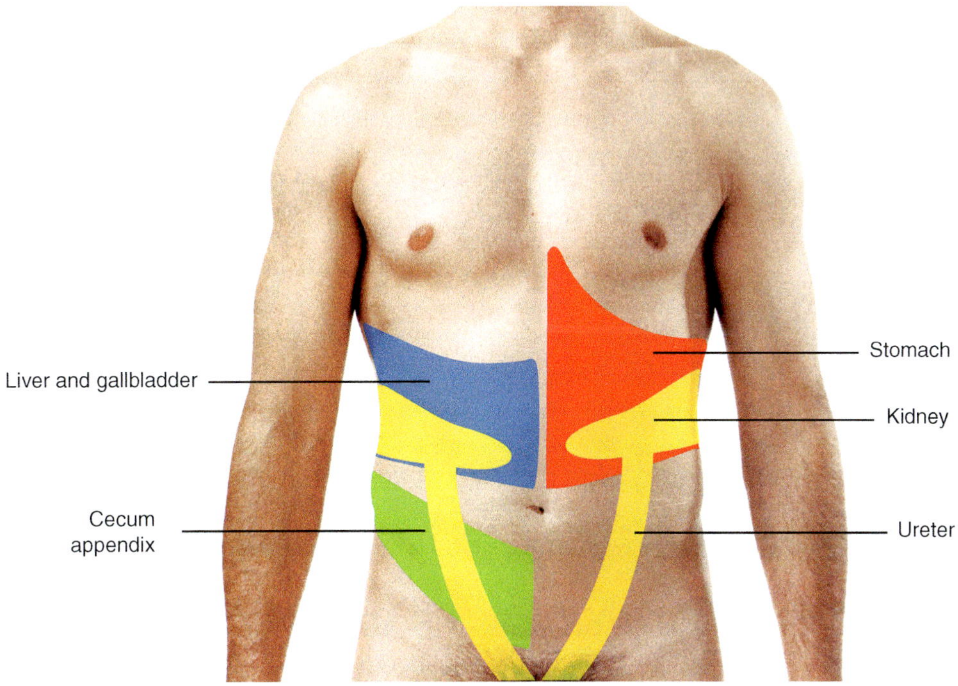

Fig. 46.13 Tenderness sites of common abdominal diseases

46.5.3 Palpation of Organs

46.5.3.1 Palpation of Liver

Single Hand Palpation

This method is more popular. Closing four fingers and straightening the metacarpophalangeal joint, the examiner puts the right hand roughly parallel to costal margin and on the right side of abdomen, estimating the lower part of the inferior border of the liver or percussing that of the liver dullness. As the patient exhales, the examiner presses down on the abdominal wall and deeply palpates the edge of liver; as he inhales, the examiner slowly lifts the fingers and examines downward movement of the liver edge toward the costal margin. Repeating it as required and aided by the patient's deeper abdominal breathing, the doctor gradually moves his fingers toward costal margin until the liver edge or costal margin is palpated. The liver edge should be palpated respectively in the right midclavicular line and anterior median line, and its distance with the costal margin as well as root of the xiphoid process should also be measured separately in centimeters during quiet respiration (Fig. 46.14).

Bimanual Palpation

Keeping the right hand at the same position as single hand palpation, the examiner holds the patient's right waist with his left hand and places it on the coastal region with thumb open. On palpation, the examiner pushes the left hand upward in order to make the inferior border of liver adhere closely to anterior abdominal wall and restricts expansion of the right lower chest to increase amplitude of diaphragmatic downward movement. Therefore, the liver having moved down is more likely to touch the right fingers on inhalation, thus rendering palpation more effective (Fig. 46.15).

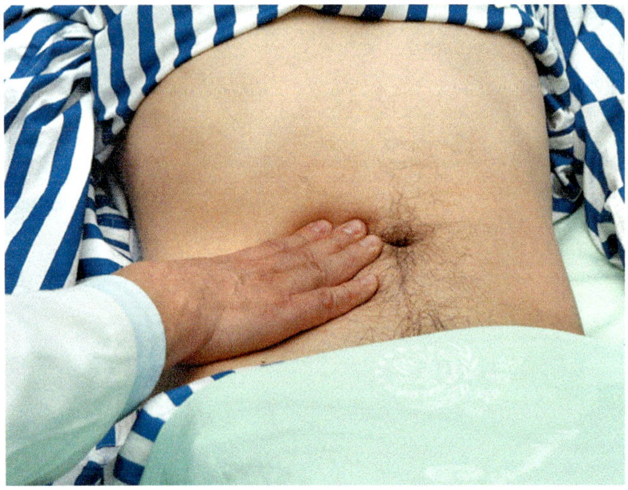

Fig. 46.14 Direction of fingers in liver palpation

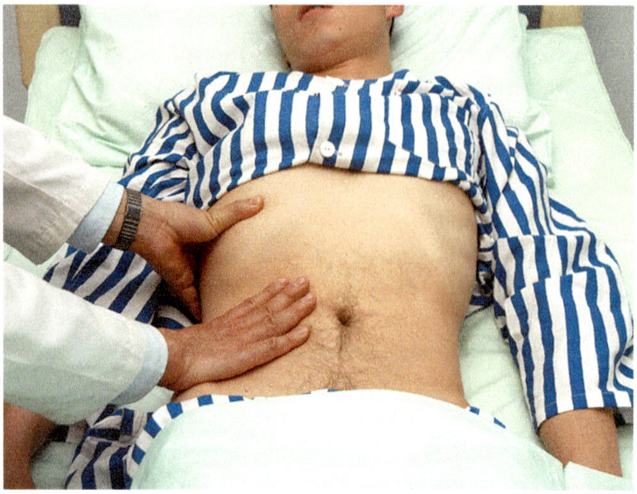

Fig. 46.15 Technique for liver palpation by bimanual palpation

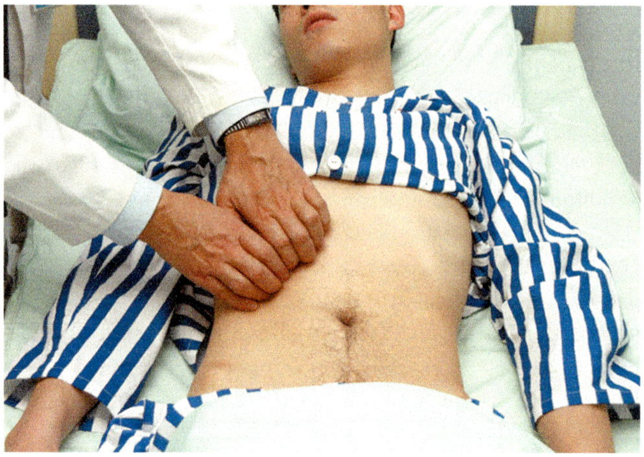

Fig. 46.16 Technique for liver palpation by hook method

Hook Method

This method is recommended for children and patients with thin and soft abdominal wall. During palpation, the examiner stands at the patients' right side of shoulder, faces his feet and rests both hands on the right lower chest with the second to fifth fingers of both hands flexing side by side and adopting the shape of a hook. After the patient is told to breathe deeply, the examiner further flexes his finger joints with each deep inhalation, so that the inferior border of the liver can be easily felt by the finger pulp during its downward movement. This maneuver can also be performed alone with the right hand (Fig. 46.16).

Once the liver is palpated, the following contents shall be described in detail:

Size

Ordinarily the adult's liver is not palpable below the costal margin. However, the inferior border of it can be felt less than 1 cm below the costal arch when slender patients with flabby abdominal wall take a deep inhalation. The inferior border of the liver touched under the xiphoid is mostly within 3 cm, while that felt under the root of the xiphoid process of slender patients, whose epigastric angle is sharp, can reach up to 5 cm, but it still will not exceed the middle and upper 1/3 junction between the root of xiphoid process and umbilicus. If the above-mentioned criteria are exceeded, yet the liver is soft with a smooth surface and there is no tenderness, it should be considered that the liver has descended. At this time, it is advisable to percuss the upper border of liver. If the upper border also descends correspondingly but the liver span remains normal, it will indicate the descent of liver; however, if the upper border is normal or elevates, it will suggest hepatomegaly.

The descent of the liver is common in visceroptosis, emphysema and the descent of the diaphragm caused by large pleural effusions in the right lateral.

Hepatomegaly can be diffuse and localized. Diffuse hepatomegaly occurs in hepatitis, hepatic congestion, hepatic cirrhosis at early stage, Budd-Chiari syndrome, leukemia and schistosomiasis etc. Localized hepatomegaly appears in liver abscess, liver neoplasms and hepatic cyst, etc.

The shrunken liver is encountered in acute or subacute severe hepatitis and advanced portal cirrhosis etc.

Texture

The texture of the liver is generally classified into three grades: softness, toughness (medium stiffness) and hardness. Normally the texture of liver is soft and tender, just like the pouted lip. In acute hepatitis and fatty liver, the texture is slightly tough, while in chronic hepatitis and hepatic congestion, the liver is usually as tough as apex nasi. In liver cirrhosis, the quality of the liver is hard, yet in liver carcinoma, the quality is hardest and as hard as one's forehead. When fluid is discovered in the liver abscess or cyst, the liver texture may exhibit cystic, and fluctuation may be palpated in patients with large and superficial abscess or cyst.

Edge and Surface

On palpation of the liver, it should be noted whether the edge is thin or thick and is regular or irregular, whether the surface is smooth or not, and whether there is any node or not. The normal liver shows well defined edges with uniform thickness and a smooth surface. Liver with rounded edge is frequently seen in fatty liver or hepatic congestion, while liver with irregular edges and rough surfaces, manifesting uneven nodules, is found in hepatocarcinoma, polycystic liver and hepatic hydatid disease. The surface of a liver showing prominent masses appears in giant hepatocellular carcinoma or liver abscess, and liver manifesting marked lobulated form occurs in hepatic syphilis.

Tenderness

Normally the liver may not be palpated as tenderness results, unless the hepatic capsule is inflamed or pulled by enlargement of itself. Mild diffuse tenderness is seen in hepatitis and hepatic congestion, localized severe tenderness is usually found in a relatively superficial liver abscess (often in the right intercostal space), and tenderness accompanied by percussion pain is encountered in deep liver abscess.

Pulsation

Normally the liver and enlarged liver resulting from inflammations and tumors are not accompanied by any pulsation. As long as the enlarged liver has not compressed abdominal aorta or the right ventricle has not yet enlarged to push down the liver, any pulsation will also not be palpated. Once the pulsation is felt, attention should be paid to its direction, that is, whether it is unidirectional or expansile. The former, unidirectional pulsation, is usually caused by liver conduction of the pulsation of abdominal aorta. If you place your hands on the surface of the liver, you will feel your hands are pushed upward and downward. The latter, expansile pulsation, is the pulsation of liver per se, and occurs in tricuspid valve insufficiency. That's because contractive pulsation of the right ventricle conduces to the liver through the right atrium and then inferior vena cava. If you place your hands on the surface of the liver or place both hands respectively on the front and back sides of it, you will have the opening-closing sensation.

Liver Friction Sensation

On examination, the examiner places the right palm surface lightly on the patient's hepatic region and tells him to take abdominal breathing, which will not give rise to a friction sensation in normal cases. However in perihepatitis, the liver surface and its neighboring peritoneum will become rough due to fibrinous exudate, between which the mutual friction can be palpated by hand, called liver friction sensation. This liver friction sound can also be heard on auscultation.

Hepatojugular Reflux

When right heart failure leads to hepatic congestion and enlargement, by compressing the hepatic region in the right upper abdomen, a rough estimate of the right heart function can be made according the degree that the jugular vein has distended. The patient is asked to stay in bed with a pillow under his head and breathe quietly with mouth open, avoiding breathlessness of Valsalva. In case of patients with distention of the jugular vein, the head of the bed should be elevated 30-45 degrees for the purpose of making distended jugular vein at the root of neck. Placing the right palm surface firmly on the hepatic region in the right upper abdomen, the examiner applies gradual pressure lasting for 10 seconds

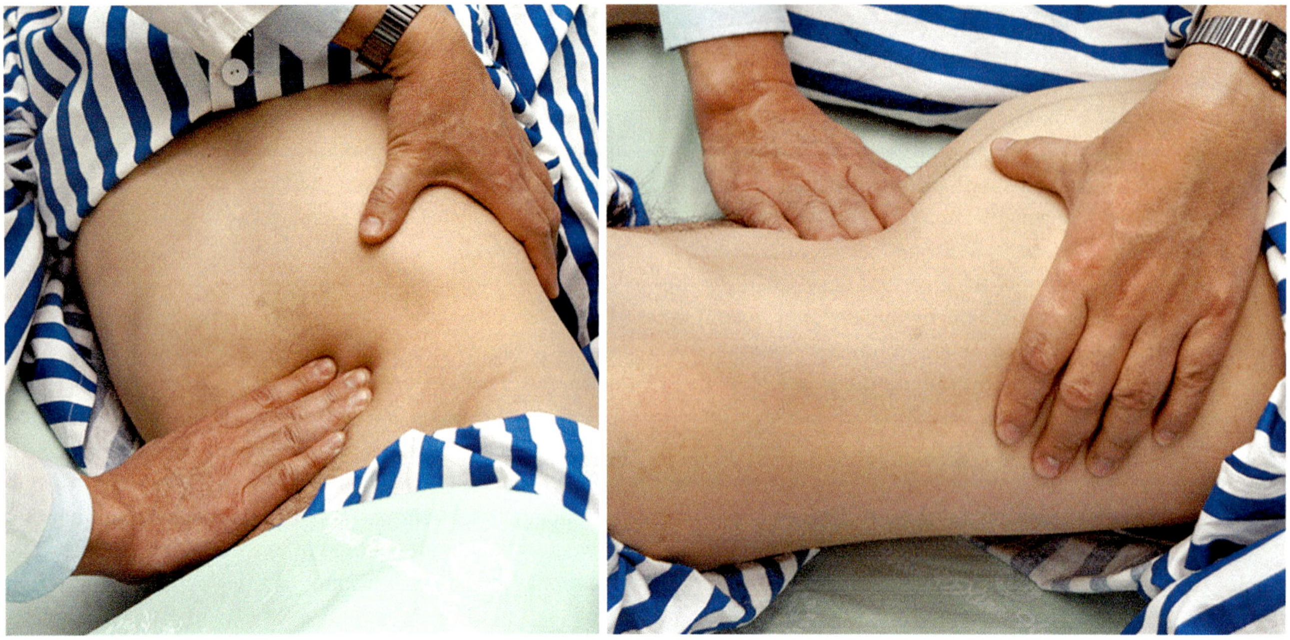

Fig. 46.17 Technique for spleen palpation

and meanwhile, observes whether there is any distention of jugular vein. Normally there is no distention of the jugular vein, or only temporary distention at the beginning of pressure, but it quickly drops to normal level. The distention of the jugular vein in patients suffering from right heart failure is persistent and obvious, it declines following stoppage of compression of the hepatic region (at least 4 cm H_2O), referred to as positive hepatojugular reflux. It is also a vital sign of right heart dysfunction at early stage, pulmonary hypertension and pericardial effusion.

Liver Thrill

If there is suspicion of liver hydatid cyst, the examiner can press the cyst site with middle three fingers of the left hand, with the middle finger exerting more pressure and the other two fingers less. Then he should use the middle finger of the right hand to repeatedly tap that of the left, and keep his fingers motionless for a while after each tapping. At this point, the examiner would have a subtle tremor sensation in his other two fingers, which is brought about by impingement of most daughter cysts on the cyst wall. This test has a low positive rate but special diagnostic significance.

46.5.3.2 Palpation of Spleen

The normal spleen is not palpable unless it manifests in a downward displacement due to visceroptosis, or left pleural effusion and descent of the diaphragm in air accumulation. If the spleen is obviously enlarged and superficially located, it will be found with right hand palpation, while bimanual palpation that is more popular clinically should be applied when an enlarged spleen is located deeply. Firstly, the patient takes the supine position and keeps both legs slightly flexed, and then the doctor uses the left hand to bypass the patient's anterior abdomen, places the palm on the 9-11th ribs below the left chest, exerting pressure to move the posterior aspect of the chest anteriorly in order to limit thoracic movement, with thumb together. Meanwhile, he places his right palm flat on the umbilicus from which palpation starts and keeps it roughly vertical with the left costal arch, which is similar to the maneuver used to palpate the liver. Under the cooperation of the patient's respiration, the doctor gradually pushes the right hand upward to feel the spleen tip, till the left costal margin (Fig. 46.17). If the slightly enlarged spleen cannot be palpated in supine position, the patient should then be rolled toward the right with both lower limbs flexed, which is a more conducive posture for the spleen to be touched with both hands.

Furthermore, the doctor can also stand at the left side of the patient's shoulder and palpate the spleen edge in the left costal margin with both hands through the hook method.

Measurement and recordings of spleen enlargement (Fig. 46.18):

Line I refers to the distance between the crossing point of the left midclavicular line and left costal margin and the inferior border of spleen, which is often expressed as centimeters (the same below) and is only measured in a slightly or moderately enlarged spleen.

Line II refers to the distance between the crossing point of the left midclavicular line and left costal margin and the most remote point of the spleen, which should be generally longer than line I.

Line III refers to the distance between the right border of the spleen and the anterior midline. If the spleen exceeds the

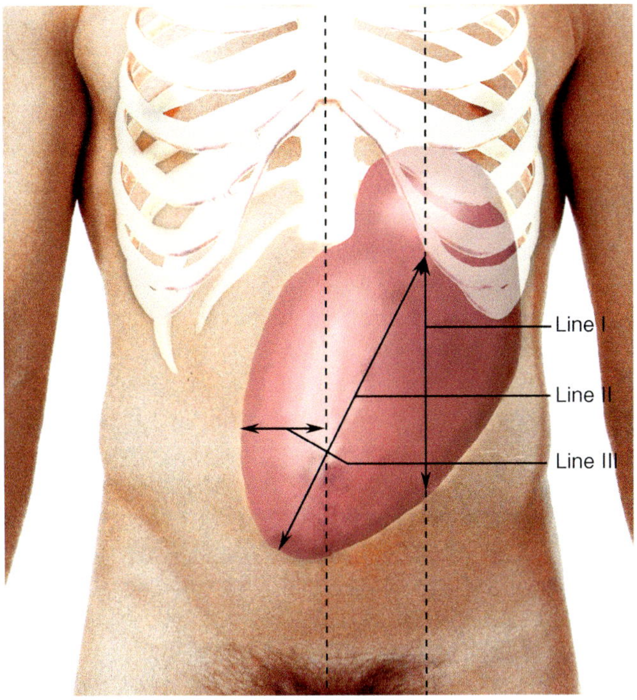

Fig. 46.18 Technique for measuring splenomegaly

anterior midline, the mark "+" is used to indicate the maximum distance; if not, the mark "-" is used to indicate the shortest distance.

In clinical practice, splenomegaly is usually classified into three levels. In a slight enlargement, the spleen edge is not more than 2 cm below the costal border; in a moderate enlargement, the lower edge of spleen is more than 2 cm below the costal border but above the umbilical horizontal line; in a severe enlargement, i.e. megalosplenia, the spleen edge is over the umbilical horizontal line or anterior midline. Line II and line III should be measured additionally and presented schematically when the spleen is markedly enlarged.

As in palpating the liver, attention should be paid not only to splenic size, but also to its texture, edge and surface, as well as the presence of tenderness and friction sensation etc., which usually suggest some causes of splenomegaly. Splenic notch, as its morphological feature, contributes to differential diagnosis.

Slightly enlarged spleen is frequently encountered in acute and chronic hepatitis, typhoid fever, miliary tuberculosis, acute malaria, infective endocarditis and septicemia, ordinarily exhibiting a soft texture; moderate splenic enlargement is commonly seen in hepatic cirrhosis, sequelae of malaria, chronic lymphocytic leukemia, chronic hemolytic jaundice, lymphoma and systemic lupus erythematosus, generally presenting a hard texture; severe enlargement of the spleen with smooth surface occurs in chronic myelocytic leukemia, myelofibrosis, Kala-azar and chronic malaria. Spleen with nodules on its surface appears in lymphoma and malignant histiocytosis. When there is cystic sensation in the surface of spleen, it suggests splenic cyst. When there exists splenic tenderness, it reveals splenic abscess and infarction. In perisplenitis or infarction of spleen, there is friction sensation accompanied by obvious tenderness due to fibrinous exudate in splenic capsule and its involvement of parietal peritoneum.

46.5.3.3 Palpation of Gallbladder

Under normal circumstances, the gallbladder cannot be palpated because it is hidden below the liver. However, it may be felt at the outer border of rectus abdominis below right costal margin through a single slipping palpation or hook method when an enlarged gallbladder exceeds the liver edge and costal margin. The enlarged gallbladder being generally pear-shaped or oval, has a smooth surface and higher tension, which is usually tender and moves up and down with respiration. As associated with accentuated tenderness, it is commonly seen in acute cholecystitis; as with gallbladder enlargement yet without tenderness, it occurs in periampullary carcinoma; as with solid enlargement of the gallbladder, it can be found in cholecystolithiasis or carcinoma of gallbladder.

The gallbladder enlargement differs with the nature of diseases. Sometimes the gallbladder is inflamed but not enlarged, or has not enlarged below the costal margin, so that it cannot be found by palpation. In this case, gallbladder tenderness will be detected. The examiner should place his left palm on the patient's right lower chest with the thumb pulp hooked at the gallbladder point under right costal margin (Fig. 46.19), and then ask the patient to take a deep, slow inspiration. During inspiration, as the inflamed gallbladder descends, it will impact the hard-pressing thumb, resulting in pain known as gallbladder tenderness. If the patient complains of pain and experiences inspiratory arrest, it is indicative of positive

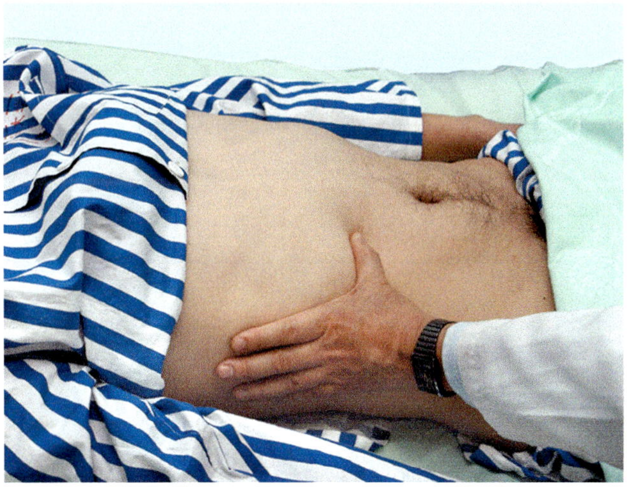

Fig. 46.19 Technique for examining Murphy's sign

Murphy's sign. Owing to biliary obstruction caused by oppression of carcinoma of the head of the pancreas to the common bile duct, jaundice will progressively deepen and the gallbladder will also enlarge significantly without tenderness, referred to as *Courvoisier's law*.

46.5.3.4 Palpation of Kidney

The kidney is usually palpated bimanually when the patient takes the supine or erect position. For palpation of the right kidney in decubitus position, the examiner requires the patient to flex both legs and take deep breath. Standing at the right side of the patient, the examiner holds the right waist from behind with his left palm and places the right palm flat on it, carrying out deep palpation along the right upper quadrant with the ulnar border of the hand approximately parallel to right costal margin. As the patient inhales, the kidney is palpated with the help of both hands of the examiner (Fig. 46.20). The lower pole of the kidney may be felt as a smooth and round structure, while the kidney retained between two hands can be sensed as fabiform with the patient being uncomfortable or nauseated in this case. For palpation of left kidney, the examiner holds the left waist from behind with his left hand crossing the front of the patient and places the right palm horizontally on the left waist, palpating bimanually as the method above described. If the patient has a thicker abdominal wall or is poorly cooperated, the doctor will have difficulty in pressing toward the posterior abdominal wall with his right hand, so that the following maneuver will be applied to palpate. When the patient inhales, the doctor supports forward the lower back with his left hand and feels right hand pushed against if the kidney descends in between; in contrast, squeezing toward the left hand with the right fingers, the doctor will also have the same feeling in his left hand during the descent of kidney. Under the circumstance that kidney is not palpated in decubitus position, the doctor should instruct the patient to stand beside the bed and then palpate it bimanually at the side of the patient. In nephroptosis or wandering kidney, it is more likely to be palpated in erect position.

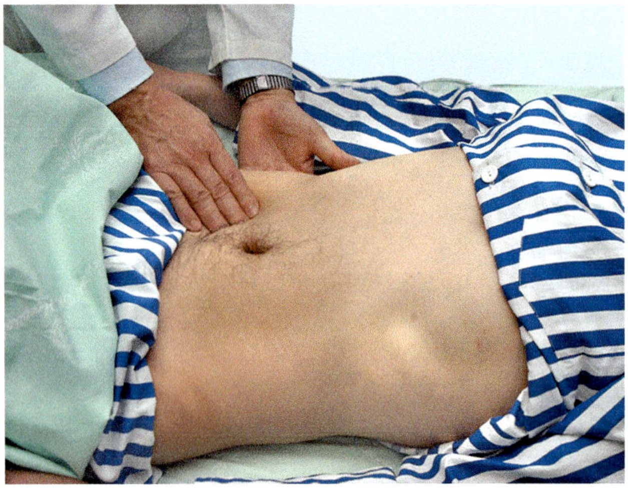

Fig. 46.20 Technique for kidney palpation

Generally the kidney is not palpated, but sometimes the lower pole of the right kidney may be felt in normal patients. It is more easily palpated in the slender, nephroptosis, wandering kidney or compensatory enlargement of it. During deep inspiration, if more than half of the kidney is felt, nephroptosis will be considered. Wandering kidney refers to the condition that nephroptosis is evident and the kidney can move in all directions in the abdominal cavity. Nephromegaly is observed in hydronephrosis or pyonephrosis, tumor of kidney and polycystic kidney etc. In the case of inflammation of the kidney and urinary tract or other diseases, tenderness point will occur in corresponding places: (a) hypochondriac point (pronephron point): it is located in the anterior end of the 10th rib with right side slightly lower, equivalent to the position of renal pelvis; (b) point of upper ureter: it is located at the umbilical plane and in the lateral border of rectus abdominis; (c) point of middle ureter: it is located at the level of anterior superior iliac spine and in the lateral border of rectus abdominis, equivalent to the position of the second narrow part of ureter; (d) vertebrocostal point: it is the apex of the crossing angle (costospinal angle) between the 12th rib on the back and spinal column; e. lumbocostal point: it is the apex of the crossing angle (lumbocostal angle) between the 12th rib and the lateral border of psoas (Fig. 46.21).

Vertebrocostal point and lumbocostal point are primary tenderness sites in some inflammatory diseases of the kidney, such as pyelonephritis, renal abscess and tuberculosis of kidney. Tenderness in hypochondriac point also has implications for renal lesions. Point of the upper ureter or point of the middle ureter appears tenderness, suggesting ureteral calculus, tuberculosis or purulent inflammation.

46.5.3.5 Palpation of Bladder

Hidden in the pelvic cavity, an empty bladder is normally not palpable. Only a full bladder beyond the superior margin of the pubis can be palpated in the middle lower abdomen generally through single slipping palpation. After the patient lies on his back and flexes knees, the doctor begins to palpate with his right hand toward the pubis from umbilicus. The enlarged bladder usually caused by accumulation of urine, showing oval-shaped or round, is palpated as cystic but cannot be pushed away with the hands. On compression, the bladder feels distended and there is the desire to urinate. An extremely full bladder is felt as hard but smooth. Enlargement of the bladder will shrink or disappear following urination or catheterization, by which it can be distinguished from pregnant uterus, ovarian cysts and rectal masses.

Bladder expansion occurs most frequently in urine retention resulting from urethral obstruction (such as prostatic

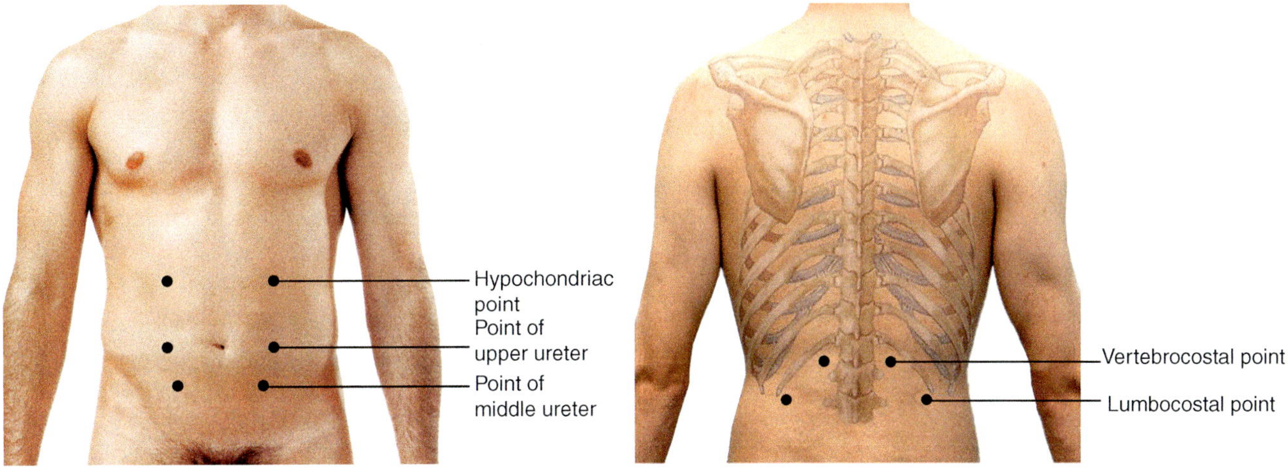

Fig. 46.21 Tenderness points of diseases of the kidney and urinary tract

hypertrophy or cancer) and myelopathy (such as paraplegia). It also appears in comatose patients, patients following anesthesia of lumbar vertebrae or sacral vertebrae and surgery and patients with local pain after surgery.

46.5.3.6 Palpation of Pancreas

The pancreas is deeply located in retroperitoneum and soft, thus it cannot be palpated. In epigastric region that is equivalent to the position of the first to second lumbar vertebra, the head and neck of pancreas are approximately situated in the right of midline, while the tail of the pancreas is in the left. There are transverse zonal tenderness and muscle tension in the middle of epigastric region or in left upper quadrant, and involving the left waist indicating pancreatic inflammation; there is an abrupt onset with the left waist being blue due to ecchymoma, revealing hemorrhagic necrotizing pancreatitis. If the transverse cord-like mass that is hard but has no mobility can be palpated in the upper abdomen, chronic pancreatitis should be considered; if the pancreas presents as a hard lump with a rough surface, suspicious of the presence of nodules, pancreatic carcinoma is possible. However, it should be noted that masses in the area need to be distinguished from gastric tumors because the stomach is in front of pancreas.

46.5.4 Abdominal Masses

In addition to above-mentioned organs, masses may also be palpated in abdomen, including enlarged or ectopic organs, inflammatory masses, cysts, enlarged lymph nodes, benign and malignant tumors, gastric calculus and intestinal fecal masses etc., which therefore should be given attention so as to differentiate. Firstly, normal organs should be distinguished from pathological masses.

46.5.4.1 Structures in Normal Abdominal Palpation

Xiphoid Process

The xiphoid process gradually experiences ossification and becomes more rigid, at the same time its flexibility also decreases with age, which can be palpated in epigastric region.

Rectus Abdominis

For those with well-developed abdominal muscles or athletes, the fleshy part of the rectus abdominis can be palpated in the middle and upper area of abdominal wall as hard, slightly round or square bulges, while tendinous intersections may be felt as transverse grooves. Both of them are easily mistaken for abdominal mass or the hepatic edge.

Lumbar Vertebrae

For the emaciated, and patients with soft abdominal walls, the mass of bone-like hardness may usually be palpated in the midline near the umbilicus. The mass protruding forward from the posterior abdominal wall is known as the vertebral body of lumbar L_4—L_5 anterior arch or S_1 protrusion of the sacral promontory, which is more likely to be misinterpreted as the posterior abdominal wall tumor by beginners.

Sigmoid Colon

Normal sigmoid colon can frequently be palpated through slipping palpation, even if there is storage of feces within it. The sigmoid colon, a smooth and cord-like structure, can be pushed by the fingers without tenderness.

Transverse Colon

In someone with normal weight or underweight, the smooth and soft transverse colon can be palpated in epigastric region and pushed by slipping palpation, showing a transverse and strip-like structure with the middle part drooping. At times, it even may drop to the umbilicus or below, exhibiting a U-shape.

Cecum

For the majority of people, the cecum can be palpated slightly medially above the McBurney point in the right lower quadrant, except for those with over-thick abdominal wall. Normally, it is felt as the cylindrical shape and its lower part, a blind end of piriform enlargement, is slightly movable and non-tender with a smooth surface.

Abdominal Aorta

On deep palpation along the left-inclined side of abdominal midline, the pulsating abdominal aorta can be found. Patients, especially the slender, may suffer from mild discomfort, which should not be considered as abnormality but should be noted to differentiate with abdominal aortic aneurysm or abdominal mass.

Right inferior Pole of Kidney

It can be palpated in right lumbar region of the slender and is located in a deeper position with a rounded edge.

46.5.4.2 Abnormal Masses

On palpation of the abdomen, besides above-described masses, the rest should be regarded as abnormal, which are mostly of pathologic significance. The following points should be noted when these masses have been palpated.

Site

Masses in various parts are often derived from organs of that area. For example, masses in the middle of the epigastrium usually are gastric or pancreatic neoplasms and cysts or gastric calculus; masses below the right costal margin are frequently associated with the liver and gallbladder.

Size

For any palpated mass, its length, width and antero-posterior diameter (thickness) should all be measured, with the latter being roughly estimated when it is difficult to be measured. In this situation, dynamic observation is recommended.

Morphology

Once the mass is palpated, attention should be paid to its shape, contour, edge and surface conditions. A regular and round mass with a smooth surface favors benignity; irregular and hard mass with a rough surface is more likely to favor malignant tumor, inflammatory or tuberculous mass.

Texture

If the mass is solid, its texture may be flexible, medium-hard or hard, which is seen in tumor and inflammatory or tuberculous infiltrative block, such as gastric cancer, hepatocarcinoma and ileocecal tuberculosis etc. If the mass is cystic, its texture will be soft, which occurs in the cyst and abscess, such as ovarian cyst and polycystic kidney etc.

Tenderness

Marked tenderness usually appears in inflammatory masses. Tumor tenderness associated with organs can be either severe or mild.

Mobility

If the mass moves up and down with respiration, it is suggestive of the liver, spleen, stomach and kidney or its mass. Since the gallbladder attaches to liver and the transverse colon connects to stomach by gastrocolic ligament, the mass also takes up and down movement with breathing. Local inflammatory mass or abscess and tumor in the posterior abdominal wall are generally unable to move.

Pulsation

Arterial pulsation can be seen or palpated in the abdomen of the emaciated. If apparent expansion accompanied by expansile pulsation, and sometimes even tremor can be palpated around the medioventral line, aneurysm of the abdominal aorta or its branches should be taken into consideration.

46.5.5 Fluid Thrills

Fluid thrill refers to the sense of fluctuation caused by hands slapping the abdomen when massive free fluid exists in the abdominal cavity. With the patient lying on his back, the examiner places the palmar surface of one hand closely on one flank of the patient's abdominal wall, and keeps four fingers of the other hand closed and flexed, and then taps the opposite flank with the fingertip (or palpate it with the fingertip impinging on abdomen). In the presence of a large amount of ascites, the palm attaching closely to the abdominal wall will feel as being impinged by a fluid wave, known as fluctuation. To prevent transmission of vibration of the abdominal wall to the contralateral, an assistant should place the ulnar edge of one hand against the medioventral line (Fig. 46.22). This method is utilized only when there is a large amount of fluid, usually more than 3000-4000 ml. Therefore the fluid thrill is not so sensitive as shifting dullness.

46.5.6 Succusion Splash

If a substantial amount of fluid and air remain in the stomach, *succusion splash* will occur on palpation. With the patient taking the supine position, the doctor keeps one ear

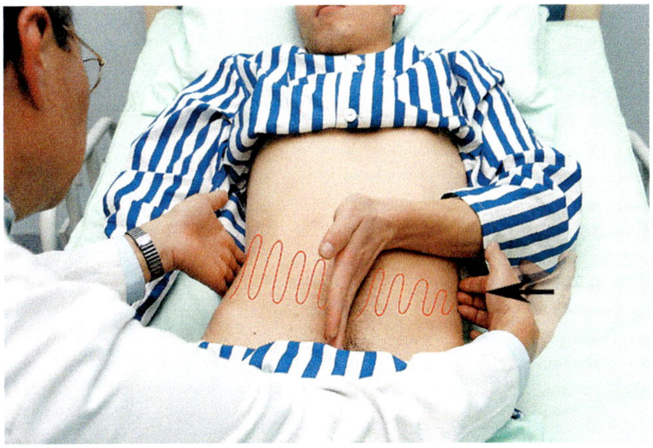

Fig. 46.22 Technique for testing fluid thrills

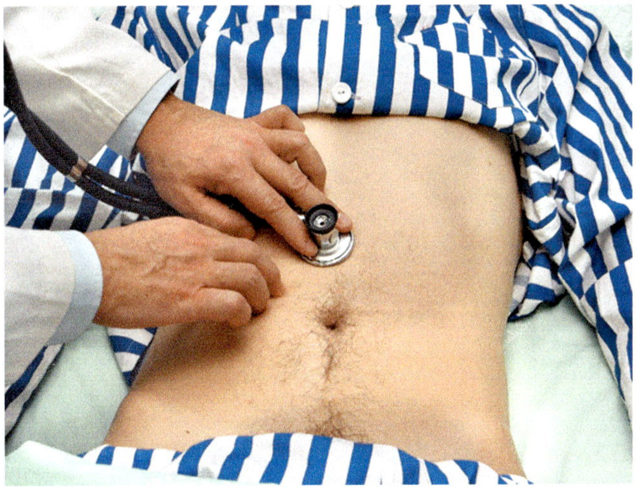

Fig. 46.23 Technique for examining succusion splash

close to the epigastric region and meanwhile, vibrates the abdomen through ballottement, by which the impacting sound between air and fluid can be heard. The doctor can also place the diaphragmatic head of stethoscope on the upper abdomen with the other hand shaking the patient from one side, or do some impacting vibration on the stomach in order to elicit succusion splash (Fig. 46.23). In normal subjects, this is positive after a meal or drinking plenty of fluids. However, if the sound is still positive on a morning empty stomach or lasts for 6-8 hours after the meal, it indicates impaired gastric emptying, such as pyloric obstruction or gastric dilatation.

Key Terms

1	Frog belly	蛙腹
2	Scaphoid abdomen	舟状腹
3	Gastral or intestinal pattern	胃型或肠型
4	Peristalsis	蠕动波
5	Bowel sound	肠鸣音
6	Scratch test	搔刮试验
7	Traube semilunar space	胃泡鼓音区
8	Shifting dullness	移动性浊音
9	Puddle test	水坑试验
10	Ruler pressing test	尺压试验
11	Peritoneal irritation sign	腹膜刺激征
12	Hepatojugular reflux	肝颈静脉回流征
13	Murphy's sign	Murphy征
14	Courvoisier's law	Courvoisier定律
15	Fluid thrills	液波震颤

Study Questions

1. Describe the Cullen's sign and its clinical significance.
2. How to measure and record the spleen enlargement?
3. What should be noted in palpation of the liver?
4. Describe the examination method of Murphy's sign and its clinical significance.
5. What internal organs can be palpated in a normal abdomen?

Suggested Websites

1. http://cc.scu.edu.cn/G2S/Template/View.aspx?action=view&courseType=0&courseId=1887
2. http://cc.scu.edu.cn/G2S/Template/View.aspx?action=view&courseType=0&courseId=6

47 Physical Examination of Anus, Rectum and Genitals

Yi Liu and Rui Zeng

47.1 Section 1: Anus and Rectum

The terminal portion of the digestive tract is composed of the rectum, anal canal and anus. The rectum is a continuation of the sigmoid colon and ends in the anal canal, and its total length is about 12–15 cm. The anal canal is about 3–3.5 cm long. The orifice at the bottom of the anal canal is called anus which is verged by mucosa with increased pigmentation at the perianal skin. The anal canal has internal and external sphincter which form the anal ring. The anal ring is marked by the skin folds. The dentate line is located at 2 cm above the anal ring, which is composed of anal columns. The voids between anal columns are called the anal crypts. The epithelium of anus is squamous epithelium that changes to mucosal epithelium at the level of the dentate line. The dentate line is also the demarcation line of the rectum and anal canal. There are nearly 85% of ano-rectal diseases occurred in this area. The anterior wall of the rectum in the male is adjacent to the prostate, in the female, it is adjacent to the vagina and uterus.

A digital anal and rectal examination is safe and easy. It may be used to find many important clinical signs. The data shows that 42.2% of rectal carcinoma is located at the distal 7 cm of the anus, so the correct digital rectal examination is crucial to the early diagnosis of rectal cancer. In the rectum and anus examination patients often have some discomfort and fear. Therefore, it is very important for physicians to have a thorough discussion with patients in advance about the necessity of the examination of the rectum and anus. It not only can release patient's fear, but also can obtain patient's cooperation. It is essential to have patients relaxed and in correct position and physicians must be calm and gentle using right posture and maneuver in order to smoothly complete the inspection and to obtain the optimal results.

Y. Liu
Department of General Surgery, Anhui Medical University, Hefei, China

R. Zeng (✉)
Department of Cardiology, Sichuan University, Chengdu, China

47.1.1 Exam Positions

Patient position is very important for *anorectal examination*. Based on the physical status of patients and specific inspection requirements, the five commonly used patient positions are discussed below:

47.1.1.1 Knee Elbow Position (Fig. 47.1)

A patient places flexed elbows on the examination table and the chest closes to the surface of the table, has two knees flexed at 90° and kneels down on the table, raises the buttocks. This position is the most commonly used to check the prostate and seminal vesicle; also used for rigid sigmoidoscopy and anoscopy.

47.1.1.2 Left-Lateral Recumbent Position (Fig. 47.2)

A patient is lying on his/her left side with right leg flexion, the upper knee and thigh drawn towards the belly, left leg straight, buttocks on the right side of the examination table. The doctor stands behind the patient to perform the exam. This position is commonly used in digital rectal examination

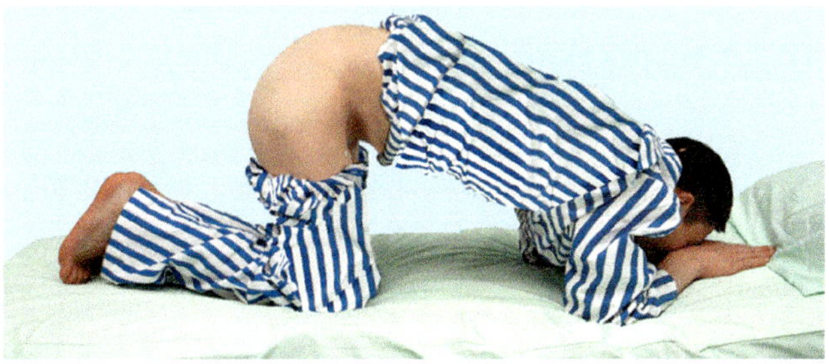

Fig. 47.1 Elbow knee position

X.-H. Wan, R. Zeng (eds.), *Handbook of Clinical Diagnostics*, https://doi.org/10.1007/978-981-13-7677-1_47

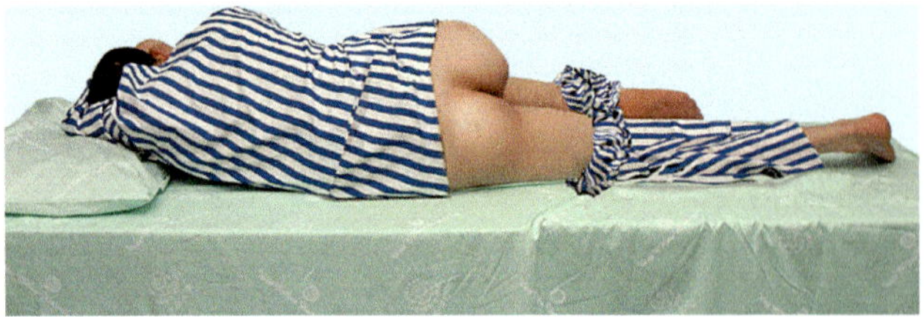

Fig. 47.2 Left lateral position

and colonoscopy examination, especially suitable for senior, very sick and female patients.

47.1.1.3 Supine Position and Lithotomy Position

A patient is lying on his/her back on the examination table with the hips elevated, the thighs apart, the knees flexed and elevated and two legs in abduction. This position is commonly used in the rectovesical pouch inspection, as well as in bimanual rectal examination which means the right index finger in the rectum, the left hand on the hypogastrium to check pelvic organs or lesions.

47.1.1.4 Kneeling-Squatting Position

A patient takes squatting position in which the body weight is on the feet but the knees and hips are flexed as using squat toilets in defecation, holding the breath and exertion. This position is suitable for inspection of rectal prolapse, hemorrhoids and rectal polyps.

47.1.1.5 Bending Forward Position

A patient bends forward with feet standing slightly apart and puts hands on the exam table for support. This position is commonly used in the inspection of the anus. The findings of the digital anal-rectal examination should be recorded according to the clock orientation and the patient position should also be recorded. For example, the locations of 12 o'clock and 6 o'clock of knee elbow position are totally opposite to supine position.

The examination methods of anus and rectum are mainly inspection and palpation, supplemented by endoscopy.

47.1.2 Inspection

The buttocks should be stretched out and physician should observe the skin color and wrinkling of sacrococcygeal anus and perianal area. Normally, the color of perianal skin is dark, the wrinkles radiate and become deeper with constriction action, while they become shallower with defecation action. The physician should pay attention to where there is the perianal skin lesion or injury, pus and blood, mucus, anal fissure, scar, external hemorrhoids, fistula orifice, ulceration, abscess and pinworms in children.

47.1.2.1 Anal Atresia and Stenosis

Anal atresia and stenosis are common in newborns with congenital malformations, but they also can be caused by infection, trauma or surgical scar.

47.1.2.2 Anal Trauma and Infection

Anal trauma or scar is more commonly caused by injury or postoperative scarring. The swelling and tenderness around the anus are often caused by perianal abscess.

47.1.2.3 Anal Fissure

An *anal fissure* is a longitudinal and spindle shaped full thickness of skin tear or infectious ulcer in anal canal distal to the dentate line and is most commonly located in the posterior midline of anal canal. Patients feel increased sharp with defecation and often inhibit defecation because of fear of the pain, resulting in dry stool with fresh blood on the surface. The physician will feel apparent tenderness during anal digital palpation.

47.1.2.4 Hemorrhoids

Hemorrhoids are swollen and inflamed venous mass caused by expansion or varicose of internal or external hemorrhoidal venous plexus in lower rectal submucosa or anal edge subcutaneous area. They are common ailments in adults who are susceptible to the symptoms of bloody stool, hemorrhoidal prolapse, pain or itching. There are three types of hemorrhoids: internal, external and mixed.

1. Internal hemorrhoids are located above the dentate line and are caused by the varicose of superior rectal veins. The surface of Internal hemorrhoids is covered by lower rectal mucosa and a soft purple-red mass can be detected in the anus. The mass may bulge out of anus during defecation;
2. The external hemorrhoids are located below the dentate line and are caused by the varicose of inferior rectal vein. The surface of external hemorrhoids is covered by anal skin and a soft purple-red mass can be detected outside of the anus.
3. The mixed hemorrhoids are caused by the expansion, varicose and admixture of internal and external hemorrhoid venous plexus. They are located both above and below the dentate line, where the part above the dental line is covered by rectal mucosa and the part below the dental line is covered by anal skin. The mixed hemorrhoids have the characteristics of both external and internal hemorrhoids.

47.1.2.5 Anorectal Fistulae

Anorectal fistula is also called anal fistula (archosyrinx). It is a granulation tunnel connecting rectum, anus to an opening on the perianal skin. Anal fistula is composed of internal orifice, fistula duct and external orifice. It is usually caused by the anus/rectum abscess, tuberculosis and Crohn's disease. It is not easily to heal. The external orifice of anal fistula can be found in the perianal skin and the internal orifice can be detected in the anus or rectum with induration. It is important to determine the location of the internal orifices for the diagnosis and treatment of anal fistula.

47.1.2.6 Rectal Prolapses

Rectal prolapse (proctoptosis) is also called hedrocele which means eversion either mucosal or complete layer of anus, rectum, even sigmoid colon wall outside of the anus. The patient should take the squatting position, the physician may inspect whether there are the protrusions outside of the anus and a purple-red globular protrusion is easily seen when patient holds breath and strains in defecation position. This protrusion suggests the rectum partly prolapse (rectal mucosa prolapse). If the protrusion shows oval lumps with circular folds on the surface, it suggests the rectum completely prolapse (rectal full-thickness prolapse).

47.1.3 Palpation

The palpation of anus and rectum is usually called digital *ano-rectal examination*. This method is simple and convenient with important diagnostic value for early detection of ano-rectal cancer (there are about 75% cases of rectal cancer can be detected by digital ano-rectal examination). Digital examination is an important diagnostic method for not only anal and rectum diseases, but also pelvic diseases such as appendicitis, iliac fossa abscess, prostate and seminal vesicle lesions, uterus and fallopian tube lesions, etc.

The patient should take the position such as knee-elbow position, left-lateral position and supine position based on the patient specific condition and clinical merit. Physician should wear gloves and coat right index finger with proper amount of lubricant such as soap, vaseline, liquid paraffin etc. for palpation. Physician first places the index finger on the external surface of the anus and gently massage to relax the anal sphincter muscles, and then slowly and gently insert the index finger into the anus to make a full circle examination of rectum and anus. (Fig. 47.3) During anal and rectal digital examination, please look for the tension of anus and sphincters, the characteristics of inner wall of the rectum and anal canal, and pay attention to the tenderness or pain

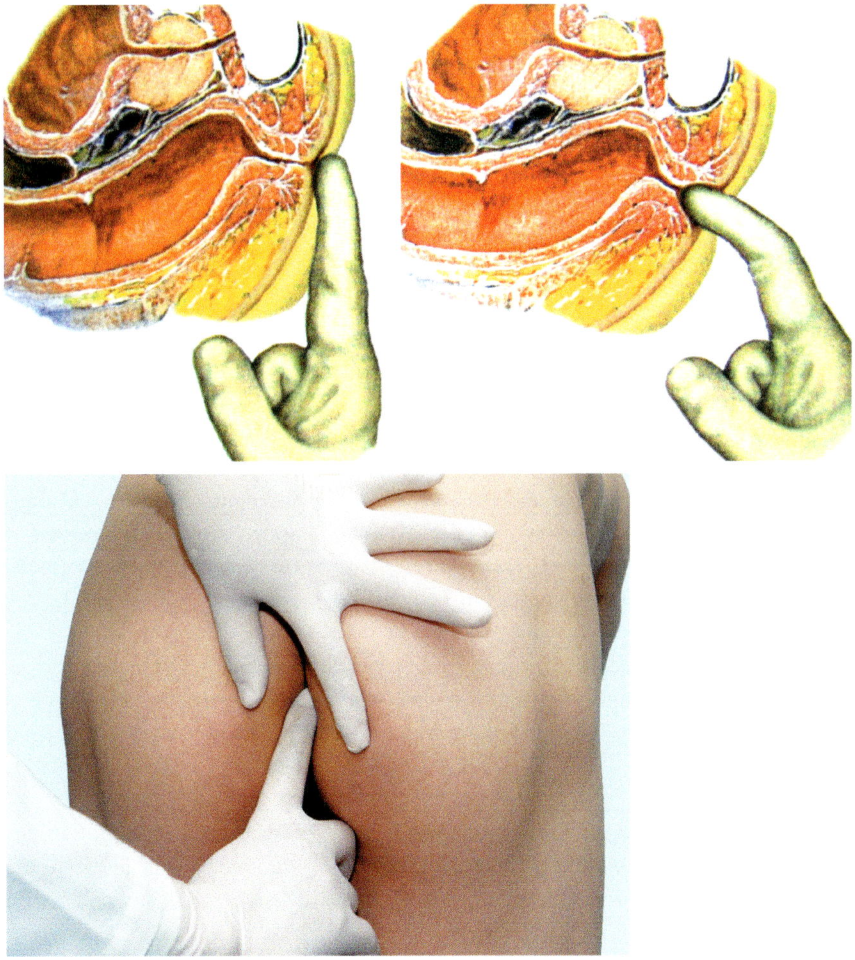

Fig. 47.3 Digital rectal examination

and smoothness of mucosa, mass and its mobility and fluctuation. The prostate should be palpated in male patient and the cervix should be palpated in female patient, the uterus and fallopian tube should be palpated as well by bimanual examination. The doctor should also check whether the gloves are contaminated by blood or mucus after pulling out of the finger.

Digital rectal examination often shows following abnormalities:

1. Extreme tenderness and pain is found in the anal fissure and infection.
2. Tenderness with fluctuation is found in the anal canal and perianal abscess.
3. Soft, smooth and elastic mass usually is rectal polyps.
4. Hard and uneven surface of a mass suggests rectal cancer.
5. Gloves contaminated by mucus, pus or blood suggest inflammation or tissue destruction, and the doctor should take the smear or bacteriological examination to help diagnosis if necessary.

47.1.4 The Rectum and Sigmoid Colon Endoscopy

The rectum and sigmoid colon endoscopy is mainly used in rectum and sigmoid colon examination. Rectoscope is a rigid endoscope, while sigmoidoscope has gradually replaced by fiberendoscope. The mucosa of normal rectum and sigmoid colon appears pink color. If there are mucosal congestion, ulcers, bleeding, exudation, and so on during endoscopy, the inflammation should be considered. For all the lesions, the physician should pay attention to the location, size and characteristics, etc.

47.2 Section 2: Male Genital Organs

The male reproductive organ is divided into two parts: the external genitalia including penis and scrotum and the internal genital organ mainly composed of reproductive gland, reproductive ducts and accessory gland. Testis is reproductive gland and reproductive ducts are connected by epididymis, vas deferens, ejaculatory duct and urethral canal. Accessory gland is mainly composed of gland prostate, seminal vesicle and so on. The main functions of the male genitalia include urination, hormone secretion and reproduction.

Male genital organs change with age. With growth and puberty, the shape and size of penis, scrotum, testis, and the color of the external genital organ will gradually change. During childhood, there is no pubic hair, the penis, scrotum and testis take shape of the juvenile. Between 9 and 13 years old, testis and penis gradually increases in sizes, pubic hair gradually grow, genital skin gradually become darker than surrounding parts of the skin. It takes about 3–5 years for male genital organs to fully develop from pre-puberty to adult form. When examining male genital organs, attention should be paid to the relationship between age and genital development, the following description is mainly about examination of adults.

When examining male genital, pay special attention to left and right side comparison, which can eliminate the interference brought by false symptoms and reduce errors of subjective judgment. When patient condition permits, always ask patient to stand. For prostate examination, ask patient to stand and stoop down to the examination table or take a position with both elbows and knees on the table. If needed, patient can also lie down with the lower limbs abduction and the lower part of the body fully exposed. The examination should include inspection, palpation and scrotum mass transillumination test. The sequence of the examination is external genital organ: penis first and then, scrotum, internal genital organ: testis, epididymis, vas deferens and prostate.

47.2.1 Pubic Hair

Male pubic hair is coarser than head hair and has a diamond distribution, It extends along the midline in a narrow strip to the abdominal and back to perianal region in some people. Senior pubic hair becomes sparse and greyish. Pubic hair may be lost or absent and like the distribution of pubic hair of female (inverted triangle, DEL) in some patients especially those suffering from endocrine diseases.

47.2.2 Penis

Penis is the cylinder at the front-end, including three parts: glans, body and tail. Normal adult penis is about 7–10 cm, composed of three corpus cavernosum: one corpus cavernous of urethra and two corpus cavernous of penis. Penile skin is thin and flexible, and skin vein of penis can be seen clearly under normal conditions. When corpus cavernosum congests, penis becomes thicker and harder, this is called the erection.

47.2.2.1 Prepuce

The skin distal to the neck of penis is folded inward to cover the head of penis (prepuce). Adult foreskin should not obscure urethral meatus, when retracted, penis glans should be exposed, otherwise, it is called *phimosis*, which is mainly caused by congenital stricture of prepuce orifice or inflammation, trauma induced adhesion. If the foreskin is longer than the glans penis, but when retracted, the urethral meatus and glans can still be revealed, this is called *prepuce redundant*. The prepuce redundant or phimosis may lead to infection and incarceration of urethral external meatus or the glans penis, and may even become one of the factors of penile cancer.

47.2.2.2 Penis

The sensitive bulbous structure at the distal end of penis is called glans or glans penis. At the junction of the head and the neck of penis, there is a shallow circular groove, called neck of penis or corona glandis. When carrying out examination, the glans penis and the neck of penis should be revealed, if the foreskin is too long, retract it or ask the patient to retract it, and restore it after examination to prevent the incarceration of glans. The observation includes the color of the surface, level of congestion, edema, secretions, scars, ulcers and nodules of the glans penis, etc. The glans penis of a normal person should be red, smooth, without redness and swelling. There may be some precipitant looking like white dried paste inside prepuce, at glans and neck, which is called smegma. The index finger, middle finger, ring finger and little finger of both hands may surround penis in the direction of root to glans during palpation (Fig. 47.4), pay attention to whether there are tender spots and nodules. Asymptomatic patients, especially young adults, should not ignore the palpation of penis as well.

47.2.2.3 Urethra

It is the main focus to observe the size and location of urethra meatus. The urethral meatus is normally located in the midline anteroinferior part of glans. In order to check the external opening of urethral meatus, which is about 1–2 mm in depth, please use thumbs and index fingers to open it up. The normal mucous membrane of urethral meatus is ruddy in color, clean, no pus or exudation, and no pain from touch or tenderness. Please press the urethra from the root of penis along the ventral urethra to its meatus for palpation. If there is urethral calculus, a solid mass may be localized. When self-reported urethral secretions are not being seen, the examiner should squeeze and press the urethra meatus from the root of penis with thumb (on the ventral side of penis) and index finger (on the dorsal side of penis), as a result, there may be excrement discharged from the urethra meatus. The examiner should take specimen by inserting sterile cotton swab in the urethra (Fig. 47.5) for smear and bacterial culture. Please pay attention to the color and characteristics of the discharge or excrement. For healthy subject there is no excrement (excrement is usually used for solid waste) discharged from the urethra by squeezing and pressing.

47.2.2.4 Common Abnormal Findings During Penis Examination

Penis size and Shape

If the penis of an adult is too small (baby type), then he may have pituitary dysfunction or gonadal dysfunction. When penis is too large during childhood (adult type), it is called the symptom of "precocious puberty". In the true precocious puberty, the patient has premature secretion of the

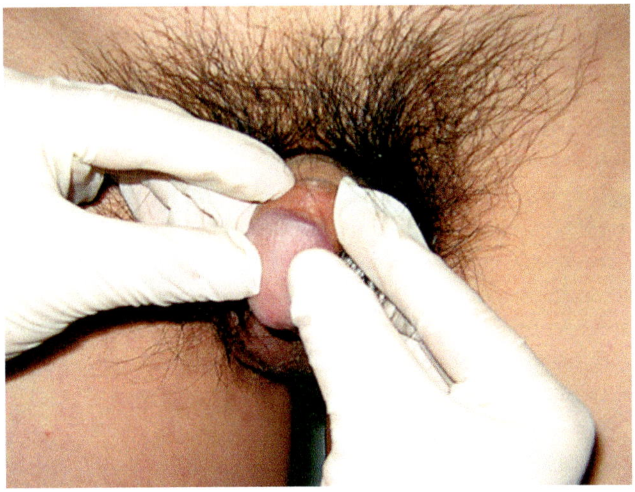

Fig. 47.4 Penis palpation

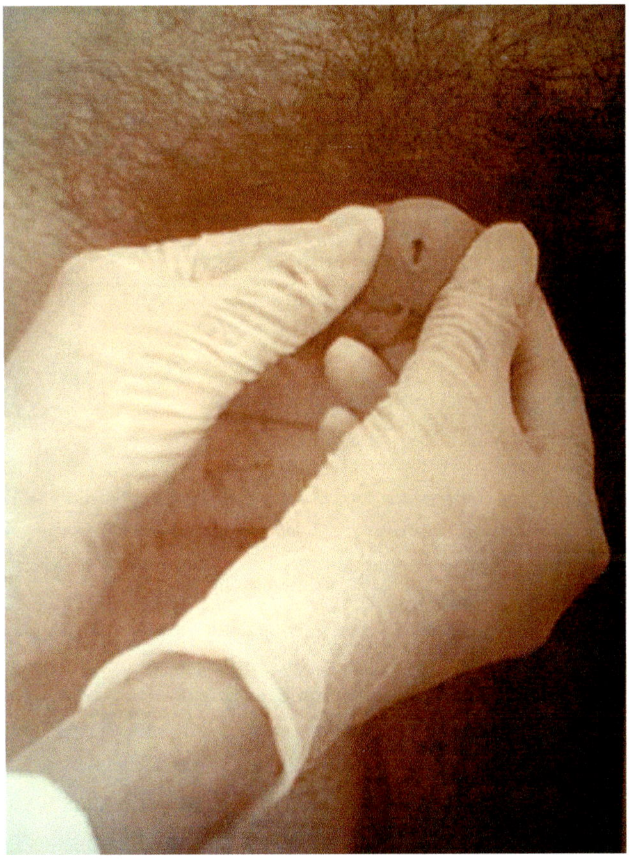

Fig. 47.5 Urethra meatus inspection technique

gonadotropic hormone; while in the pseudo precocious puberty, the patient has Leydig's cell tumor. Sperms are not produced in pseudo precocious puberty patients. Penis bends with erectile pain is seen in Peyronie disease. Penis edema can either be the part of the systemic edema or be caused by an obstruction of pelvic vein or lymph flow. A large amount of ascites can also cause penile swelling.

Glans and Corona

If there are hardened nodules with dark red ulcer, easy to bleeding or fused into cauliflower shape, a possible *penile carcinoma* should be taken into consideration. If a single oval hardened ulcer (called *chancre*), leaving a scar after healing, is found at the corona of penis, one should take it as an important sign of syphilis. Condyloma acuminatum is the manifestation of human papillary virus infection, commonly taking place at penis corona, sometimes it may occur at the other parts of penis. Genital herpes simplex virus infection is caused by the corresponding virus, which can occur at any parts of penis. Circinate balanitis (a skin inflammation of penis) can happen in Reiter's syndrome.

Urethral Meatus Position

Urethral meatus position may vary, it is commonly located at phallic ventral, which is called *hypospadias*, the case of urethral meatus location at phallic dorsolateral is called *upper urethral cracking*, which is rare; the case of red urethral meatus with discharge or ulcer and tenderness, is commonly seen in infections caused by urethritis; milky discharge flows out from the urethra meatus of the patient who has *gonorrhea urethritis*.

Blunt Trauma

It typically happens during traffic accidents. Penis and scrotum have butterfly shaped hematoma, suggesting a urethra rupture.

47.2.3 Scrotum

Scrotum is a continuation of abdominal wall, this pouch wall is composed of multilayer tissue. Scrotum has pigmented skin and folds, a small amount of pubic hair, full of sweat glands and sebaceous gland. The two halves of the pouch are separated by a septal fold of dartos, each half contains a testis, epididymis and spermatic cord inside. When the ambient temperature is low, or the temperature of the examiner's hand is low, or patient is nervous, scrotum can contract and get thickened, resulting in changes in appearance. A normal scrotum is asymmetrical, with left side at a slightly lower position. During inspection, the examiner should lift the scrotum, so that the back side can be seen, pay attention to the color of the scrotum, check whether there is rash, sebaceous cysts, edema, etc. Palpation should be done simultaneously with both hands, namely, two thumbs are placed at the front and the remaining fingers at the back of the scrotum (Fig. 47.6). Observe the two sides for symmetry. Palpation can also be done at one side, the side of examination is usually placed between the thumb, index finger and middle finger of the examiner.

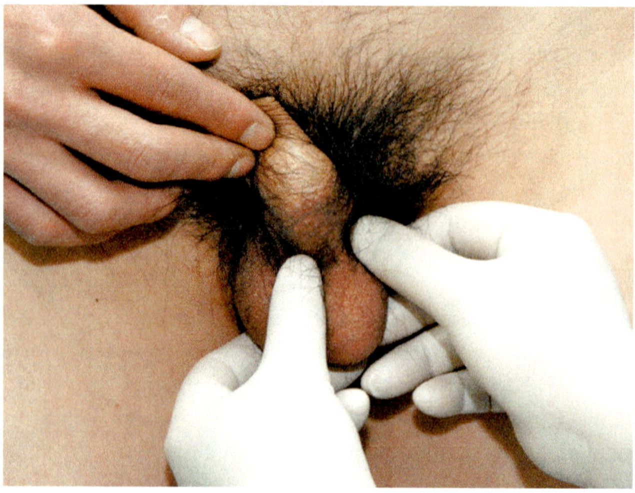

Fig. 47.6 Palpation of the scrotum

47.2.3.1 Testes

Testes are ovoid organs that produce sperm, with one at the left side and one at the right side. The normal testis is about 5 cm long, 2–3 cm thick, with smooth and flexible surface. Generally, left testicle is slightly lower than the right one. Each testis should be separately checked, use one hand to secure testis and the other to palpation, and two sides comparison should also be carried out. Pay attention to the size, shape and hardness, bitterness, and nodules, under normal circumstances, pressure testes will produce a sense of uncomfortableness.

47.2.3.2 Epididymis

Epididymis is the organ that stores sperm and promotes sperm to mature. Epididymis is located at the posterolateral of testis, the upper inflated end is the head, the lower small end looking like a sac cone is the tail, which connects to the spermatic cord. Approximately 7–10% of adults have congenital transversion of the testes, therefore, the epididymis is located in the front of the testes. Under normal circumstances, make palpation to check the size and shape of epididymis on both sides and to check for the symmetry as well.

Abnormal findings of scrotum and its contents.

Scrotum

- *Edema of scrotum*: Scrotal tissue is loose, very prone to edema, which can be part of systemic edema, or caused by local factors such as local inflammation or allergic reaction, venous blood or lymph flow blockage; Tension ascites can lead to significant swelling of scrotum; The retroperitoneal hemorrhage (such as abdominal aortic aneurysm rupture) causes non traumatic penile scrotal ecchymosis, also known as blue genital sign of Bryant.

- *Chyloderma*: Scrotal swelling, rough skin, thickening of the elephant dermoid, are known as chyloderma or scrotum elephantiasis. It is often seen in lymphatic inflammation or lymphatic obstruction caused by Filariid. Lymphogranuloma venereum caused by chlamydia trachomatis, can also lead to elephantiasis in advanced stage.
- *Scrotum hernia*: Scrotal hernia refers to the bowel or mesenteric and other intra-abdominal organs, which is down to scrotum and form groin hernia via the inguinal canal. The symptoms are unilateral or bilateral scrotal swelling mass with cystic sense of touch. Sometimes, it can be retreated in abdominal cavity with patient lying down position or pushed with hands, while coughing or other causes to increase intraperitoneal pressure can make it descend to scrotum again. The examiner uses one hand to hold the hip of the patient, places the index finger of the other hand at the scrotum which is above the testis, and then insert a finger into the external inguinal ring and felt a coughing impulse when patient coughs if there is hernia. If the bowel movement sounds can be heard during auscultation of scrotal hernia, it indicates that hernia contents are an intestine.
- *Hydrocele*: Scrotal swelling, painless by touch, a water balloon feeling, and always located in the front of the testis, these are mostly known as testicular hydrocele. During *transillumination test*, hydrocele is orange-red colored semi-translucent, which is called positive transillumination test, while substantive tissue scrotal hernia or testicular cancer is opaque. Those can be served as a parameter for differential diagnosis. Transillumination test is simple and easy to perform in the darkroom, put pen flashlight tightly over scrotal skin (avoiding light leakage at the contact edge between the flashlight and the skin), shed light from the back of the mass or cyst and observe from the front (Fig. 47.7). Or make a cylinder with non-transparent paper, put one end of the cylinder on the swollen scrotum, shed light with a flashlight to the scrotum at the opposite side, and observe the transmittance from the other end of the cylinder.
- *Others*: Scrotal eczema can lead to the thickening of scrotal skin and make it look like moss with small scales, or make skin dark red, debauched dissipated erosion, with a large amount of serofluid exudation, sometimes forming soft callus, accompanied by intractable itching. Cutaneous hemangiomas is a small red papules, also known as Fordyce spots, normally occurs in men over the age of 40, but in children, its appearance is associated with a congenital metabolic disease called Fabry disease. Fournier disease is a very threatening infectious disease caused by mixed infection of both anaerobic and gram negative aerobic bacteria, manifesting as testis, penis, perineal or perianal ulcer and severe black necrosis.

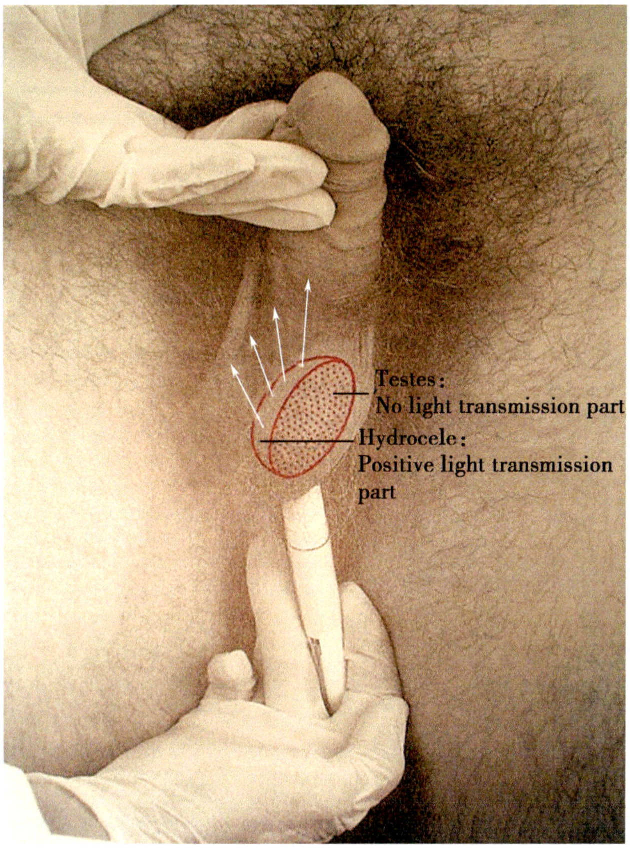

Fig. 47.7 Testicular light transmission test

Testis

- Acute testicular swelling, pain, and obvious tenderness are the commonly caused by *acute orchitis*, trauma, or epidemic mumps, gonorrhea and other inflammation, but they rarely develop into the fester. The chronic testicular swelling and pain are mainly caused by tuberculosis.
- When the length of testis is smaller than 4 cm, it is called testicular atrophy. The unilateral atrophy is often caused by trauma, and a careful review of the patient's history can obtain some clue. Small and tough bilateral testes can be seen in Klinefelter syndrome (patients are usually young and lanky), alcohol sclerosing atrophy, AIDS related testicular atrophy, rare trauma or epidemic mumps orchitis sequela and varicocele compression atrophy etc. Small and soft bilateral testes can be found in gonadal function decline caused by the insufficient gonadotropin secretion, such as obesity related reproductive incompetence syndrome.

- Swollen, hard and enlarged testis with nodules, with or without tenderness, suggests *testicular tumor* or leukemia cell infiltration. Among testicular tumors, germ cell tumor is often seen in young patients, while testicular lymphoma is more common in older patients. The earlier the diagnosis, the better the treatment of these two testicular tumors. Therefore, when the testicular swelling and pain can't be quickly alleviated or controlled by antibiotic therapy, the testicular tumor should be considered.
- When one or both of testes do not drop into the scrotum (undescended) or seclude in the abdomen, inguinal canal or phallic root ministry and perineum, it is known as *cryptorchidism*. During palpation, examiner should carefully look for testes in other locations if they are not found in scrotum. The abnormally localized testes are usually smaller and softer than normal ones. Cryptorchidism on one side is more common, while bilateral one is seen in occasion. Bilateral cryptorchidism can affect the development of reproductive organs and the secondary sex characteristics. Sometimes in normal children, exposure to coldness or strong contraction of cremaster muscles may make the testis temporarily hidden in the upper part of scrotum or in inguinal canal. During examination, the examiner may use hand to push the testis into the scrotum or ask the child to cough to make the testis drop into the scrotum. No testis detected is commonly seen in congenital anorchia caused by sex chromosome anomalies. It can be either unilateral or bilateral, for patients with bilateral cryptorchidism, their reproductive organs and secondary sex characteristics do not develop.

Epididymis

- Sperm cyst (*spermatocele*): It is usually located at the upper pole of epididymis, soft and cystic like in palpating, connecting to epididymis, left-right asymmetry and containing milky semen. It is often found by patient self-inspection. Transillumination test can be used for identification. Epididymal cyst, a painless and fluid-filled cyst, may occur in any parts of epididymis which are often seen in multiple and bilateral form. The liquid type hygromas itself is not important, but clinical differentiation should be made between substantive and inflammatory mass.
- Chronic epididymitis: A swollen and enlarged epididymis with nodules and a little tenderness may be palpated in chronic epididymitis. Acute epididymitis is often expressed in obvious pain. Enlarge and swollen epididymis may or may not be palpated, but it often accompanied by urethritis that caused by *Neisseria gonorrhoeae* or *Escherichia coli*. If epididymis palpation shows nodular lumps without tenderness, accompanied by bead-like thickening vas deferens, which is often related to epididymal tuberculosis. Tubercular lesions can adhere to scrotal skin and fistula after ulceration is not easy to heal. Primary epididymis tumor is very rare.

47.2.4 Prostate

The prostate is lying just inferior to the bladder, about 2 cm posterior to the symphysis pubis and is the substantive accessory gland surrounding the base of the urethra. The shape is like a chestnut, but is slightly flatter, the superior base is wide and big, and the inferior apex is slim and small, the posterior surface is slightly flat, the median part has a vertical shallow furrow, dividing the main portion into a left and right lobe, urethra vertically passes through the center of prostate, prostate excreting tube opening is located at the prostatic urethra. When examining prostate, patient may stand in bent-over-the-table position and hold the container to collect prostate liquid for further checkup (see prostate checkup and massage method). Patient may also take knee-elbow position on the desk. The examiner cover a finger glove (or glove) on right hand index finger with lubricant, gradually insert index finger into the anus and palpate towards the ventral (Fig. 47.8). For normal adult, the prostate is 4 cm away from the anus, the diameter is less than 4 cm, and protruding in the rectum is less than 1 cm. During palpation, the examiner can feel the elastic tenacious prostate with no tenderness, the left and right lobes are symmetrical in both shape and size, and the median furrow can be palpated as well. The prostate palpation and massage can be done simultaneously in order to obtain the prostatic fluid. The method is as following: massage prostate with index finger forwardly and inwardly a few times on each side, then glide and squeeze along the median

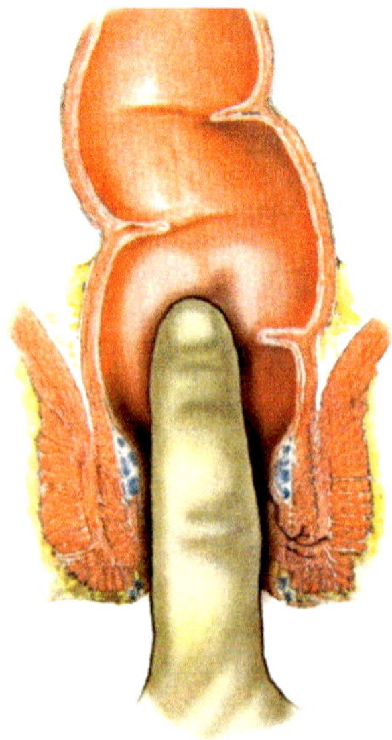

Fig. 47.8 Prostate palpation

furrow towards the urethra meatus, the prostate liquid can be seen flowing out the urethra meatus, and the specimen should be collected for further examination.

In the case of *prostate hyperplasia*, the median furrow becomes shallower or disappears. In the case of benign prostatic hyperplasia, the prostate is swollen and resilient with smooth surface, no tenderness or adhesion. Prostatic hyperplasia may be limited to the anterior lobe and cannot be palpated through rectum palpation. Patients in this case may have urethral compression which leads to dysuria, but the size of the prostate may be normal through rectal palpation. Therefore the possibility of prostate hyperplasia cannot be rule out in this situation. In diffuse or focal enlargement of the prostate with obvious tenderness, the patient is often found having acute prostatitis or prostatic abscess, the prostate massage to get purulent prostatic fluid is helpful for this diagnosis. For the prostatic nodules with or without prostate enlargement, the following differentials should be considered: prostate cancer, benign prostatic hyperplasia, prostatic calcification, prostate infarction and granuloma of prostatitis etc.

47.2.5 Spermatic Cord

Spermatic cord is a soft tubular structure, the cord extends from the external inguinal ring to the tail of epididymis. It consists of the vas deferens, cremaster, arteries, veins, spermatic nerves, lymphatic vessels, etc. The cord is symmetrically positioned in both left and right scrotum and superior to the head of the epididymis, and is soft with no tenderness in palpation. Palpation of the spermatic cord is the best to perform when patient is in the upright standing position, lift patient's penis, but do not lift too high in order to avoid the skin tightening and affect the exam. Examiner gently picks the scrotum up on the midline and the spermatic cord sits between the thumb and index finger, holds the scrotum with the rest of the fingers, checks the whole cord from the epididymis to the external inguinal ring and pays attention to whether there is nodules, swelling and tenderness. The hard cord of 2–4 mm in diameter inside the spermatic cord is the spermaduct.

Common abnormal manifestations of the spermatic cord examination: The beaded swelling of the spermatic cord is often seen in vas deferens tuberculosis; Local red and swelling skin with compressing pain is an acute inflammation of spermatic cord; The spermatic cord thickening and swelling with positive testis elevation test (Prehn sign), i.e. increased pain when patient's testis is elevated, suggests the torsion of the spermatic cord; Palpable induration of the spermatic cord near the epididymis is usually caused by Filariasis; The earthworm-like clusters of spermatic cord is varicocele, which is caused by blood stasis and expansion of spermatic vein plexus with negative transillumination test. The severe varicocele can be seen by naked eye inspection. When varicoceles seen on the both sides of spermatic cord, it can reduce the fertility; A collection of fluid along the spermatic cord forms *hydrocele of cord* that lies superior to the testis and has a positive transillumination test. This soft cystic mass along the spermatic cord needs to be identified from inguinal hernia. The hydrocele of cord usually doesn't need to be treated unless it is too large.

47.3 Section 3: Female Genital Organs

Female genital organs are divided into two parts: one part is the external genitalia, including mons pubis, labium majus, labium minus, clitoris and vaginal vestibule. The other part is the internal organs, including the vagina, uterus and uterine adnexa, which is composed of fallopian tubes and ovaries. The main function of female genital organs is reproduction.

Female genitalia changes with the age and is related to the development of breast. Usually breast develops at 8–13 years old, while pubic hair develops at 8–14 years old, and the average age of the beginning of puberty is about 11 years old, spans at least 1.5–6 years and on the average of 3 years to the state of maturity.

The female genital examinations include inspection, palpation and vaginal speculum examinations. Except for patients with urinary incontinence, the bladder should be emptied and defecation should be encouraged before the examination. The patient is generally taking the lithotomy position so that the buttocks are at the edge of the examination table, the head is slightly raised and hands are flatted on the body side or on the abdomen. The doctor standing just between the patient legs will face the patient to perform the examination. Urinary fistula patients should take knee-chest position for exam. Doctors should ask patient to gently exert abdominal pressure in order to relax sphincter muscles when inserting vaginal speculum or performing the digital vaginal and rectal examination. Gynecological examination should be avoided during the time of period. If vaginal bleeding has to be checked, the examinations should be done with sterile gloves and equipment after disinfection of the vulva. Generally women without sexual life history should be checked only by anal abdominal exam and pay attention to prevent cross infection.

47.3.1 External Genital Organs

Firstly, observe the development of the vulva and distribution of pubic hair, deformity, edema, inflammation, ulcer, vegetations, or mass etc., pay attention to whether there are some abnormal appearances on the color, thickness and atrophy of the skin and mucous membrane. Secondly, separate the minus

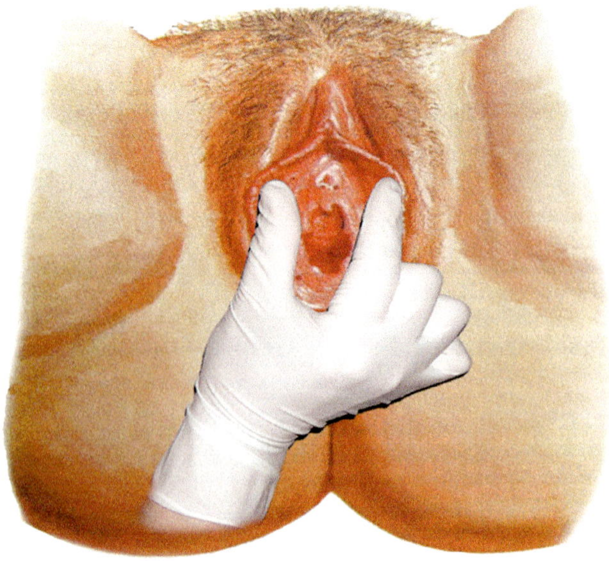

Fig. 47.9 Female external genital inspection

labia with the thumb and index finger of one hand to expose the vestibule and urethra, the vaginal os and hymen to check whether there are anomalies (Fig. 47.9). It is necessary to ask the primipara or multipara women to take a deep breath and hold it or cough to inspect the bulging of anterior or posterior vaginal wall and prolapse of uterus as well as stress urinary incontinence, etc.

47.3.1.1 Mons Pubis

Mons pubis, a prominence formed by the pad of fat that overlies the pubic symphysis and it begins to grow pubic hair during puberty. The distribution of normal pubic hair is the tip downward triangle. The density, thickness and color can vary in individuals and in racial groups. The pubic hair is sparse or absent in the cases of gonadal dysgenesis or hypogonadism; while in the conditions of hyperandrogenism such as in polycystic ovary syndrome, masculine tumors or hyperadrenocorticism, the pubic hair will be thick and diamond shaped distribution as men.

47.3.1.2 Labium Majora

Labium majora is a pair of longitudinal round skin folds and is rich in fat and blood vessels etc. Pubic hair starts to grow at puberty. Both ridge sides of labium major are naturally closed in nullipara and separated in multipara. The labium major becomes atrophy during the time of menopause. Local injuries easily form haematomas; red and swollen are the signs of the inflammation of vulva.

47.3.1.3 Labium Minora

The labium minora are two thin brown skin folds without hair, medial to the labium major and rich in nerve endings. The labia minora on both sides are often closed and covered vaginal vestibule, and extend posteriorly to form the fourchette. Swollen, redness and pain of the labium minor is common in inflammation. Local skin depigmentation is common in vulvar dystrophy and vitiligo. Cancerous possibility should be considered if the nodules and ulceration seen on the vulval surface.

47.3.1.4 Clitoris

The clitoris is a bulging part between the junction of the labium minora and anterior commissure of the labium majora, it is the erectile homologue to the penis, which is composed of the corpora cavernosa and is rich in nerve endings. The length of the clitoris generally does not exceed 2.5 cm, it is smaller in patients with gonadal dysgenesis; while it is bigger in androgen excess or hermaphrodism patients.

47.3.1.5 Vaginal Vestibular

The rhombus space between the lines of attachment of the labia minora is called the vestibular, where the urethra meatus is anteriorly situated and the vaginal orifice is the posterior boundary. The greater vestibular glands lie on the each side of the viginal orifice and the gland size is similar to soybean. When the greater vestibular gland has inflammation it will be red, swelling, painful or pus discharging. Hymen lies the vaginal orifice, its opening shape, size and thickness vary depend on age, parity and sexual experience. The hymen is mostly intact without sex life, there is hymen cracks for the married and only remnant marks for the parous women.

47.3.2 Internal Genital Organs

47.3.2.1 Exam Method

Vaginal Speculum Exam

Select an appropriate size of vaginal speculum with the two blades closed and the front-end coated with saline or lubricant, use thumb and index finger of one hand to separate the labium minora, the other hand inserts the speculum diagonally at 45° angle along the posterior vaginal wall slowly into the vagina, push superoposteriorly rotating clockwise at 45° and gradually open the blades while keep them parallel to each other until completely expose the cervix (Fig. 47.10). Inspect the vagina and cervix, then do vaginal cervical discharges or cell smear examination (Fig. 47.11). Finally, slowly withdraw the speculum after closing the two blades.

Bimanual Pelvic Exam

Gently insert the index and middle fingers of your gloved and lubricated hand into the vagina along the posterior vaginal wall. Place your other hand on the abdomen and press downward toward following the patient breath. Using the

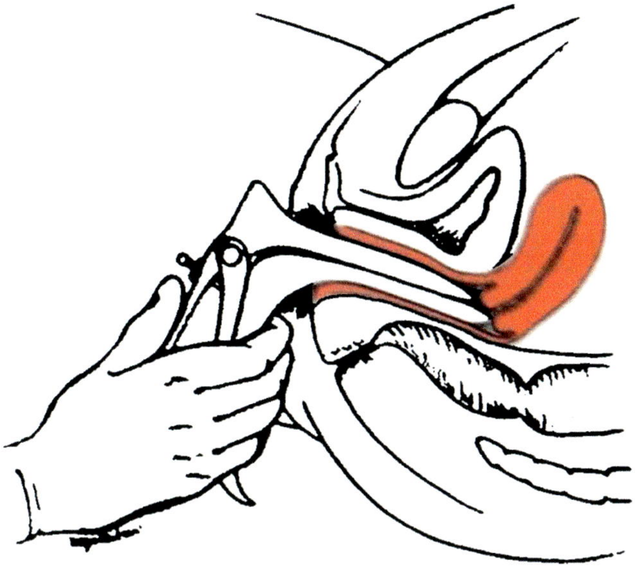

Fig. 47.10 Vaginal speculum exam

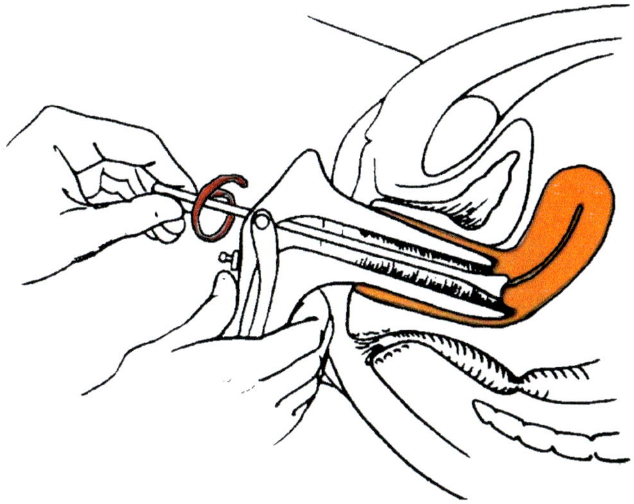

Fig. 47.11 Collection of vaginal and cervical discharges or cells

palmar surface of your fingers palpates the vagina, cervix and pelvic organs systematically (Figs. 47.12 and 47.13).

Rectovaginal Exam

The *rectovaginal exam* is often used as a supplement of a bimanual exam. Gently introduce the index and middle fingers of your gloved and lubricated hand into the vagina and the rectum respectively. Place your other hand on the abdomen of patients. Palpate the uterine posterior wall, rectouterine pouch, uterosacral ligament and bilateral pelvic posterior wall. It is particularly useful for the conditions of retroverted uterus, suspected endometriosis and malignant tumor. (Fig. 47.14).

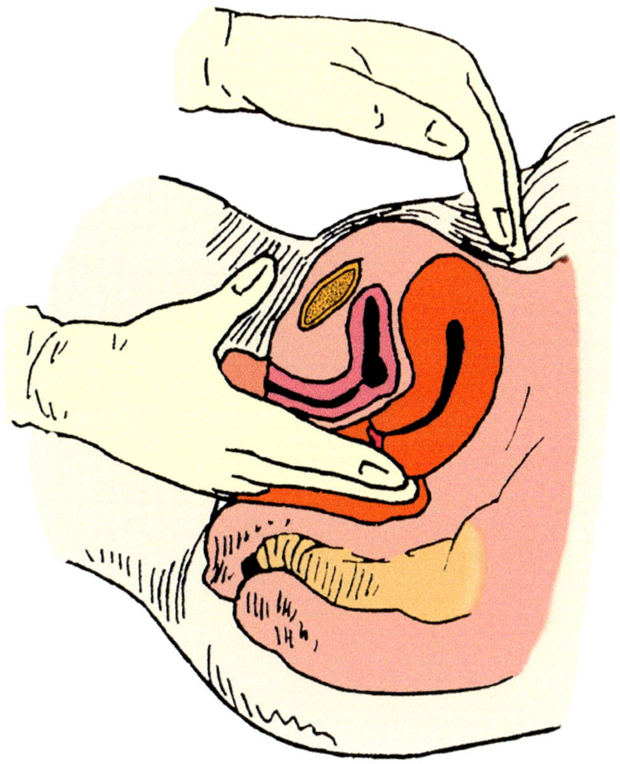

Fig. 47.12 Bimanual pelvic exam for uterus

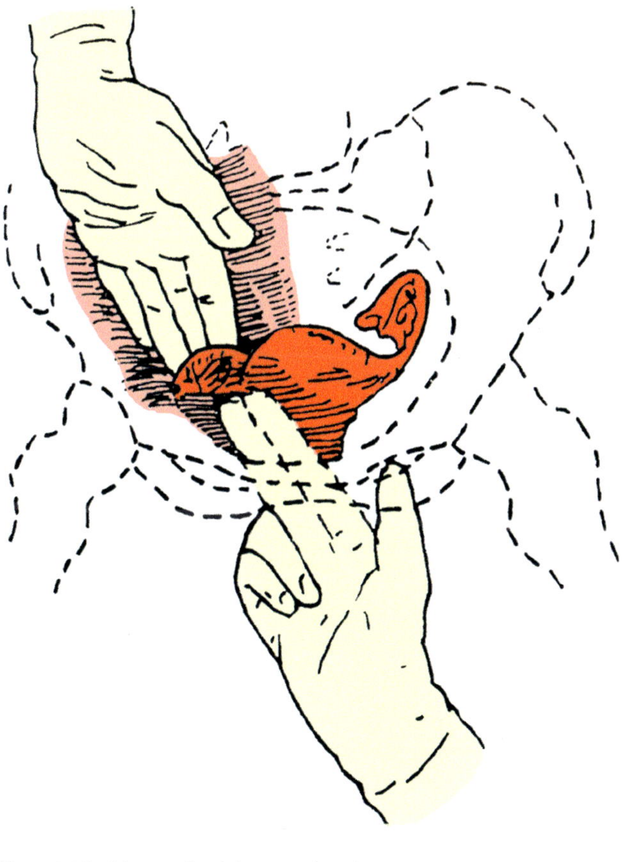

Fig. 47.13 Bimanual pelvic exam for adnexa

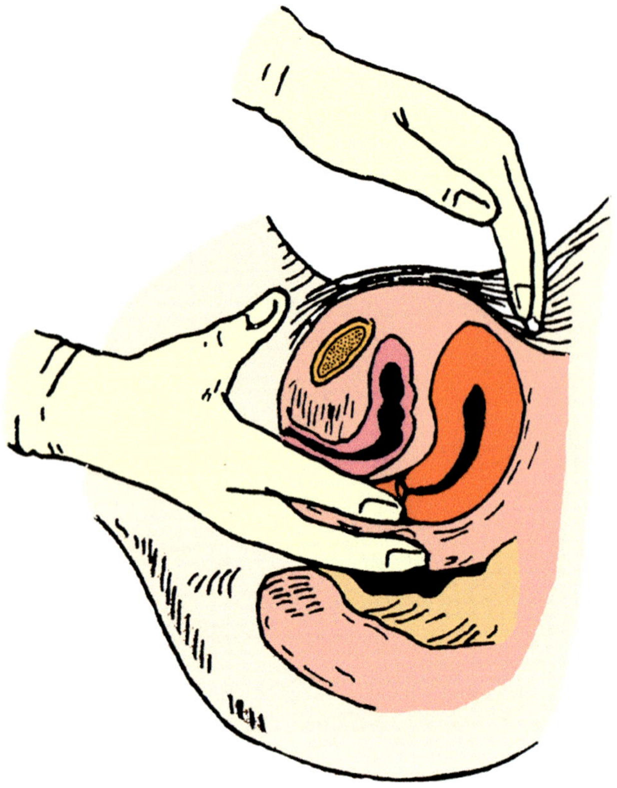

Fig. 47.14 Rectovaginal exam

Rectoabdominal Examination

Gently introduce the index finger of your gloved and lubricated hand into the rectum and place your other hand on the abdomen for assisting. *Rectoabdominal examination* is usually used for the unmarried, vaginal atresia or other inappropriate situations, where the vaginal examination is unsuitable. However the rectoabdominal examination is far less informative than the bimanual pelvic examination or rectovaginal exam.

47.3.2.2 Internal Genital Organs

Vagina

The vagina is an elastic, muscular canal that is slightly shallower on the dorsal and ventral parts, and is rich in venous plexus. The dorsal and ventral walls are usually touching each other. The vaginal wall of reproductive woman has lots of folds that have great stretch. The mucous membrane is pink. For both young girls and postmenopausal women, the vaginal mucous membrane is very thin and has a fewer folds with a little stretch. During examination, pay attention to its elasticity, any degree of obstruction, depth, mucous membrane color, folds, deformity, hyperaemia, haemorrhage, ulcer, scar, mass and so on. Pay attention to the amount, color, smell and characteristics of vaginal secretions, and abnormal leucorrhea should take smear examination.

Uterus

The uterus is an upside-down pear-shaped hollow organ and sits in the center of the pelvic cavity. The upper part is called uterine corpus and the lower part is called the uterine cervix. Uterine corpus to cervix ratio is 1–2 in infants and 2–1 in adults. The external os of the cervix is round in the nulliparous women and transverse slit in the parous women due to reproduction, which is called the anterior and posterior lips of the external os. Doctors should pay attention to the cervical size, color, external shape, hardness, erosion, cracks, extroversion, vegetations, mass or contact bleeding etc. If there is lifting or rocking pain when doctors uplift or swing the cervix, it is called cervical lift or swing pain and it is the manifestation of pelvic inflammatory diseases or pelvic accumulation of blood. The patients should be advised to have the cervical smear examination or cervical secretions examination. The manifestation of cervicitis are congestion, erosion even pus overflow, Patients with contact bleeding should be alert to the possibility of malignant tumor.

During the bimanual examination, coordinate fingers in vagina uplifting and fingers on abdomen pressing downward harmonically to palpate the uterine position, size, shape, hardness, activity, mass or tenderness. The uterus is normally positioned in anteflexion and anteversion (Fig. 47.15). The angle of flexion refers to the angle between the corpus and cervix. Anteflexion means the two longitudinal axes are bending forward, where the two longitudinal axes are bent backward is called retroflexion (Fig. 47.15). The angle of version refers to the longitudinal axis formed between the corpus and body. The anteversion refers to the corpus leaning forward toward the pubis (Figure15) while the retroversion refers to the corpus leaning backward toward sacrum. Normal adult uterus is about 7.5 cm long, 4.5 cm wide, 2.5 cm thick. Normally, the uterus is smooth, movable and without tenderness. The uterine will increase in size and be tougher in palpation after childbirth. Physiological enlargement of uterine is seen in pregnancy while pathological enlargement is seen in various tumors.

47.3.2.3 Uterine Accessories

Uterine accessories includes both ovaries and fallopian tubes. After palpated the uterine, move the fingers in vagina to one side of the vaginal fornix, place the other hand on the same side abdomen at the level on iliac crest and press down and gradually slid downward in coordination with the fingers vagina to palpate whether there are lumps, thickness or tenderness. Pay attention to the location, shape, texture, motion, tenderness and the relationship with the surrounding organs if the lump palpated.

The normal fallopian tubes are a pair of slender and curved tubular organs about 8–14 cm long. Normally the surface of the tubes is smooth, no tenderness and can not be palpated. The manifestations of tubal inflammation are

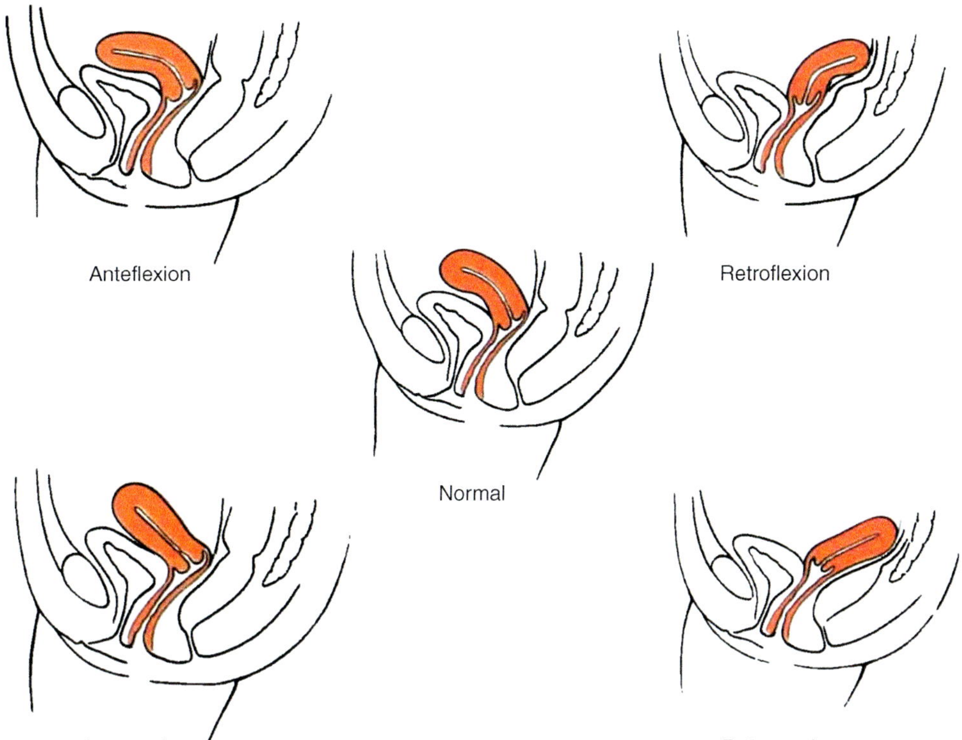

Fig. 47.15 Schematic diagram of a variety of uterine positions

swelling, thickening or nodules, obvious tenderness, and it can also lead to adhesion and fixation with the surrounding tissue or organs, especially common in acute and chronic pelvic inflammation or tuberculosis. Obviously enlarged tube is called hydrosalpinx or pyosalpinx.

Ovaries are a pair of flat oval gonads, the size of an adult female ovary is about 4 cm × 3 cm × 2 cm (length, width, thickness) and the surface is smooth and soft. Sometimes the normal ovary can be palpated in women with a thin abdominal wall and have a sense of soreness. The ovaries become smaller and harder because of atrophy in postmenopausal women. Ovarian enlargement is commonly seen in ovarian mass or inflammation. Ovarian cyst torsion patients have severe pain and obvious tenderness at the twisting part.

Key Terms

1	Anal atresia and stenosis	肛门闭锁与狭窄
2	Anal fissure	肛裂
3	Hemorrhoid	痔疮
4	Anorectal fistula	肛管直肠瘘
5	Rectal prolapsed	直肠脱垂
6	Ano-rectal examination	直肠指诊
7	Prepuce redundant	包皮过长
8	Penile carcinoma	阴茎癌
9	Chancre	下疳
10	Hypospadias	尿道下裂
11	Edema of scrotum	阴囊水肿
12	Scrotum hernia	阴囊疝
13	Hydrocele	阴囊积水
14	Transillumination test	透视检查法
15	Bimanual pelvic exam	双合诊

Study Questions

1. What are the commonly used positions of the anorectal examination?
2. A digital rectal examination including what content?
3. What are the abnormal changes in the digital rectal examination?
4. What are the common manifestations of abnormal penis?
5. What are the common methods of the female internal genital inspection?

Suggested Websites

1. http://v.youku.com/v_show/id_XOTUwNzc0Njg=.html
2. http://www.56.com/u78/v_OTcxMTk5NDc.htm156.com
3. http://ocw.tufts.edu/Course/24/Lecturenotes

48 Physical Examination of the Musculoskeletal System

Lie Dai and Rui Zeng

Musculoskeletal system consists of bones, skeletal muscles, ligaments, tendons, cartilages and other connective tissues, and joints are the fundamental functional unit. The primary methods used for physical examination of musculoskeletal system are inspection and palpation. Percussion and auscultation are only used in special situations such as percussion pain of vertebrae, auscultation for bone crepitus. The examination should include assessment of muscle strength and range of motion and maneuvers to test joint function and stability. Both active movements (where the patient moves the joint themselves) and passive movements (where the examiner moves the joint) should be performed. Notice the symmetry, looking for symmetry of involvement and noting any joint deformities or malalignment of joints or bones. Examination should also include assessment of surrounding tissues, noting skin changes, subcutaneous nodules and muscle atrophy, and assessment of inflammation especially redness, swelling, warmth and tenderness. Use the back of your fingers to compare the involved joint with its unaffected contralateral joint, or with nearby tissues if both joints are involved.

The examiner should perform physical examination gently to avoid painful experience of patients. If the joint has been injured, consider an X-ray before attempting movement. Following trauma or suspected cervical injury, the cervical spine must always be immediately immobilized in a rigid collar prior to any movement or examination of the patient.

48.1 Vertebral Column

The vertebral column consists of 33 vertebrae arranged in five regions: seven cervical (C), twelve thoracic (T), five lumbar (L), five sacral (S) and four coccygeal.

L. Dai
Department of Rheumatology and Immunology, Sun Yat-Sen University, Guangzhou, China

R. Zeng (✉)
Department of Cardiology, Sichuan University, Chengdu, China

48.1.1 Vertebral Surface Landmarks

Vertebral landmarks are useful in determining the location of lesions. Moving inferiorly from the inion, C2 is the first spinous process. Running inferiorly down the neck the first big bump is usually C7 which is the most prominent and more conspicuous vertebral landmark when the neck and back are flexed. The spinous process of T3 is approximately at the level of the medial aspect of the scapular spine. T7 is at the level of inferior angle of the scapula. A horizontal line joining the highest points of the iliac crests passes through the tip of the L4 spinous process and the L4-L5 intervertebral disc. A horizontal plane between the posterior superior iliac spine crosses between L5 and S1 processes (Fig. 48.1).

48.1.2 Vertebral Column Examination

Before examination, the patient should be undressed to expose the vertebral column. The patient should stand with heels together, knees straight, and hands dropped down naturally.

48.1.2.1 Posterior Inspection

1. **Vertebral Column**
   First, examine whether the vertebral column is straight at the midline of the back. Scoliosis is characterized by an abnormal lateral curvature that is accompanied by rotation of the vertebrae. The curve is usually in an "S" or a "C" shape. Scoliosis is typically classified as either functional or structural. The former could be caused by various conditions such as poor sitting posture during childhood, disc herniation, polio sequelae or one leg being shorter than the other. Structural scoliosis could be caused by rickets, chronic pleural thickening, pleural adhesions, shoulder deformities or other diseases and it cannot be corrected by changing postures.

X.-H. Wan, R. Zeng (eds.), *Handbook of Clinical Diagnostics*, https://doi.org/10.1007/978-981-13-7677-1_48

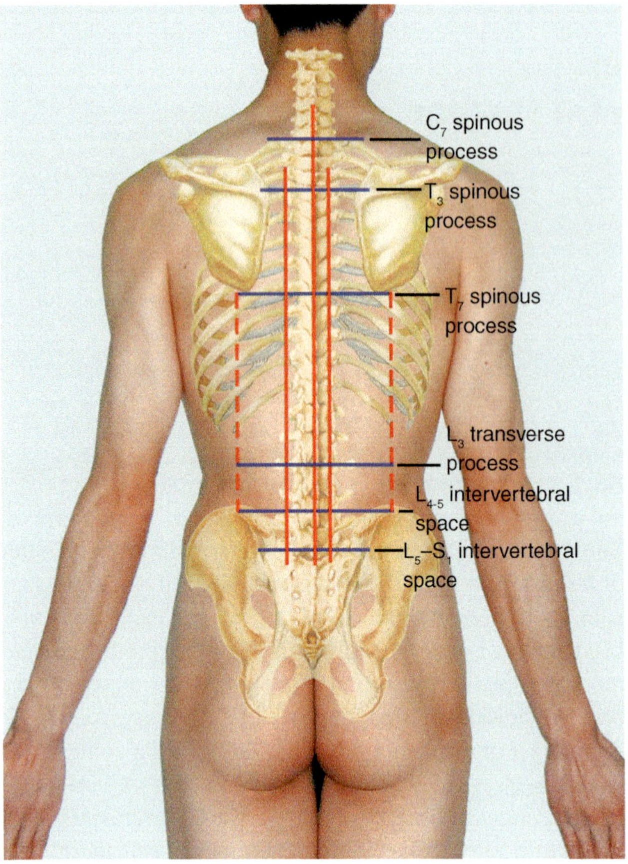

Fig. 48.1 Landmarks of vertebral column

2. **Back Muscles**
   Back muscles bulge on both sides of the vertebral column in normal circumstances. However, back muscles usually undergo atrophy in people who hold longstanding bending position or lack of exercise, and spinous processes present as a central bulge. These patients are at high risk for kyphosis and back ligament strain. It should also be noted that whether the erector spinae is asymmetrical, atrophy or spasm.
3. **Voluntary Movement**
   There are three basic types of movement of the entire vertebrae: flexion or extension, lateral bending and axial rotation. The cervical and lumbar vertebrae are more mobile than the other parts of the vertebrae. Shoulders should be fixed during the cervical vertebrae examination. The ranges of motion of cervical and lumbar vertebrae are shown in Fig. 48.2.

To evaluate thoracic rotation, the examiner rotate the patients' trunk by pulling the shoulder anteriorly and then the hip posteriorly with pelvis fixed. The amount of chest expansion is measured from deep expiration to full inspiration at the level of the fourth anterior costa. The normal chest expansion measurement is more than 5cm. Loss of the chest expansion is usually seen in ankylosing spondylitis.

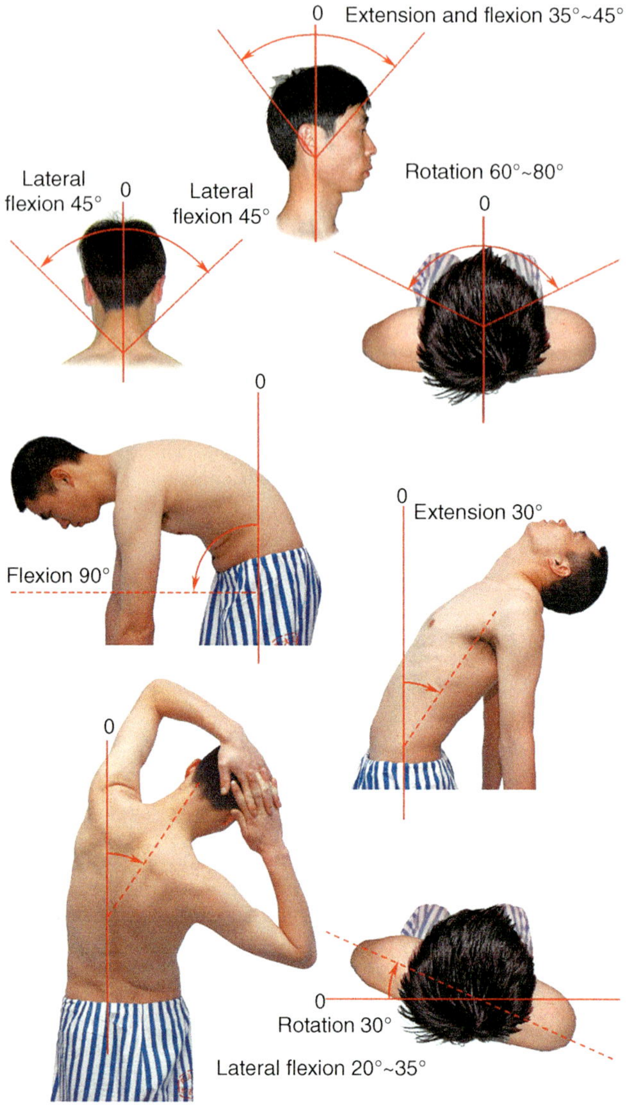

Fig. 48.2 The range of motion of cervical and lumbar vertebrae

48.1.2.2 Lateral Inspection

When viewed laterally, the vertebral column presents four distinct curves with a natural "S" shape. The thoracic and sacral kyphoses are concave anteriorly, whereas the cervical and lumbar lordoses are concave posteriorly.

1. **Kyphosis**
   Kyphosis is characterized by an abnormal increase in the thoracic curvature. The vertebral column curves posteriorly, which is also known as gibbus. Thoracic vertebrae bend backward in various degrees, sometimes accompanied with collapsed chest. Kyphosis is mainly caused by rickets in children, while it may be caused by thoracic vertebral tuberculosis or spinal osteochondritis in adolescents. Postural kyphosis is typically noticed during adolescence and caused by abnormal posture or weakening muscles and ligaments in the back. In adult, ankylosing

spondylitis usually leads to kyphosis. The most common cause of kyphosis in elderly is vertebral compression fractures due to osteoporosis. Traumatic thoracic fracture is a common cause of kyphosis in all age group.

2. **Lordosis**

   Lordosis is referred to the inward curvature of the lumbar and cervical vertebrae. Many physical conditions or disorders can cause lordosis, such as pregnancy, ascites, spondylolisthesis, congenital hip dislocation and hip flexion deformity.

48.1.2.3 Spinal Tenderness and Percussion Pain

Instruct the patient to take a prone position so that paraspinal muscles are relaxed. The examiner presses his right thumb along paraspinal muscles or along spinous processes to detect muscle or vertebral pain. If there is tenderness in certain parts, the examiner should locate the exact site by searching for the vertebral landmarks. Tenderness at paraspinal muscles indicates muscle strain. Tenderness at transverse processes of lumbar vertebrae indicates psoas strain as the psoas sheath is attached to the lumbar transverse processes.

There are two methods to perform percussion in vertebral column: (a) Direct percussion: Tap each spinous process directly by using a hammer or finger. (b) Indirect percussion: Instruct the patient to take the sitting position, the examiner puts his left hand on the patient's head and then taps the back of left hand by his right fist's hypothenar. Pain elicited by percussion may reveal spinal tuberculosis, fractures or disc herniation.

Tenderness in vertebrae usually suggests that superficial lesion while percussion pain indicates a deep lesion. For example, percussion elicits more serious pain than palpation in vertebral tuberculosis.

48.1.2.4 Special Tests of the Vertebrae

1. **Lindner's test**

   Instruct the patient to take sitting position with straight legs and then the examiner slowly flexes the patient's head forward. Any pain in lumbar vertebrae or even radiating to leg indicates lumbar nerve root compression.

2. **Straight leg raising test**

   With the patient lying down on his or her back on an examination table or exam floor, the examiner lifts the patient's leg with straight knee (Fig. 48.3). Normal person is able to lift the limb for more than 70° without pain. If the patient experiences sciatic pain when the straight leg is at an angle less than 30°, it suggests diseases such as sciatica, lumbar disc herniation or lumbosacral nerve root inflammation. In order to make this test more specific, the ankle can be dorsiflexed which will increase the stretching of the nerve root and dura. This is called Lasègue sign.

3. **Lumbosacral joint test or pelvic rotation test**

   The patient is in supine position with knees and hips extremely flexed. This lifts the buttocks and keeps the lumbar flexed (Fig. 48.4). If the patient experiences pain, called lumbosacral joint test positive, it suggests soft tissue strain of low back or lumbosacral disorders. In patient with disc herniation, the test is negative.

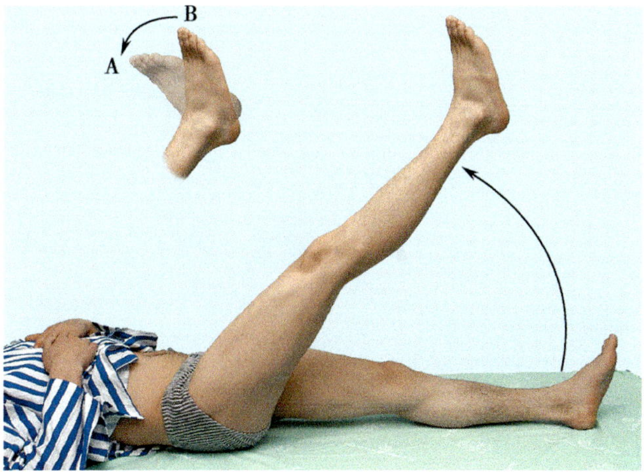

Fig. 48.3 Straight leg raising test

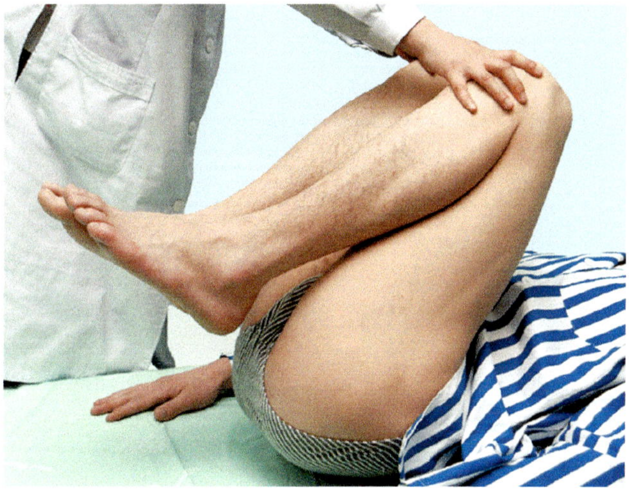

Fig. 48.4 Lumbosacral joint test

4. **Hip abduction and external rotation test or "4" test**

   The examiner moves the leg into 45° of flexion, then externally rotates and abducts the leg so that the ankle rests proximal to the knee of the straightening contralateral leg. If pain is elicited on the contralateral side posteriorly around the sacroiliac joint, it suggests disorders in that joint. If pain is located in the inguinal area, it indicates myofibrositis of vastus medialis muscles, tendon or muscle injury while the sacroiliac joint is normal (Fig. 48.5).

5. **Ely's test**

   Instruct the patient in prone position with knee extremely flexed (Fig. 48.6). In that case, femoral nerve and the anterior femoral muscles are pulled. If radiating pain emerges in anterior thigh, the test is positive which indicates femoral nerve irritation, tightness of the rectus femoris muscle, psoas abscess, spinal ankylosing, quadriceps contracture or sacroiliac joint disorder.

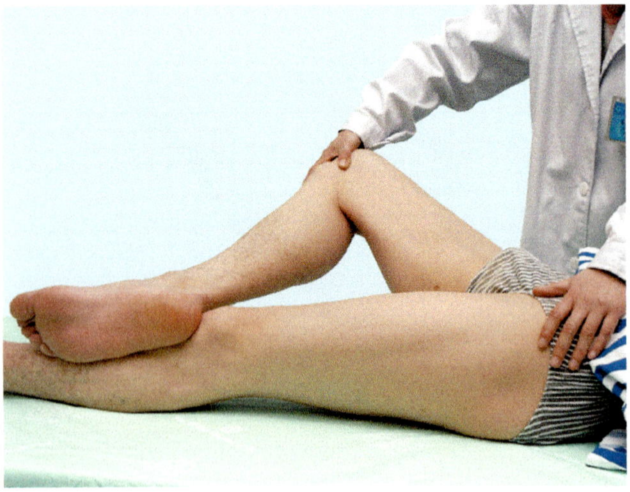

Fig. 48.5 Hip abduction and external rotation test

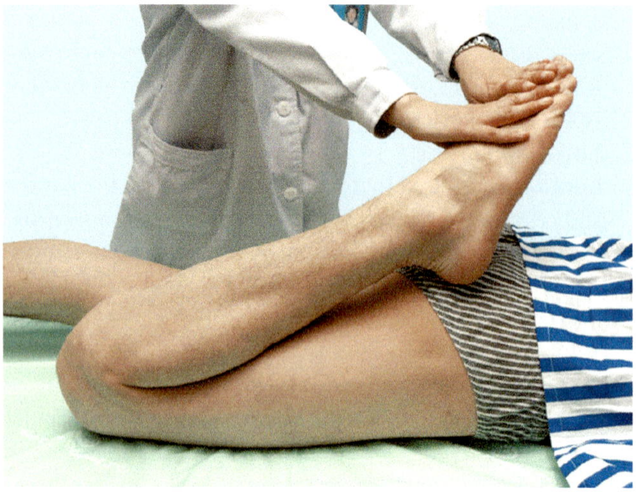

Fig. 48.6 Ely's test

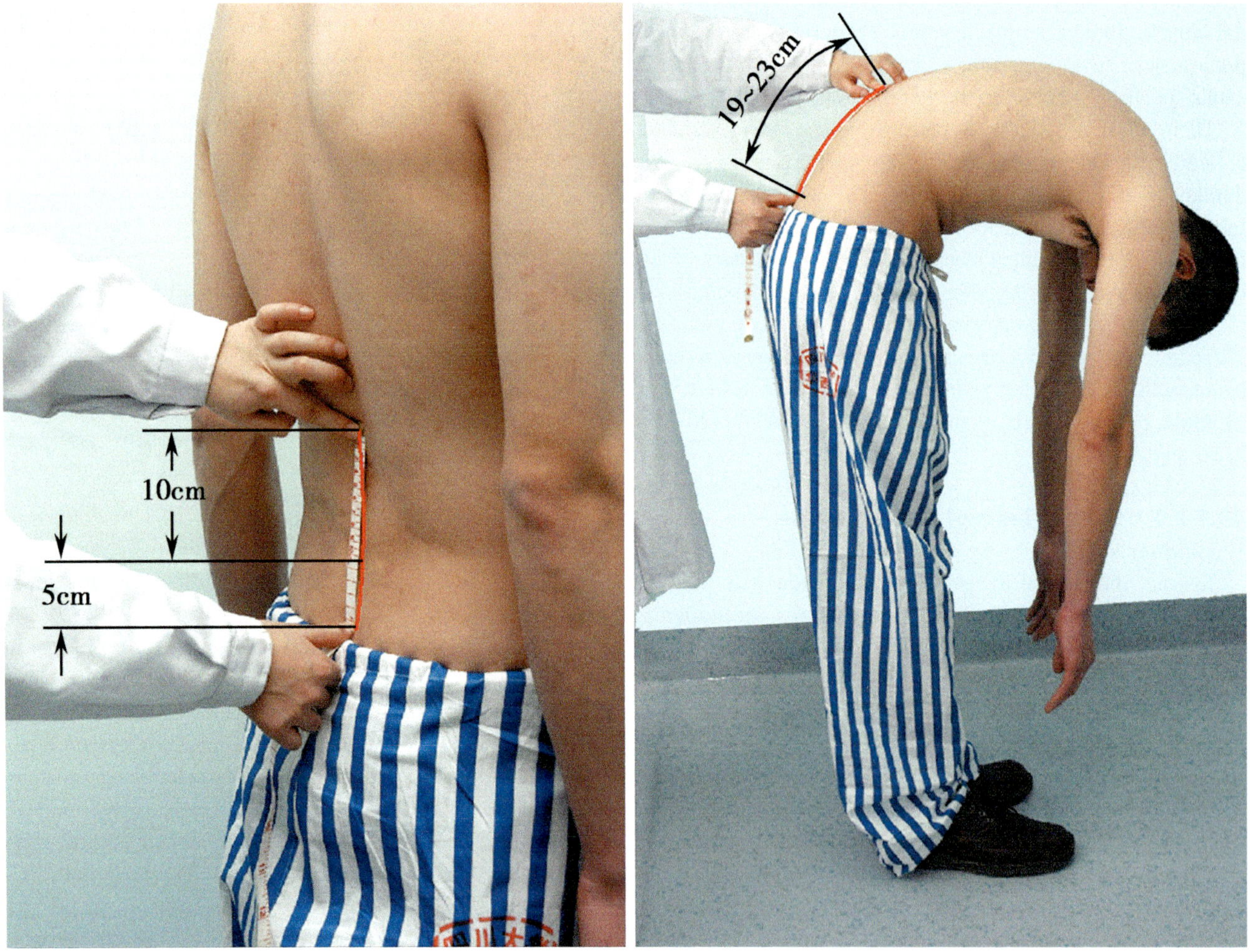

Fig. 48.7 Schöber test

6. **Schöber test**

   The purpose of the Schöber test is to examine the range of lumbar flexion. In this test, a mark is made at the level of the posterior iliac spine on the vertebral column. Two points are marked: 5 cm below and 10 cm above this mark (for a total of 15 cm distance). The patient is then instructed to touch his toes without knee flexion (Fig. 48.7). If the increase in distance between the two points is less than 4 cm, it indicates limitation of lumbar flexion which is commonly seen in patients with ankylosing spondylitis.

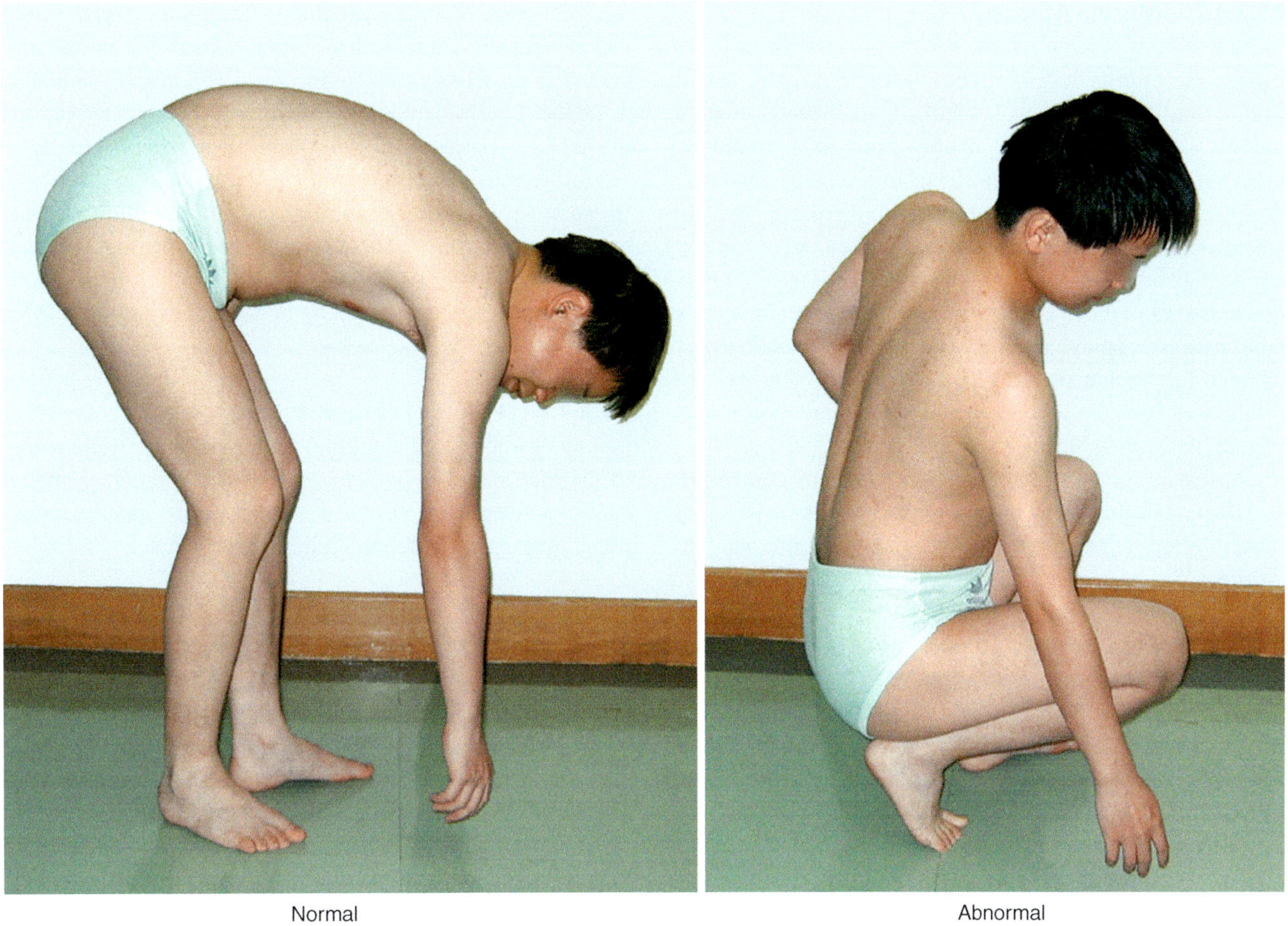

Fig. 48.8 Bend and pick up test

7. **Bend and pick up test**
   The aim of the test is to examine anterior flexion movement of the vertebrae. Ask the patient to pick up an item on the ground. Patient with disorder in lumbar vertebrae flexes knees and hips with straightening the back to pick up the item (Fig. 48.8).

48.2 Limbs and Joints

48.2.1 General Principles

Physical examination of limbs and joints mainly use inspection and palpation. Examiner should inspect for evidence of swelling, atrophy, redness and deformity, observe skin, hair distribution, veins and fingers (toes), and look for any rash, ulcers, boils, gangrene, syndactyly or other abnormal signs. The range of motion should be assessed both actively and passively. Assess temperature by palpating the skin with the dorsum of the hand. Symmetrical cold limbs may indicate critical illness or shock state. Asymmetry skin temperature and pulse intense may reveal peripheral artery stenosis including radial artery, dorsal artery and popliteal artery.

Muscle strength is usually evaluated and recorded in a systematic fashion. It is wise to compare both sides. Muscle strength is often rated on a scale of 0/5 to 5/5 as follows:

- 0/5: no contraction.
- 1/5: muscle flicker, but no movement.
- 2/5: movement possible, but not against gravity (test the joint in its horizontal plane).
- 3/5: movement possible against gravity, but not against resistance by the examiner.
- 4/5: movement possible against some resistance by the examiner.
- 5/5: normal strength.

48.2.1.1 Acromegaly

Acromegaly is the result of excessive production of growth hormone (GH) by an adenoma in the anterior pituitary gland. GH stimulates proliferation of cartilage, periarticular connective tissue and bone. The signs and symptoms of acromegaly include enlarged hands and feet, enlarged facial features, thickened skin, excessive sweating and body odor. In children, it is called gigantism.

48.2.1.2 Muscle Atrophy

Muscle atrophy is the wasting or loss of muscle bulk. In palpation, the muscle will be flabby. Muscle atrophy usually occurs from lack of physical activity, myositis or neurogenic atrophy. Myogenic atrophy results from inflammatory or viral myositis, inherited muscle disorders (e.g. Duchenne muscular dystrophy or glycogen storage diseases), myasthenia gravis or drug-induced myopathy. Neurogenic muscle atrophy occurs when there is an injury or disease of the nerve that connects to the muscle, which includes brainstem motor neurons injury, spinal anterior horn cells or peripheral nerve damage (e.g. acute poliomyelitis, peripheral neuritis). The differences between myogenic and neurogenic muscle atrophy are listed in Table 48.1.

Muscle atrophy may be masked by thick subcutaneous fat in infants and the following signs are helpful for detecting muscle atrophy: low muscle tone, flabby muscle and limb weakness.

48.2.1.3 Fracture and Joint Dislocation

Fracture means broken bone. The signs and symptoms of fracture include tenderness, swelling, bruising, discolored skin around the affected area, abnormal movement, angulation or limb shrink. A dislocated joint may be visibly deformed or out of place, swollen or discolored and immovable.

48.2.1.4 Varicose Veins

Varicose veins are swollen and enlarged veins that usually occur in the lower limbs. The varicose veins are lumpy, bulging or twisted in appearance. Other signs include swollen feet and ankles, dry skin and color changes in the lower leg. In some cases, inflammation of the skin or skin ulcers may appear.

48.2.1.5 Edema

Both inspection and palpation are needed to look for edema. Notice the symmetry of edema. Symmetric edema is a feature of generalized edema which is more prominent in lower limbs compared to upper limbs. Unilateral limb edema is mostly caused by the local venous or lymphatic drainage insufficiency. The former is found in venous thrombosis, paralysis or neurological disorders. The latter can be found in lymphatic obstruction, such as filariasis. In patients suffering from filariasis, the lymph vessels expand and rupture, causing lymph fluid spilling over and thickening of the skin. Lymphatic obstruction produces elephantiasis, characterized by non-pitting edema of lower limbs.

48.2.1.6 Palmar Erythema

Palmar erythema is a condition with reddening of the palms in the thenar and hypothenar eminences. Palmar erythema can be a feature of chronic liver disease or appears sometimes in pregnancy, due to high estrogen level.

Acropachy

The fingertips appear bulbous with unusually curved and rounded fingernails with Lovibond's angle >180° (Fig. 48.9). Clubbing may affect the fingers and toes. It often occurs as a sign of underlying disorders including respiratory diseases (e.g. lung cancer, bronchiectasis, pleural tumors, lung abscess, empyema, pulmonary hypertrophic osteoarthropathy), cardiovascular diseases (e.g. cyanotic congenital heart disease, infectious myocarditis, subacute infective endocarditis) or malnutrition caused by malabsorption syndrome, Crohn's disease, ulcerative colitis or liver cirrhosis. Unilateral clubbing may reveal ipsilateral subclavian artery aneurysm.

Koilonychia

Koilonychia is a disorder that occurs in the fingernails with a concave formation of the fingernail and striped rough surface (Fig. 48.10). It can be a sign of iron-deficiency anemia and amino acids metabolic disorders, occasionally rheumatic fever.

Table 48.1 Comparison of myogenic and neurogenic muscle atrophy

	Myogenic atrophy	Neurogenic atrophy
Distribution	Usually proximal and symmetrical (except for spinal muscles)	Segmental or distal
Tendon reflexes	Normal, or sometimes diminish or no reflex in later stage	Early diminish or no reflex
Sensory disturbances	No	Usually occurs
Fasciculation	No	Yes
Electromyography	Myogenic changes	Neurogenic changes
Serum muscle enzymes	Usually elevated	Normal or mildly elevated
Muscle biopsy	Myogenic changes	Neurogenic changes

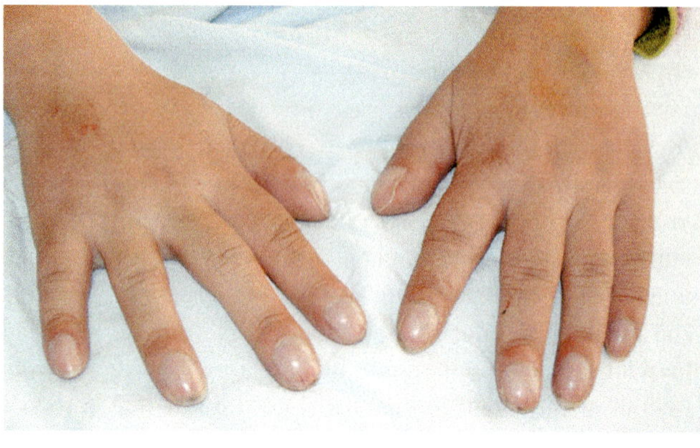

Fig. 48.9 Acropachy

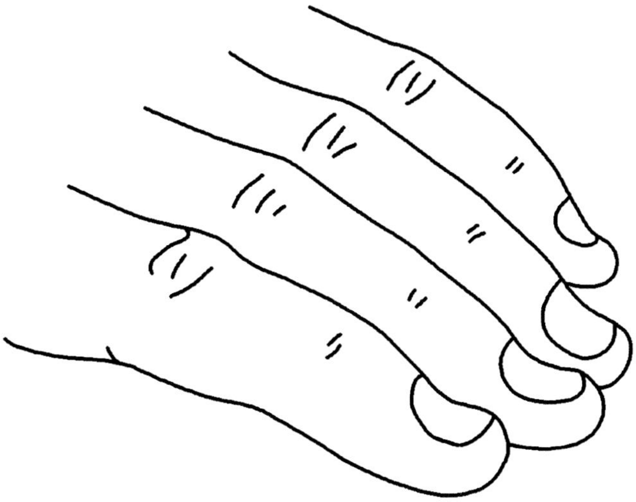

Fig. 48.10 Koilonychia

48.2.2 Joints Examination

Examiners should pay attention to joint appearance, structure and function.

48.2.2.1 Joints of Upper Limbs

Neck, shoulders, elbows, wrists and hands are closely linked in anatomy as well as physiology and pathology. These parts need to be considered as a whole.

Shoulders

When examining the shoulders, it is important to have the patient remove enough clothing so that both shoulders can be viewed and compared completely. Observe any asymmetry and any evidence of movement restriction. Inspect the contour of sternoclavicular and acromioclavicular joints to search for any evidence of swelling or deformity.

The range of motion in the shoulders should be assessed both actively and passively. Adduction is measured by having the patient touch the opposite ear with elbow close to anterior chest wall. Flexion, abduction and external rotation are measured by having the patient's hand reach behind the head and touch the opposite ear. Conversely, internal rotation and adduction of the shoulder should be tested by having the patient's hand touch the inferior aspect of the opposite scapula from the back.

Besides local lesions in the shoulder, pain in the shoulder may result from neck nerve root irritation due to compression or inflammation. Visceral disorders may also refer the pain to the shoulder, known as referred pain. There is no tenderness in the shoulder and no restriction of motion in these disorders.

Special tests of shoulders include: (a) Dugas test: It is a simple clinical test for diagnosis of the dislocated shoulder. When the hand of the affected side is placed on the opposite shoulder, the elbow cannot touch the chest, called positive Dugas test. (b) Painful arc: Painful arc is the pain that occurs in the shoulder as the patient raises the arm out to the side and up to patient's ear. In rotator cuff lesions, the painful arc is located at 60°–120° of abduction, as rotator cuff rubs with acromion. In acromioclavicular joint diseases, the painful arc is located at 150°–180° of abduction (Fig. 48.11).

Elbows

When examining the elbows, it is important to compare both sides. Compare the size of the elbows, looking for asymmetry. Keynotes for the elbow examination:

- When the elbow joint is extended, the tip of the olecranon and the humeral epicondyles should lie on a straight line. When the elbow is flexed, the olecranon descends until its tip forms the apex of an approximately equilateral triangle, of which the epicondyles form the angles at its base. These normal relationships are dismissed in dislocation of the elbow joint and arthritis. However, these relationships will not change in case of humeral fracture.
- The carrying angle is formed by the upper and lower arm in the anatomic position. It is normally 10°–15°. When distal part of the forearm points laterally with an angle more than 15°, it is called cubitus valgus. When distal part of the forearm points medially with an angle less than 0°, it is called cubitus varus.
- Look for the evidence of elbow lateral movement, which indicates collateral ligaments laxity or broken, or condylar fracture.
- Brachioradialis joint is located in the radial side of elbow olecranon, showing as a dip. The "dip "will disappear with tenderness in case of brachioradialis arthritis or fracture of the radial head. Radial head dislocation manifests as a prominent olecranon. Fusiform elbow and fullness around triceps tendon in flexion indicate effusion or hemorrhage. Rheumatoid nodules are usually found on the extensor surface of the elbow.

Wrists and Hands

- Wrists: Compare side to side and look for deficits in the range of motion. Wrist motion can reach dorsal extension for about 35–60° and palmar flexion 50–60° without causing pain. Radial or ulnar deviation of the wrist can reach up to 30°. Ask the patient to hold their wrists in complete flexion by pushing the dorsal surfaces of both hands together, then in complete extension by pushing the palm of both hands together (Fig. 48.12). Limitation of any motion is a feature of wrist arthritis (e.g. rheumatoid arthritis, wrist tuberculosis.), wrist fracture or dislocation.
- Hands: Hands are vulnerable to mild injury. The skin of the palm is thick and connected to the skeleton by a layer

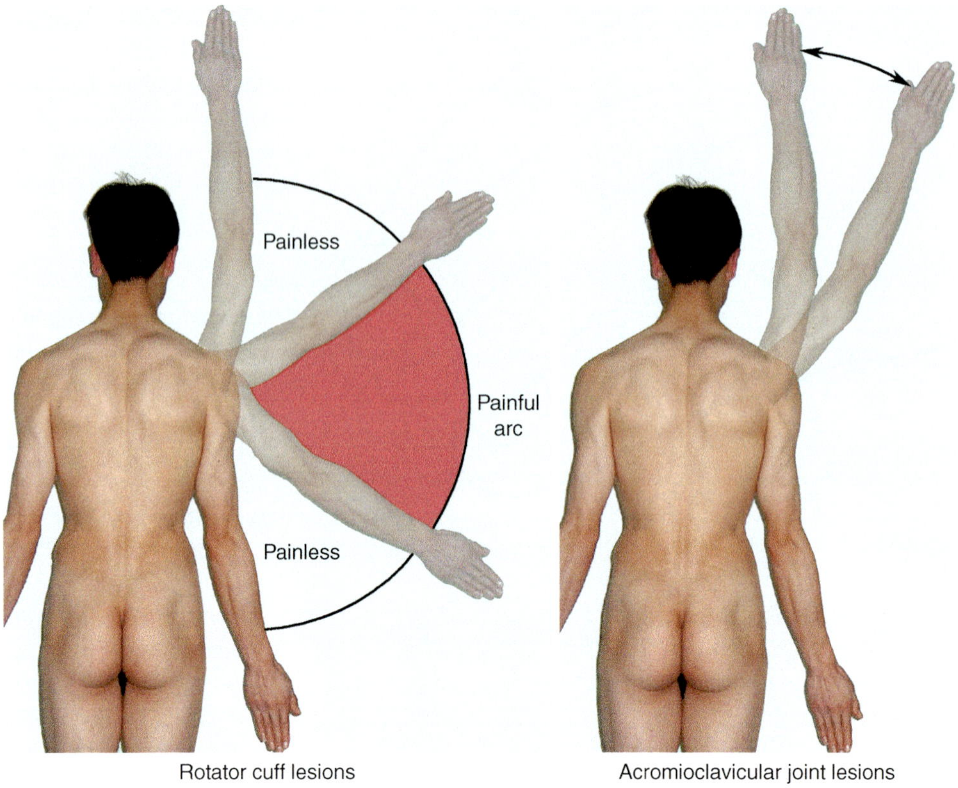

Fig. 48.11 Painful arc

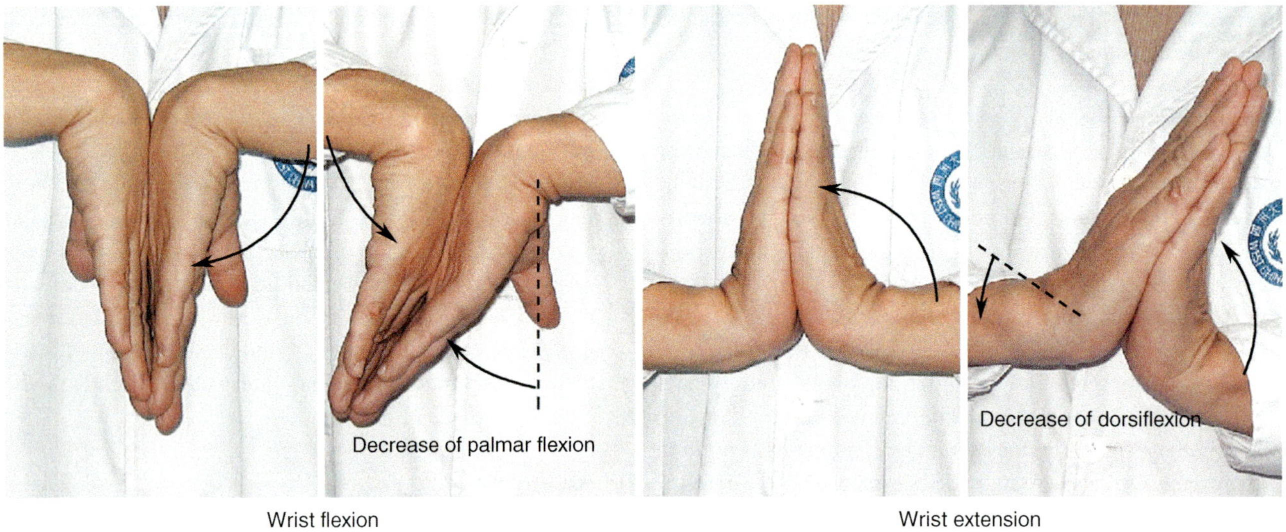

Fig. 48.12 Wrist flexion and extension test for comparison

of fibrous connective tissue (fascia), while the skin of the dorsum is thin and movable so that fingers can flex. The lymphatic tissue is located in the dorsum of the hand. That is why the dorsum swells more significantly than the palm in case of hand inflammation.

When the hand remains in resting position, the wrist is in 15° dorsiflexion and the phalanges are slightly flexed. The thumb is in partial opposition and forward. In hand deformity or tendons rupture, this normal position changes.

The functional position of the hand is that wrist is in 30° dorsiflexion and 15° ulnar deviation, the thumb is abducted and opposite to the pads of the fingers, the proximal interphalangeal joints are flexed, a shape just like holding an egg. If the patient can make a fist and extend fingers quickly, hand function is normal.

48.2.2.2 Joints of Lower Limbs

Hip Joints

When examining the hip joints, the examiner should look for evidence of asymmetry, inspect scars or sinus around the joint, and confirm whether there is abnormal apophysis or collapse. Ask patient to stand with legs together. Inspect from the anterior side to see whether the anterior superior spines are on the same plane, and from the lateral side to see whether there is an abnormal bulge on the buttock, whether plicae are in the same plane, any notable gluteus atrophy or proliferation.

- Internal and external rotation: Hip lesions firstly present as abnormal rotation motion, especially internal rotation combined with activity limitation. Methods to exam rotation:
  - Unilateral hip measurement: Place the patient in supine position with legs straight. Examiner holds the affected thigh then rotates internally and externally. In case of hip contracture with restricted leg extension, the examiner can bend both hip and knee joints up to 90°, using the lower leg as a lever to perform hip internal and external rotation. Pelvis should be fixed to prevent errors (Fig. 48.13). In a prone position with hip extension and knee flexion, compensatory movement of the pelvis is easily found when taking internal and external rotation exams.
  - Bilateral hip measurement: Place the patient in supine position with hips and knees flexed. Check internal rotation by separating feet and holding knees together. External rotation is checked by separating knees and holding feet together (Fig. 48.14). Limitation of internal or external rotation can be found in hip tuberculosis, osteoarthritis, septic arthritis, rheumatoid arthritis and ankylosing spondylitis. However, internal rotation increases and external rotation decreases in congenital hip dislocation.
- Adduction and abduction:
  - Unilateral examination: With the patient in supine position, examiner holds anterior superior iliac spine to immobilize the pelvis by one hand. The examiner then holds the ankle, straightens the leg and abducts lower limb using the other hand to measure abduction movement. The examiner then adducts it to the contralateral leg which can be touched up to the middle-third of the thigh in normal condition.
  - Bilateral examination: Place the patient in supine position with straightening legs. Examiner stands at the end of the bed to hold patient's heels and takes lower limbs apart to test abduction, intersects them to test adduction (Fig. 48.14). Abduction limitation can be found in coxa vara, posterior dislocation and inflammatory diseases of the hip. Adduction limitation can be found in iliotibial band contracture.
- Flexion and extension: Place the patient in supine position and use following three sequential steps to compare bilateral hips: (a) Bend left knee and take left hip fully flexed, then observe the extent of right hip extension. Normally when left knee touches to the chest, right hip can maintain the straight position. (b) Keep left hip fully flexed, and make right hip fully flexed (pay attention not to make pelvic anterior tilt) to compare any differences in the extent of hips flexion. (c) Keep right hip fully flexed, extend the left hip as far as possible and observe how far it can be extended.
- Hyperextension test of hip joint: Place the patient in prone position, examiner immobilizes the pelvis by one hand, holds the ankle to lift the lower limb by the other hand. In normal condition, the hip can extend up to about 15°. Limited extension suggests hip contracture or inflammation.
- Special tests of hip joints: (a) Thomas sign: Hip flexion contracture may be compensated by lumbar lordosis. When supine with hip and knee fully flexed, the examiner's hand is placed under the patient's back to check whether lumbar lordosis is removed during full flexion of the hip. The contralateral hip should then be observed.

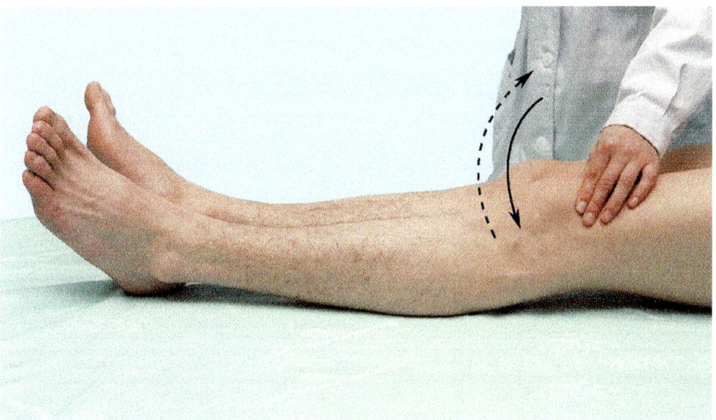

Examination on extension position

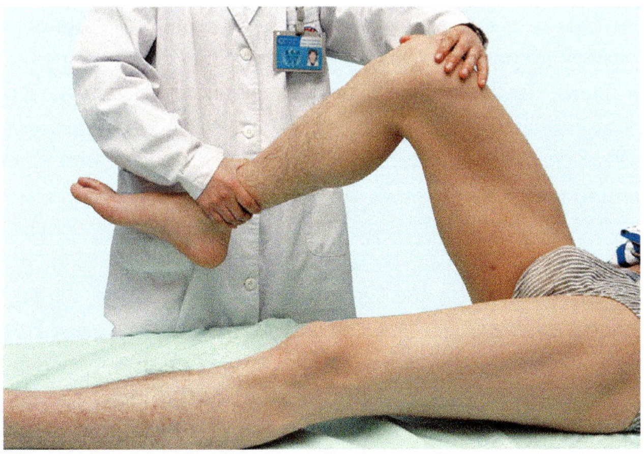

Examination on flexion position

Fig. 48.13 Unilateral hip measurement of internal and external rotation

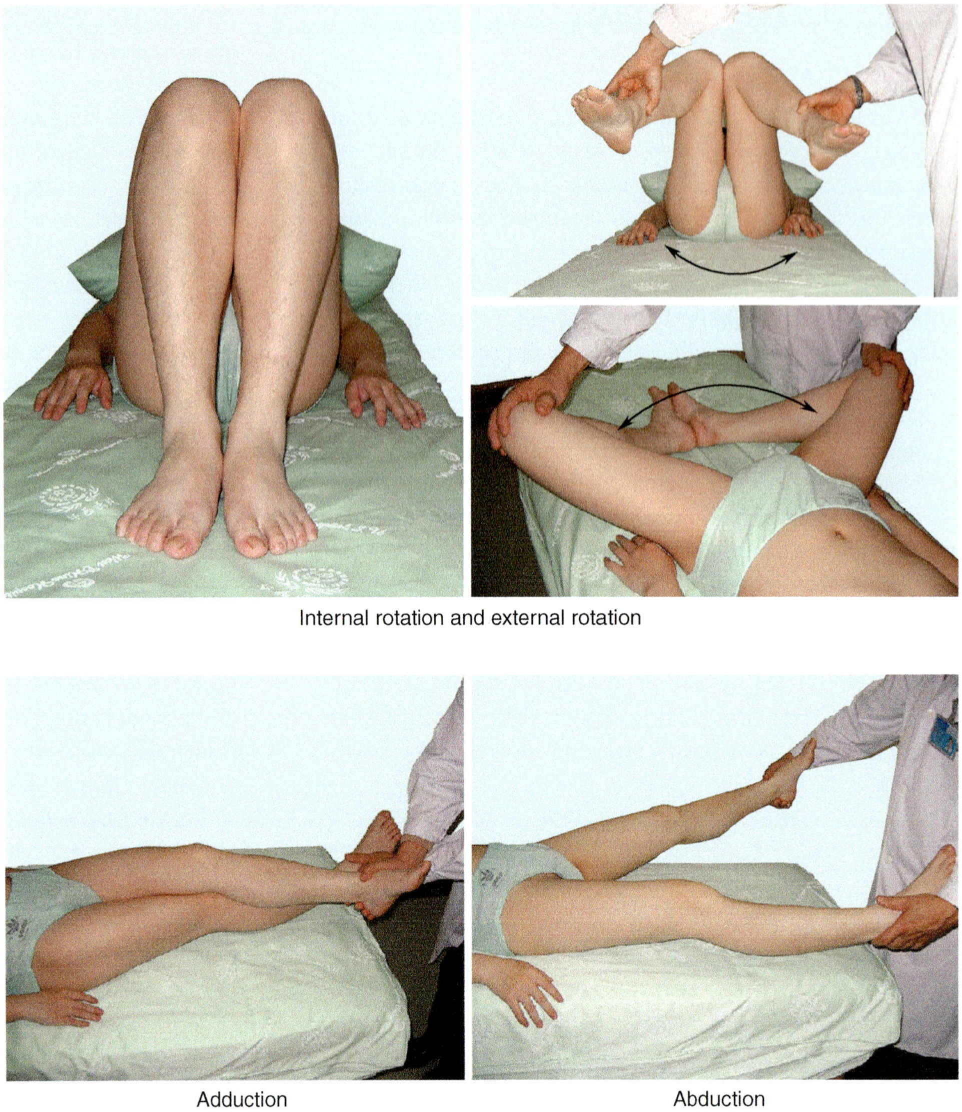

Fig. 48.14 Bilateral hip measurement

If there is a fixed flexion deformity, this leg will be forced off the couch. Then record angle between bed and limb (Fig. 48.15). (b) Hip weight-bearing function test (Trendelenburg test): Ask the patient to stand alternately on each leg alone. The examiner assesses the hip and gluteal muscle strength of the standing side. In a negative test, the pelvis remains stable or even rises. In a positive test, the pelvis will dip on the contralateral side. (Fig. 48.16). A positive result indicates congenital or traumatic hip dislocation, gluteus medius or minimus paralysis.

Knees

Take the examination in standing position, with legs close together. Normally, bilateral knees and ankles can close together simultaneously. If ankles close together but knees are separated, it is called genu varum (bowleg) (Fig. 48.17). If knees close together but ankles are separated, it is called genu valgum (knock-knee) (Fig. 48.17). The range of motion in knees is about 0–150° and under passive movement, the range of motion can be increased about 5–10°. In knee flexion, the heel can reach the buttocks. Normally no frication sounds are heard when knees flex or extend. In flexion contracture, the knee is restricted in extension. If the knee is over-extended, it is called genu recurvatum (Fig. 48.17). Observe whether there are abnormity gaits, squat, jump and single-leg jump.

In knee disorders, quadriceps muscle may atrophy because of disuse, especially the medial head. In knee flexion, the fovea is found on the lateral side of the patellar tendon, known as "elephant eyes". Disappearance of fovea or any projection indicates swollen joints, except in obese women.

Special tests of knee joints include: (a) Ballotable patella test: The patient is positioned in supine position with the involved knee extended. The examiner slides hand down the patient's thigh, compressing the suprapatellar pouch. This forces any elusion behind the patella. Two or three fingers of

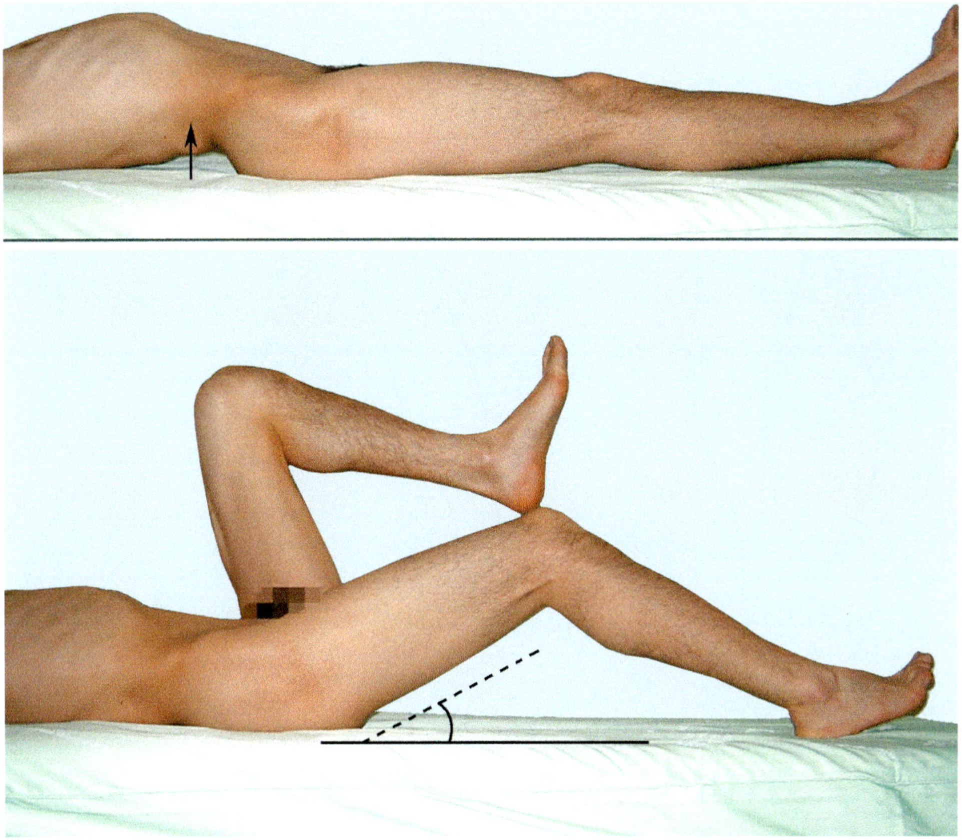

Fig. 48.15 Thomas sign

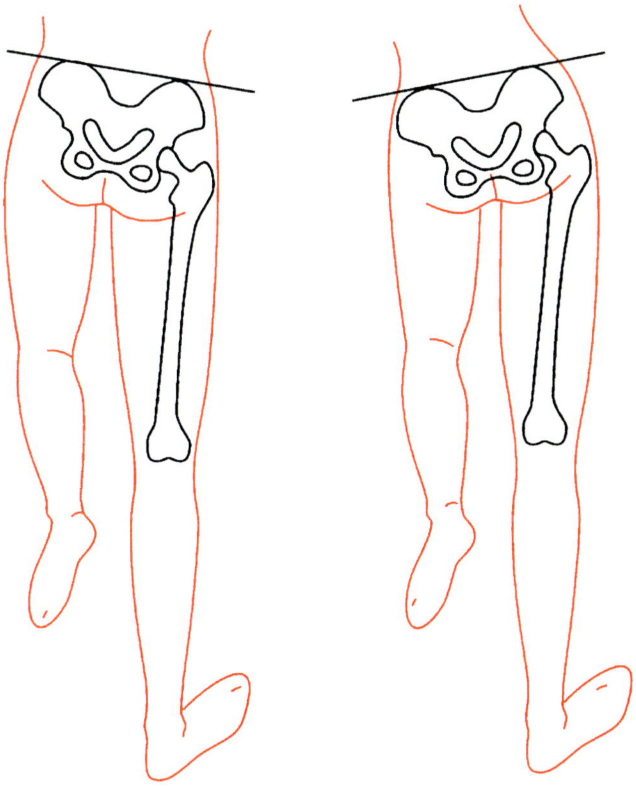

Fig. 48.16 Hip weight-bearing function test

the other hand push the patella down gently. In a positive test the patella will bounce and tap (Fig. 48.18). (b) Patella pressure grinding test: To exam whether patellar articular cartilage surface is smooth. The patient is positioned in supine position or seated with the involved knee extended. The examiner places the web space of his hand just superior to the patella with pressure. The test is positive if the patient feels pain when the patella is pushed up, down, left, right, with or without fricatives. In patella joint degenerative disease, rough-sand sense and friction sound are detected with pain.

Ankles and Feet

Ankles and feet should be fully exposed by taking off shoes and socks and rolling trousers up to the knees. Observe the shape and position of the feet and ankles, the arch height and signs of ankle swelling. Fullness on either side of the Achilles' tendon suggests the possibility of ankle effusion. The footprint is critical to measure the arch shape, burden point of the foot and foot width. Ankle motion is mainly dorsiflexion and toe flexion.

Common foot deformities are shown in Fig. 48.19:

- Flatfoot (pes planus): The normal height at the apex of medial longitudinal arch is approximately 1cm when standing. A finger can be inserted under the arch. In mild

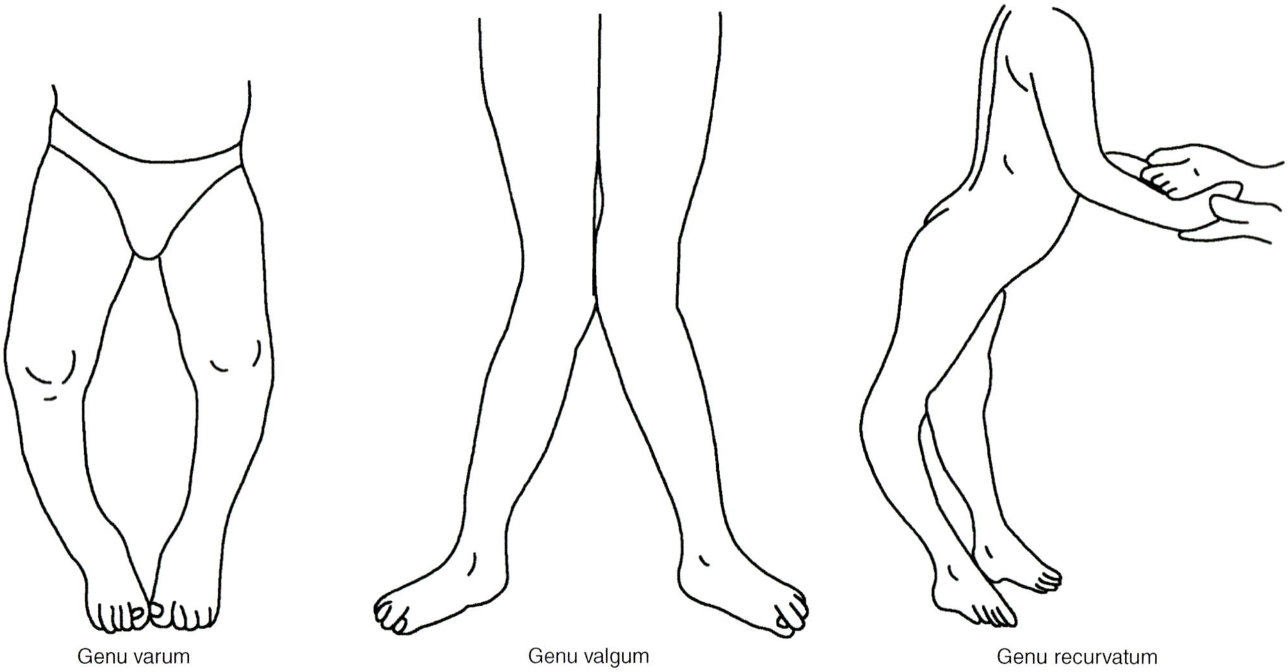

Fig. 48.17 Knee deformities

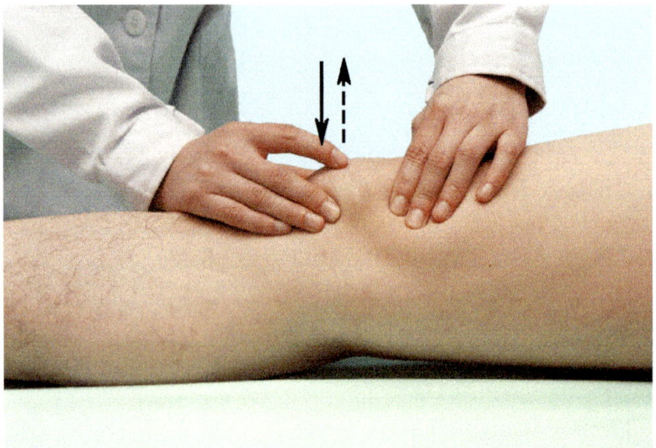

Fig. 48.18 Ballotable patella test

flatfoot, the arch of foot decreases and finger can't be inserted into the arch although the arch hasn't touched the ground yet. In severe cases, arches of the foot collapse, the entire sole of the foot completely contacts with the ground with talar-head bulging and foot valgus deformity.

- Clubfoot (Talipes equinovarus): The affected foot appears to be rotated internally at the ankle. Patients with an untreated clubfoot usually walk on the forefoot with the Achilles tendon contracture. It is mainly caused by paralysis of tibialis anterior muscle.
- Talipes varus: When standing or walking, lateral foot bears the weight, with heel and Achilles tendon deflect inside. Footdrop and varus are often co-existence.
- Talipesvalgus: On the contrary to varus, the medial longitudinal arch disappears, medial foot bears the weight, with heel and Achilles tendon deflect outside due to paralysis of tibialis posterior muscle.
- Talipes calcaneus: Heel bears the weight and sometimes forefeet can't touch the ground. The ratio of heel and forefoot will change because of compensatory widened heel. It is often caused by paralysis of gastrocnemius and soleus muscle.
- Talipes cavus: Characterized by increased foot longitudinal arch, dropped metatarsal head, abnormally shortened plantar soft tissue. Arched foot is often secondary to muscle paralysis due to polio and spina bifida.

Key Terms		
1	Scoliosis	脊柱侧凸
2	Kyphosis	脊柱后凸
3	Straight leg raising test	拉塞格征
4	Wright-Schober test	瑞-舒测试法
5	Acropachy	杵状指
6	Dugas test	杜加斯征
7	Thomas sign	托马斯征
8	Ballotable patella test	浮髌试验

Study Questions

1. Describe special examinations of the vertebrae.
2. Classify muscle strength.
3. What is Thomas sign?
4. What is ballotable patella test?

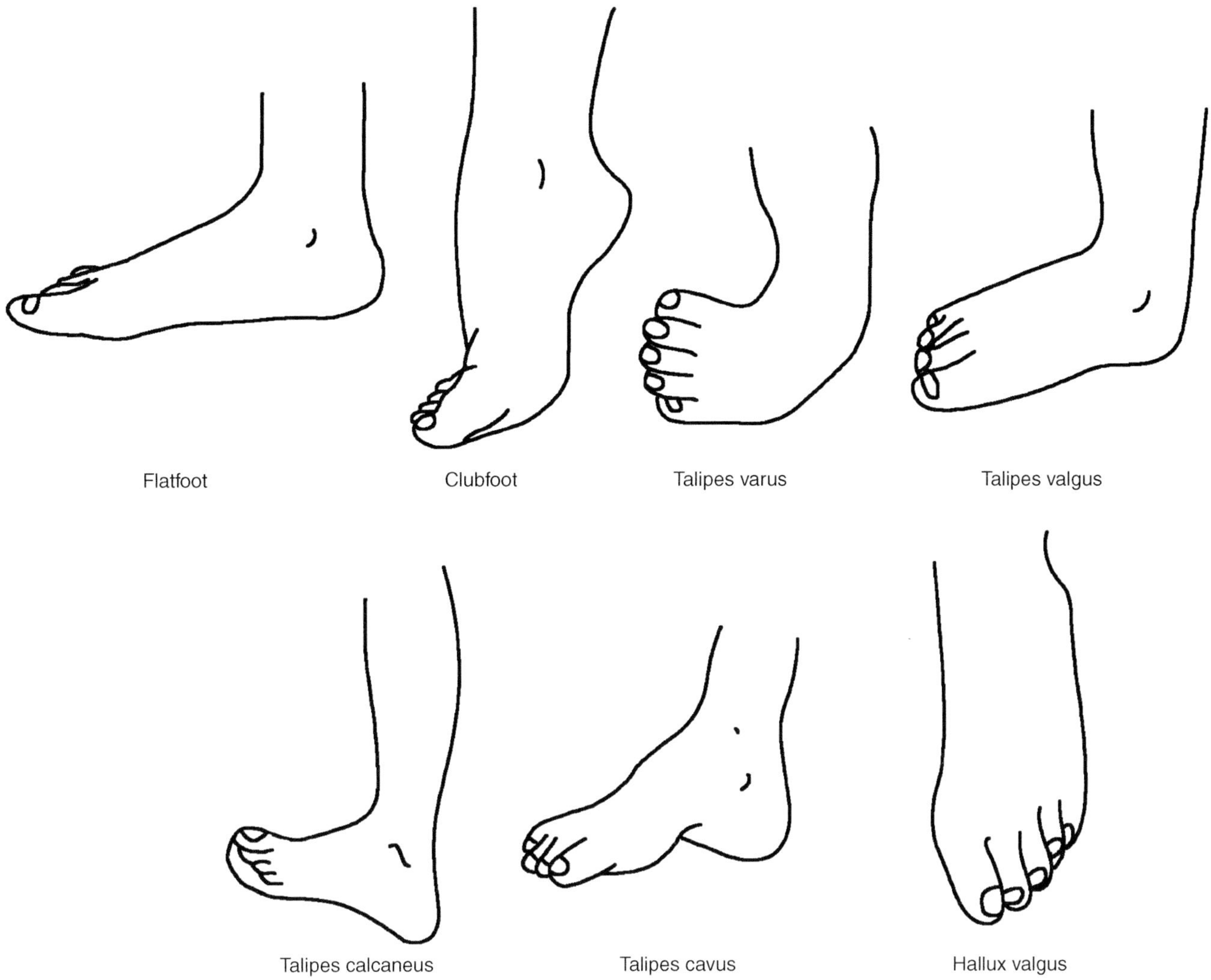

Fig. 48.19 Common foot deformities

Suggested Websites

https://meded.ucsd.edu/clinicalmed/joints.htm
http://www.osceskills.com/e-learning/modules/musculoskeletal-medicine/

49 Physical Examination of the Neurological Examination

Jianfang Ma and Rui Zeng

The neurological examination includes the following items: high brain function, cranial nerves, sensory function, motor function, reflexes, coordination, gait and autonomic function. As neurological examination is complicated and extremely important for neurological anatomy localization, it should be performed in sequential and carefully interpreted to obtain a high accuracy of the findings.

49.1 High Brain Function

The requirement of high brain function examination depends on the relevance of the patients' complaints. Simple observation of the patient during the interview can give the examiner an idea whether the patient needs to be exclusively examined of high brain function (sometimes referred as mental status). A full mental status test includes several domains: Level of consciousness, attention, language, memory, constructional ability, higher cognitive functions and related cognitive functions. Several scales have been developed for clinical evaluation of mental status. Among them, mini-mental status examination has been shown an easy and practical bed-side screening scales for mental status examination. Please see "suggested reading" for more detail information on this section.

49.2 Cranial Nerves

Totally, there are 12 pairs of cranial nerves. These 12 pairs of cranial nerves should be examined sequentially, independently and compared carefully.

J. Ma
Department of Neurology, Shanghai Jiaotong University, Shanghai, China

R. Zeng (✉)
Department of Cardiology, Sichuan University, Chengdu, China

49.2.1 Olfactory Nerve

Before assessment of the ability to smell, it is important to make sure that the patient is able to inhale and exhale through the open nostril. Let the patient close his eyes. Then the examiner presses one nostril to close it and presents a small test bottle filled with something that has a distinct, common odor (e.g. coffee, cigarette) to the open nostril. A person with normal olfactory function should be able to identify the odor at approximately 10 cm away accurately. Bilateral olfactory problems often indicate the nasal mucosa lesions while unilateral olfactory problem localizes the lesion to olfactory nerve. The olfactory nerve dysfunction can also be found in severe brain trauma, frontal tumor and meningitis.

49.2.2 Optic Nerve

This nerve carries visual impulses from the eye to the optical cortex of the brain. Testing optic nerve involves following three phases (see section of Eye Examination in Chap. 3 of Part III):

49.2.3 Ocular Nerve, Trachlear Nerve and Abducens Nerve

In order to form a single image in retina, six eye muscles innervated by these three cranial nerves move in concert. In addition, ocular nerve also raises the eyelid and mediates constriction of the pupil. Examiner stands in front of the patient (30 cm ahead) and asks the patient to follow his/her finger with their eyes while keeping his head in one position, in the direction of up, down, left, right, left-up, left-down, right-up and right-down. Then the examiner brings his own finger directly towards the patient's nose to look accommodation which is referred to cross-eyed and constrict of the pupil.

X.-H. Wan, R. Zeng (eds.), *Handbook of Clinical Diagnostics*, https://doi.org/10.1007/978-981-13-7677-1_49

Lesion in these three cranial nerves can cause double vision (diplopia) because in-coordination of eye movement results in discordant images in retina. Lesion in abducens nerve cause lateral rectus dysfunction and the eye cannot move laterally. Lesion in trochlear nerve cause superior oblique muscle dysfunction and eye movement to down-lateral side is impaired. If there is ocular nerve lesion, ipsilateral eyelid drops (referred to as ptosis), and eye movements to median, up or down side are impaired, with dysfunction in accommodation and pupil reflex.

49.2.4 Trigeminal Nerve

This nerve has both motor and sensory components.

1. **The sensory limb of trigeminal nerve** has three major branches: ophthalmic, maxillary, and mandibular, dominate the sensation of face skin, mucosa inside nose and mouth. Ask the patient to close their eyes, test the sensation of touch (cotton), pain (needle) and thermal (warm and cold tube) in three branches of trigeminal nerve.
2. **The motor limb of trigeminal nerve innervates Temporalis and Masseter muscles**, both important for closing the jaw. Place your hands on both Temporalis muscles which are located on the lateral aspects of the forehead. Then ask the patient to tightly close their jaw to test the strength of Temporalis muscles. Place your hands on both Masseter muscles which are located just in front of the Tempero-Mandibular joints (point where lower jaw articulates with skull). Then ask the patient to tightly close their jaw, or move their jaw from side to side, to test the strength of Masseter muscles.
3. **Corneal reflex:** The ophthalmic branch of trigeminal nerve also receives sensory input from the surface of the eye which is part of corneal reflex. Pull out a wisp of cotton. While the patient is looking straight ahead, gently brush the wisp against the lateral aspect of the sclera (outer white area of the eye ball). This should cause the patient to blink. Blinking also requires that facial nerve function normally, as it controls eye lid closure. Direct corneal reflex refers to eye lid closure after stimulating the ipsilateral corneal while indirect corneal reflex refers to eye lid closure after stimulating the contralateral corneal. Trigeminal nerve lesion is highly suspected when bilateral corneal reflex is lost. When direct corneal reflex is lost while indirect corneal reflex conserved, facial nerve palsy is the probable lesion.
4. **Jaw reflex:** Ask the patient to open his mouth slightly, the examiner puts his thumb on the jaw and hits the thumb with the hammer to find the jaw closed tightly.

49.2.5 Facial Nerve

This nerve innervates facial expression muscle, taste sensations in the anterior 2/3 parts of the tongue, lachrymal and salivary secretion.

1. **Motor function:** First look at the patient's face. It should be symmetrical: the same amount of wrinkles on either side of the forehead, equal nasolabial folds, similar height of the corners of the mouth. Ask the patient to wrinkle their eyebrows and then close their eyes tightly. You should not be able to open the patient's eyelids. Ask the patient to smile. The corners of the mouth should rise to the same height and equal amounts of teeth should be visible on either side. Ask the patient to puff out their cheeks. Both sides should puff equally and air should not leak from the mouth.

   The pattern of weakness or paralysis of facial nerve palsy will differ depending on central or peripheral lesions of facial nerve. Central facial nerve palsy: The patient had symmetrical wrinkle of forehead on both sides. However, the patient would be unable to effectively close their eye or raise the corner of their mouth contralateral to the lesion. Peripheral facial nerve palsy: The patient would not be able to wrinkle their forehead, close their eyes or raise the corner of their mouth on the lesion side.
2. **Taste sensation:** Ask the patient to stick out the tongue, the examiner dips a little bit of solution (e.g. vinegar, salt, sugar) on anterior 2/3 part of one side of the tongue and asks the patient to point to the right word on a paper written the different name of tastes. The patient should taste one solution at one time and clean his mouth between each of them.

49.2.6 Acoustic Nerve

Acoustic nerve carries sensory innervations of cochlea and vestibular functions.

1. **Cochlea function:** Ask the patient to close his eyes. Examiner whispers a few words from just behind one ear or rubs his fingers together. The patient should be able to hear the word or sound. These tests are rather crude. For more precise quantification, special equipment and training are required (see ear examination in Sect. 4 in Chap. 3 of Part III).
2. **Vestibular nerve:** The main symptoms and signs of vestibular nerve lesion are vertigo (sensation of environment spinning, often accompanied by nausea and vomiting), nystagmus (back and forth movements of the eyeballs) and imbalance (unsteady gait that leans to the lesion side).

49.2.7 Glossopharyngeal Nerve and Vagus Nerve

Both nerves had motor and sensory components, innervating the movement of palate, pharyngeal and upper esophagus, pharyngeal sensation and taste sensation of posterior 1/3 part of the tongue.

1. **Motor function:** Check any swallow difficulty or choking. Then ask patient to open his mouth and say, "ahhhh," to raise the palate upward. The examiner should look at the uvula to see whether it stays in the middle part or deviates to one side. If both palates could not raise upward, bilateral nerve palsy are suspected.
2. **Gag reflex:** Ask the patient to open his mouth. The examiner gently brushes it against the posterior pharynx, which will generate a gag in normal people. Loss of gag reflex can be seen in bilateral nerve palsy or some normal elderly.
3. **Sensory function:** The examiner gently touches the palate or the pharyngeal mucosa by cotton to check any sensation change. Taste sensation on the posterior 1/3 of the tongue is tested in the same way described in facial nerve.

49.2.8 Accessory Nerve

Accessory nerve innervates the Trapezius muscle which permits shrugging of the shoulders and Sternocleidomastoid muscle which permits turning the head laterally. Ask the patient to shrug while the examiner provides resistance on the either shoulder. Accessory nerve palsy will cause weakness/absence of movement on ipsilateral side. Ask the patient to turn into your hand while you provide resistance against the patient's cheek. The accessory nerve palsy will cause the head to turn to one side.

49.2.9 Hypoglossal Nerve

Hypoglossal nerve innervates the tongue movement. Ask the patient to stick their tongue straight out of their mouth and search for any fasciculation, atrophy or deviation. Central lesions cause the tongue deviation to the contralateral side of the lesion without early tongue fasciculation or atrophy. Peripheral lesions cause the tongue deviation to the lesion side with early tongue fasciculation or atrophy.

49.3 Sensory Examinations

Some basic principles should be kept in mind before starting sensory examination. (a) The patients should remain alert and examiner needs to explain the patients about why and how to do the sensory tests; (b) A quiet environment is required for better feeling of different sensation; (c) Ask the patient to close their eyes to avoid visual clues; (d) Start from the lesion site to the normal, compare the sensation between left and right, upper and down, distal and proximal part; (e) When examining the patients with consciousness impairment, examiner can only evaluate the sensation changes by judging the reaction of the patients after sensory stimulates (e.g. painful facial expression, withdrawal limbs, etc.)

49.3.1 Sensory Examination

49.3.1.1 Spinothalamics (Light Sensation)

1. Pain: Ask the patient to close his eyes. Use a disposable needle or the sharp and blunt ends of a safety pin to slightly touch the skin of the patient and ask whether the patient feels the sharpness.
2. Temperature: Ask the patient to close his eyes. Use hot (40–50 °C) or cold (5–10 °C) tubes to slightly touch the skin of the patient and ask whether he can feel hot or cold.
3. Crude touch: Ask the patient to close his eyes. Use the ends of cotton to touch the skin of the patient and ask whether he can feel the touch or not.

49.3.1.2 Dorsal Columns (Deep Sensation)

1. **Proprioception (position):** Ask the patient to close his eyes. Grasp both sides of the toe at the interphalangeal joint with one hand and move the toe up or down (flexion or extension) slightly (a millimeter or two). Then ask the patient whether he can feel the movement and the direction of the movement. Similar testing can be done on the fingers, ankle or wrist if necessary.
2. **Vibration:** You will need a 128 Hz tuning fork to perform vibration test. Grasp the tuning fork by the stem and vibrate it by striking the forked ends against the floor. Place the vibrating forks on the joint of the patient and ask if they can feel the vibration and tell as soon as it stops.

49.3.1.3 Complex Sensation

It is also known as cortical sensation which includes point localization, two-point discrimination, stereognosis and graphesthesia. More information is available in "Suggested reading".

49.3.2 Sensory Terminology

Disturbing sensory afferent pathways can cause variable sensory complaints including allodynia, dysesthesia, hyperesthesia, allesthesia and pain. Destruction of sensory system can lead to hypesthesia or sensory loss. Pain-innervation system dysfunction will cause pain which is usually classified into following patterns: local pain, radiating pain, diffused pain and referred pain.

49.3.3 Interpreting Results of Sensory Testing

Different pattern of sensory changes, corresponding to certain neuroanatomy-based lesion, is listed in the following:

1. **Neuropathy:** symmetrically, stocking and glove-like sensory impairment in polyneuropathy, sensory impairment confining to a simple peripheral nerve in mononeuropathy (e.g. radial nerve palsy).
2. **Plexopathy:** patchy loss of pain, e.g. lumbosacral plexopathy.
3. **Radiculopathy:** pain or paresthesias, distributed as dermatomal pattern (e.g. band-like in thorax region).
4. **Posterior Horn Sensory Impairment:** pain and temperature sensory loss with intact touch and deep sensation, often refers to as dissociated sensory impairment.
5. **Myelopathy:** completely or incompletely sensory loss under the level of spinal lesion.
6. **Brainstem:** light or deep sensory loss in ipsilateral face and contralateral body, also named as crossed sensory impairment.
7. **Thalamus:** sensory loss contralateral to the lesion, including facial and body sensation.
8. **Cerebral:** cortex lesion, especially parietal or posterior frontal, can cause a sensory loss of position sensation. In addition, two-point discrimination, stereognosis, graphesthesia are commonly impaired.

49.4 Motor Examinations

Normal motor function requires interconnected system including cortex, brainstem, spinal cord, cerebellum and basal ganglion, sensory pathways and other neurological systems. Lesion in cortico-spinal tract will result in weakness of upper motor neuron (UMN) pattern or spastic paralysis. Lesion in basal ganglion will result in muscle tone changes and display involuntary movements. Lesion in cerebellum will cause ataxia or imbalance. Lesion in peripheral nerve system will lead to weakness of low motor neuron (LMN) pattern. The characteristics of UMN and LMN weakness are listed in Table 49.1.

49.4.1 Muscle Strength

1. The grade of muscle strength: Muscle strength refers to the power of muscles when it contracts to its great extent and is tested when the patient holds a position and tries to resist the examiner's attempt. It is commonly evaluated by the British Medical Research Council methods which grades muscle strength into a scale of 0–5 (Table 49.2).
2. Neuroanatomy localization of paralysis (weakness of muscle)
   - Cortical: usually presents with contralateral monoplegia;
   - Internal capsule: presents with hemiplegia, hemiparathesis and hemianopsia;
   - Brainstem: presents with crossed paralysis;
   - Spinal cord: Lesions above the cervical enlargement will cause UMN tetraplegia. Lesions in cervical enlargement result in LMN weakness in upper limbs and UMN weakness in lower limbs (paraplegia). Lesions in thoracic spinal cord cause paraplegia in lower limbs. Lesions in lumber spinal cord result in LMN weakness in lower limbs;
   - Anterior horn: presents with LMN weakness of muscles innervated by the lesion, usually with fasciculation;
   - Anterior root: presents with LMN weakness of muscle innervated by the lesion;
   - Neuropathy: presents with LMN weakness innervated by the lesion.

Table 49.1 Differentiation between UMN and LMN weakness

	UMN weakness	LMN weakness
Involving muscles	Muscles of one limb or more limbs	Single or multiple muscle groups
Muscle wasting	No early wasting in paralyzed muscle except for disuse atrophy	Early wasting in paralyzed muscles
Muscle tone	Spasticity	Decreased muscle tone (flaccid paralysis)
Deep tendon reflex	Increased or hyperactive	Diminished or no reflex
Pathologic signs	Positive	Negative
Electrophysiological tests	No signs of muscle denervation and normal nerve transduction	Signs of muscle denervation and abnormal nerve transduction

Table 49.2 Grading of muscle strength

Grade	Muscle strength
0/5	No movement
1/5	Slight flicker of muscle, though not enough to move the structure to which it's attached
2/5	Voluntary movement which is not sufficient to overcome the force of gravity
3/5	Voluntary movement capable of overcoming gravity, but not any applied resistance
4/5	Voluntary movement capable of overcoming "some" resistance
5/5	Normal strength

49.4.2 Muscle Tone

When a muscle group is relaxed, the examiner tries to move the joint through its normal range and feels the resistance during this movement. The resistance is referred as muscle tone.

1. **Increased muscle tone:**
   - Spasticity: Tone increases mostly in the beginning of the joint movement or if the examiner moves the joint more quickly. This is also named as clasp-like increased muscle tone (feeling of sudden giving-way) and the typical finding of an UMN lesion.
   - Rigidity: Tone remains increased to the same degree during the entire joint movement or regardless of how quickly the joint is moved. This is also named as pipe-like increased muscle tone and the typical finding of basal ganglion lesion (e.g. Parkinson's disease). When a tremor coexists with rigidity, it can produce cog-wheel rigidity as the examiner may feel a ratchet-like resistance similar to cog- wheeling during the joint movement.
2. **Decreased muscle tone:** This occurs in the lesion of lower motor neuron lesion, cerebellum and muscle.

49.4.3 Coordination

To maintain a functional movement, not only normal muscle strength is required, but also coordination among related muscles. The coordination requires interplay and balance involving different movement systems from cerebellum, vestibular, sensory pathways and cerebral extrapyramidal parts. Any lesion in these parts, especially cerebellum will result in the inaccuracy of any intentional voluntary movement which is also named as ataxia. Lesion in cerebellum commonly presents with ataxia and gait changes (see Chap. 3 of PART III). The common tests for examining ataxia are listed in Table 49.3.

Table 49.3 Tests for coordination

Name of test	How to test	Interpretation
Finger-to-nose	Ask the patient extend his arm and try to touch his nose by the tip of his index as accurately, quickly and smoothly as possible. Test again when the patients close their eyes	Cerebellar dysfunction: abnormal finger-to-nose test either eyes open or closed Deep sensory dysfunction: normal finger-to-nose test when eyes open but abnormal when eyes closed
Finger-nose-finger	Ask the patient extend his arm and try to touch his nose by the tip of his finger, then to the examiner's finger, and back to the nose again	Cerebellar dysfunction
Heel-to-knee	Ask the patient to place a heel on the opposite knee, then slide it down the front of the shin to the great toe. Test it again when eyes are closed	Cerebellar dysfunction: unable to maintain the balance either eyes open or closed Deep sensory dysfunction: unable to maintain the balance only when eyes closed
Rapid alternating movement	1. Ask the patient to pat the knee with the palm and then the back of hand as quick as possible 2. Ask the patient to pronate and supinate one hand on the other hand as quick as possible 3. Ask the patient to touch the thumb to each finger as quick as possible	Any slowing down of speed or problems in posture indicates coordination or extrapyraminal dysfunction
Romberg test	Ask the patient to put his feet together, stretch his arms in the front, and try to maintain the balance Test again when the patient close his eyes	Cerebellar dysfunction: unable to maintain the balance either eyes open or closed Deep sensory dysfunction: unable to maintain the balance only when eyes closed

49.4.4 Involuntary Movements

It refers to abnormal involuntary movements when patient remains alert, commonly caused by dysfunction of extrapyramidal system (basal ganglia), which include tic, myoclonus, dystonia, tremor, chorea and athetosis. More information is available in "Suggested Reading".

49.4.5 Other Muscle Abnormal Movements

It refers to abnormal involuntary muscle movements including spasm or cramp (commonly seen in hypocalcemia, hypomagnesemia or tetanus), nocturnal cramps, fasciculation (quick muscle twitch due to muscle fibers contraction, seen in anterior cell spinal diseases or radiculopathy), myokymia (sustained vermiform movement usually involving face or limbs, especially oculi muscles).

49.5 Reflexes

Neurological reflex evaluates the integrity of a local nerve circuit that consists of five components: sensory receptor, afferent nerve, nerve centre, efferent nerve and effector. It is usually less affected by the consciousness of the patients but requires a considerate cooperation from the patient.

The examiner asks the patients to be relaxed and compares the results between both sides as minor asymmetries can have a diagnostic significance. The major purpose of reflex examination is to differentiate central from peripheral nerve system.

49.5.1 Superficial Reflex

Superficial reflex is elicited by the skin or mucosal stimulus. Only unilateral absence is regarded as abnormal. Bilateral superficial reflex absence does not have a diagnostic value in most situations.

1. **Abdominal reflex:** Ask the patient to lie on his back and have the abdomen relaxed with the knee flexed slightly. Then quickly stroke the abdominal skin towards umbilicus horizontally laterally to medially from three directions (see Fig. 49.1). The response of abdominal reflex is the contraction of the abdominal muscle with umbilicus deviating to the stimulus side. Loss of abdominal reflex suggests Thorax spinal lesions: upper part refers to T7-8, middle part to T9-10 and low part to T11-12.

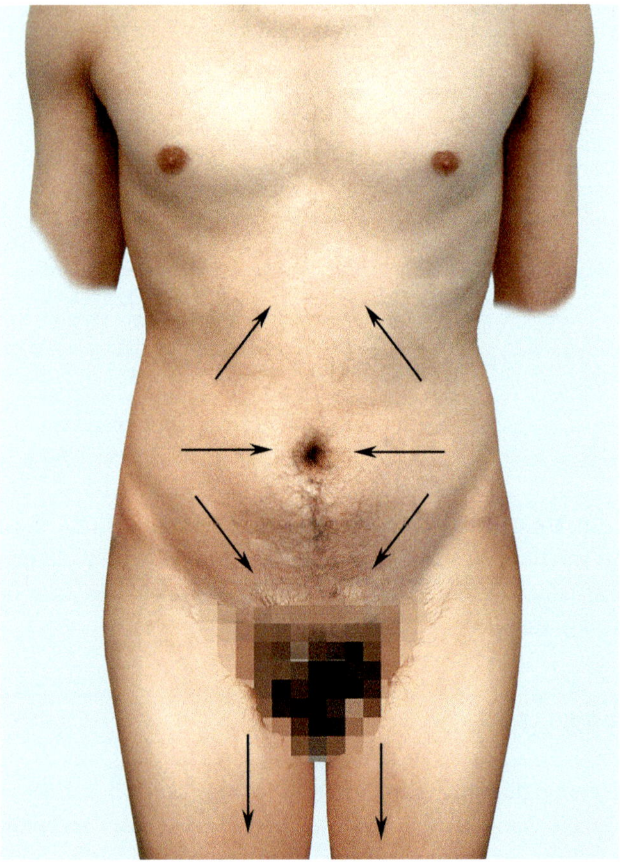

Fig. 49.1 The examination of abdominal reflex and cremasteric reflexes

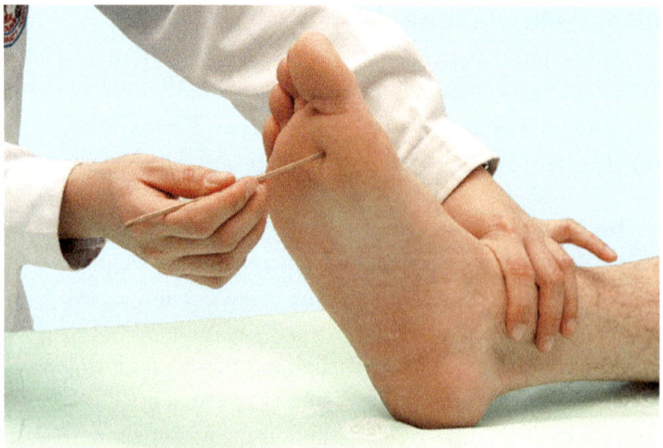

Fig. 49.2 The examination of planter reflex

2. **Cremasteric reflex:** Stroke the inner side of the thigh of the patient (only men). The response is the elevation of the testicle on the stimulus side (see Fig. 49.1). Unilateral absence of cremasteric reflex suggests ipsilateral cortical spinal tract lesions of lumber spinal L1-2.
3. **Plantar reflex:** Stroke the sole from the heel to the ball of the foot and then curve towards the big toe. The response is plantar flexion. The loss of plantar reflex indicates sacral spinal S1-2 dysfunction (see Fig. 49.2).
4. **Anal reflex:** Ask the patients to lie on the left or right side. Stroke the skin in the perianal area. The response is the contraction of anal sphincter. The loss of anal reflex suggests the lesion in sacral spinal S4-5 or anococcygeal nerve.

49.5.2 Deep Tendon Reflex

Deep tendon reflex is elicited by stretching tendon and is commonly graded into the following scale: no/absent, 1+(diminished), 2+(normal), 3+(increased/brisk without clonus) or 4+(hyperactive/abnormal brisk with clonus).

1. **Biceps reflex:** Ask the patient to sit or lie on his back with elbow semiflexed. The examiner puts his thumb or index on the biceps tendon, taps it by reflex hammer and causes quick flexion of the elbow (see Fig. 49.3). This reflex centre is cervical spinal C5-6.
2. **Triceps reflex:** Ask the patient to sit or lie on his back with elbow semiflexed. The examiner holds the patient's forearm and taps the triceps tendon which is located 2.5–5 cm above the ulna's olecranon process. The positive sign is quick extension of the elbow (see Fig. 49.4). This reflex centre is cervical spinal C6-7.
3. **Brachioradialis reflex:** Ask the patient to sit or lie on his back, elbow semiflexed and forearm semipronated.

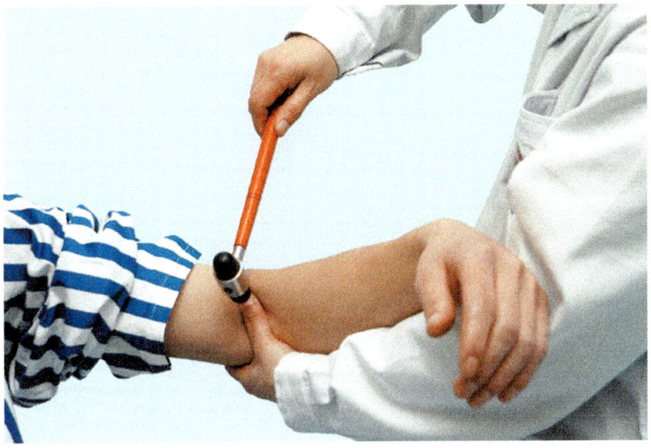

Fig. 49.3 The examination of biceps reflex

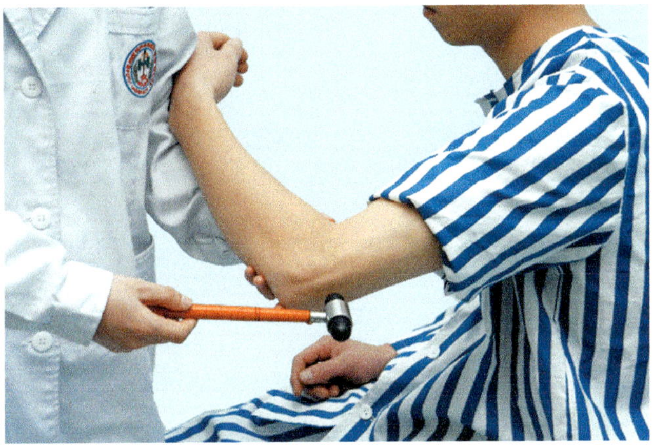

Fig. 49.4 The examination of triceps reflex

The examiner strikes the styloid process of radius which is located 2.5–5 cm above the wrist. The response is elbow flexion, forearm supination and finger flexion. This reflex centre is cervical spinal C5-8.

4. **Patellar reflex:** Ask the patient to sit with his legs dangling off the side of the bed or lie on his back with his knee in minor flexion. The examiner strikes the quadriceps tendon which is located beneath the patellar. The positive sign is the knee extension (see Fig. 49.5). This reflex centre is lumber spinal L2-4.
5. **Achilles tendon reflex (ankle reflex):** Ask the patient to lie on his back with knee and hip in flexion. The examiner tries to dorsiflex the ankle and strikes on the Achilles tendon which is located on the posterior aspect of the calcaneus. The positive sign is ankle extension. This reflex centre is sacral spinal S1-2.
6. **Clonus:** It refers to repetitive jerks after a single strike. Sustained clonus always indicates abnormalities in corticospinal tract.
   - Ankle clonus: Ask the patient to lie on his back. Then examiner pushes the ankle dorsiflexion quickly and hardly. The positive sign is repetitive and sustained ankle jerks (see Fig. 49.6).
   - Patella clonus: Ask the patient to lie on his back. The examiner pushes down the patella with his thumb and index hardly and quickly. The positive sign is repetitive and sustained patellar jerks (see Fig. 49.7).

49.5.3 Abnormal Reflex

These reflexes are only positive in children under two-year old. They will reappear only when corticospinal tract gets impaired. The positive sign is dorsiflexion of the big toe with the fanning of the rest toes. This is always abnormal and termed as pathological reflex.

1. **Babinski sign:** Hold the ankle and stroke the sole of the foot from the heel to the ball of the foot (see Fig. 49.8).
2. **Oppenheim sign:** Push hard downwards from knee to ankle along the shin of the leg (see Fig. 49.9).
3. **Gordon sign:** Give pressure to the gastrocnemius muscle.
4. **Chaddock sign:** Hold the ankle and stroke the lateral surface skin of the foot from the heel to the toes.
5. **Hoffmann sign:** Ask the patient to sit or lie on his back with his hand in pronated position and middle finger hyperextended. Flick the patient's nail downwards by the examiner's thumb quickly and strongly. The positive sign is the flexion of the patient's thumb (see Fig. 49.10).

49.5.4 Menigeal Signs

These are signs indicating meningeal irritation and can be positive in the following disorders, e.g. meningitis, subarachnoid hemorrhage, etc.

1. **Nuchal rigidity:** Ask the patient to lie on his back. Put one hand under his head and the other hand on his chest, and then try to put the patient's chin to the chest. In normal people, chin can reach the chest except for some elderly, obese peoples and diseases such as cervical osteoplytosis, cervical muscle strain, neck trauma and severe rigidity of extrapyramidal disorders. The positive sign is the resistance of neck to be fully flexed.
2. **Kernig sign:** Ask the patient to lie on his back with both his hip and knee flexed to 90° on one side. Try to extend his leg at the knee on this side another 45° to a total degree of 135°. The positive sign is the resistance of leg extension within a degree of 135°, usually resulting in pain or flexion of the other leg (see Fig. 49.11).
3. **Brudzinski sign:** Ask the patient to lie on his back. Put one hand under his head and the other hand on his chest, and then try to flex his neck. The positive sign is the flexion of the patient's hips and knees (see Fig. 49.12).

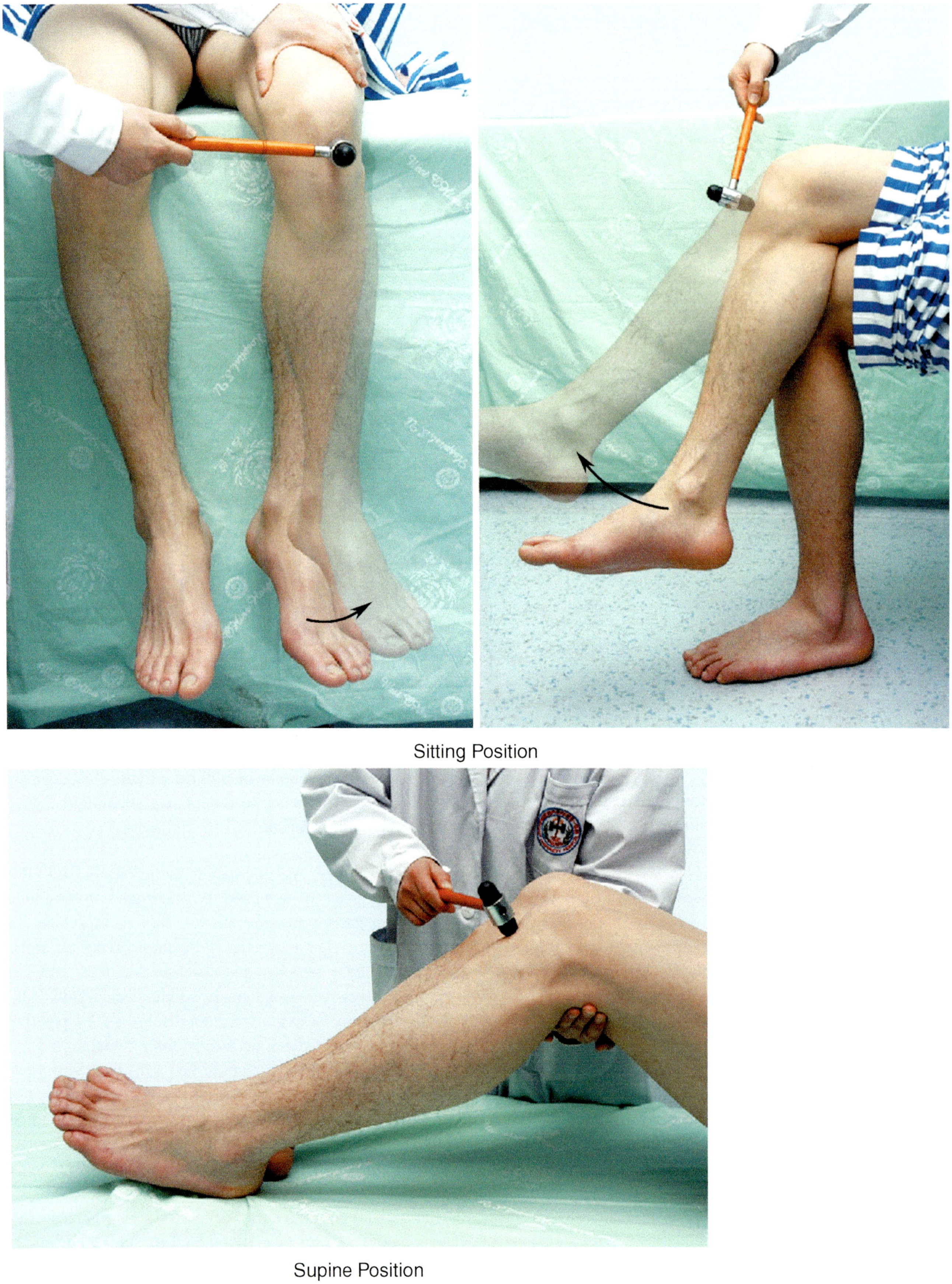

Fig. 49.5 The examination of patellar reflex

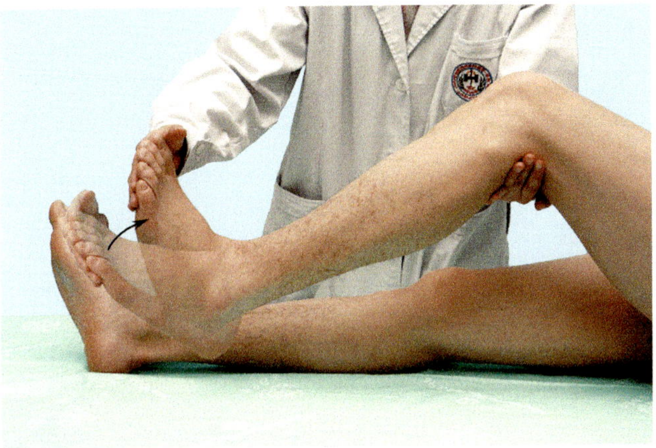

Fig. 49.6 The examination of ankle clonus

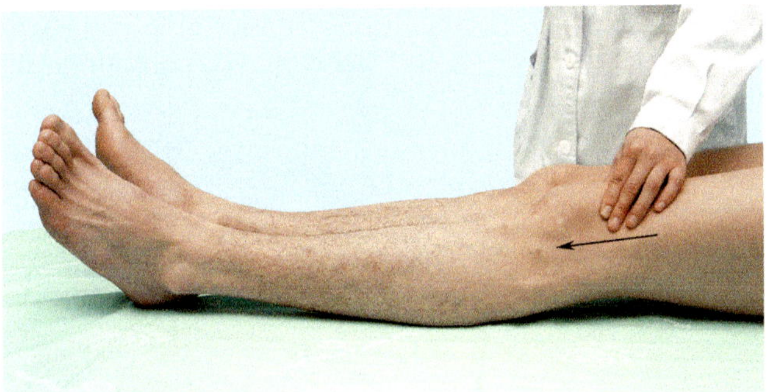

Fig. 49.7 The examination of patella clonus

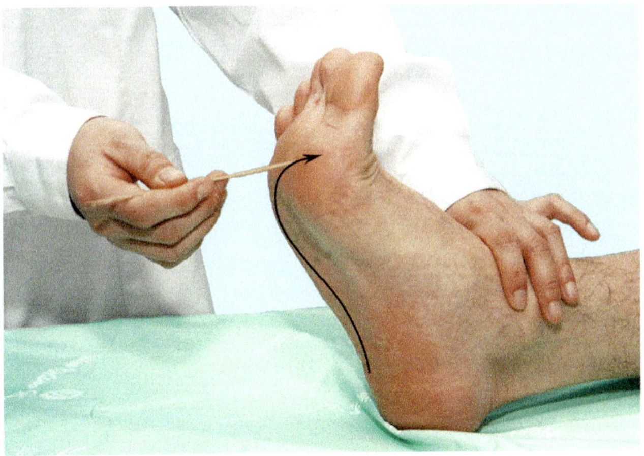

Fig. 49.8 The examination of Babinski sign

49.6 Autonomic System Examination

Autonomic function is composed of sympathetic system and parasympathetic system both of which interplay with each other to maintain the normal function of vessels, endocrines and various human organs. Examination of autonomic system includes general inspection on skin, mucosa, hair, nail and sweating condition. Several tests can be used in clinical to examine the function of autonomic system, such as oculocardiac reflex, orthostatic test, dermographism, pilomotor reflex, sweating test and valsalva maneuver.

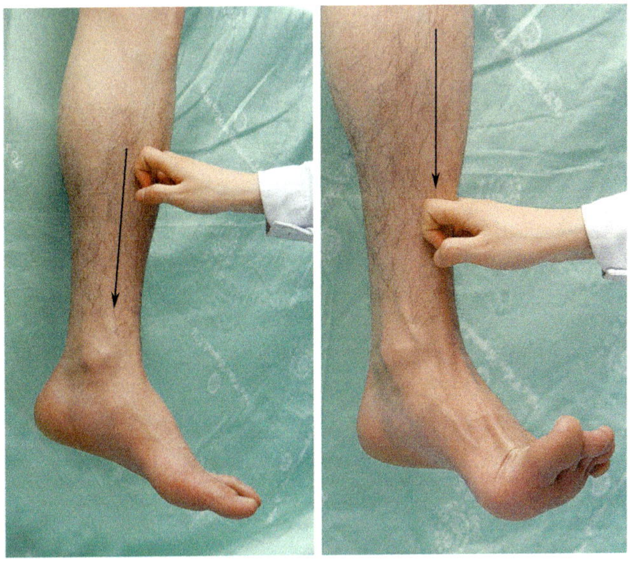

Fig. 49.9 The examination of Oppenheim sign

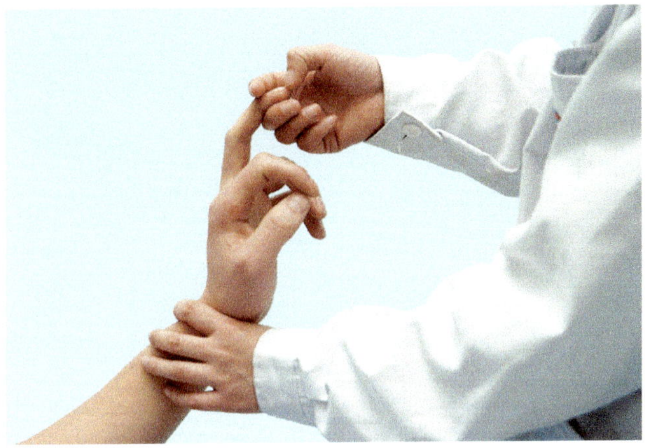

Fig. 49.10 The examination of Hoffman sign

Key Terms		
1	Diplopia	复视
2	Corneal reflex	角膜反射
3	Facial nerve palsy	面神经麻痹
4	Spastic paralysis	痉挛性瘫痪
5	Flaccid paralysis	弛缓性瘫痪
6	Cogwheel rigidity	齿轮样强直
7	Ataxia	共济失调
8	Superficial reflex	浅反射
9	Deep tendon reflex	腱反射
10	Pathological reflex	病理反射

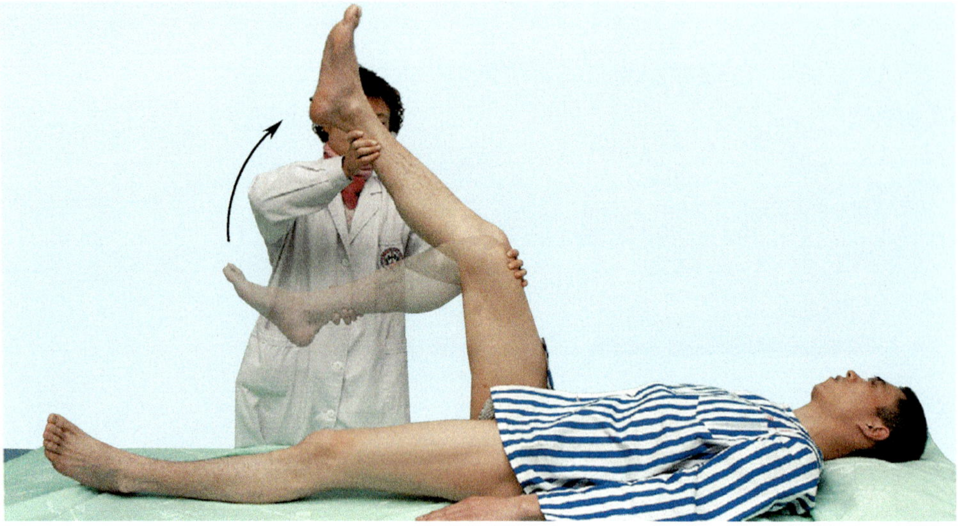

Fig. 49.11 The examination of kernig sign

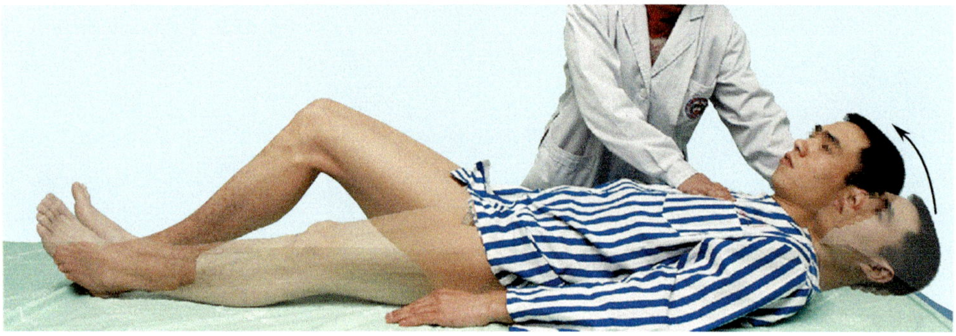

Fig. 49.12 The examination of brudzinski sign

Study Questions

1. How to assess the grade of muscle strength?
2. How to differentiate rigidity from spasticity?
3. Describe the characteristics of different sensory impairment pattern in regarding to neurological localization.
4. Describe the characteristics of different movement impairment pattern in regarding to neurological localization.
5. What are meningeal signs?

Suggested Readings

Biller J, Gruener G, Brazis P. DeMyer's the neurologic examination: a programmed text. 6th ed. Columbus: McGraw-Hill Education/Medical; 2011.

Strub RL, Black FW. The mental status examination in neurology. 4th ed. Philadelphia: F.A. Davis Company; 2003.

Complete Physical Examination

50

Rui Zeng

50.1 Basic Requirements of Complete Physical Examination

Complete physical examination is an essential skill for every clinician and medical student. It is also an important part of the evaluation and assessment of the basic clinical skills of the doctors. After subsection learning of the system examination, students should learn how to mastery, comprehensive application. For specific cases, physical examination should be systematic and sequenced completed from head to foot. Its basic requirements are as follows:

1. **The content of complete physical examination should be comprehensive and systematic** which is in order to collect enough objective data, play a role in screening examination, also facilitate to complete medical records as specified requirements. In addition, physical examination is usually carried out after history taking, the inspectors have already known the focus examination. Therefore, focused examination of the organs must be more in-depth and meticulous. In general, it should include all required contents in systematic teaching, which makes complete physical examination for each case is not mechanically repeat screening, but focused examination based on comprehensive and systematic requirements.
2. **The order of complete physical examination should be from head to foot.** We emphasizes a reasonable and logical sequence, not only could maximally ensure medical efficiency and speed, but also could greatly reduce patient's discomfort and unnecessary postural changes, also it is easy to complete the examination. In order to the examination convenience, certain organs, such as skin, lymph nodes, nervous system, has to be taken sectional examination and unified record.
3. **Follow the basic principles and contents of complete physical examination, you could also been allowed to your own habits.** Appropriate adjustments to some examination sequence can be implemented. Such as thyroid palpation is always been done behind the patients. Therefore, supine patients can be added in seat position during the examination of back. In order to have a comprehensive understanding of pulmonary signs, you should immediately check the back after the examination of anterior chest. The better sequence of abdominal examination should be inspection, auscultation, percussion and palpation. For the examination of limbs, upper limbs are usually from hands to shoulders, while lower limbs should be carried out from near to far.
4. **Physical examination should pay particular attention to the principle of flexibility.** In some specific cases, such as emergency and severe cases, may need simple physical examination then start to rescue and treat, complementary information could be collected after patients in stable condition, not sitting patients, Back examination need only been done at lateral position to those patients who could not seated. Anus rectum, external genital examination should check only if necessary, special attention should also be paid to protect the privacy of patients during the process.
5. **The order of complete physical examination:** Supine position: General examination/vital signs→Head and neck→Anterior and lateral chest (Heart and lung)→(Seated position) Back (Include lung, spine, kidney, sacral area)→(Supine position) Abdomen→Upper and lower limbs→Anus rectum→External genital→Nervous system→Standing position.

   Seated position: General examination/vital signs→Upper limbs→ Head and neck→Back (Include lung, spine, kidney, sacral area)→(Supine position) Anterior and lateral chest (Heart and lung)→Abdomen→Lower limbs→Anus rectum→External genital→Nervous system→Standing position.

R. Zeng (✉)
Department of Cardiology, Sichuan University, Chengdu, China

X.-H. Wan, R. Zeng (eds.), *Handbook of Clinical Diagnostics*, https://doi.org/10.1007/978-981-13-7677-1_50

6. **The method of complete physical examination is the enrichment and extraction of systematic examination, with good skills to ensure standard and reasonable, properly applied.** Such as thyroid palpation, different methods depend on different positions. Percussion shifting dullness for ascites examination should be supine. Explain first to achieve understanding before instruments will be used to. Appropriate exposure, then recovery after examination.
7. **Emphasize on deliberation, evaluation, inquiration and verification while examination.** The knowledge and experience of the doctors are helpful to understand normal limits for objective examination result and clinical significance. In order to make a correct judgment and analysis, you should always notice to compare during examination. Gentle action, not to make the patients feel pain.
8. **Appropriate communication with patients during examination.** Self introduction, and we also should notice that doctor-patient relationship and communication, not only could be harmonious for doctor-patient relationship, but also complementary for medical history. The patient's health education and mental support could also be expressive in the examination process. Examination process should have a good professional attitude, caring and considerate patients, respect their privacy.
9. **The schedule and time of examination.** In order to avoid the examination discomfort or burden for patients, it should be completed in 30–40 min.
10. **At the end of the examination should be a simple conversation with the patient, indicating important findings, patients should also pay attention to the matter or the next treatment plan.** But beginners should understand their professional responsibilities, grasp the sense of propriety, do not easily explain for some uncertain signs, so as to avoid the mental heaviness of patient, or cause disturbance to the medical work.

50.2 Complete Physical Examination Checklist

50.2.1 General Examination/Vital Signs

——1. Prepare and count instruments

——2. Introduce yourself to patient, usually last name and title and have a little conversation to relax the patient and to judge mental state

——3. Observation of the general state, include development, nutrition, face, expression and consciousness, etc.

——4. Wash hands before starting examination

——5. Measuring body temperature

——6.Palpate radial (wrist) pulses for at least 30 seconds and record

——7. Palpate both radial (wrist) pulses simultaneously for symmetry

——8. Measure respiratory rate for at least 30 s and record

——9. Measure blood pressure on right arm twice and record

50.2.2 Head and Neck

——10. Observe scalp (parting hair, and observing hair density, color, luster and distribution)

——11. Palpate skull

——12. Inspect both eyes and eyebrows

——13. Visual screening

——14. Observe cornea, sclera and conjunctive by gently moving lower eyelids down,

——15. Observe lacrimal puncta

——16. Observe sclera and bulbar conjunctiva by gently elevating upper eyelid while patent looks down

——17. Check crn VII upper division: wrinkle forehead or forced eyelid closing

——18. Evaluate extraocular muscle function in both eyes in six directions (left, upper left and lower left, right, upper right, lower right)

——19. Observe pupillary direct response to light

——20. Observe pupillary indirect response to light

——21. Check for convergence reflex

——22. Observe the auricles and post-auricular regions bilaterally

——23. Palpate the auricles and post-auricular regions bilaterally

——24. Palpate temporomandibular joint for tenderness and movement

——25. Use proper technique to check auditory acuity separately in each ear (Finger friction or watch used)

——26. Inspect and palpate external nose

——27. Observe nasal vestibule and septum

——28. Test patency by inhaling through each nostril separately while the opposite nostril is he held occluded

——29. Palpate maxillary sinus for swelling and tenderness

——30. Palpate frontal sinus for swelling and tenderness

——31. Palpate ethmoid sinus for swelling and tenderness

——32. Observe lips, buccal mucosa, teeth, gums and tongue

——33. Observe the buccal mucosa, teeth, gums and floor of mouth by tongue blade

——34. Inspect tonsils and oropharynx by tongue blade

——35. Observe midline protrusion of the tongue (crn XII)

——36. Show teeth, puff out cheeks or purse lips (lower division of crn VII)

——37. Test contraction of masseter (jaw) muscle or forced opening of mouth against resistance (motor division crn V)
——38. Test for facial sense of pain and touch (must check at least 2 out of 3 sensory divisions for crn V)
——39. Expose neck correctly to observe appearance and skin of neck
——40. Observe the configuration and skin of neck, also the jugular vein and the carotid pulse.
——41. Examine movement of cervical spine, include flexion, extension, lateral bending and rotation.
——42. Test rotation of patient's head against resistance or check resistance of shrugged shoulders (crn XI)
——43. Palpate preauricular nodes (front of ears)
——44. Palpate post-auricular nodes (back of ears)
——45. Palpate occipital nodes (base of skull)
——46. Palpate submaxillary nodes (by bending finger under patient's jaw)
——47. Palpate submental nodes (by bending finger under patient's chin
——48. Palpate anterior cervical nodes (superficial group under mastoid and the front of sternomastoid muscle)
——49. Palpate posterior cervical nodes (behind sternomastoid muscle)
——50. Palpate supraclavicular nodes (by bending finger above patient's collarbone)
——51. Palpate thyroid cartilage
——52. Palpate isthmus of thyroid with and without swallowing
——53. Palpate thyroid gland (lobes) with and without swallowing
——54. Gently palpate carotid artery (bilaterally)
——55. Palpate the position of trachea
——56. Auscultate of the neck (thyroid, vascular murmur)

50.2.3 Anterior and Lateral Chest

——57. Expose chest
——58. Observe configuration, symmetry, skin and movements of chest
——59. Palpate left breast as the following areas: super-internal, super- lateral, infer-internal, infer-lateral and nipples.
——60. Palpate right breast as the following areas: super-internal, super-lateral, infer-internal, infer-lateral and nipples.
——61. Palpate axilla lymph nodes on left by right hand
——62. Palpate axilla lymph nodes on right by left hand
——63. Palpate flexibility and tenderness of chest
——64. Palpate bilateral respiratory movements (upper, middle, lower and symmetry)
——65. Palpate bilateral tactile fremitus (upper, middle, lower and symmetry)
——66. Palpate pleural friction fremitus
——67. Percuss apex pulmonis bilaterally and symmetrically.
——68. Percuss anterior and lateral lung fields (top to bottom, outside to inside, bilateral comparison).
——69. Auscultate apex pulmonis bilaterally and symmetrically.
——70. Auscultate anterior and lateral lung fields (top to bottom, outside to inside, bilateral comparison).
——71. Vocal resonance (upper, middle, lower and symmetry)
——72. Observe apex and precordium impulse (view tangentially).
——73. Palpate apical area with palm and fingertips.
——74. Palpate precordial area with palm.
——75. Percuss relative dullness of the left heart.
——76. Percuss relative dullness of the right heart.
——77. Auscultate mitral area (frequency, rhythm, heart sound, murmurs).
——78. Auscultate pulmonary area (heart sound, murmurs)
——79. Auscultate aortic area (heart sound, murmurs)
——80. Auscultate second aortic area (heart sound, murmurs)
——81. Auscultate tricuspid area (heart sound, murmurs)
——82. Auscultate with diaphragmatic type of stethoscope, bell type as the complementary.

50.2.4 Back

——83. Patient is seated in a chair
——84. Expose the back correctly
——85. Inspection the spinal column, contour of thorax and breathing movement
——86. Palpate thoracic expansion and symmetry
——87. Palpate bilateral tactile fremitus
——88. Palpate pleural friction fremitus
——89. Have patient cross arms in front and touch opposite shoulder
——90. Percuss bilateral posterior chest
——91. Percuss posterior lung fields comparatively and symmetrically
——92. Percuss bilateral movement range of the inferior lung boundary(Scapular line)
——93. Auscultate bilateral posterior chest
——94. Auscultate pleural friction rub
——95. Examine bilateral vocal resonance
——96. Palpate spinous processes one by one (check for scotiosis and tenderness)
——97. Test for percussion pain of spinal column by direct method

——98. Test vertebrocostal and costolumbar point for tenderness by pressure
——99. Test vertebrocostal point for percussion pain by fist percussion

50.2.5 Abdomen

——100. Expose abdomen completely from below breasts to above pubis
——101. Place pillow under head, bend knees, arms at side, have patient breathe normally
——102. Observe abdominal shape, symmetry, skin, umbilical and abdominal breathing
——103. Auscultate for bowel sounds for at least 1 min
——104. Auscultate for vascular murmurs of abdomen
——105. Percuss abdomen
——106. Percuss upper bound of liver
——107. Percuss lower bound of liver
——108. Check the percussion pain of liver
——109. Percuss shifting dullness (umbilicus level)
——110. Palpate superficially (Palpate all areas of abdomen counter- clockwise from left lower quadrant)
——111. Palpate deeply (Palpate all areas of abdomen counter-clockwise from left lower quadrant)
——112. Train patients to do deep abdominal breathing 2–3 times
——113. Palpate liver at midclavicular with monomanual method
——114. Palpate liver at midclavicular line with bimanual method
——115. Palpate liver at midsternal line with bimanual method
——116. Hepatojugular reflux
——117. Murphy sign or gallbladder tenderness sign
——118. Palpate spleen with bimanual method.
——119. Palpate spleen with patient rolled toward his right side.
——120. Palpate kidney's with bimanual method.
——121. Test for pain or light touch on abdominal wall.
——122. Abdominal reflex

50.2.6 Upper Limbs

——123. Expose upper limbs
——124. Inspect skin and joints of upper limbs
——125. Inspect hands and fingernails
——126. Palpate metacarpophalangeal and interphalangeal joints
——127. Check the movement of fingers
——128. Check for distal muscle strength
——129. Palpate wrist
——130. Check the movement of wrist
——131. Palpate olecranon process and epicondyles
——132. Palpate epitrochlear lymph nodes
——133. Check the movement of elbow
——134. Check for muscle strength at flexion and extension
——135. Expose shoulder
——136. Inspect both shoulders
——137. Palpate both shoulders
——138. Functional examination
——139. Test for sense of pain or light touch in at least 2 or 3 positions of upper limbs
——140. Check biceps reflex
——141. Check triceps reflex
——142. Check radial reflex
——143. Check Hoffmann sign

50.2.7 Lower Limbs

——144. Expose lower limbs
——145. Inspect skin and joints of lower limbs
——146. Check lumps or hernia in groin.
——147. Palpate transverse group of superficial groin lymph nodes
——148. Palpate longitudinal group of superficial groin lymph nodes
——149. Femoral artery (groin)
——150. Check flexion, internal/external rotation of the hip
——151. Check proximal muscle strength (flexion of hips)
——152. Palpate the knee joint and check floating patella test
——153. Check flexion of the knee joint
——154. Check the patellar clonus
——155. Palpate ankle joint including Achilles tendon
——156. Check for pitting edema
——157. Dorsalis pedis artery (top of foot)
——158. Check movement at ankle joint (dorsiflexion-plantarflexion)
——159. Check for distal muscle strength
——160. Check movement at subtalar joint (eversion-inversion)
——161. Flexion of toes (curl toes) and extension of toes (straighten toes)
——162. Test for sense of pain or light touch in at least 2 or 3 positions of lower limbs
——163. Test position sense in both feet
——164. Check patellar reflex
——165. Check Achilles tendon reflex
——166. Check ankle clonus
——167. Check Babinski sign
——168. Check Oppenheim sign
——169. Check Kernig sign
——170. Check Brudzinski sign
——171. Check Lasegue sign

50.2.8 Anus and Rectum (Check Only If Necessary)

——172. Ask patient at left lateral position, right leg flexion
——173. Observe anus, perianal area and perineal region
——174. Put on gloves, test digital rectal examination by index finger with lubricant.
——175. Observe secretions of the finger

50.2.9 External Genital (Check Only If Necessary)

——176. Explain the need for inspection, eliminate concerns, protect privacy
——177. Confirm the bladder has been emptied and ask the patient at supine position
Male:
——178. Inspect pubic hair, penis, coronary sulcus, glans and prepuce
——179. Inspect orificium urethrae externum
——180. Inspect scrotum, cremasteric reflex as necessary
——181. Palpate bilateral testis, epididymis and spermatic cord
Female:
——178. Inspect pubic hair, mons pubis, labia majora and labia minora, clitoris
——179. Inspect urethral orifice and vaginal orifice
——180. Inspect mons pubis, labia majora and labia minora
——181. Palpate paraurethral glands, bartholin gland

50.2.10 Coordinate Movement, Gait and Movement of Lumbar Spine

——182. Ask patients to stand up
——183. Finger to nose test (with open or closed eyes)
——184. Rapid alternating movement
——185. Perform Romberg test
——186. Check gait (arms swinging at side)
——187. Flexion of lumbar spine
——188. Extension of lumbar spine
——189. Lateral bending of lumbar spine
——190. Rotation of lumbar spine

50.3 Key Physical Examination

The previously mentioned physical examination is very important for starters because it act as a screening tool for those without chief complaints. It is also indispensable for building a complete medical record. However, in every day medical work, after acquiring health history and forming a diagnostic hypothesis, doctors are well aware of the involved organ and type of lesion.

Physical examination done on this basic knowledge is usually very focused with the intention of finding the cause for the patient's symptoms and confirming the diagnosis. In other words, the purpose is to exclude diseases of small likelihood and attain evidence for the diagnosis based on information acquired from health history taking. Problem-focused physical examination is carried out in the same order as complete physical examination, but should be adjusted logically according to the position and physical condition of the patient to minimize discomfort.

The content of physical examination should encompass specific exams in various systems and special techniques. If the patient complains of an abdominal mass, doctors should confirm the complaint and all characteristics of the mass during physical exam. Problem-focused physical examination is an advanced and refined method especially suitable for outpatient or emergency settings, as well as for patients admitted by chief residents who have limited effort and time. Special attention should be paid to:

1. Vital signs should be acquired first, including temperature, pulse, respiration and blood pressure.
2. The specific exams in physical examination is done selectively but the sequence is consistent regardless of the position of the patient (sitting or decubitus).
3. Comprehensive examination including inspection, palpation, percussion and auscultation should be carried out in depth in critical systems.
4. Special examinations can be done for a more definite diagnosis.
5. Confirmation of all doubts should be implemented during the examination, with attention paid to negative signs to exclude diseases of small possibility.
6. When the original hypothesis fails to explain new findings in physical examination, repeated history taking should be done to propose a new hypothesis, followed by associated examinations.

50.4 Physical Examination for the Elderly

The twenty-first century will witness the increase in the proportion of senior citizens over the age of 65. Medical practitioners of all specialties except pediatrics will see a growing number of elderly patients. Changes related to aging process and pathological conditions should be properly distinguished, and more skills are required in physical examination.

50.4.1 Be aware of Changes Related to Aging Process in the Elderly

1. Decline in vision, audition, and memory.
2. Reduction in skin elasticity.
3. Slightly blunted pupil light reflex, declined capacity of gazing upwards, arcus senilis.
4. Dominant systolic murmurs, slightly increased systolic pressure within the normal range.
5. Increased sagittal diameter of thorax related to cyphosis and collapsed vertebral body, crepitus in auscultation without structural disease.
6. Declined peristalsis of GI tracts.
7. Atrophy of genitals (labia vulvae and vagina for female and testicles for male).
8. Enlarged prostate.
9. Mild atrophy of muscles.
10. Slower gait and smaller steps.

50.4.2 Special Considerations for Physical Examination for the Elderly

1. Regular examinations are necessary, but the elderly may suffer from immobility due to changes in bone and joint. Physicians should be more considerate and use more time, patience and carefulness in physical examination.
2. The contents and order of physical examination for the elderly is not different from that of the adults. Vital signs are very important.
3. Examination methods should be flexible. E.g. Effectively evaluating intelligence and memory in a talk, getting information from family members and caregivers and etc.
4. Mental status can be evaluated with three "A"s—general status (appearance), emotion (affect) and language, behavior (appropriateness). Time, Place and person orientation can also be evaluated in a talk.
5. Pay attention to the degree of loss in visual acuity and hearing. There is usually difficulty in distinguishing whispered or high pitched voices.
6. Change in S1 and occurrence of S3 in cardiac examination may indicate pathological changes.
7. Blood pressure is ideally measured in both arms with the patient in different positions including sitting, decubitus, and standing, so that compensative capacity of the circulation is taken into consideration.
8. Note vascular murmurs in abdominal auscultation, and widened abdominal aorta in palpation, normally it does not exceed 3.5 cm in diameter.
9. In neurological examination, note weakened ankle reflex; slightly diminished deep reflections and muscle strength.
10. When bone and joint changes are evident, osteoarthritis should be differentiated; gait should be carefully observed; locomotory function can be evaluated along with analysis of daily living skills.

50.5 Physical Examination in Special Population

Sometimes due to limits of the patients' conditions and position, psychological or physiological defects, they cannot satisfactorily cooperate with the doctor with conventional methods and order for physical examination. Doctors need to consider changing the order, or use alternative methods.

50.5.1 Physical Examination for Patients with Mental Retardation

Patients with mental disorders may have difficulty cooperating due to incapability of understanding doctor's intention, unpleasant experience of the past, and fear or inability to adapt to doctor's examination.

Particular patience should be given at this time. Creating a comfortable environment, protecting patient's privacy, allowing a close family or health provider to stay at the site can often reduce the patient's concerns and strengthen cooperation. Examination should be conducted in a slow, gentle, and delicate way, and can be divided into separate sections when necessary. Carefully observe patient's movement and response to determine the focus of examination. Similar to examining a child, invasive or feared procedures should be left to the final part, so as not to affect key parts of the examination.

50.5.2 Physical Examination for Patients with Emotional Disorders or Mental Illnesses

Patient's noncooperation and hostility may impede the examination. Sometimes experienced staff or family members can comfort patients and encourage the patient to cooperate with doctors. For whom comprehensive or focused examination is absolutely necessary, examination can be carried out with sedatives or appropriate constraints.

50.5.3 Physical Examination for Patients with Physiological Defects

Examination should be conducted in a slow and gentle way, with flexible methods and order. Lifting, turning over, and changing positions of the patient may require help from an assistant. Special attention should be paid to the organ systems associated with the patient's chief complaints and history of present illness. Order of examination should be flexible.

1. Comprehensive physical examination for bedridden patients should sometimes be conducted solely in decubitus position. The examiner needs to change his own position to complete the entire examination. As for a patient who cannot sit up or stand, examination of the fundus of the patient's left eye sometimes has to be conducted with the examiner standing at the cranial end of the patient examining with his right eye.
2. Examination of the head and neck, heart and lungs, upper and lower extremities for a patient in a wheelchair are all the same as that for a normal patient in sitting position. Examination of abdomen, rectum, genitalia, lower back, and hip cannot be satisfactory. If examination of these parts is necessary, the patient should be transferred to the examining table before examination is conducted.

50.5.4 Poor Examining Conditions

When conducting physical examinations at a patient's home, doctors need to bring with necessary equipment. Note that bed is usually lower than examining table. Try to adjust to get sufficient light. It is best to have an assistant or family member at the site to give some help.

If the patient is not compromised in activity and cooperation, generally physical examination can be completed without difficulty, otherwise an assistant is needed to help to turn the patient over or to fix his position. After the examination. doctors should note that all used disposable equipment are to be bagged and disposed as instructed, and other instruments should be fully cleaned and disinfected for second use.

Key Terms		
1	Key physical examination	重点体格检查
2	Elderly	老年人
3	Special population	特殊人群
4	Complete physical examination	全身体格检查

Study Questions

1. What are the whole contents of complete physical examination?
2. How to use basic skills to complete physical examination for elderly?
3. How to use basic skills to complete physical examination for special population?
4. What are the differences between key physical examination and complete physical examination?

Suggested Readings

Bickley LS. Bates' guide to physical examination and history taking. 10th ed. Philadelphia, PA: Lippincott Williams & Wilkins; 2009.

Swartz MH. Textbook of physical diagnosis. 7th ed. Philadelphia, PA: Elsevier; 2014.

Wan X. Diagnostics. 8th ed. Beijing: People's Medical Press; 2013.

Wan X. Clinical dignostics. 3rd ed. Beijing: People's Medical Press; 2015.

Part IV

Auxiliary Examination

Basic Knowledge of Electrocardiogram (ECG)

51

Rui Zeng

51.1 Section 1: The First Sight of ECG

This is a normal standard 12-leads ECG (Fig. 51.1). What can you see when you get a first sight of this ECG?

First, you will find that there are a lot of square boxes; Second, you will find that there are many confusing waves; Finally, you may also find that there are some Roman numerals(I, II, III) as well as some combinations of letters and numbers (aVR, aVL, aVF,V_1, V_2, V_3, V_4, V_5, V_6).

Therefore, in order to fully appreciate the world of ECG, we first need to accomplish some preparation, in other words, to get familiar with ECG. Let's start with the boxes.

51.1.1 What's the Connotation of the Boxes?

All the boxes are squares with 1 mm on a side. The horizontal line of the boxes (horizontal ordinate) represents time. The length of time in each box can vary, depending on the constant speed of the graph paper. Normally when the graph paper moves at a constant speed of 25 mm/s, one box represents 0.04 s (40 ms); when the graph paper moves at a constant speed of 50 mm/s, then one small box represents 0.02 s (20 ms), and the rest can be done in the same fashion. The vertical line of the box (vertical ordinate), otherwise, represents voltage, 0.1 mV per small box normally (Fig. 51.2).

Every 25 boxes (5 × 5) contribute to a large box, so the large box is also a square, each of which represents 0.2 s (200 ms) on the horizontal ordinate and 0.5 mV on the vertical ordinate (Fig. 51.2).

This chapter is reprinted with permission from: Rui Zeng, Dingke Wen, Zhanhao Su et al, Basic Knowledge of ECG. In the book: Graphics-sequenced interpretation of ECG. ISBN: 978-981-287-953-0. Springer, 2016.

R. Zeng (✉)
Department of Cardiology, Sichuan University, Chengdu, China

51.1.2 What Are the Confusing Waves?

After boxes, we came to see the confusing waves. Before we explain the waves, we should review some basic cardiac electrophysiology.

The electrical impulses is derived from a special pacemaking area in the right atrium called sinoatrial (SA) node and then triggers the contraction of heart in course of its gradual conduction. Figure 51.3 shows the whole process of how the impulse is produced by the SA node and spread to the entire heart. The impulse would first move through right and left atrium, then reach the atrioventricular (AV) node through the conduction of internodal pathways. After the impulse having reached the AV node, the depolarization would be delayed for a while. Finally the impulse moves to stimulate the ventricular muscle through the bundles of His and the left and right bundle branches. It's noteworthy that the SA node has no stable resting potential and it has automaticity, meaning it possess the feature of automatic depolarization and repolarization thus acting as the pacemaker of the heart. Normally, the cardiac muscles, conduction system aside, are unable to depolarize automatically, they can only be stimulated by the impulse from the other part of the heart.

51.1.2.1 The Depolarization and Repolarization of Heart

When at resting state, for a cardiac muscle cell specifically, the positively charged ions are located at the outer side of the cell membrane and the negatively charged ions are located at the inner side of the cell membrane, therefore rendering the cell at a state of equilibrium described as positive outside and negative inside or polarized (Fig. 51.4a). When the cell membrane is stimulated by the outer electric activity, the negatively charged ions move inward, to alter the state to negative outside and positive inside. This process is called depolarization (Fig. 51.4b). At the recovery phase of cardiac muscle cells, the positively charged ions, again, move back to the outside of the cell membrane, and the negatively charged ions move to the inside. Thereby the cell returns to a

X.-H. Wan, R. Zeng (eds.), *Handbook of Clinical Diagnostics*, https://doi.org/10.1007/978-981-13-7677-1_51

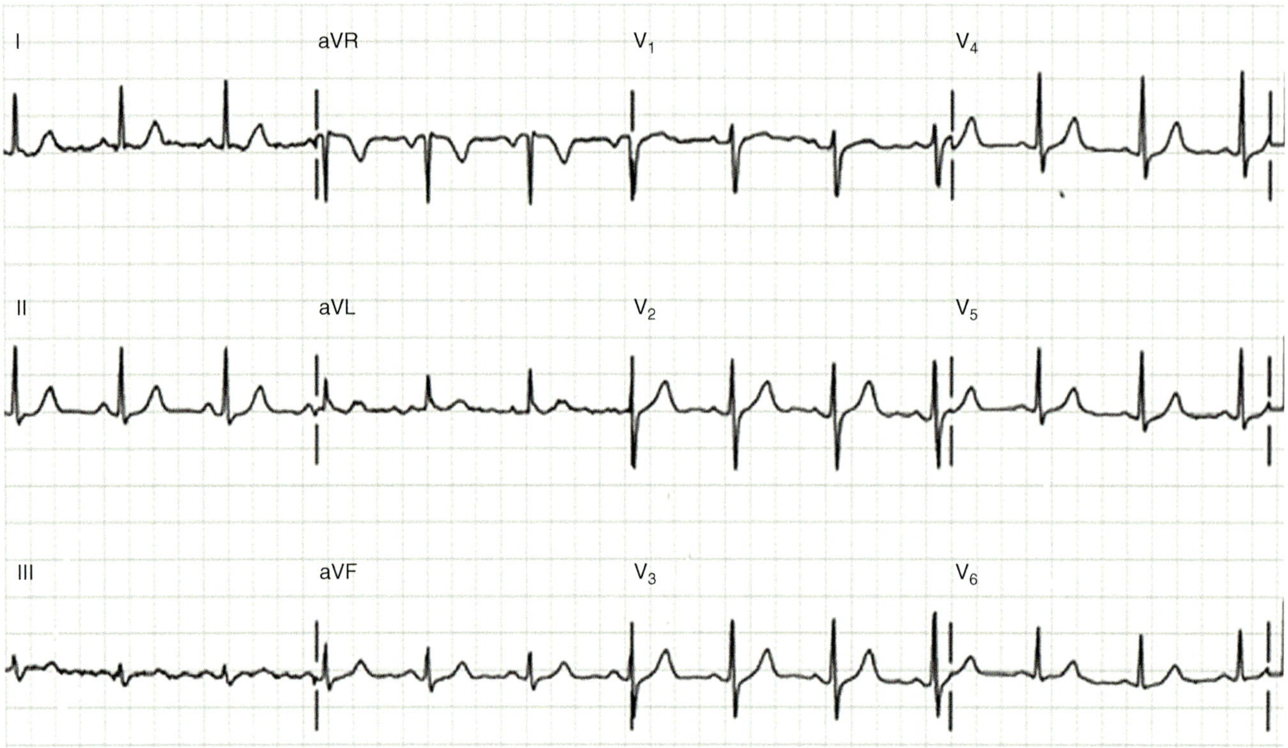

Fig. 51.1 Normal standard 12-leads ECG

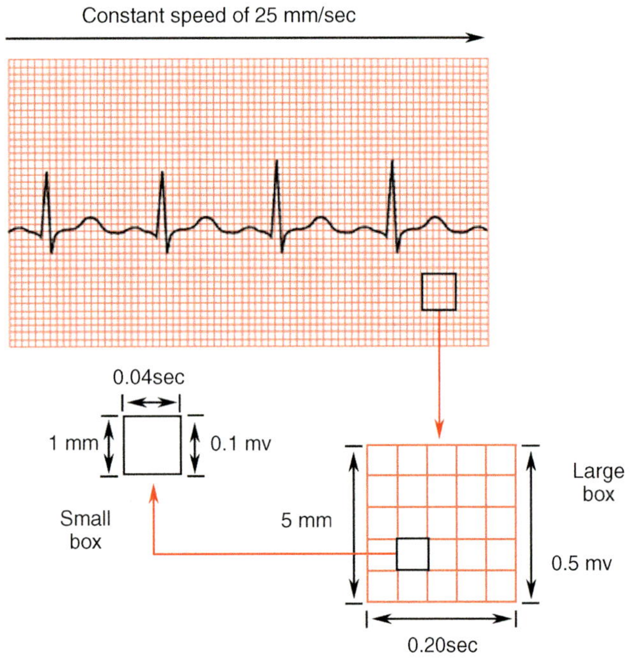

Fig. 51.2 The connotation of the boxes at 25 mm/s paper speed

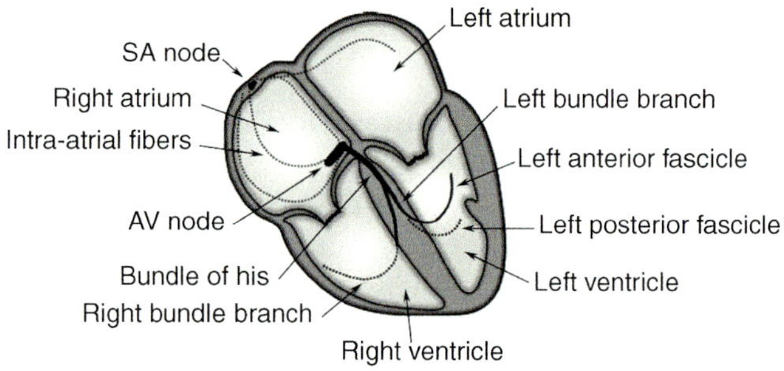

Fig. 51.3 Cardiac electrical conduction

state of outward whereas the positively charged ions move electrical equilibrium. This process is called repolarization (Fig. 51.4c). When the depolarization wave moves toward the electrodes, the galvo-recorder would detect and record a wave that is upward (positive) (Fig. 51.5a). When the depolarization wave moves away from the electrodes, the galvo-recorder would record a downward (negative) wave (Fig. 51.5b). And when the depolarization wave has some distance from the location of electrodes, a small deflection would be recorded (Fig. 51.5c); that is one of the reasons for low voltage occurrence in the ECG.

51.1.2.2 Resting Potential of Myocardial Cell

The resting potential of cardiac muscle cell is the potential difference between the inside and outside of the cell membrane when the cardiac muscle cell is not stimulated by the outside electrical activities (at the resting state). The theory can be explained as follows: At resting state, the concentration of K^+ inside the cell is 30 times higher than that of the outside (the concentration of Na^+ outside the cell is 30 times

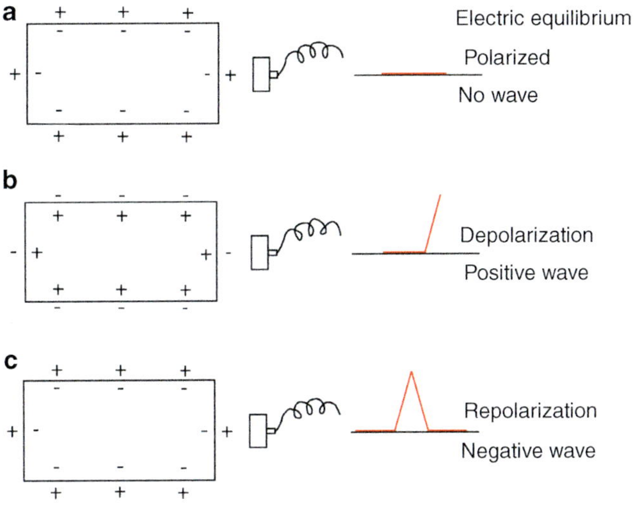

Fig. 51.4 Polarization, depolarization and repolarization of cardiac muscle cell

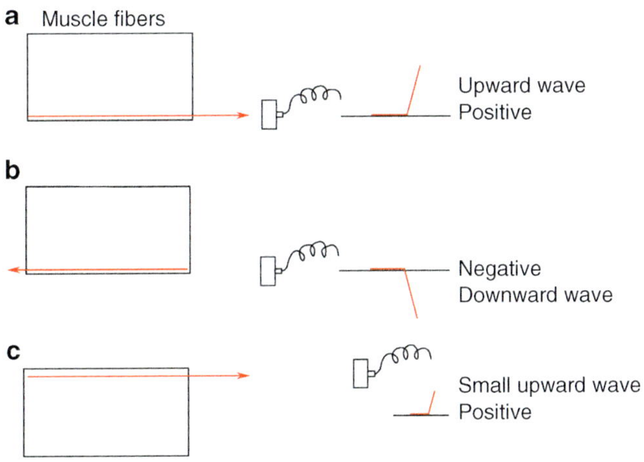

Fig. 51.5 Relationship between current flow direction and ECG wave pattern

higher than that of the inside). In addition, the cell membrane has a relatively high permeability to K^+, and a relatively low permeability to Na^+ and organic negatively charged ions A^-. As a result, K^+ could diffuse from inside of the membrane to the outside under the concentration difference (concentration gradient) whereas the negatively charged ions A^- could not diffuse with K^+ in the opposite direction. With the process of K^+ moving out, the membrane would slowly form a potential difference which is negative inside and positive outside. Such potential difference would slow down the process of K^+ further moving out, until reaching a point when the potential difference and the concentration difference of K^+ balance out. Then the moving stops and this potential difference between the inside and outside of the membrane is called the resting potential (Fig. 51.6). Normally, the resting potential of cardiac muscle cell is −90 mV.

51.1.2.3 Action Potential of Cardiac Muscle Cell

If the cell is stimulated properly on the basis of resting potential, a rapid and transient fluctuation of the membrane potential will be triggered. Such fluctuation in the membrane is called action potential. Action potential is the sign of cardiac excitation.

Action potential of cardiac muscle cell can be divided into four phases (Fig. 51.7) as phase 0, phase1, phase2, and phase 3 according to the change of potential. The mechanism is as follows: when the cardiac cell receives a certain level of stimuli, the stimuli would trigger the opening of Na^+ channel in the cell membrane and increase of Na^+ inflow. Under the dual effect of both the electric gradient and the concentration gradient, Na^+ move inside the cell membrane rapidly and result in a rapid increase of potential inside which is higher than the outside (+30 mV). The cell membrane is then at a positive inside and negative outside

Fig. 51.6 Resting potential of cardiac muscle cells

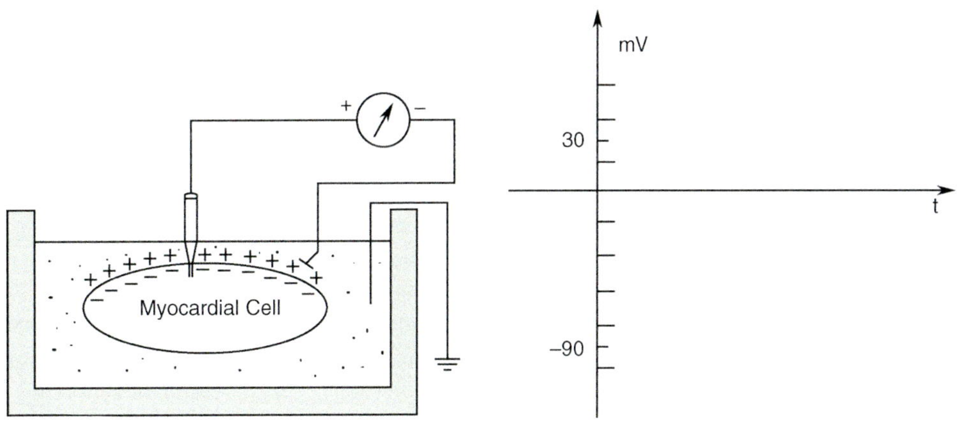

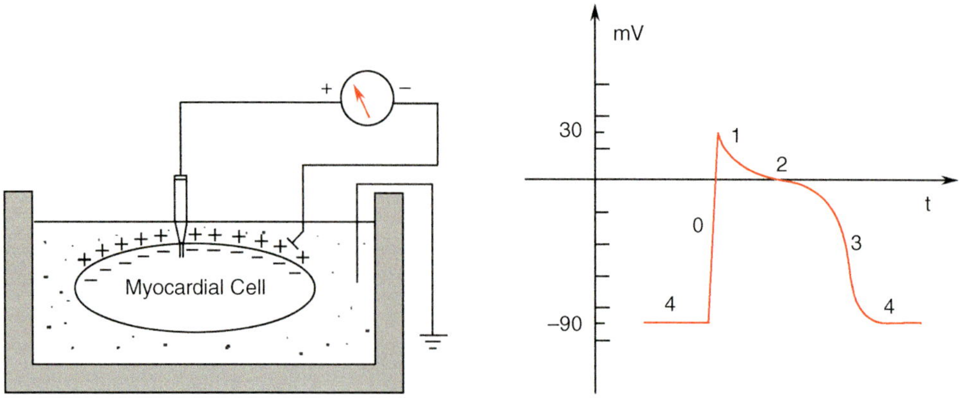

Fig. 51.7 Action potential of cardiac muscle cells

depolarized state. This process is the phase 0 of action potential. Na^+ channel is fast channel, activation and inactivation both happen in very short time, and when the cell depolarization reaches a peak, the potential inside will decline with the closing and inactivation of Na^+ channel, that is, the repolarization process of cardiac muscle. The repolarization process is rather slow, including Phase 1, Phase 2, and Phase 3. At phase 1, the cause for action potential waveform is the outflow of K^+; The waveform at phase 2 is relatively flattened so it is called the plateau phase or the slow recovery state, the mechanism of this plateau is mainly the relatively balanced state of outflow (K^+) and inflow (Ca^{2+}) of ions; The action waveform of phase 3 is rather steep. With the inactivation of Ca^{2+} channel and massive opening of K^+ channel, the process of repolarization accelerates apparently (the rapid recovery phase), and eventually recover to the previous negative inside and positive outside state, otherwise, the resting state.

51.1.2.4 Conduction of Action Potential

The action potential could travel around the cell without attenuation, which is a very important feature. When a spot of cell is stimulated and produces impulse, this part of the cell membrane presents a depolarization state that is "positive inside and negative outside," whereas the adjacent cell membrane presents a polarized state that is "negative inside and positive outside," and the potential difference occurs between them (Fig. 51.8). The potential difference renders "local current" between the two parts. When the local current begins to move, it results in the elevation of membrane potential in the adjacent cell membrane (the potential difference between the inside and outside of the membrane decreased). When the membrane potential reaches the threshold potential, it will excite the adjacent part to form action potential. In such case, one part of excitation in the membrane can travel through the whole cell membrane by the local current, producing new action potential successively until the whole cardiac cell is excited.

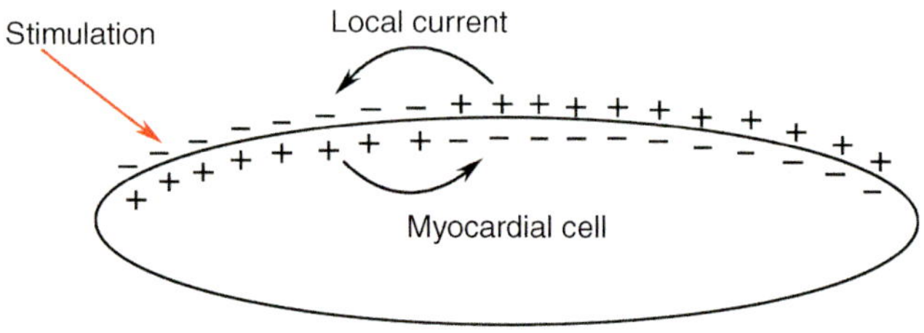

Fig. 51.8 Conduction of action potentials

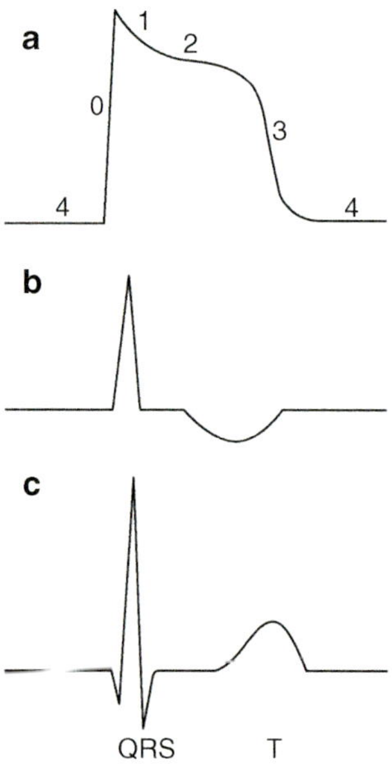

Fig. 51.9 Action potential of cardiac muscle cell and corresponding waveform. (**a**) Inner cell potential changes in one single cell, (**b**) Outer cell potential changes in one single cell, (**c**) The waveform of ECG is the potential changes of all cardiac muscle cells

51.1.2.5 Relationships of Depolarization, Repolarization and Waveforms on ECG

The recording of action potential is actually the recording of inner cell potential changes during the process of depolarization and repolarization in one single cell (Fig. 51.9a); What is recorded in the Fig. 51.9b is the outer cell potential changes of one single cell during the process of depolarization and repolarization; The waveform of ECG is the potential changes of the whole heart (all cardiac muscle cells) during the process of depolarization and repolarization.

51.1.3 Roman Numerals and the Meaning of Combinations of Characters and Numerals

51.1.3.1 The Conventional 12-Leads

The Roman numerals (I, II and III) in ECG, and several combinations of characters and numerals (aVR, aVL, aVF, V_1, V_2, V_3, V_4, V_5, V_6) represent the leads on ECG. It consists of three standard leads (I, II and III), three augmented leads (aVR, aVL, aVF) and six chest leads (V_1, V_2, V_3, V_4, V_5, V_6).

Standard leads, or bipolar limb leads (Fig. 51.10):

- First standard lead, or Lead I, in which left upper limb is connected to positive electrode and right upper limb connected to negative electrode.
- Second standard lead, or Lead II, in which left lower limb is connected to positive electrode and right upper limb connected to negative electrode.
- Third standard lead, or Lead III, in which left lower limb is connected to positive electrode and left upper limb connected to negative electrode.

Augmented unipolar limb leads (Fig. 51.11):

- Augmented right upper limb lead, or Lead aVR, in which electrodes are placed on right upper limb.
- Augmented left upper limb lead, or Lead aVL, in which electrodes are placed on left upper limb.
- Augmented left lower limb lead, or Lead aVF, in which electrodes are placed on left lower limb.

Chest leads: As known as V leads, are also unipolar leads. (Fig. 51.12):

- Lead V_1: Electrode is placed in the fourth intercostal space to the right of the sternum.
- Lead V_2: Electrode is placed in the fourth intercostal space to the left of the sternum.

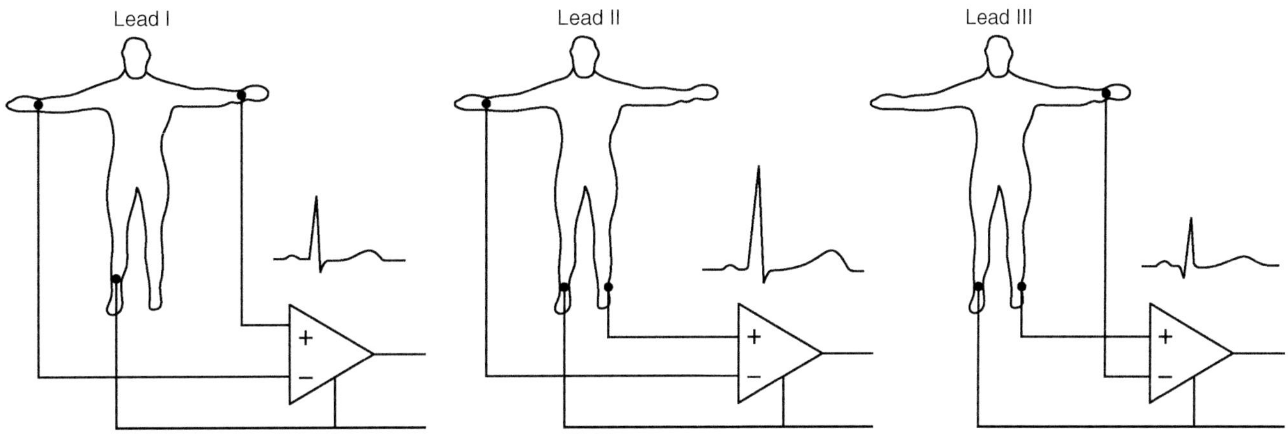

Fig. 51.10 Electrode placement of standard limb leads

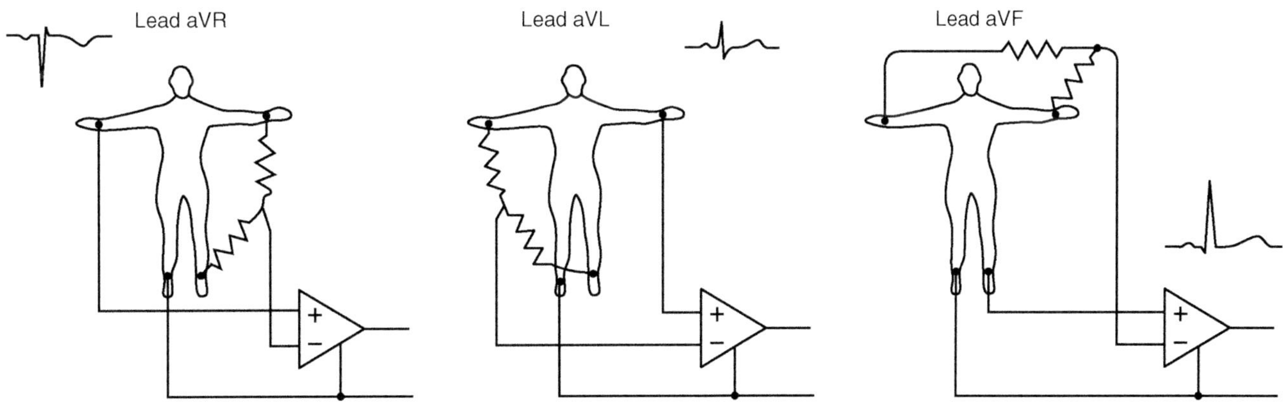

Fig. 51.11 Electrode placement of augmented unipolar limb leads

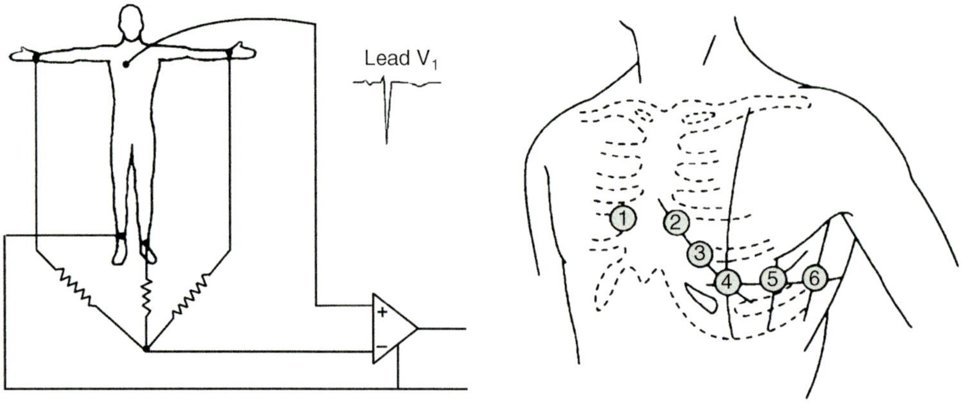

Fig. 51.12 Electrode placement of chest leads

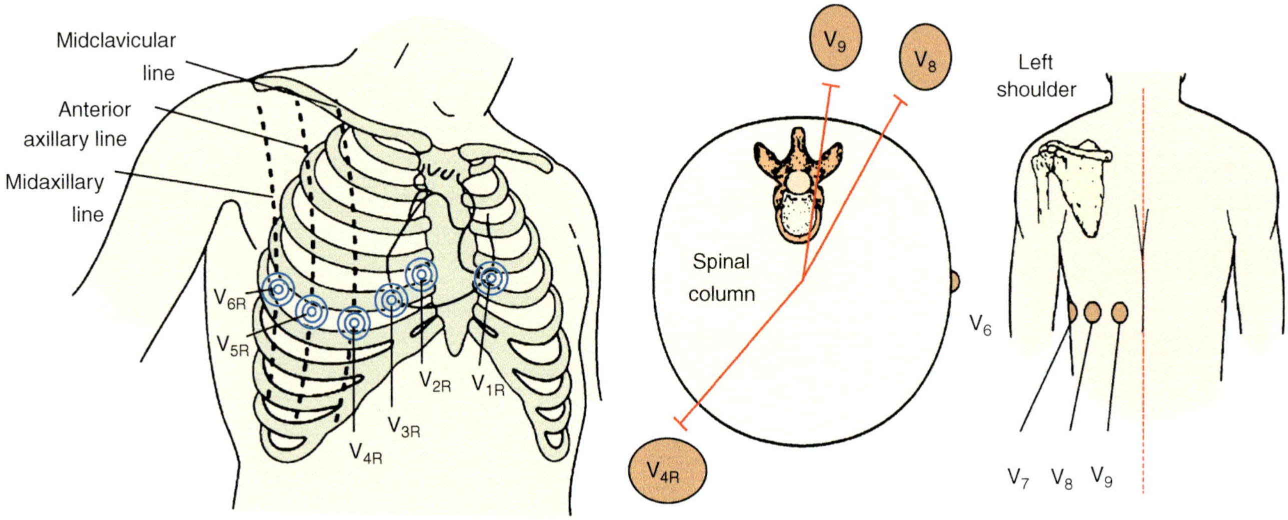

Fig. 51.13 Electrode placement of right-sided chest leads and posterior leads

- Lead V_3: Electrode is placed in the midpoint between V_2 and V_4.
- Lead V_4: Electrode is placed in the fifth intercostal space in the midclavicular line.
- Lead V_5: Electrode is placed at the intersection of left anterior axillary line and V_4 electrode level.
- Lead V_6: Electrode is placed at the intersection of left middle axillary line and V_4 electrode level.

51.1.3.2 Other Special Leads

Right-Sided Chest Leads (Fig. 51.13)

Chest Leads V_1 to V_6 are placed at the same position on the right chest, and thus labeled as V_{1R} to V_{6R}. Right-sided chest leads are mainly used to make clinical diagnosis of right ventricular hypertrophy, dextrocardia and right ventricular infarction.

Posterior Leads (Fig. 51.13)

Electrodes are placed at intersections of V_4 level and posterior axillary line, left scapular line and left of spinal column, with each labeled as posterior leads V_7, V_8 and V_9 respectively.

An 18-Leads ECG

In certain clinical situation, an 18-leads ECG will be adopted, including three right-sided chest leads (V_{3R}, V_{4R} and V_{5R}) and three posterior leads (V_7, V_8 and V_9) besides the conventional 12 leads.

51.1.3.3 The Axis

The axis of a certain lead is defined as an imaginary line extending from negative electrode to positive electrode of the lead. Usually, an arrowhead is used to represent the positive electrode. Axes are mainly categorized as limb leads (Fig. 51.14) and chest leads (Fig. 51.14). For example, in lead I, positive electrode is placed on left upper limb and negative electrode on right upper limb. Therefore, the axis for Lead I starts from right upper limb to left upper limb (from negative to positive), and the direction is shown in Fig. 51.14. In lead II, positive electrode is placed on left lower limb and negative electrode on right upper limb. Therefore, the axis for Lead II starts from right upper limb to left lower limb (from negative to positive), and the direction is shown in Fig. 51.14. Following the method discussed

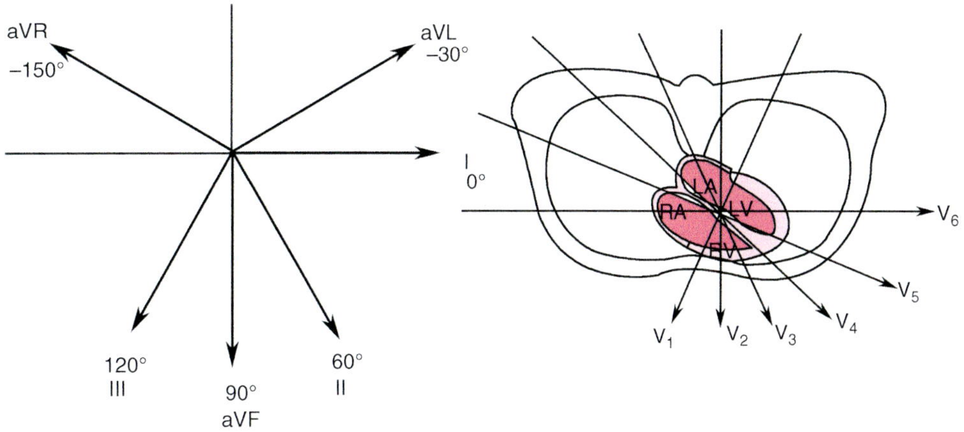

Fig. 51.14 Hexaxial reference system and cardiac axes in horizontal plane

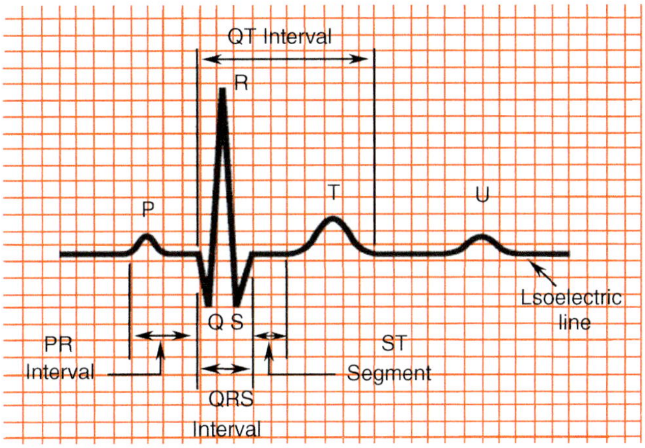

Fig. 51.15 Waves and segments in ECG

above, you could try to work out directions of the rest of axes by yourself.

Axes for limb leads are in cardiac frontal plane, indicating distribution of vectors in the frontal plane and is called hexaxial reference system. Axes of chest leads are in cardiac horizontal plane, indicating distribution of vectors in the horizontal plane.

51.2 Section 2: Configuration and Representation of Waves and Segments in ECG

Electrical impulse discharged from sinoatrial node activates atria and ventricle and sequentially causes depolarization and repolarization, producing a series of potential differences on the body surface, which are recorded as ECG (Fig. 51.15). Waves in ECG are labeled as P, Q, R, S, T and U, all of which were defined during early ECG development. Among all the waves, P, T and U waves are single deflection, while Q, R and S are grouped together to form QRS complex.

51.2.1 P Wave

P wave is the first deflection in a group of waves. It represents left and right atrial depolarization. P wave is upright (including rounded, notched, double-peaked, tall-peaked), or may have biphasic and inverted morphology (Fig. 51.16).

51.2.2 PR Interval

PR Interval refers to the interval from the beginning of P wave to the beginning of QRS Complex, and measures the time during which depolarization begins in atrium and travels through internodal pathways, atrioventricular junction, bundle of His, left and right bundle branch and their fascicles and Purkinje fibers to depolarize ventricles.

51.2.3 QRS Complex

QRS complex is a group of deflections that has greater amplitude and consists of Q, R and S waves. It represents depolarization in left and right ventricles. A typical QRS complex includes three consecutive deflections. The first negative deflection is called Q wave, the first positive deflection is called R wave and the negative deflection after R wave is called S wave, altogether comprise the QRS complex.

Occasionally, a positive deflection follows S wave and thus is called R′ wave (R-prime). If R′ wave occurs, then a negative deflection follows, and it's called S′ wave. If its amplitude is less than 0.5mv, then the wave is represented by lowercase letters q, r and s. If its amplitude is greater than or equal to 0.5mv, then the wave is represented by capital letters Q, R and S. Common configurations of the QRS complex are in Fig. 51.17.

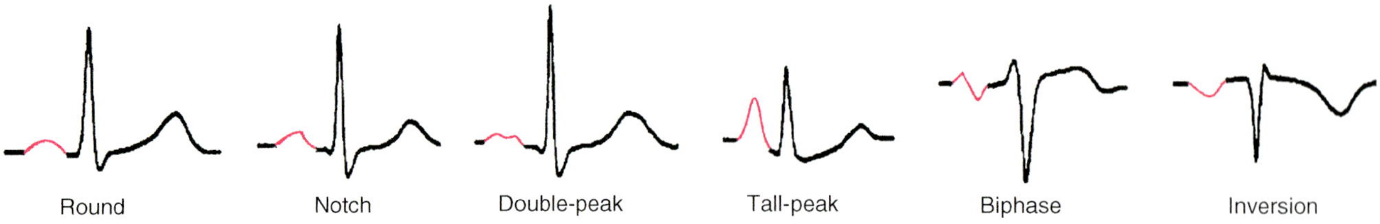

Fig. 51.16 Common configuration of P wave

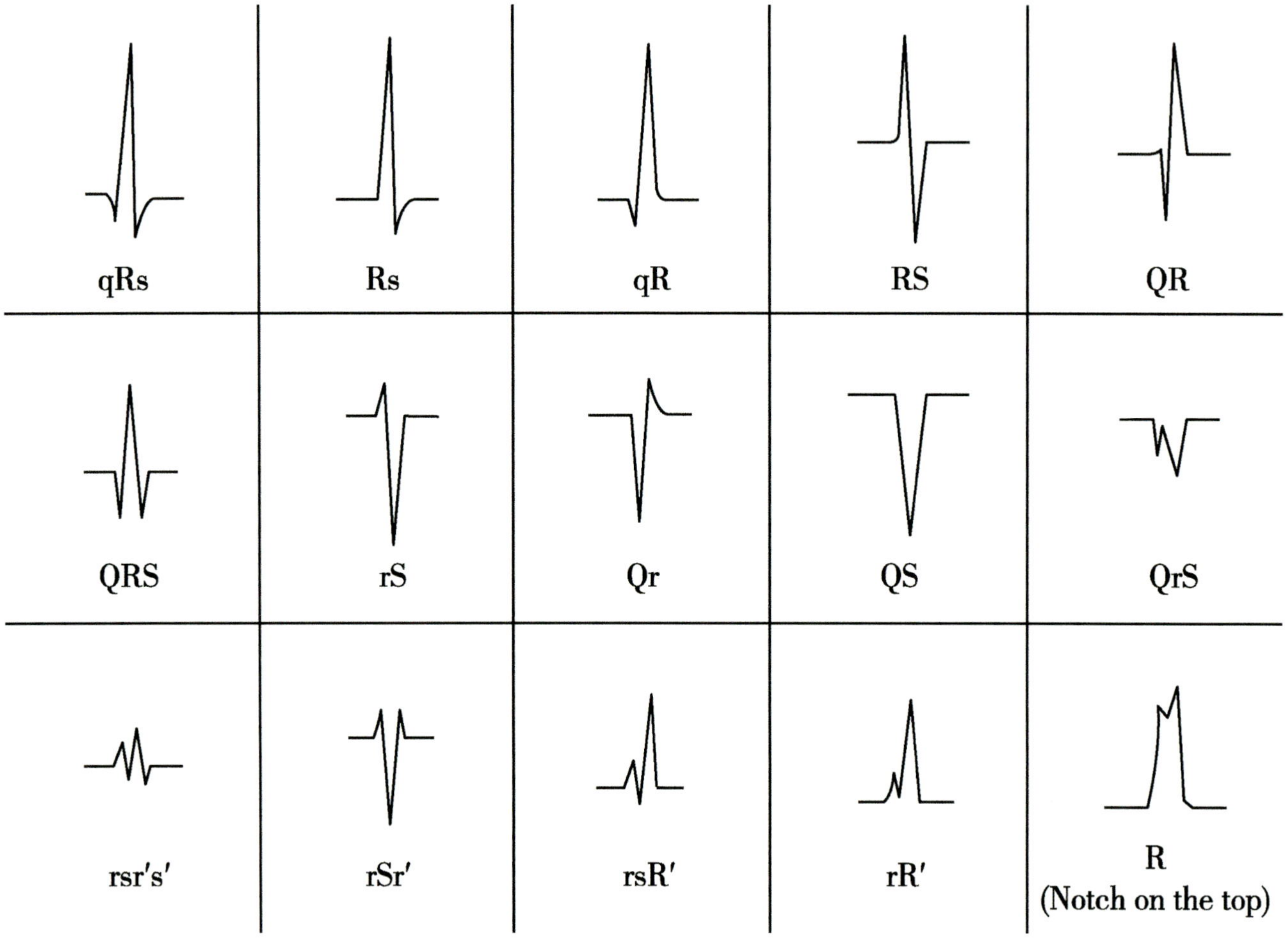

Fig. 51.17 Common configurations of the QRS complex

51.2.4 ST Segment

ST segment is the line that connects the end of QRS complex and the beginning of T wave, representing the slow process of ventricular depolarization. See Fig. 51.18 for the common variants of ST segment.

51.2.5 T Wave

T wave is a deflection that follows ST segment and represents rapid repolarization across the ventricle. Like P wave, T wave has multiple variants: upright, notched, flattening, positive-negative biphasic, negative-positive biphasic and inverted. See Fig. 51.19.

51.2.6 QT Interval

QT interval measures the time from the beginning of QRS complex to the end of T wave, representing the whole process of ventricular depolarization and repolarization. QT interval is frequently affected by heart rate. When heart rate is between 60 and 100 bpm, duration of QT interval is

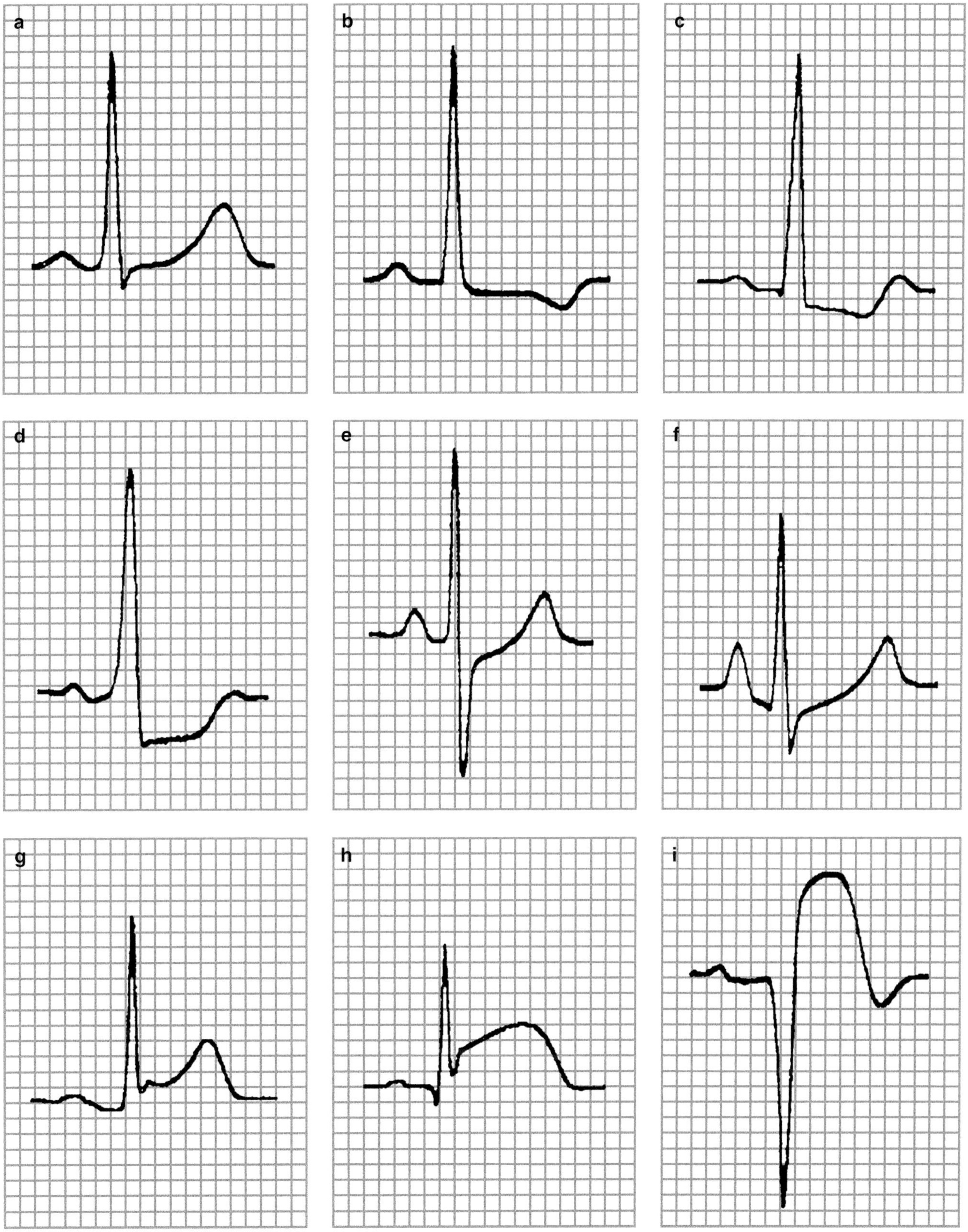

Fig. 51.18 Common deviations of ST Segment. (**a**) Normal ST segment, (**b**) Horizontal ST depression, (**c**) Down-sloping ST depression, (**d**) Horizontal ST depression, (**e**) J Point depression (J point is the point between the end of QRS complex and the beginning of ST segment), (**f**) Up-sloping ST depression, (**g**) Concave ST elevation, (**h**) Convex ST elevation, (**i**) Convex ST elevation

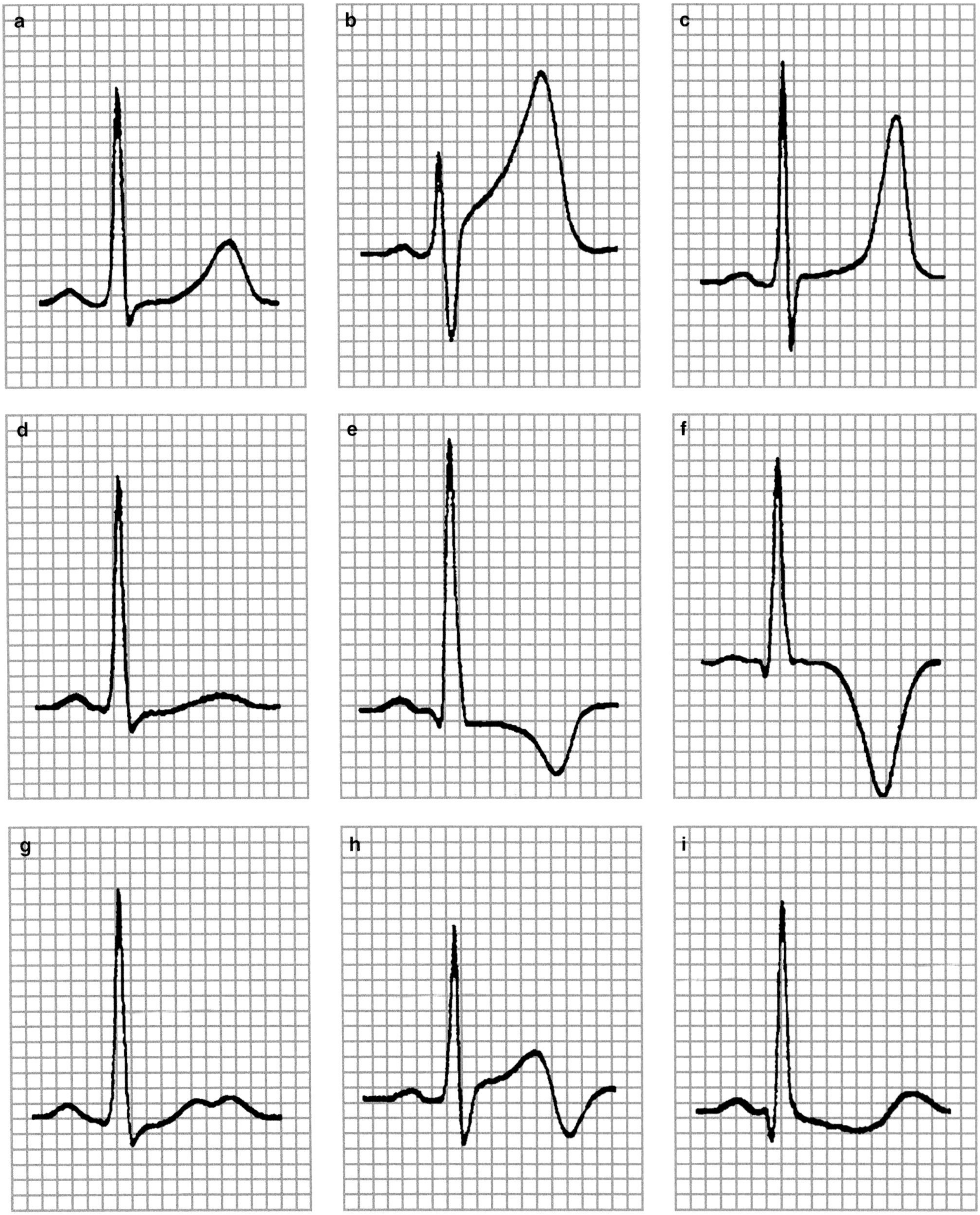

Fig. 51.19 Common deviations of T WAVE. (**a**) Normal T wave, (**b**) Peaked T wave, (**c**) Tall peaked T wave, (**d**) Flattening T wave, (**e**) Asymmetrically inverted T wave, (**f**) Symmetrically inverted T wave, (**g**) "Camel Hump" T wave, (**h**) Positive-negative biphasic T wave, (**i**) Negative-positive biphasic T wave

0.32–0.44 s. To eliminate its effect on QT interval, we can calculate a corrected value of QT interval (QTc) by the following equation: $QTc = QT/\sqrt{RR}$, which represents the QT interval at 60 bpm.

51.2.7 U Wave

U wave is a small deflection that follows T wave, and its generating mechanism remains unknown. More details will be discussed later.

52 Graphics-Sequenced Interpretation of ECG

Rui Zeng

After learning the basics of ECG in previous sections, now we come to the part learning how to interpret ECG. Based on experience of years of clinical teaching, the author had summarized a simple and practical study method—Graphics-Sequenced Interpretation of ECG. There are two key words here, one is ECG Graphics, which means understanding the mechanisms that cause normal and abnormal ECG tracing and memorizing them based on Graphics. Another one is Sequence, which means interpreting an ECG tracing following the order that it is generated (P wave, PR interval, QRS complex, ST segment, T wave, QT interval, U wave). In this way, analysis of ECG can be quite easy and would not miss any significant diagnostic information. In following study, we will learn how to use this method to interpret ECG. In general, when you come across an ECG tracing, you should follow these steps:

- **Step 1: Calculating heart rate in regular or irregular rhythm**
- **Step 2: Analyze P wave**
- **Step 3: Analyze PR interval**
- **Step 4: Analyze QRS complex**
- **Step 5: Analyze ST segment**
- **Step 6: Analyze T wave**
- **Step 7: Other ECG variants**

52.1 Section 1: Calculating Heart Rate in Regular or Irregular Rhythm

52.1.1 Regular Rhythm

When the rhythm is regular in an ECG tracing, heart rate is determined by two successive PR intervals. In previous sections, we have studied the significance and function of boxes, now let us review this part. In every horizontal axis, a small box represents time, which stands for 40 ms; 5 × 5 small boxes comprise a large box, which stands for 200 ms; 5 large boxes grouped together count exactly 1 s. See Fig. 52.1.

Therefore, based on the understanding of boxes, when the rhythm is regular we can calculate heart rate by counting

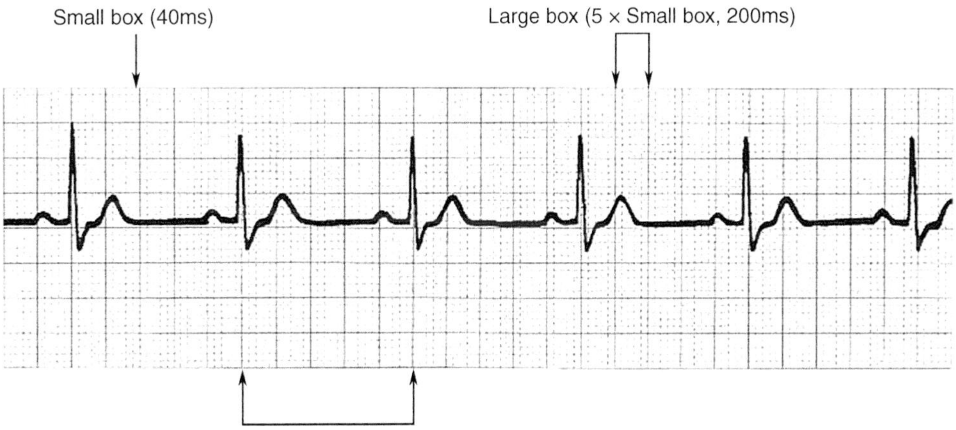

Fig. 52.1 Review basic information of boxes

This chapter is reprinted with permission from: Rui Zeng, Fengrui Cheng, Lixia Deng et al, P Wave. In the book: Graphics-sequenced interpretation of ECG. ISBN: 978-981-287-953-0. Springer, 2016.

R. Zeng (✉)
Department of Cardiology, Sichuan University, Chengdu, China

X.-H. Wan, R. Zeng (eds.), *Handbook of Clinical Diagnostics*, https://doi.org/10.1007/978-981-13-7677-1_52

the boxes. See Fig. 52.2 for more details. For example, the time of one large box is 0.2 s, the heart rate could be calculated by 60/0.2 = 300 bpm, two large box is 60/0.4 = 150 bpm, and so on.

52.1.2 Irregular Rhythm

When the rhythm is irregular in an ECG tracing, we could first count heart beats in 6 s, and then multiply the count by 10 to get heart rate. For example in Fig. 52.3, the count of heart beat in 6 s is 10, then the heart rate is: 10 × 10 = 100 bpm.

52.2 Section 2: Analyze P Wave

The P wave is the first deflection in the P-QRS-T complex, representing the potential changes produced by the depolarization of the right and left atrium.

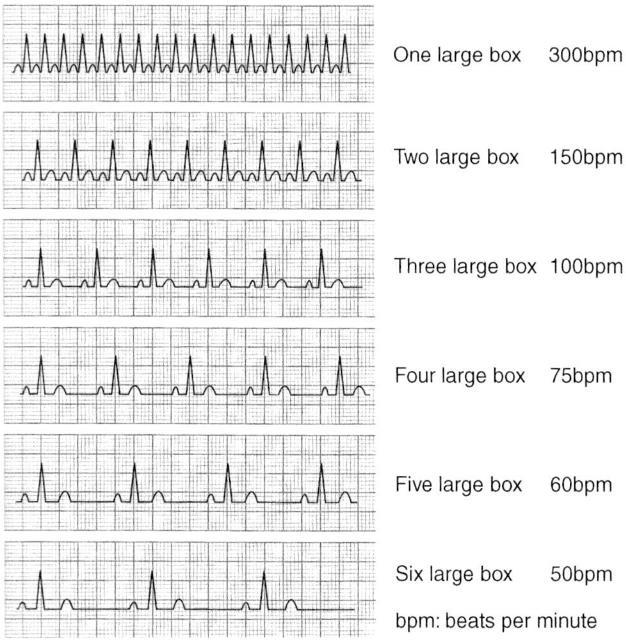

Fig. 52.2 Heart rate and corresponding boxes in regular rhythm

52.2.1 Sinus P Wave

Normal sinus P wave generate from the sinus node, which is located at the junction of the superior vena cava and the right atrium. The sinus node discharges electrical impulses to activate the atrium, forming a depolarization vector in atrium, which mainly points to lower left (Fig. 52.4). Considering the hexaxial reference system and the axes of chest leads, we can see: the atrial depolarization vectors are positive in leads I, II, aVF, V_4 to V_6, following the pattern in lead II; while they are negative in lead aVR, obviously opposite to the pattern in lead II. Then we can draw a brief conclusion about the ECG features of the normal sinus P wave.

52.2.1.1 Characteristics of the Normal Sinus P Wave

1. P wave in sinus rhythm appears small, rounded, and upright in leadsI, II, aVF, V_4 to V_6.
2. Sinus P wave is inverted in lead aVR.
3. In other leads, it can be upright, inverted, or biphasic (half upright, half inverted).
4. Normal duration of sinus P wave should be less than 0.12 s, and amplitude of P wave less than 0.25 mV in limb leads or less than0.2 mV in chest leads (Fig. 52.5).

52.2.1.2 Abnormality in Frequency of Sinus P Wave

The frequency of normal P wave is 60 to100 bpm. When the frequency is less than 60 bpm, it is sinus bradycardia (Fig. 52.6); when it is more than 100 bpm, it is sinus tachycardia (Fig. 52.7).

Sinus Bradycardia

ECG Recognition (Fig. 52.6)

1. Sinus P wave is present.
2. The frequency of P wave is less than 60 bpm.
3. It may be accompanied by sinus arrhythmia.

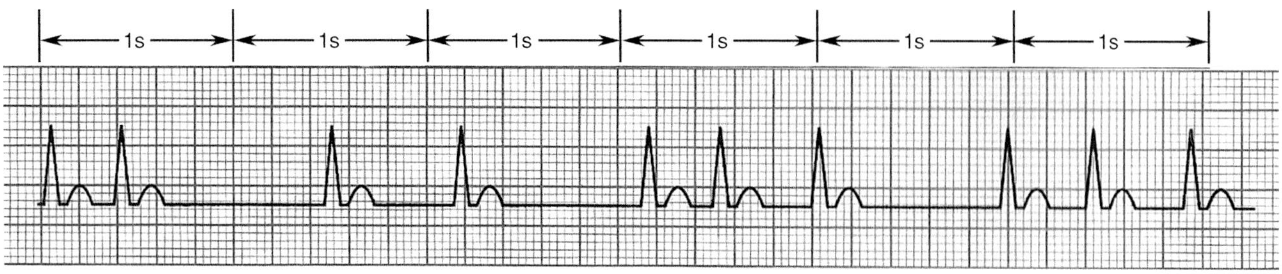

Fig. 52.3 Calculating heart rate in irregular rhythm

Fig. 52.4 Cause of the morphology of sinus P wave

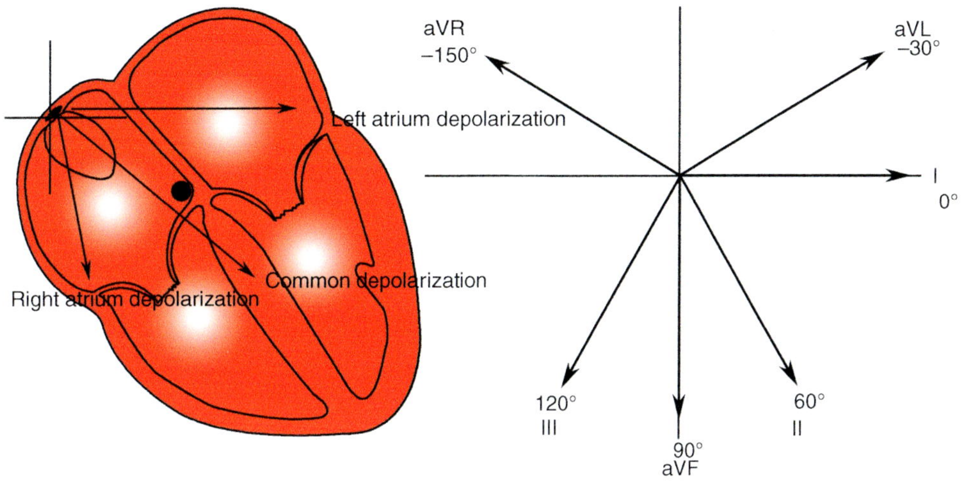

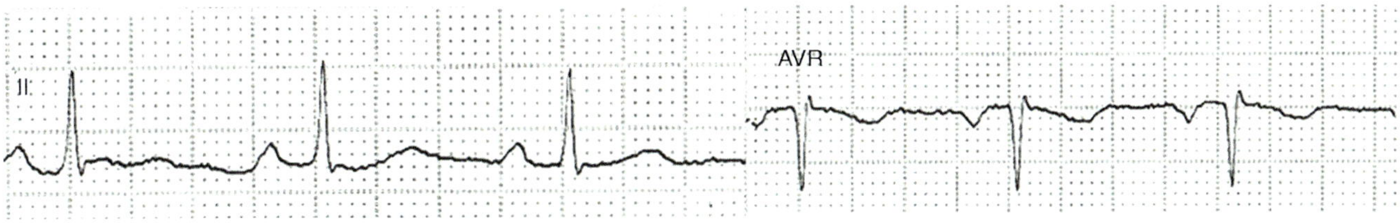

Fig. 52.5 Sinus P wave: P wave is upright in lead II, and inverted in lead aVR

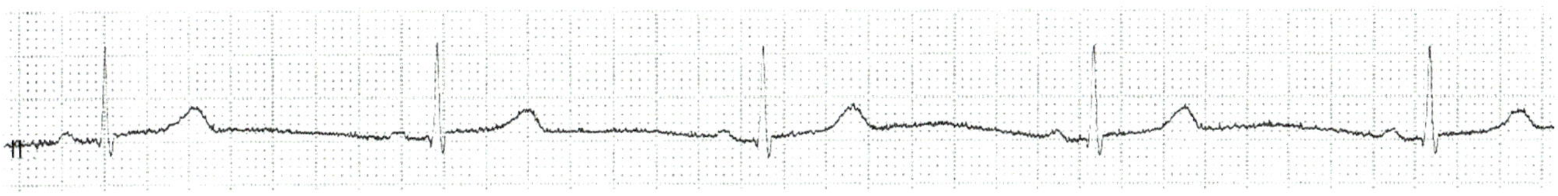

Fig. 52.6 Sinus bradycardia

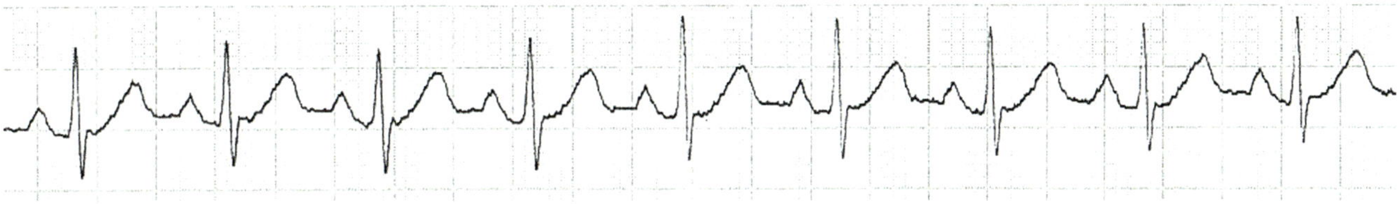

Fig. 52.7 Sinus tachycardia

Sinus Tachycardia

ECG Recognition (Fig. 52.7)

1. Sinus rhythm.
2. The frequency of P wave is more than 100 bpm or maybe higher in children

52.2.1.3 Abnormality in Voltage or Duration of Sinus P Wave

Since the sinus node is located at the junction of the superior vena cava and the right atrium, the electrical impulses discharged by the excited sinus node first activate the right atrium, then the left atrium. The depolarization of all atria is reflected by P wave on ECG; therefore, the right atrial depolarization takes the first 2/3 of P wave and the depolarization of the left atrium takes the last 2/3, which means the middle 1/3 of the P wave is the sum of synchronal depolarization of right and left atriums (Fig. 52.8).Normal P wave appears small and rounded in lead II, and positive-negative biphasic in lead V_1. Lead II and lead V_1 are regarded as the best leads to analyze the electrical activities of both atria on ECG.

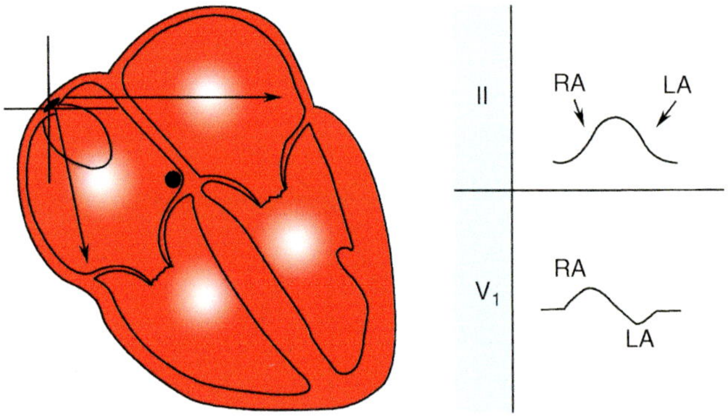

Fig. 52.8 Compositions of sinus P wave

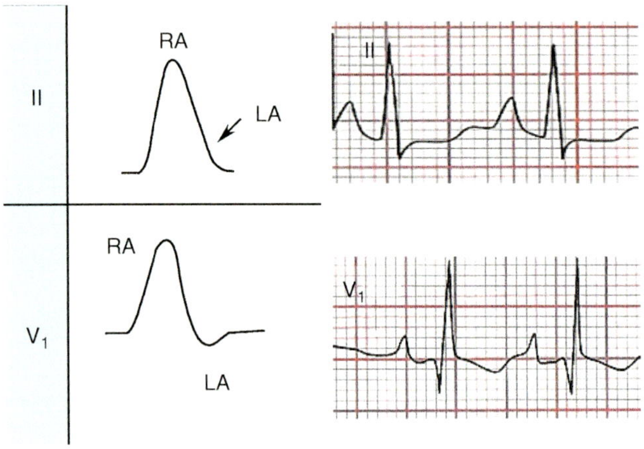

Fig. 52.9 Right atrial enlargement

Abnormality in Voltage of Sinus P Wave (Right Atrial Enlargement)

If right atrial enlargement exists, the right atrial depolarization vector which directs anteriorly to the right bottom will increase. The increased depolarization vector is closer to the positive direction of leads II, III, aVF, causing P wave to be tall and peaked and obviously increased amplitude in leads I, III, aVF.

ECG Recognition (Fig. 52.9)

1. In leads II, III, aVF, P wave is abnormally tall and peaked, and the voltage exceeds 0.25 mV (P pulmonale).
2. Electrical axis of P wave often exceeds 70°.
3. The duration of the P wave is still within normal range.

Abnormality in Duration of Sinus P Wave (Left Atrial Enlargement)

If left atrial enlargement exists, the prolonged depolarization time will broaden the P wave on ECG. Besides, as a result of the increased left atrial depolarization vector, the resultant atrial depolarization vector points left posteriorly (much closer to the direction of leads I, II, avR and avL), and opposite to the direction of lead V_1 on the horizontal plane. P wave in leads I, II, aVR, and aVL could be obvious widened and also the widening of negative portion in lead V_1 (Fig. 52.10).

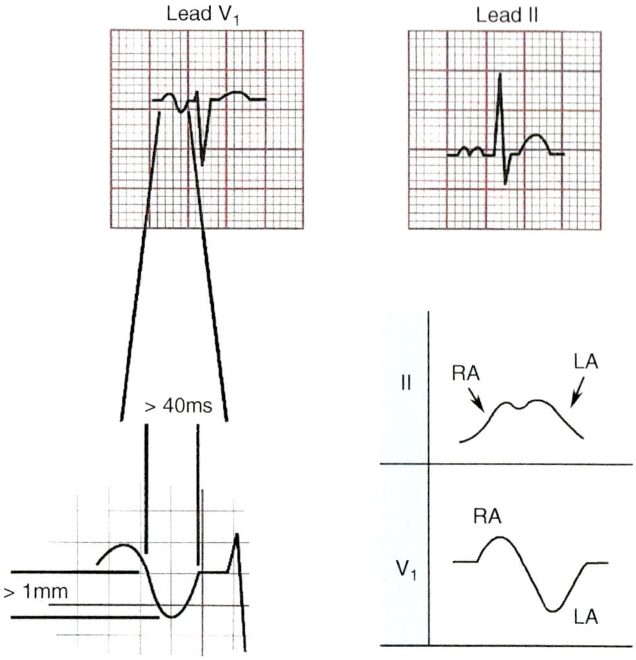

Fig. 52.10 Left atrial enlargement

ECG Recognition (Fig. 52.10)

1. P wave in leads I, II, aVR, and aVL is widened to over 0.12 s (P mitrale).
2. P waves are mostly double-peaked. The second peak is often bigger than the first one, and the duration of the P wave often exceeds 0.04 s.
3. In lead V_1, the voltage of the P wave increases to over 2 mV, and appear biphasic. The terminal negative portion were apparently widened (>40 ms) and deepened (>1 mm), which makes the Ptf-V_1 ≤ -0.04 mm·s (Ptf-V_1 is the terminal vector in lead V_1, the cross product of the negative depth (mm) and duration (s) of the P wave in lead V_1).

52.2.2 Non-Sinus P Wave

After the former discussion, readers are supposed to understand the characteristics of waveform of the sinus P wave and be able to conduct rough ECG diagnosis using the morphological features of the sinus P wave. Since the sinus P wave exists, non-sinus P wave exists correspondingly. First let's draw an overview of the morphological features of non-sinus P wave according to those of sinus P wave.

1. **Morphology of non-sinus P wave:** Though the P wave is upright in lead II and inverted in lead aVR, its morphology is different from normal sinus P wave.

2. **Manifestation of non-sinus P wave**: The P wave is inverted in lead II and upright in lead aVR. It is generated by the impulse conducted retrogradely through the atrioventricular node, then excites the atria and produces the P wave (retrograde P wave).

52.2.2.1 Morphology of Non-Sinus P Wave (Atrial P Wave)

Premature Atrial Contraction

The contraction from the atrial ectopic pacemaker that occurs earlier than expectation is called premature atrial contraction. Since it originates in the atrial ectopic pacemaker, different atrial depolarization sequence is produced comparing with sinus pacemaker. As a consequence, P wave generated under this circumstance is different from sinus ones, and in order to distinguish them, we use P′ instead.

ECG Recognition (Fig. 52.11)

1. P′ wave that occurs prematurely is different from sinus P wave morphologically.
2. P′ waves are usually followed by QRS complex with normal morphology and duration (normal anterograde conduction, Figure 52.11a); a few P′ waves are followed by wide, bizarre QRS complex (aberrant conduction, Fig. 52.11b); a few other P′ waves are followed by no QRS complex (nonconduction, Fig. 52.11c).
3. The P′-R interval is no less than 0.12 s.
4. In most cases, the compensatory pause is incomplete.

Atrial Escape Contraction

Escape contraction and premature contraction are a pair of opposite concepts; the former means the impulses are discharged later than expectation, and the latter comes earlier than expectation. The occurrence of atrial escape contraction mainly because:

1. The sinus node, for some reason, cannot discharge impulses normally (including the rate of impulses slowing down or asystole).
2. The impulses cannot anterogradely conduct due to conduction disturbances.
3. Other reasons that can cause a long pause. In this case, the downstream ectopic pacemaker will be released from the suppression of normal rates and discharge impulses in its natural cycles. When only 1 or 2 impulses are discharged by them, it is called escape contraction, and if 3 impulses or more are discharged consecutively, it is called escape rhythm.

According to different original sites, there is atrial escape contraction (rare, Fig. 52.12), junctional escape contraction (the most common type, Fig. 52.15), and ventricular contraction (common, discussed in detail in Step 4).

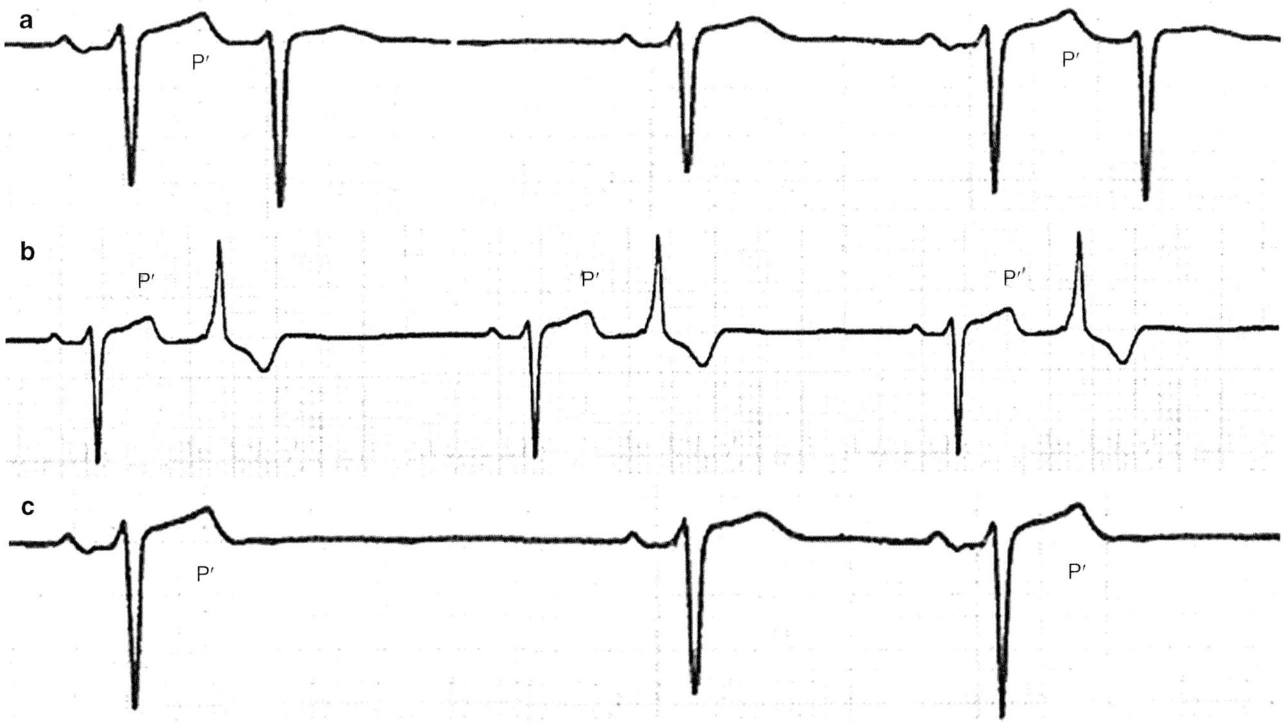

Fig. 52.11 Premature atrial contraction. (**a**) Normal anterograde conduction; (**b**) Aberrant conduction; (**c**) Non-conduction

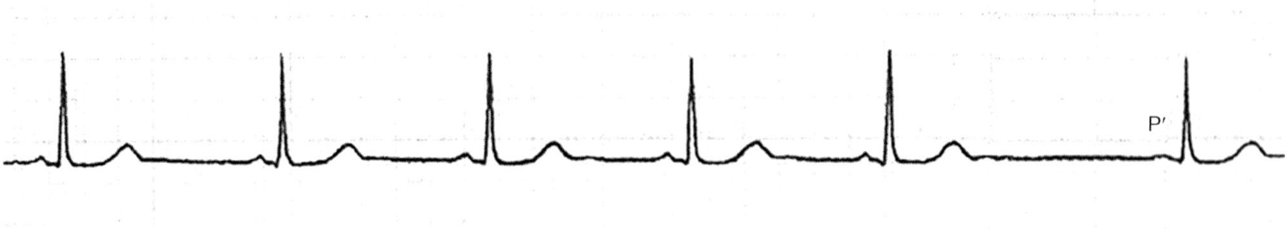

Fig. 52.12 Atrial escape contraction

ECG Recognition (Fig. 52.12)

1. P′ appears after a long pause and is different from the sinus P wave morphologically.
2. The P′-R interval is no less than 0.12 s.
3. P′ is followed by QRS complex with normal morphology and duration; wide, bizarre QRS complex is rare.
4. It is called atrial escape contraction if there are 1–2 abnormal contractions discussed above; it is called atrial escape rhythm if 3 or more such contractions are seen in a row, and the rate normally ranges between 50 and 60 bpm.

52.2.2.2 Manifestation of Non-Sinus P Wave (Retrograde P′ Wave)

Premature Atrial Contraction

Ectopic pacemaker located in lower part of the atria discharges impulses ahead of time, and produces retrograde P′ waves (Fig. 52.13).

ECG Recognition (Fig. 52.13)

1. Retrograde P′ wave which occurs ahead of time and precedes QRS complex.
2. P′ waves are usually followed by QRS complexes of normal morphology and duration (normal anterograde conduction); a few P′ waves are followed by wide, bizarre QRS complexes (aberrant conduction); a few other P′ waves are followed by no QRS complexes (non-conduction).
3. The P′-R interval is no less than 0.12 s.
4. Usually the compensatory pause is incomplete.

Premature Junctional Contraction

The impulse discharged ahead of time by the ectopic pacemaker at the atrioventricular junction is called premature junctional contraction. The junctional impulse which appears early is able to conduct anterogradely and retrogradely at the same time. Retrograde conduction activates the atria and subsequently produces retrograde P′ waves, while anterograde conduction activates the ventricles and produce QRS complexes. Due to different velocities of retrograde and anterograde conduction, the retrograde P′ wave may present before (Fig. 52.14a) or after the QRS complex (Fig. 52.14b). Mainly based on the P′-R interval and whether the compensatory pause is complete or not, we can distinguish the premature junctional contraction from the premature atrial contraction when retrograde P′ wave precedes the QRS complex. If the P′-R interval is no less than 0.12 s and the compensatory pause is not complete, it is premature atrial contraction; if P′-R interval less than 0.12 s with a complete compensatory pause, it is premature junctional contraction.

ECG Recognition (Fig. 52.14)

1. QRS complexes that occur ahead of time usually have normal morphology, or sometimes become bizarre as a result of aberrant intraventricular conduction.
2. The retrograde P′ wave may appear before the QRS complex (the P′-R interval is less than 0.12 s in adults, no more than 0.10s in children, or differs largely from the sinus P-R interval), after the QRS complex (the P′-R interval < 0.20s), or be buried in the QRS complex and difficult to distinguish (absent P wave).
3. Usually the compensatory pause is complete.

Junctional Escape Contraction

Junctional escape contraction is defined as escape contraction which originates from the junction of atria and ventricles (Fig. 52.15).

ECG Recognition (Fig. 52.15)

1. QRS complex with normal morphology and duration appears after a relatively long pause.
2. Absence of P wave or relevant P wave before most QRS complex in escape contraction. However, presence of retrograde P′ wave could be discovered before or after few QRS complexes, in which case, P′R interval is less than 0.12 s if the retrograde P′ wave is before QRS complex, and RP′ interval is less than 0.20 s if it is after.

52.2.3 Absence of P Wave

52.2.3.1 Atrial Flutter

Atrial flutter is a fast heart rhythm. The main characteristic of atrial flutter is that p waves disappear from ECG tracing in each lead, replaced by flutter waves (F waves). Atrial flutter is usually instable, it can be restored to sinus rhythm, or

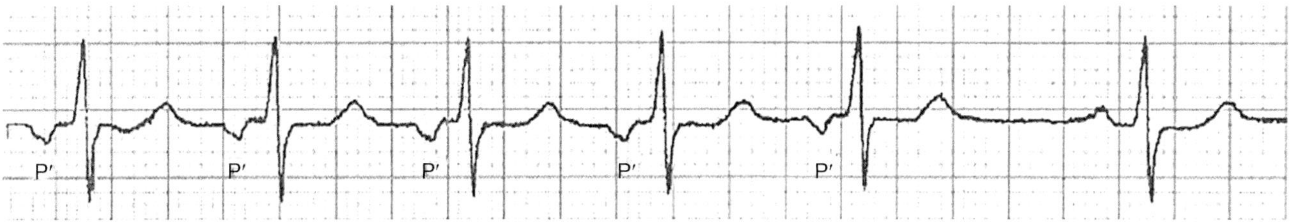

Fig. 52.13 Premature atrial contraction with retrograde P′ waves

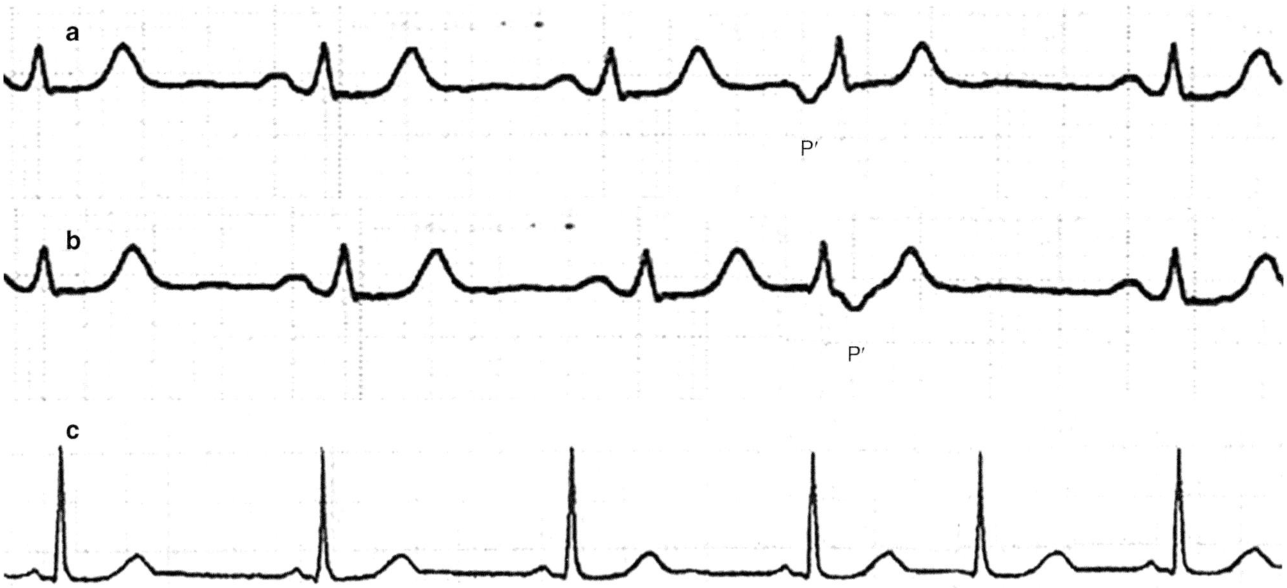

Fig. 52.14 Premature junctional contraction. (**a**) retrograde P′ waves appear before the QRS complexes. (**b**) retrograde P′ waves appear after the QRS complexes. (**c**) Retrograde P′ wave is buried in the QRS complex

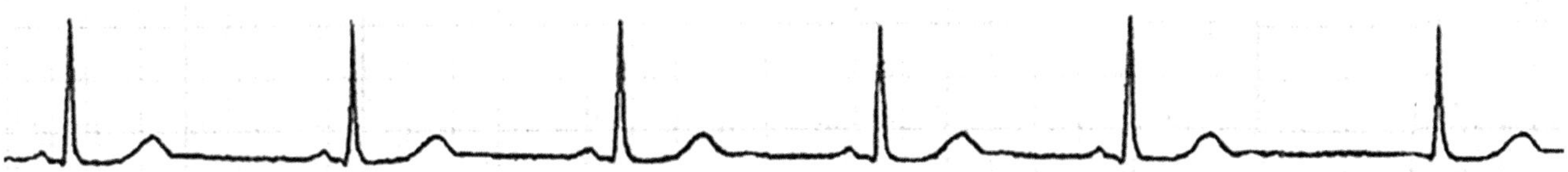

Fig. 52.15 Juncitonal escape contraction

develop into atrial fibrillation,while in some cases, atrial flutter can last for quite a long time.

ECG Recognition (Fig. 52.16)

1. P waves disappear from all leads, replaced by F waves.
2. F waves have a wavelike or saw-toothed appearance, with uniform sizes and F-F interval.
3. F waves usually have a frequency of 250–350 bpm.
4. F: R ratio is usually 2:1, so ventricular rate is 140–160 bpm.
5. QRS complex is usually normal, but can manifest aberrant intraventricular conduction, especially when the conduction ratio appears to be 2:1 and 4:1 alternatively, the heart beat which appeared in the long-short cardiac cycle might be easy to show intraventricular aberrant conduction.

52.2.3.2 Atrial Fibrillation

Atrial fibrillation, is a heart rhythm even faster than atrial flutter. Its main ECG feature is that P waves from each lead disappear and are replaced by small fibrillatory waves (f waves).

ECG Recognition (Fig. 52.17)

1. P waves disappear from every lead, replaced by f waves.
2. Fibrillatory waves are not uniform in size and appearance, nor interval, with a frequency of 450–600 bpm.

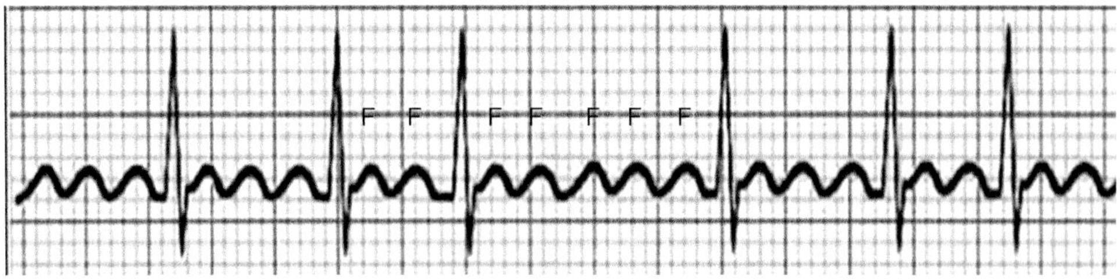

Fig. 52.16 Atrial flutter

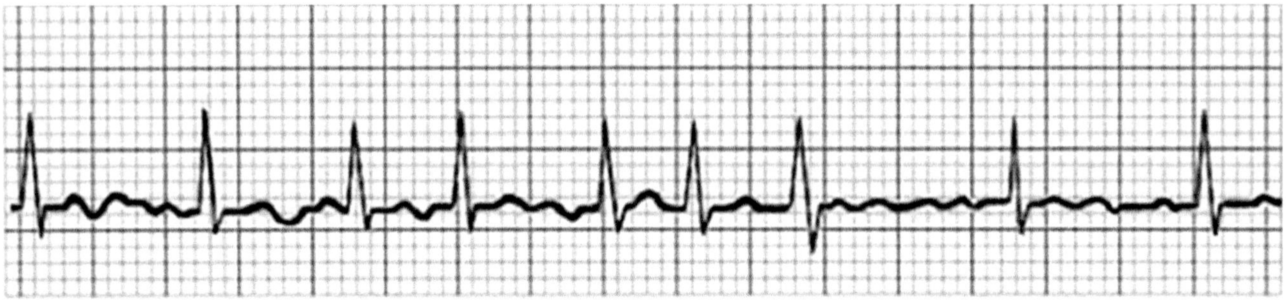

Fig. 52.17 Atrial fibrillation

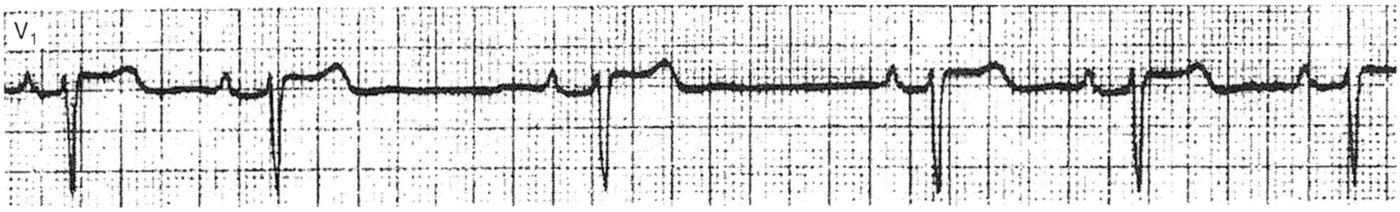

Fig. 52.18 Sinus arrest

3. RR intervals are uneven.
4. Ventricular rate usually increases, but do not exceed 160 bpm. It can be slowed down after administration of digitalis or during chronic atrial fibrillation.
5. QRS complex is normal, but because of the big fluctuation of ventricular cycle, the heart beat which appeared in the long-short cardiac cycle might be easy to show intraventricular aberrant conduction.

52.2.3.3 Sinus Arrest

Sinus arrest is also known as sinus pause, during which SA nodes stop generating electrical impulses due to certain reasons in a period of time, causing the atria or the entire heart to stop functioning. During this time, lower patent pacemakers usually discharge in place of the SA node, presenting an escape contraction or rhythm.

ECG Recognition (Figure 52.18)

1. Sinus rhythm.
2. A long PP interval appears in a regular sinus rhythm.
3. The long interval does not form a fixed ratio with the normal sinus PP interval.
4. The long interval is usually followed by an escape contraction or rhythm.

52.2.3.4 Sinoatrial Block

Although the function of sinus itself is normal, but disturbance conduction between the sinoatrial node and atria, this situation is known as sinoatrial block. Sinoatrial block can be divided into first-degree, second-degree and third-degree. While both first-degree (sinus node potentials cannot be recorded by ECG) and third degree (it cannot be differentiated with sinus arrest by ECG) sinoatrial block are unable to diagnosis by ECG, we could only make diagnosis of second degree sinoatrial block (Type I and II).

Second Degree Sinoatrial Block (Type I)

ECG Recognition (Fig. 52.19)

1. Sinus rhythm.
2. The PP interval is progressively decreased with each beat until one P wave dropped, a long PP interval appears.
3. The long PP interval is less than two times of the shortest PP interval.
4. The shortest PP interval is always present before the long PP interval.
5. Sinoatrial conduction ratio is usually at 3:2,4:3 or 5:4.

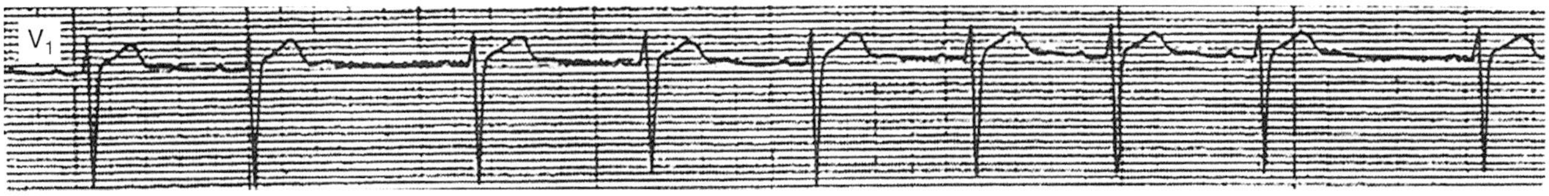

Fig. 52.19 Second degree sinoatrial block (Type I)

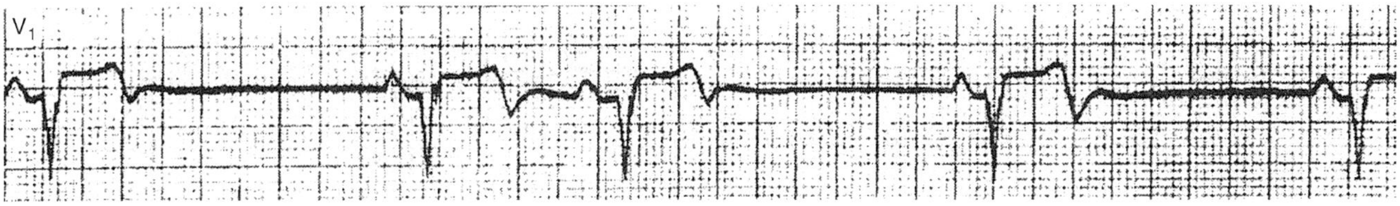

Fig. 52.20 Second degree sinoatrial block (Type II)

Second Degree Sinoatrial Block (Type II)

ECG Recognition (Fig. 52.20)

1. Sinus rhythm.
2. A long PP interval appears in a regular sinus rhythm.
3. The long interval does form a fixed ratio with the normal sinus PP interval.
4. Sinoatrial conduction ratio is usually at 3:2, 4:3 or 5:4.

52.3 Section 3: Analyze PR Interval

The PR interval is defined as the interval between the beginning of the P wave and the beginning of the QRS complex, representing the depolarization time from the atria to the ventricles.

52.3.1 The Normal PR Interval

The normal PR interval is usually between 0.12 and 0.20 s, and it is greatly affected by age and heart rate of the patient. This interval usually decreases with faster heartbeat or in early childhood while increases with slower heartbeat or in old age. Therefore, the normal range of the PR interval varies with regard to different age and heart rate of the patient (Table Table 52.1).

52.3.2 Abnormal PR Interval

Generally, a prolonged PR interval longer than 0.20 s is an indication of delayed conduction from the atria to the ventricles, and the patient is said to have atrioventricular block with different causes; shortened PR interval less than 0.12 s on the other hand, is an indication of enhanced conduction from the atria to the ventricles, which is often seen in preexcitation syndromes.

52.3.2.1 Prolonged PR Interval (Atrioventricular Block)

Atrioventricular block (AV block, AVB) is the impaired impulse conduction from the atria to the ventricles due to pathologically prolonged refractory period of some parts in the atrioventricular conduction pathways. AV block could mean delayed, incompletely or completely blocked impulse conduction.

The ECG tracing of atrial depolarization is the P wave, while the ventricular depolarization the QRS complexes. Normally, every P wave is followed by a corresponding QRS complex, and the time duration of the PR interval will not exceed a certain range. When there is an AV block, the ECG shows the association between P wave and the corresponding QRS complex is abnormal: the PR interval may prolong, or the corresponding QRS complex is absent after the P wave.

AV block can be divided into first-degree, second-degree, high-degree and third-degree according to the severity. First-degree, second-degree and high-degree are also known as incomplete AV block, while third-degree AV block is also known as the complete AV block.

First-Degree AV Block

First-degree AV block is a delay of conduction from the atria to the ventricles, characterized by the PR interval prolonged over the normal range of ECG. However, every supraventricular impulse is able to pass to the ventricles without any dropped beats no matter how long the PR interval is.

ECG Recognition (Fig. 52.21)

1. The PR interval is more than 0.20 s (>0.22 s in the elderly, >0.18 s in children under the age of 14). The PR intervals are mostly between 0.21 s and 0.35 s.
2. The PR interval is greatly affected by age and heart rate of the patient. Additionally, in patients with first-degree AV block, the PR interval is longer than the upper limit

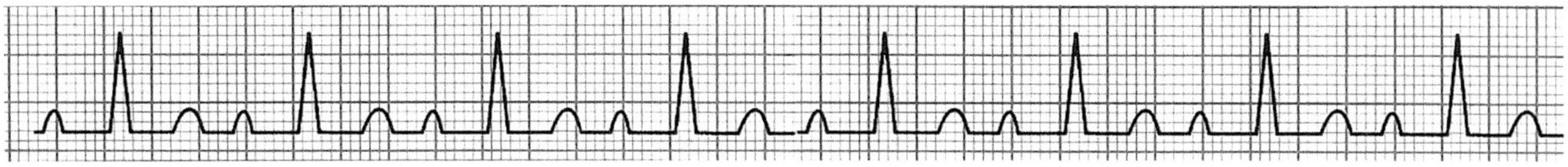

Fig. 52.21 First-degree AV block

Table 52.1 Age, heart rate and maximum of PR interval(s)

Heart rate (bpm)	<70	71–90	91–110	111–130	>130
Age (years) 18	0.20	0.19	0.18	0.17	0.16
Age (years) 14–17	0.19	0.18	0.17	0.16	0.15
Age (years) 7–13	0.18	0.17	0.16	0.15	0.14
Age (years) 1.5–6	0.17	0.165	0.155	0.145	0.135
Age (years) 0–1.5	0.16	0.15	0.145	0.135	0.125

normal range corresponding to the patient's age group (see Table 52.1).

3. On two continuous ECG examinations of a patient, the PR interval is shown to be more than 0.04 s longer than that of the previous one without obvious change in the heart rate.

Second-Degree AV Block

In second-degree AV block, the impulses from the atria to the ventricles are partly interrupted, but not every atrial impulse is able to pass through the AV node to the ventricles, which is defined as dropped beat. As shown in ECG, not every P wave is followed by a corresponding QRS complex. Second-degree AV block is first described by Wenckebach and Morbiz, and therefore it is called Wenckebach AV block or Morbiz AV block (type I and type II).

Second-Degree AV Block (Type I), or Mobitz AV Block (Type I), Wenckebach Block

Second-degree AV block (Type I), also known as Wenckebach block or Mobitz AV block (Type I), is the most common type in second-degree AV block. Second-degree AV block (Type I), which is always due to a block within the AV node or in the proximal bundle of His, is mostly a functional block with good prognosis.

ECG Recognition (Fig. 52.22)

1. The PR interval is progressively prolonged with each beat until one QRS complex dropped.
2. The P wave is regular sinus P wave.
3. After the dropped QRS complex, the PR interval is progressively prolonged again until another QRS complex dropped.
4. The ratio of conduction can be fixed or varied, the latter is more common in clinical practice.

Second-Degree AV Block (Type II) or Mobitz AV Block (Type II)

Second-degree AV block (Type II), also known as the Mobitz AV block (Type II), is relatively rare in second-degree AV block. Second-degree AV block (Type II) is mostly an organic disease, or due to a block below the AV node in the distal or branches of bundle of His. Patients with second-degree AV block (Type II) usually have poorer prognosis.

ECG Recognition (Fig. 52.23)

1. The PR interval is constant.
2. Regular P wave with abrupt QRS complex drop.
3. The QRS complexes can be normal (if the block happens in distal bundle of His) or resemble the ECG variant of the bundle branch block or fascicular block in morphology (if the block happens in bundle branch).
4. The conduction ratio can be constant or varied.

High-Degree AV Block

Atrioventricular conduction ratio, which means the ratio of P wave to QRS complex, is often used to measure the severity of AV block. When a tracing shows 4:3 block, it means only three out of four atrial impulses are able to pass to the ventricles with one impulse blocked; similarly, 4:1 block means only one out of four atrial impulses is able to pass to the ventricles with three impulses blocked. High-degree AV blocked is identified when two or more successive P wave impulses are not able to reach the ventricles.

ECG Recognition (Fig. 52.24)

1. The ECG shows 3:1 or greater conduction ratio (e.g. 4:1, 5:1 or 6:1…).
2. As a result of slow ventricular rate, Junctional or ventricular escape rhythm are often present (depending on the blocking site), which in ECG is shown as incomplete AV block.

Third-Degree AV Block

Third-degree AV block is also known as complete AV block. No supraventricular impulses can pass through the AV node to the ventricles. The atria and ventricles are driven by independent pacemakers, resulting in complete AV dissociation. Ventricular capture does not exist in third-degree AV block.

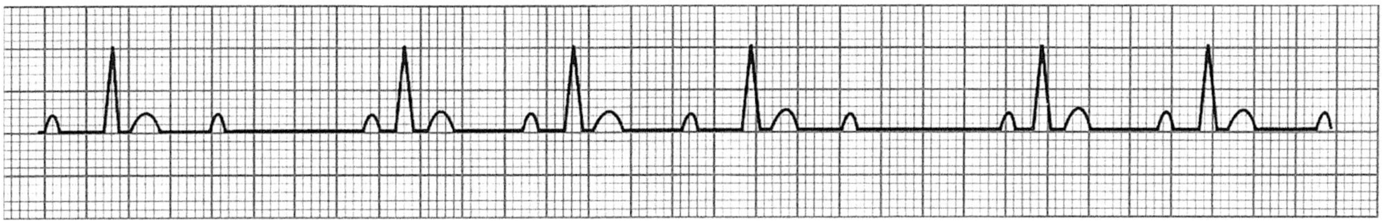

Fig. 52.22 Second-degree AV Block (Type I)

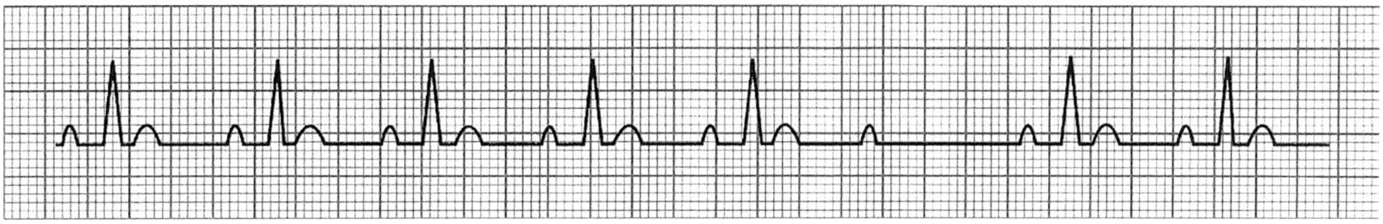

Fig. 52.23 Second-degree AV block (Type II)

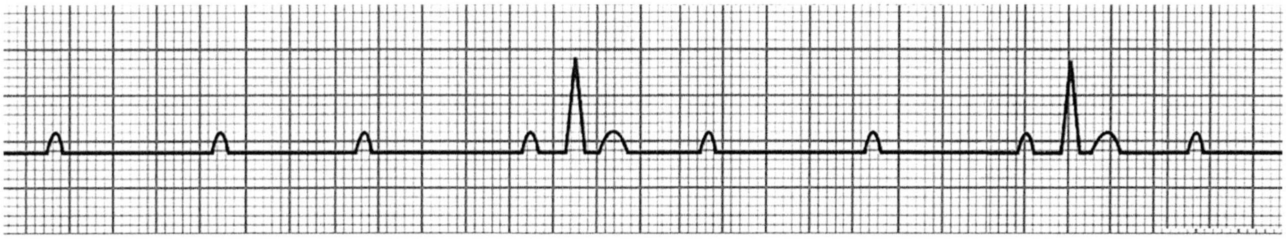

Fig. 52.24 High-degree AV Block

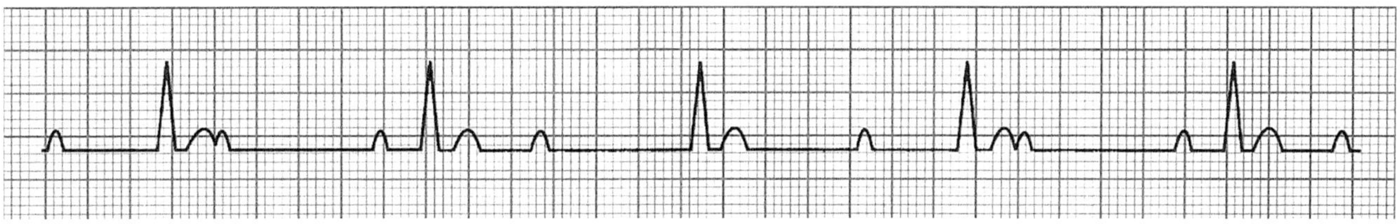

Fig. 52.25 Third-degree AV Block

ECG Recognition (Fig. 52.25)

1. The P-P intervals and R-R intervals follow to their respective pattern.
2. P waves and QRS complexes are not related.
3. P waves appear more frequent than QRS complexes, because P waves are at sinus rate (60 to 100 bpm) while the QRS complexes are at the junctional (40 to 60 bpm) or ventricular (20 to 40 bpm) escape rate.

52.3.2.2 Shortened PR Interval (Preexcitation Syndromes)

The only way by which impulses ordinarily can pass from the atria to the ventricles is through the AV node-His-Purkinje system. In the preexcitation syndromes, there exist abnormal accessory atrioventricular bundles (also known as the accessory pathway). Atrial impulses can pass through the AV node by the normal pathway or the accessory pathway. On account of the electrophysiological properties of the accessory pathway, the impulses which pass through the accessory pathway can reach the ventricles ahead of time, allowing some or all ventricular myocardial cells to be activated prematurely, and its corresponding ECG variant is called the ventricular preexcitation. Moreover, the existence of the accessory pathway has made the atrioventricular reentry possible, causing the atrioventricular reentry tachycardia (AVRT). In clinical practice, preexcitation syndrome is defined as ventricular preexcitation with paroxysmal supraventricular tachycardia (PSVT) on the ECG.

There are two major types of preexcitation syndromes: Wolff-Parkinson-White (WPW) syndrome and Lown-Ganong-Levine (LGL) syndrome.

Wolff-Parkinson-White syndrome

Wolff-Parkinson-White (WPW) syndrome is also known as the bundle of Kent syndrome. It was first reported by Wolff, Parkinson and White in 1930. In WPW syndrome, the accessory pathway has been named the bundle of Kent, which is a discrete aberrant conducting pathway located in the atrioventricular ring and connects the atria and ventricles.

ECG Recognition (Fig. 52.26)

1. The PR interval is less than 0.12 s.
2. The QRS complex longer than 0.12 s.
3. A preexcitation wave (also known as delta wave) is present at the beginning of the QRS complex.
4. The P-J interval is normal.
5. Secondary ST-T segment abnormity.
6. Some patients may experience recurrent onsets of PSVT.

Lown-Ganong-Levine syndrome

Lown-Ganong-Levine (LGL) syndrome is characterized by recurrent onsets of tachycardia clinically, while ECG shows only shortening of the PR interval with normal QRS complex between episodes of tachycardia (Fig. 52.27). It was first reported by Lown, Ganong and Levine in 1952, and therefore designated LGL syndrome. It is also known as the short PR interval syndrome because its manifestation on ECG is basically the shortening of PR interval. The existence of aberrant pathways or James fibers within the AV node is the main cause of LGL syndrome.

ECG Recognition (Fig. 52.27)

1. The PR interval is less than 0.12 s.
2. The QRS complex is normal without delta waves.
3. Some patients may experience recurrent onsets of tachycardia.

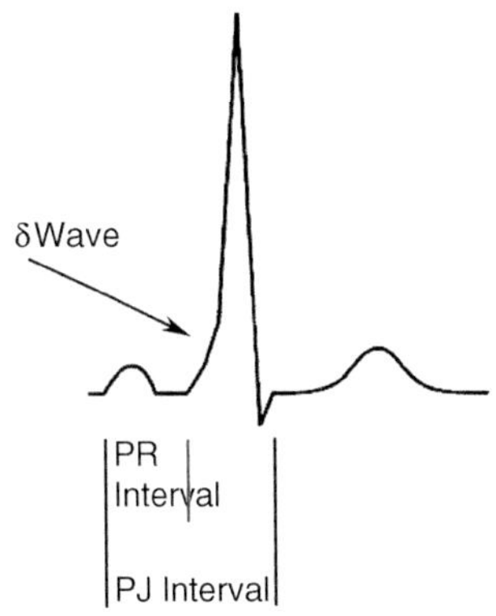

Fig. 52.26 Wolff-Parkinson-White Syndrome

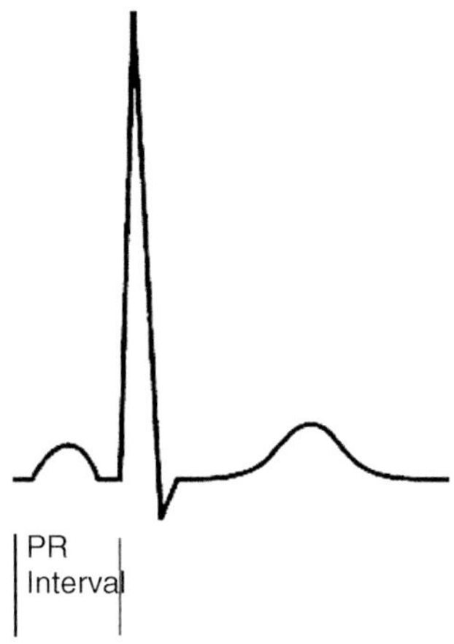

Fig. 52.27 Lown-Ganong-Levine Syndrome

52.4 Section 4: Analyze QRS Complex

52.4.1 Normal QRS Complex

52.4.1.1 Features of Normal QRS Complex and Voltage

Features of Normal QRS Complex

QRS complex is a group of waves of comparatively deep amplitude, and shows the electrical changes during left and right ventricular depolarization. The morphological features of normal QRS complex can be summarized into the main wave's direction and the morphology of Q (q) wave.

1. The main wave is positive in leads I, II and V_4 to V_6; While the main wave is negative in leads aVR and V_1.
2. From lead V_1 to V_6, R wave grows taller, S wave grows smaller, and R/S ratio becomes larger.
3. InleadsV$_1$ and V_2, there should be no Q (q) wave (QS pattern can be present). In leads aVR, aVL, III, there can be Q or q wave. In leads I, II, aVF and V_4 to V_6, Q wave should not be present (q wave is probably present).

Features of Normal QRS Complex Voltage

1. In at least one limb lead, the sum of Q, R, S voltages (sum of the absolute values) is greater than or equal to 0.5 mv.
2. In at least one chest lead, the sum of QRS voltages (sum of the absolute values) is greater than or equal to 0.8 mv.
3. R_{V5} < 2.5 mv, R_{aVL} < 1.2 mv, R_{aVF} < 2.0 mv, R_I < 1.5 mv, $R_{V5} + S_{V1}$ < 3.5–4.0 mv.
4. R_{V1} < 1.0 mv, $R_{V1} + S_{V5}$ < 1.2 mv, R_{aVR} < 0.5mv.

If you think what is mentioned above hard to memorize, don't worry and keep reading, you will find some simple drawing can help you understand and memorize these details with ease.

52.4.1.2 QRS Vector Loop

Since the myocardial cells participating in the depolarization locate in different parts of the heart, the vectors that represent their depolarization can point to different directions, when the ventricles depolarize. The way two vectors interact are if they have the same direction, they are enhanced; if they have opposite directions, they are weakened; if they form angle between 0° and 180°, the diagonal of the parallelogram is defined as their resultant vector, or mean vector (Fig. 52.28). Therefore, the interaction all the vectors have with each other at any moment can be summed into an instant resultant vector.

Since the number and the position of the myocardial cells involved in the depolarization are constantly changing, the length and direction of the instant resultant vector vary at different moment of the ventricular depolarization. If we draw a line to connect the termination of the vectors together in an order, or record the process of the changes, we can get a curve, a vector loop in three dimensional spaces (special QRS vector loop).

(A: Divide the ventricular depolarization into eight parts, record the amplitude and direction of the instantaneous complex vector; B: Draw a line to connect the termination of the vectors together in proper order and you get a QRS vector loop)

52.4.1.3 Formation of Normal QRS Complex in Limb Leads

If we place the QRS vector loop into hexaxial reference system that we've learnt before, we can easily understand the morphology of QRS complex in limb leads (Figs. 52.29, 52.30, 52.31, 52.32).

Similar to the QRS complex in all limb leads, we can understand QRS complex in all six chest leads when the vectors in QRS vector loop are projected on chest lead axes (Fig. 52.33).

After you have learned the basic information about morphology of QRS complex, let us review the features of normal QRS complex again and you could find it is easy to memorize them, also we could use them to diagnosis weird retrograde P′ wave below:

1. The main wave is positive in leads I, II and V_4 to V_6; While the main wave is negative in leads aVR and V_1.
2. From lead V_1 to V_6, R wave grows taller, S wave grows smaller, and R/S ratio becomes larger

52.4.1.4 Weird Retrograde P′ Wave (LA/RA Reversal)

When you are reading an ECG and find retrograde P′ wave (that is, inverted P wave in lead II and upright P wave in lead aVR), you are supposed to consider that misplacement of left and right arm leads could possibly happen, besides atrial or junctional premature contraction.

ECG Recognition (Fig. 52.34)

1. Apparent P′ wave (inverted P wave in lead II and upright P wave in lead aVR)
2. Right axis deviation (pseudo-right axis deviation)
3. Inversion of normal waveform in lead I, interchange of waveform between lead II and lead III, interchange of waveform between lead aVR and lead aVL, normal in lead aVF.
4. Normal pattern of R-wave progression in the chest leads (R wave grows taller, S wave grows smaller from V_1 to V_6)

52.4.1.5 Another Weird Retrograde P′ Wave (Dextrocardia)

Finally, there is yet another possibility for a retrograde P′ wave, congenital dextrocardia. The key to differentiation of dextrocardia from LA/RA Reversal is the pattern of R-wave progression in the chest leads (In the case of dextrocardia, QRS complex shows an rS pattern in all chest leads and regression in amplitude from V_1 to V_6). If retrograde P′ wave shows up with normal R-wave progression, the diagnosis of LA/RA Reversal could be made. Retrograde P′ wave with disturbed R-wave progression reveals dextrocardia.

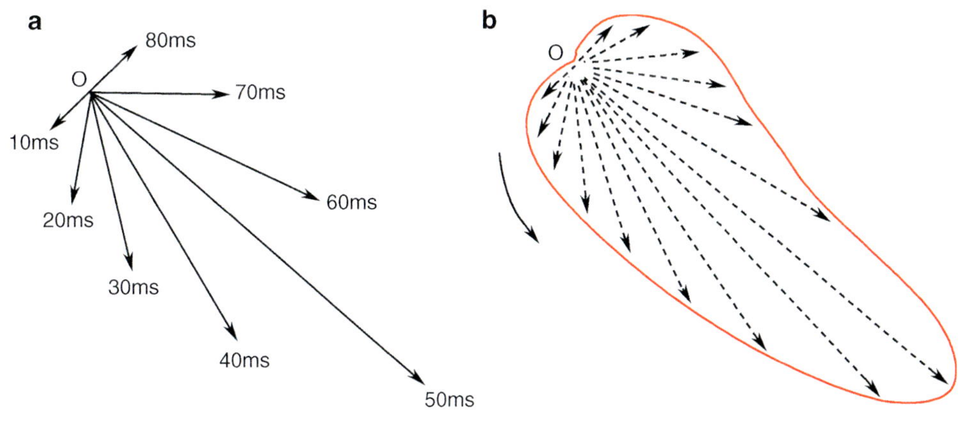

Fig. 52.28 Formation of QRS vector loop

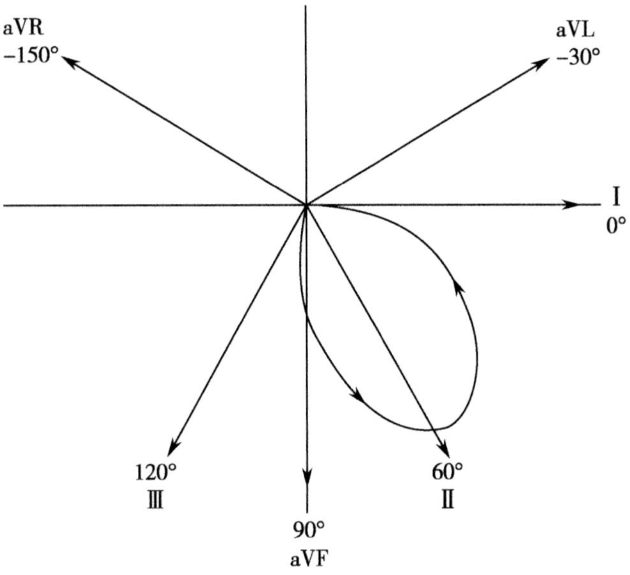

Fig. 52.29 Projection of QRS vector loop on axes in hexaxial reference system

ECG Recognition (Fig. 52.35)

1. Apparent P′ wave (inverted P wave in lead II and upright P wave in lead aVR)
2. Right axis deviation
3. Inversion of normal waveform in lead I, interchange of waveform between lead II and lead III, interchange of waveform between lead aVR and lead aVL, normal in lead aVF.
4. Disturbed R-wave progression (RS complex shows an rS pattern in all chest leads and R wave grows smaller, S wave grows taller in amplitude from V_1 to V_6)

52.4.2 Abnormal QRS Complex

52.4.2.1 Abnormalities in QRS Complex Axis

The direction of ECG axis is usually measured by the angle between the axis and the positive direction of lead I axis. The diagnosis recommended by WHO guideline regarding electric

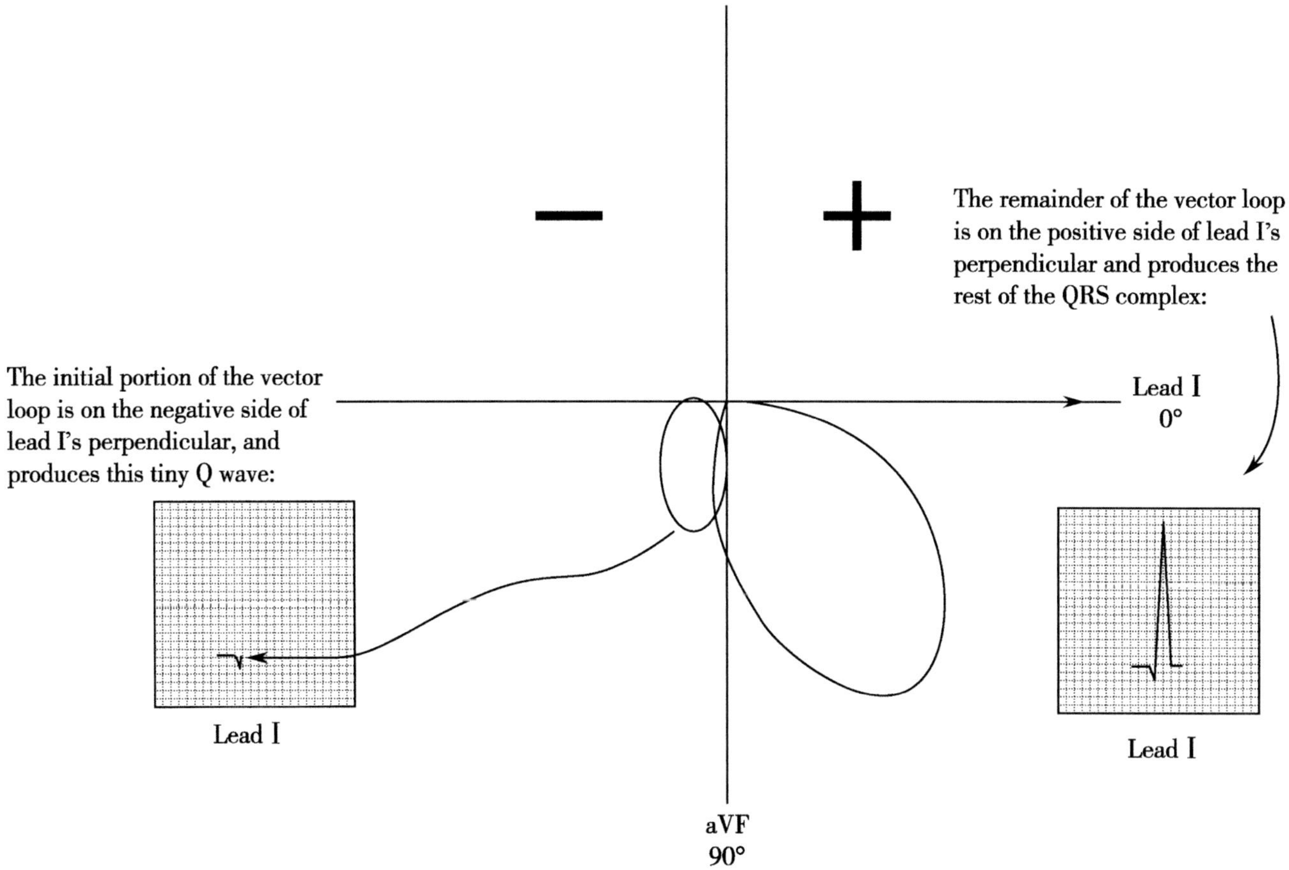

Fig. 52.30 Formation of QRS complex in lead I

Fig. 52.31 Formation of QRS complex in lead aVF

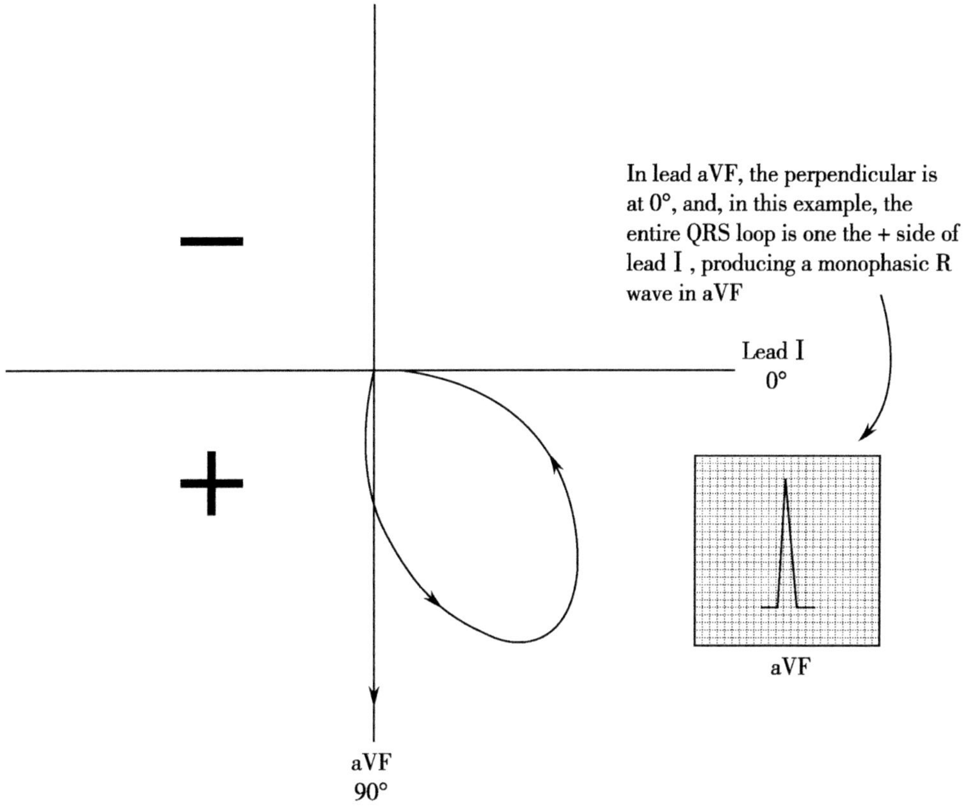

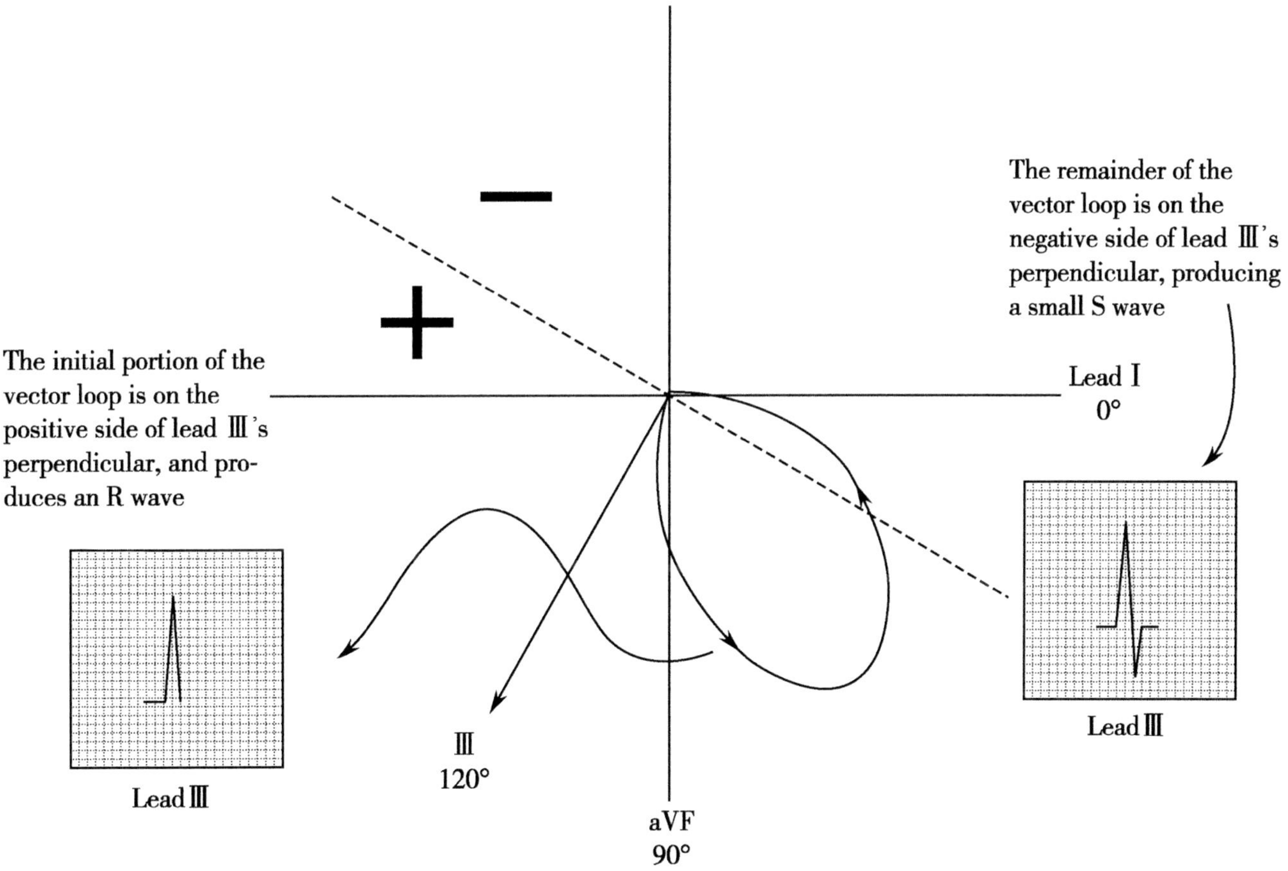

Fig. 52.32 Formation of QRS complex in lead III

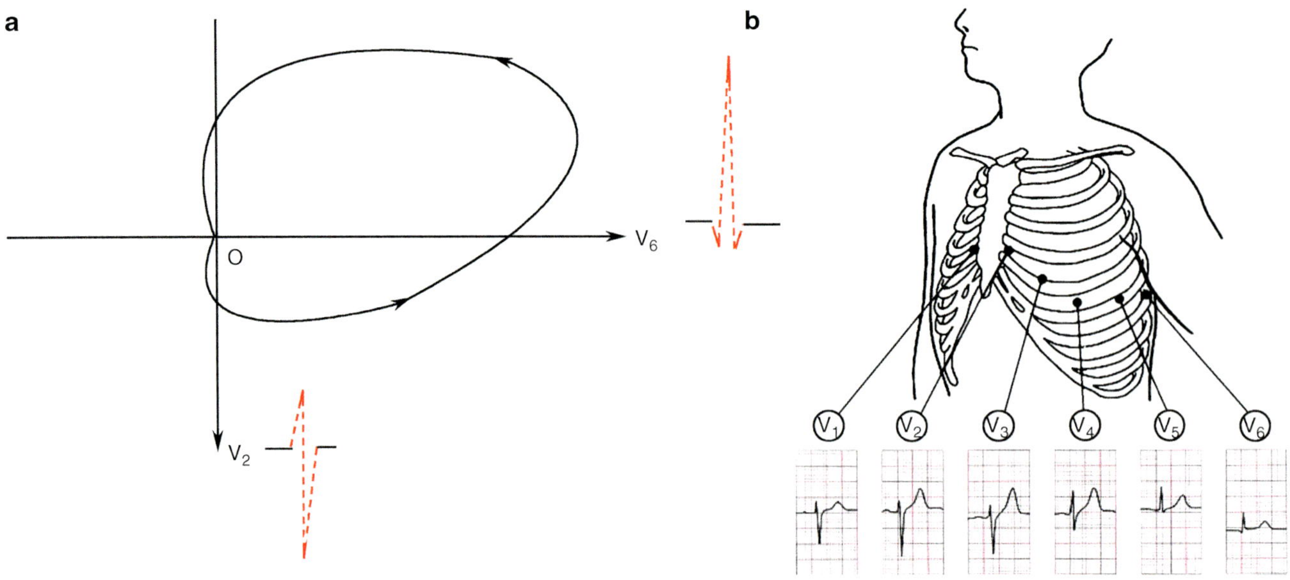

Fig. 52.33 QRS vector loop projected on chest leads axes (**a**) and morphology of QRS complex in chest leads (**b**)

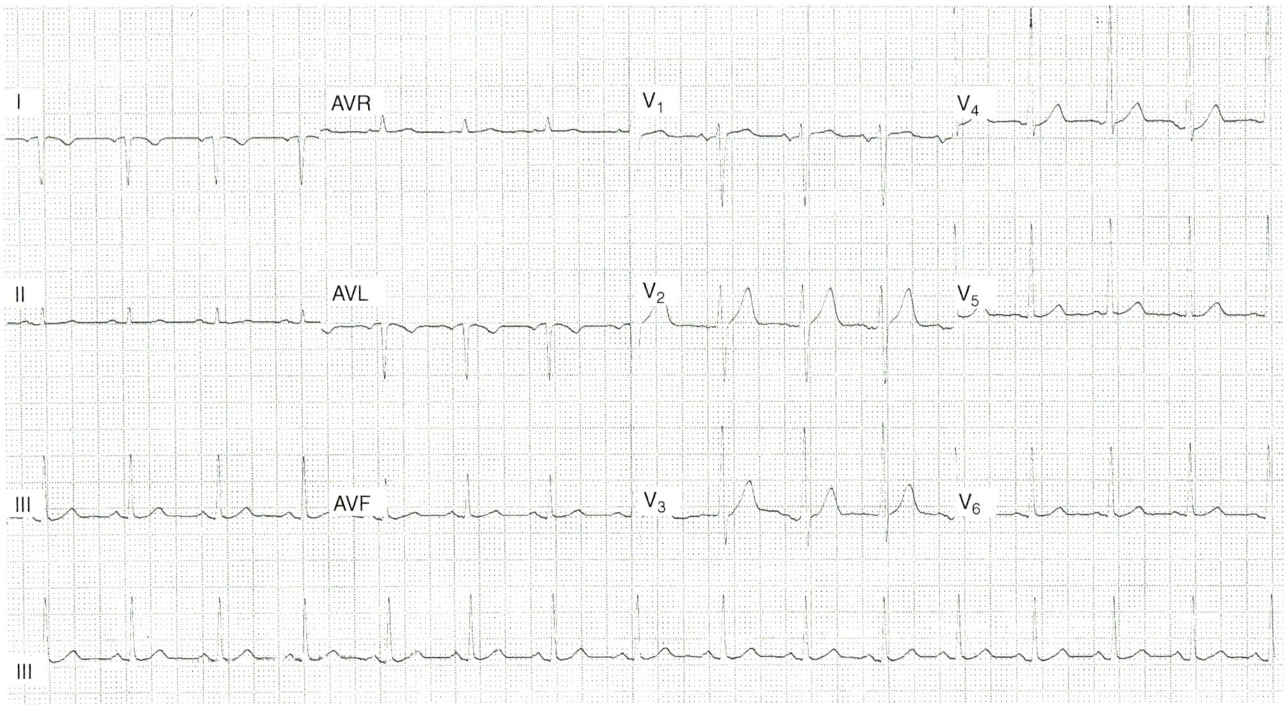

Fig. 52.34 LA/RA Reversal

axis is as follows (Fig. 52.36). To determine axis deviation, we should mainly focus on leads I and aVF.

52.4.2.2 Axis Deviation (Fig. 52.36)

No Axis Deviation

ECG Recognition

1. The cardiac electric axis lies between −30° and +90°.
2. Two common variants:

- Main wave is positive in both leads I and aVF (Fig. 52.37): For the main wave in lead I is positive, the QRS axis is in the positive direction of lead I axis, that is, in the first or forth quadrant (of the frontal plane); For the main wave in lead aVF is positive, the QRS axis is in the positive direction of lead aVF axis, in other words, in the third quadrant or forth quadrant. Therefore the QRS axis lies in the fourth quadrant (0° to +90°). It is no axis deviation.

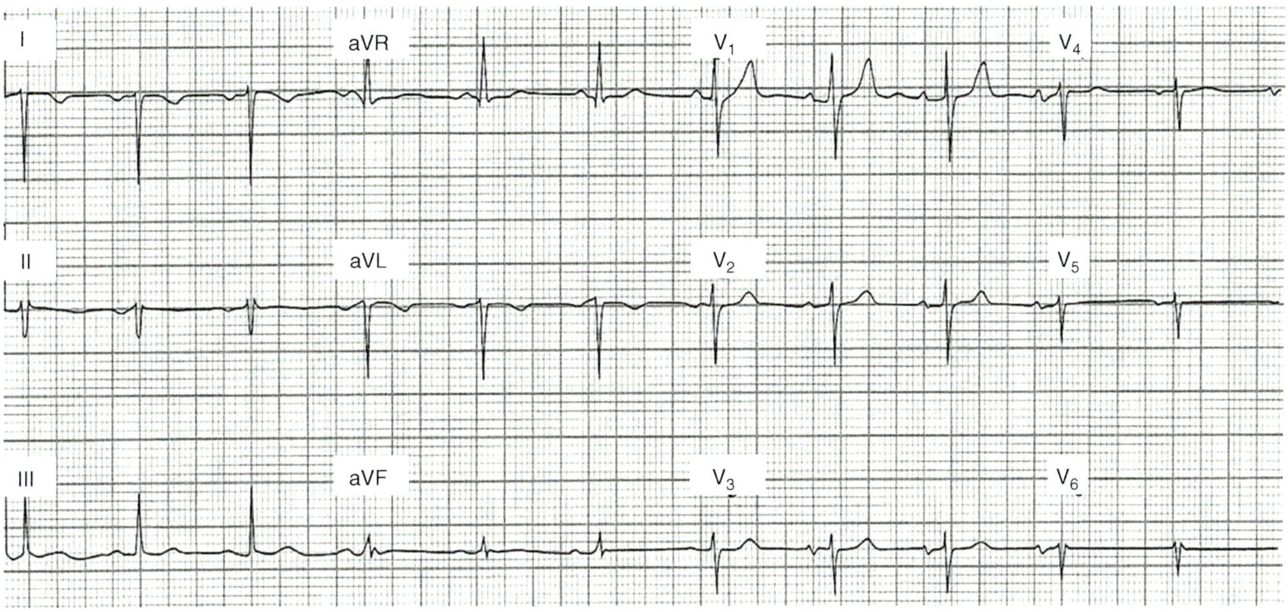

Fig. 52.35 Dextrocardia

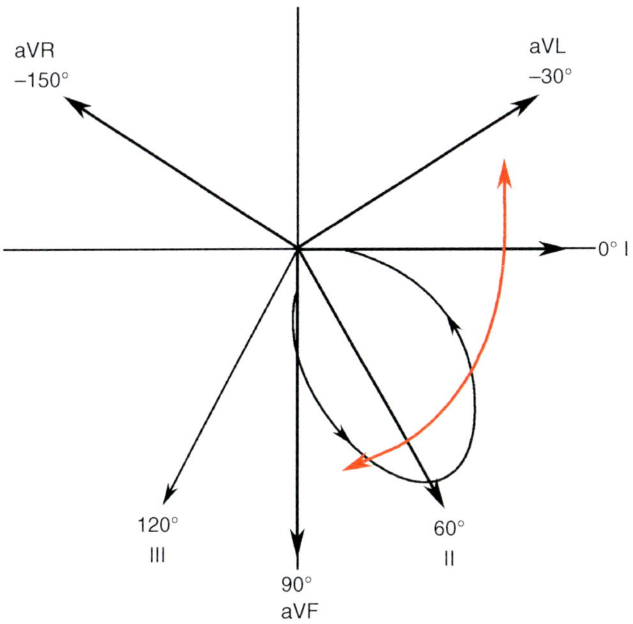

Fig. 52.36 Axis deviation. −30° to +90° no axis DEVIATION; −30° to −90° left axis deviation; +90° to +180° right axis deviation; −90° to −180° uncertain axis

- The main wave is positive in leads I and II, and negative in lead aVF (Fig. 52.38): For the main wave in lead I is positive, the QRS axis is in the positive direction of lead I axis, that is, in the first or forth quadrant; For the main wave in lead aVF is negative, the QRS axis is in the negative direction of lead aVF axis, that is, in the first or second quadrant. Therefore the QRS axis lies in the first quadrant (0° to −90°). Since the main wave is positive in lead II, the QRS axis is within 0° to −30°, in other words, it is no axis deviation.

Left Axis Deviation

ECG Recognition (Fig. 52.39)

1. The angle of cardiac electric axis lies between −30° and −90°.
2. The main wave is positive in lead I, and negative in leads aVF and II: For the main wave in lead I is positive, the QRS axis is in the positive direction of lead I axis, that is, in the first or forth quadrant; For the main wave in lead aVF is negative, the QRS axis is in the negative direction of lead aVF axis, that is, in the first or second quadrant. Therefore the QRS axis lies in the first quadrant (0° to −90°). Since the main wave is negative in lead II, the QRS axis is within −30° to −90°, in other words, it is left axis deviation.

Right Axis Deviation

ECG Recognition (Fig. 52.40)

1. The cardiac electric axis lies between +90° and + 180°.
2. The main wave is negative in lead I, and positive in lead aVF: For the main wave in lead I is negative, the QRS axis is in the negative direction of lead I axis, that is, in the second or third quadrant; For the main wave in lead aVF is positive, the QRS axis is in the positive direction of lead aVF axis, that is, in the third or fourth quadrant. Therefore the QRS axis lies in the third quadrant (+90° to +180°). It is right axis deviation.

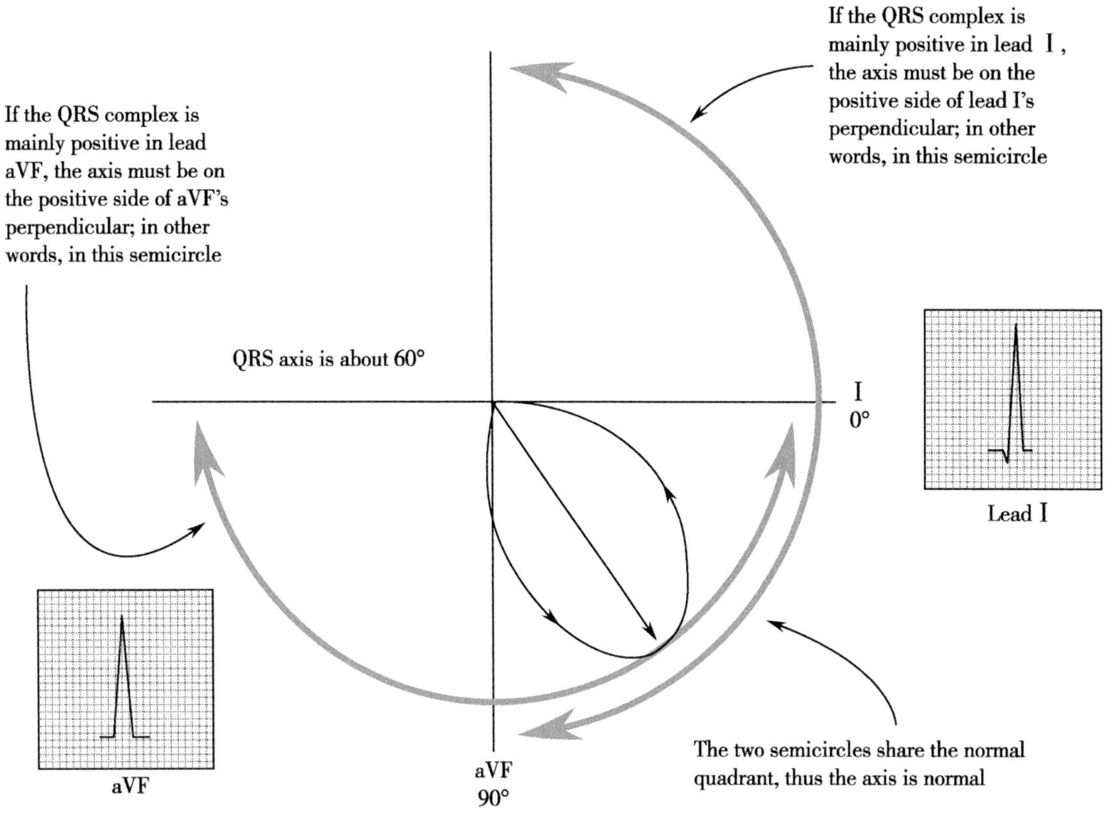

Fig. 52.37 Determination of no axis deviation (positive main wave in aVF)

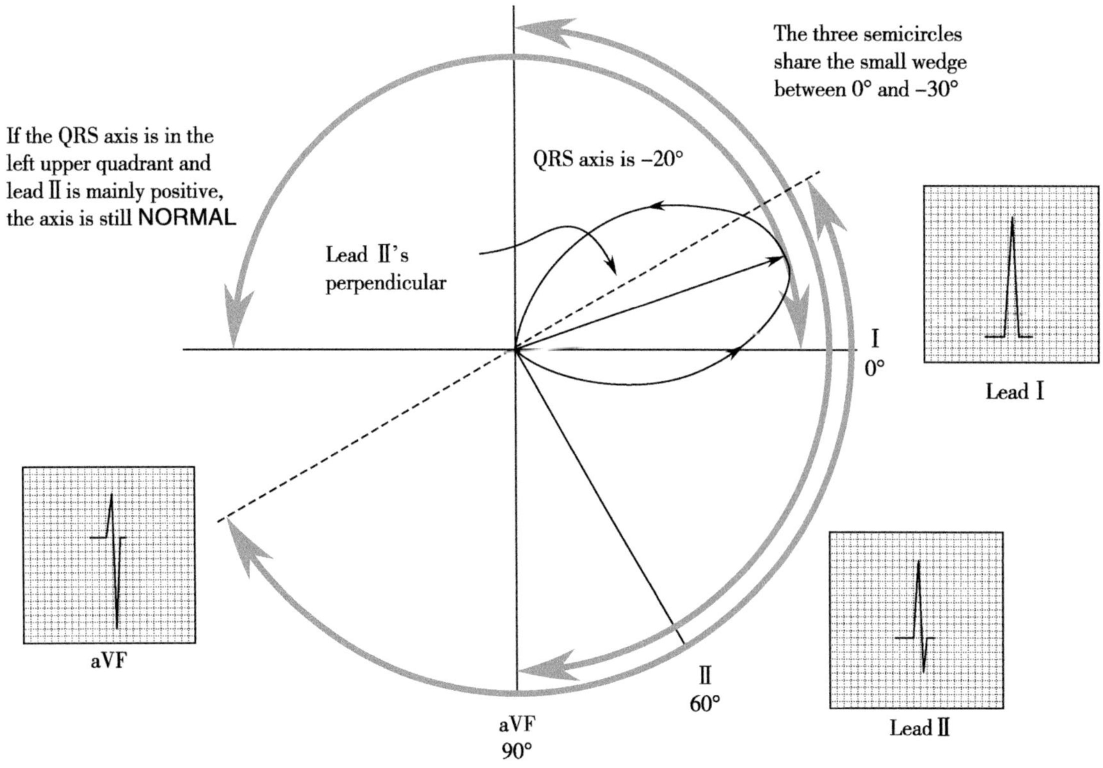

Fig. 52.38 Determination of no axis deviation (negative main wave in aVF)

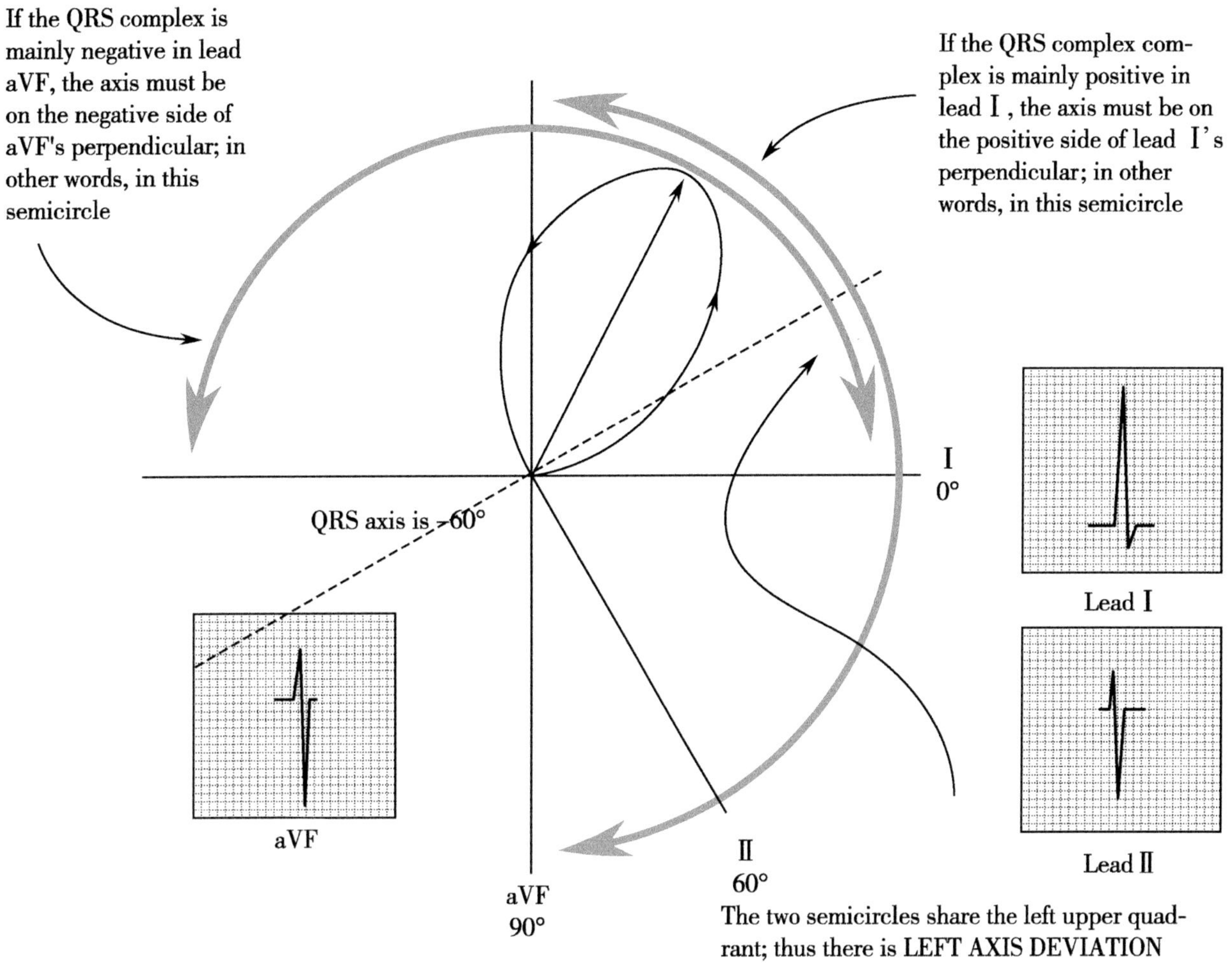

Fig. 52.39 Left axis deviation

Uncertain Axis

ECG Recognition (Fig. 52.41)

1. The cardiac electric axis lies between −90° and −180°.
2. The main wave is negative in leads I and aVF: For the main wave in lead I is negative, the QRS axis is in the negative direction of lead I axis, that is, in the second or third quadrant; For the main wave in lead aVF is negative, the QRS axis is in the negative direction of lead aVF axis, that is, in the first or second quadrant. Therefore the QRS axis lies in the second quadrant (−90° to −180°). It is uncertain axis.

The Summary of Axis Deviation (Fig. 52.42)

52.4.2.3 Abnormalities in Voltage of QRS Complex

High QRS Voltages

Left Ventricular Hypertrophy

ECG Recognition (Fig. 52.43)

1. QRS voltage changes: **R_{V5} or R_{V6} voltage is greater than 2.5 mV; R_{V5} + S_{V1}** is greater than 4.0 mV (for female is greater than 3.5 mV); R_I voltage is greater than 1.5 mV; R_I + S_{III} is greater than 2.5 mV; R_{aVL} voltage is greater than 1.2 mV or R_{aVF} voltage is greater than 2.0 mV;
2. Prolonged QRS complex duration: QRS complex duration prolonged to 0.10–0.11 s, but still less than 0.12 s;
3. Left axis deviation: most patients with left ventricular hypertrophy show mild or moderate left axis deviation;
4. Secondary ST-T change: In leads where the R wave predominates in the QRS (such as the left chest leads), the ST segment depression is greater than 0.05 mm with flat, biphasic or inverted T wave; while in the leads where the S wave predominates (such as right chest leads), ST segment elevation can correspondingly appear with tall upright T wave. An increased QRS complex voltage with ST-T change is left ventricular hypertrophy with strain.

Right Ventricular Hypertrophy

ECG Recognition (Fig. 52.44)

1. QRS complex morphology change: QRS complex shows qR pattern in V_1, R/S is greater than 1 in leads V_1 and aVR; R/S is less than 1 in lead V_5; evident clockwise transposition can be seen and QRS complex shows rS pattern from V_1 to V_4, even to V_6somtimes.

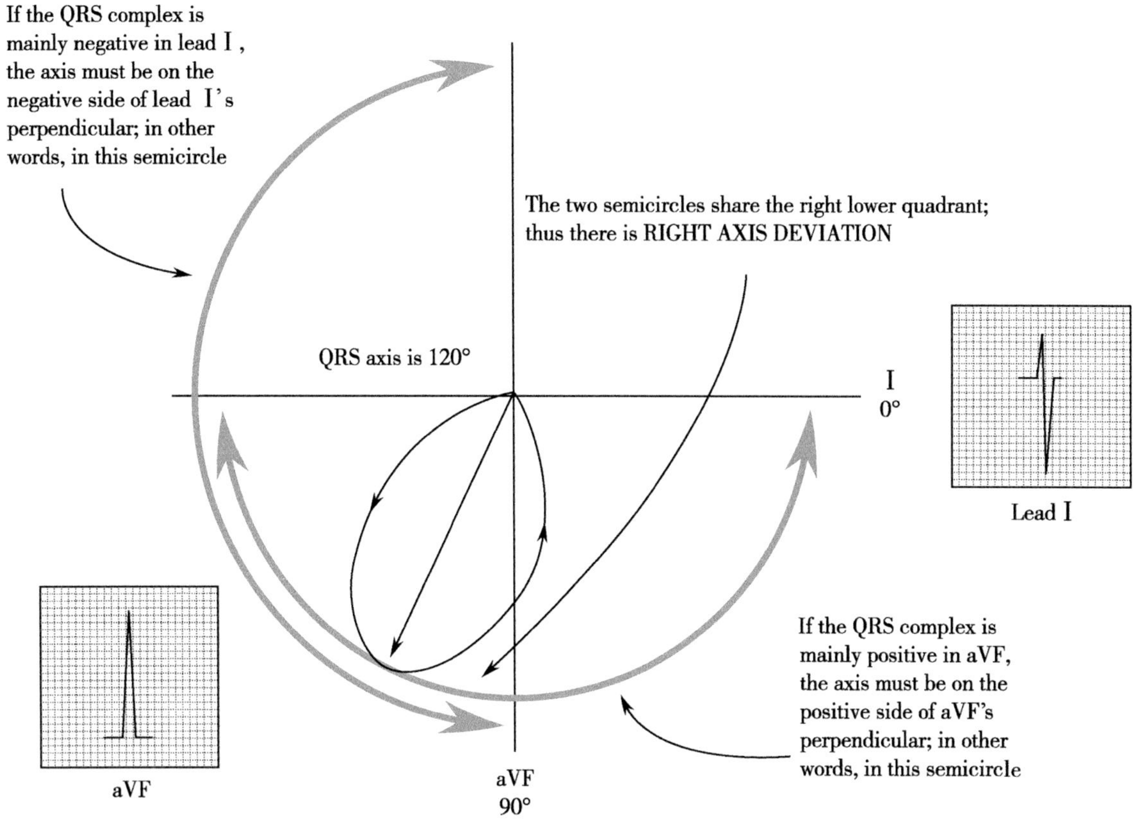

Fig. 52.40 Right axis deviation

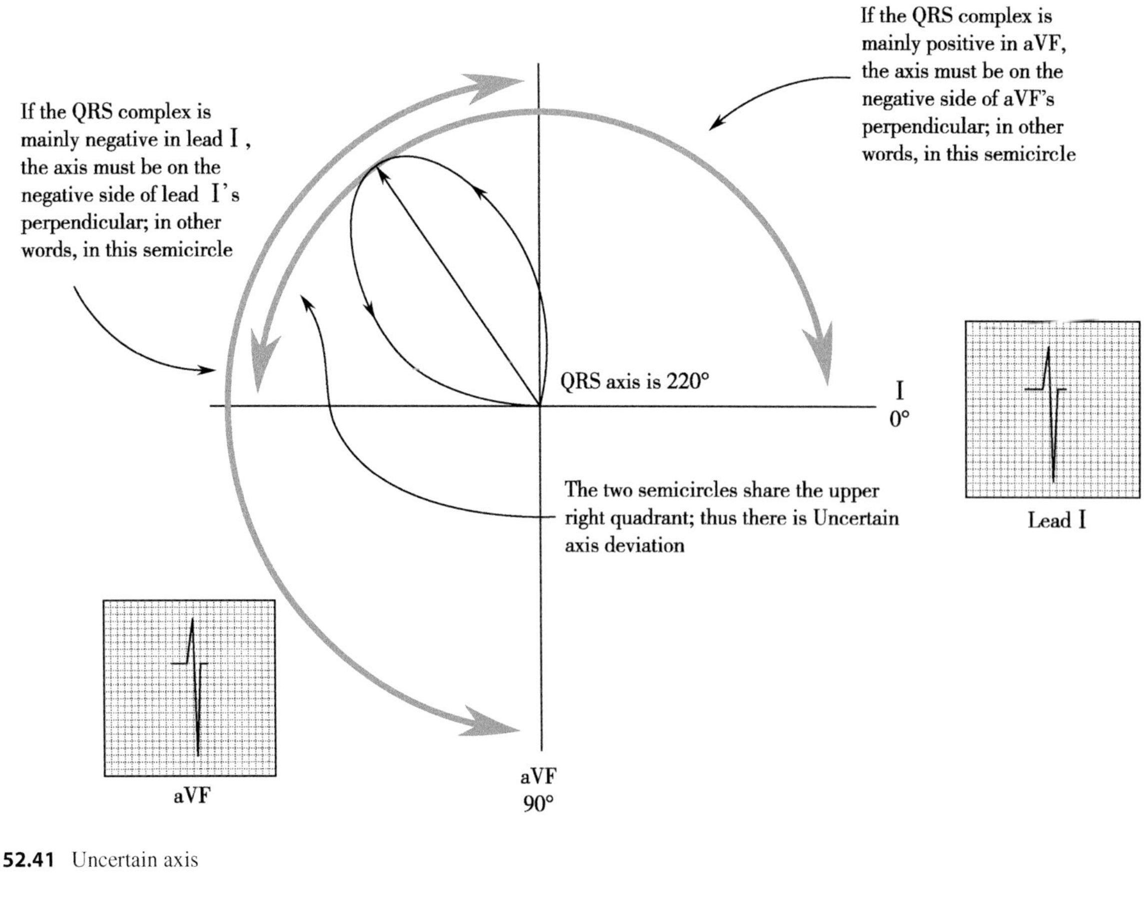

Fig. 52.41 Uncertain axis

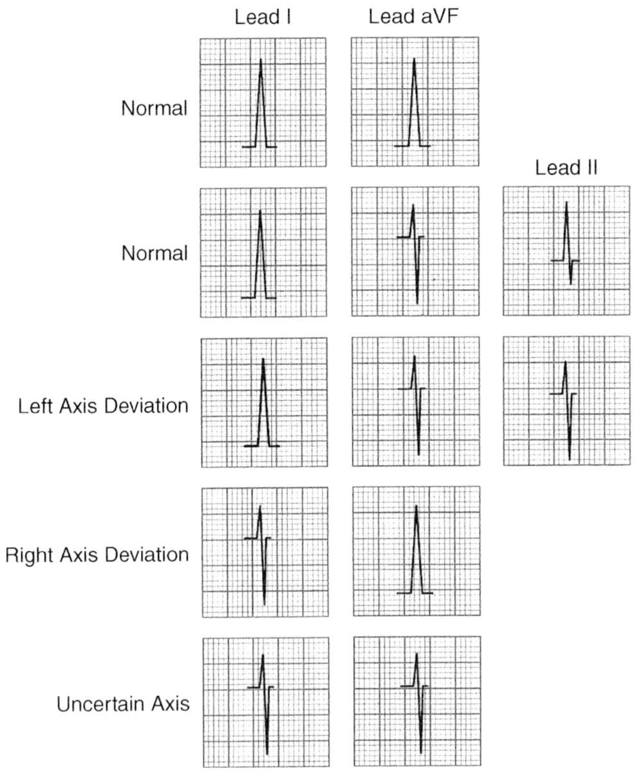

Fig. 52.42 The summary of axis deviation

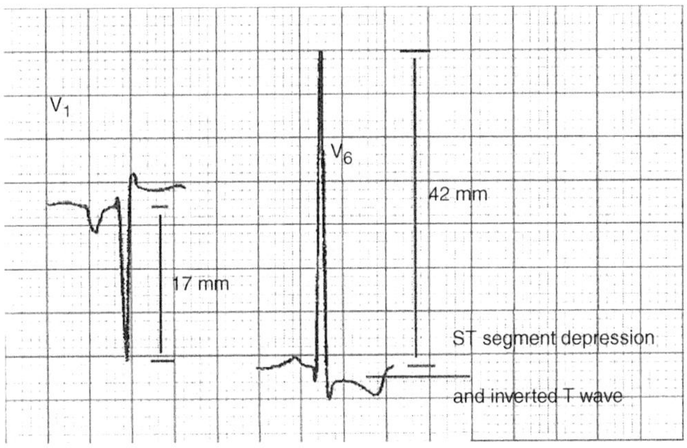

Fig. 52.43 Left ventricular hypertrophy

2. QRS complex voltage changes: **QRS complex voltage increases: Voltage in R_{V1} is greater than 1.0 mv;** R_{V1} + S_{V5} is greater than 1.2 mv; R_{aVR} is greater than 0.5mv.
3. Right axis deviation.
4. ST-T Change: ST segment is depressed with biphasic or inverted T wave in V_1. Tall R wave in lead V_1 with ST-T change is defined as right ventricular hypertrophy with strain.

Low Voltage in QRS Complex

Common causes:

1. Low voltage caused by myocardium: restrictive cardiomyopathy (amyloidosis, sarcoma etc.)

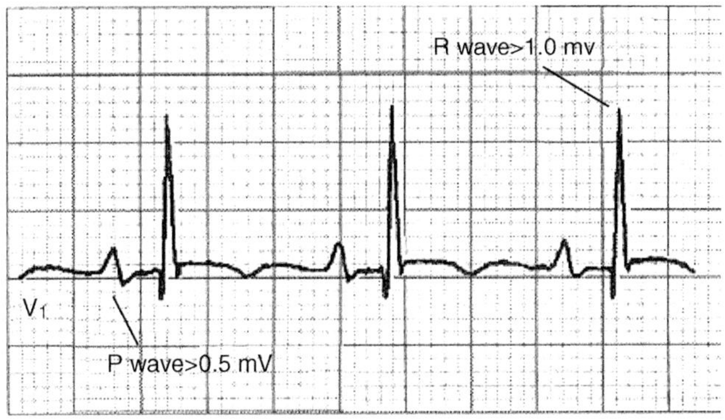

Fig. 52.44 Right ventricular hypertrophy

2. Increased impedance between tissue (myocardium) that forms voltage and leads: fat (overweight), air (COPD, pneumothorax) and water (pericardial or pleural effusion, ascites)
3. Hypothyroidism

ECG Recognition (Fig. 52.45)

1. No absolute voltage value of any QRS complexes in any chest leads≥0.8mv (known as low voltage in chest leads)
2. Or no absolute voltage value of any QRS complexes in any limb leads≥0.5mv (known as low voltage in limb leads)
3. If both limb and chest leads are present low voltage, it is known as low voltage in whole leads.

52.4.2.4 Wide QRS Complex

Wide QRS Complex has its duration greater than 0.12 s. Common causes include premature ventricular contraction, ventricular escape contraction, implantation of artificial cardiac pacemaker, W-PW syndrome, bundle branch block. Electrolyte and acid-base balance disturbances may also be included.

Premature Ventricular Contraction (PVC)

ECG Recognition (Fig. 52.46)

1. QRS complexes have wide (>0.12 s in adults and >0.10 s in children) and bizarre appearance. T wave and QRS complex are in the opposite direction.
2. No corresponding P waves are present before PVC.
3. Retrograde P′ wave may appear after the QRS complex and RP′ >0.20 s.
4. Usually a PVC is followed by a full compensatory pause. However, a non-compensatory pause is also possible.

Ventricular Escape Contraction

ECG Recognition (Fig. 52.47)

1. In combination with bradycardia, the delayed QRS wave is wide (>0.12 s in adults and >0.10 s in children) and bizarre. T wave and QRS complex are in the opposite direction.
2. No corresponding P wave are present before the escape beat.

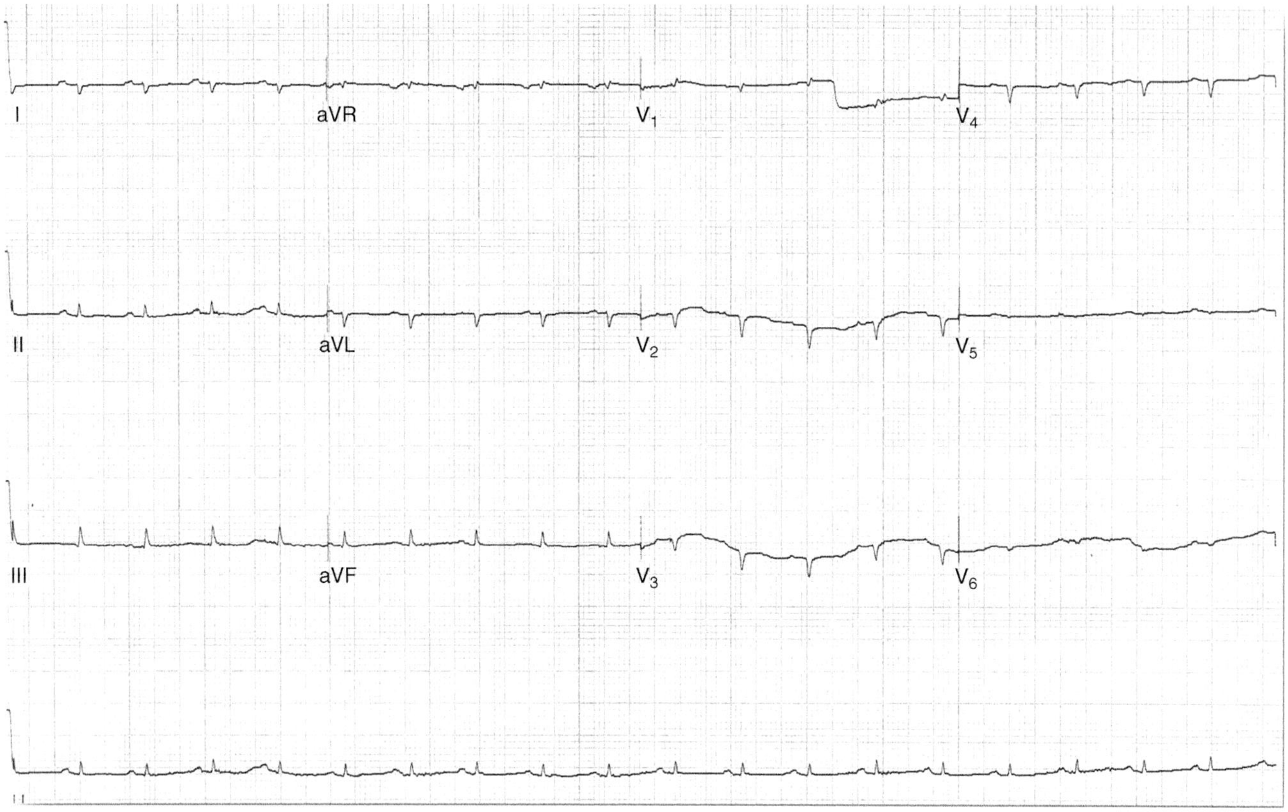

Fig. 52.45 Low QRS voltage in whole leads

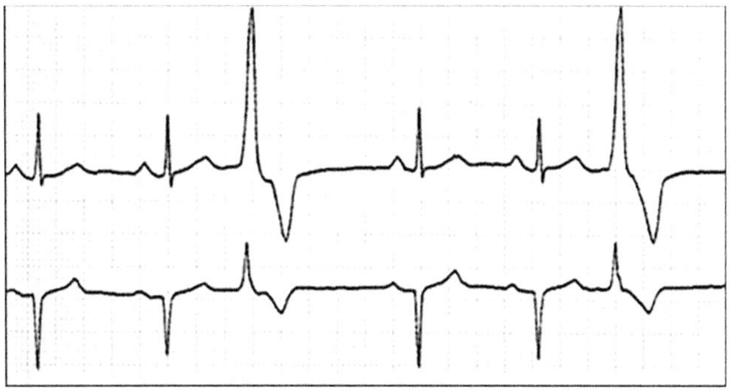

Fig. 52.46 Premature ventricular contraction

Bundle Branch and Fascicular Block

Right Bundle Branch Block (RBBB)

The sequence of depolarization changes into ventricular septum to the left ventricle to the right ventricle because of right bundle branch block. The end of QRS complex is prolonged with changed pattern (Fig. 52.48).

ECG Recognition (Fig. 52.49)

1. Complete right bundle branch block is when the duration of QRS complex is greater than or equal to 0.12 s. Otherwise is incomplete right bundle branch block.
2. QRS complex resembles rsR′ or 'M' configuration in lead V_1 or V_2.
3. S wave is broad (duration≥0.04 s) and notched in leads I, V_5 and V_6.
4. QRS complex resembles QR pattern in leads aVR with wide and notched R wave.
5. The duration of R wave in V_1 is greater than 0.05 s. ST segment is mildly depressed with inverted T wave in V_1 and V_2. T wave in leads I, V_5 and V_6 is upright.

Left Bundle Branch Block (LBBB)

The sequence of depolarization changes into ventricular septum to the right ventricle to the left ventricle because of left bundle branch block. The end of QRS complex is prolonged with changed pattern (Fig. 52.50).

ECG Recognition (Fig. 52.51)

1. Complete left bundle branch block is when the duration of QRS complex is greater than or equal to 0.12 s. Otherwise it is incomplete left bundle branch block.
2. R wave is broad, with a round peak, or notched in leads I, aVL, V_5 and V_6.
3. Left axis deviation
4. QRS complex resembles rS or QS configuration in leads V_1 and V_2. q wave disappears in leads I, V_5 and V_6.

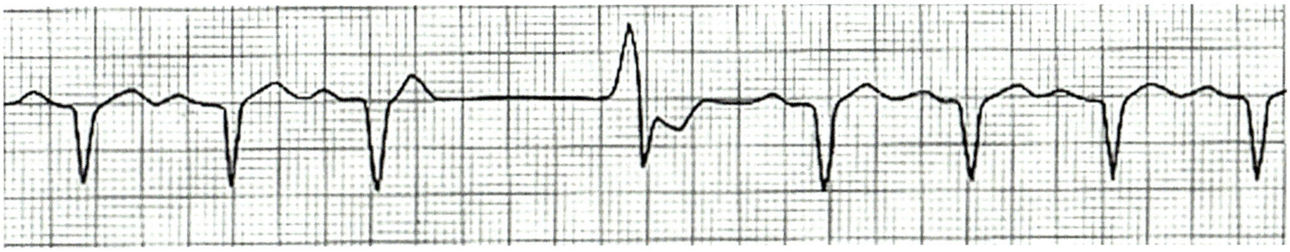

Fig. 52.47 Ventricular escape contraction

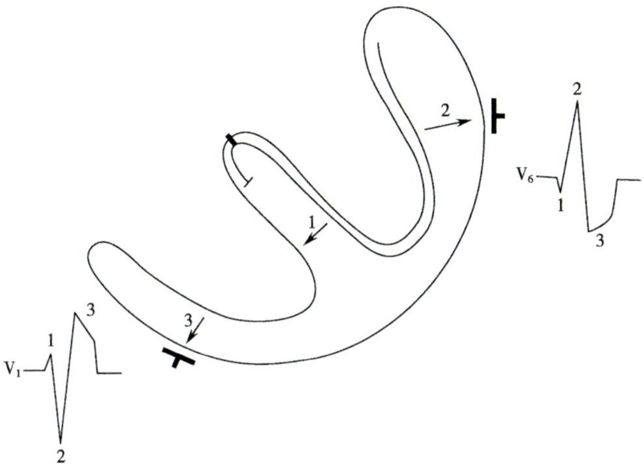

Fig. 52.48 The principle of changed pattern in QRS complex in RBBB

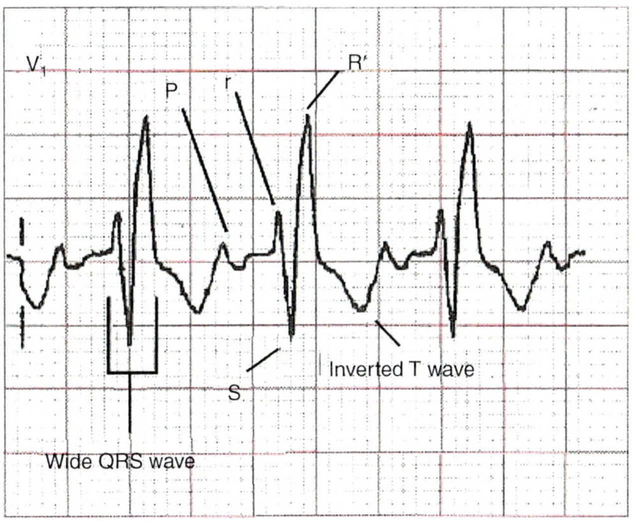

Fig. 52.49 Right bundle branch block

5. The duration of R wave is greater than 0.06 s in leads V_5 and V_6.
6. The direction of ST-T segment and QRS complex is opposite.

Non-specific Intraventricular Block

ECG Recognition (Fig. 52.52)

1. QRS complex is wide (≥0.12 s).
2. It does not have the specific patterns showed in LBBB or RBBB.

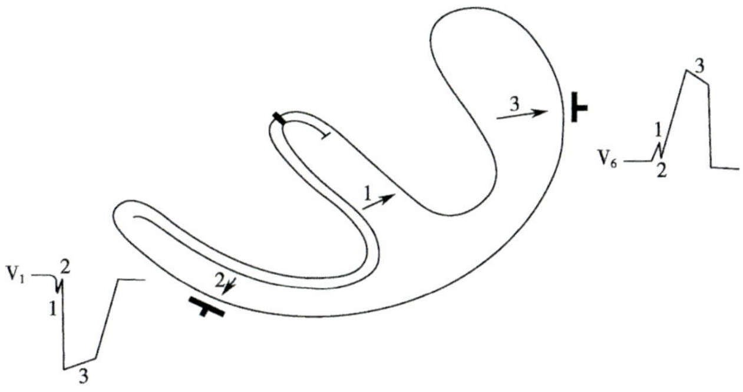

Fig. 52.50 The principle of changed pattern in QRS complex in LBBB

Left bundle branch could be divided into left anterior fascicular and left posterior fascicular. Left anterior and posterior fascicular have totally opposite axis direction (Fig. 52.53a). When left anterior fascicular block happen (Fig. 52.53b), left axis deviation could be seen; while left posterior fascicular block is present, you could find right axis deviation (Fig. 52.53c).

Left Anterior Fascicular Block (LAFB)

ECG Recognition (Fig. 52.54)

1. A left axis deviation between −30° and −90° can be seen. An axis ≥−45° is more suggestive of LAFB.
2. Leads II, III, and aVF show a rS pattern and the S wave in lead III is deeper than that in lead II. Lead aVL shows a qR pattern and the amplitude of the R wave in lead aVL is greater than that in lead I.
3. The duration of QRS complex is prolonged but is still less than 0.12 s.

Left Posterior Fascicular Block (LPFB)

ECG Recognition (Fig. 52.55)

- A right axis deviation between +90° and +180°.
- Some rS patterns are seen in leads I and aVL, and qR patterns are seen in leads III and aVF. The duration of the Q wave is less than 0.025 s.
- The amplitude of the R wave is greater in lead III than that in lead II
- The duration of QRS complex is less than 0.12 s.

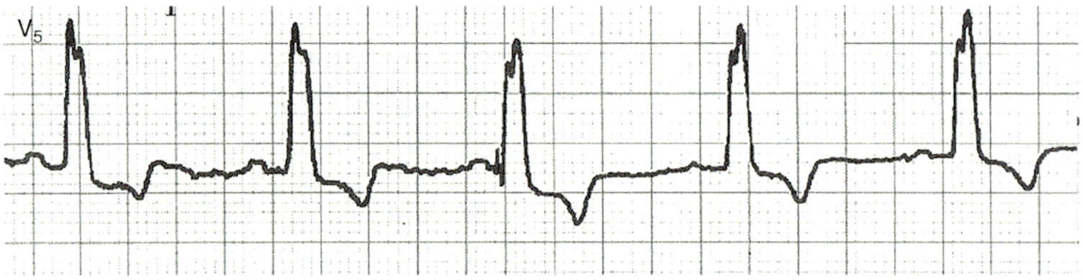

Fig. 52.51 Left bundle branch block

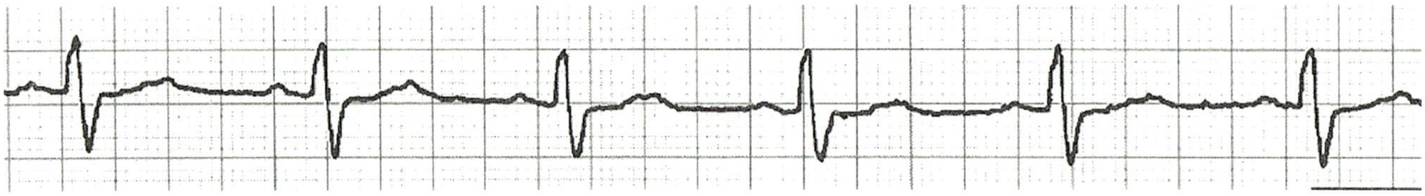

Fig. 52.52 Non-specific intraventricular block

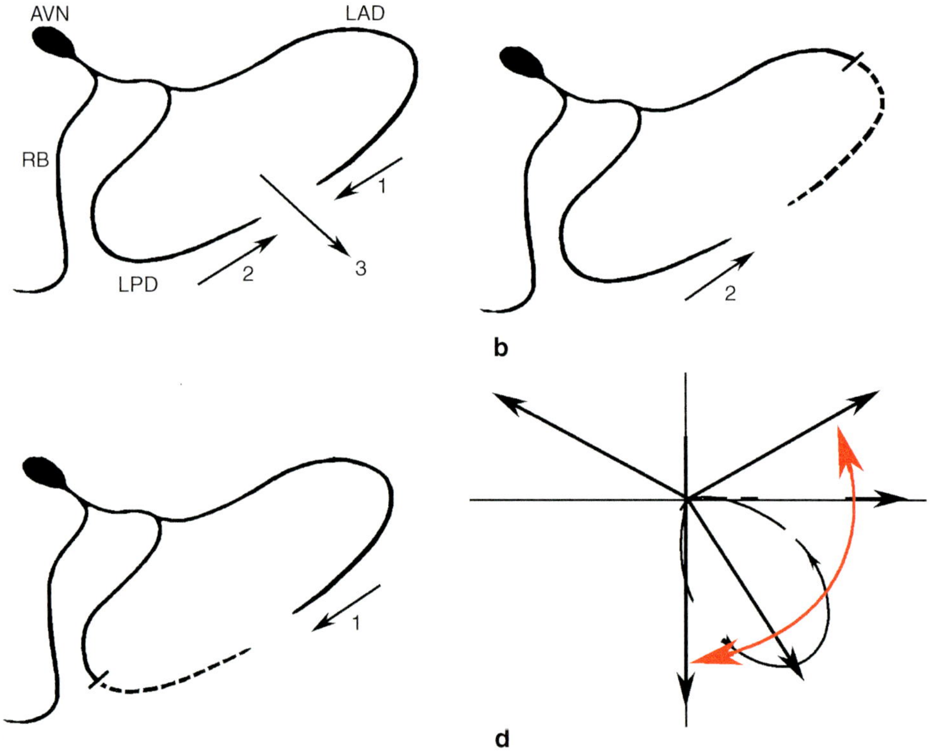

Fig. 52.53 The principle of axis deviation in fascicular block

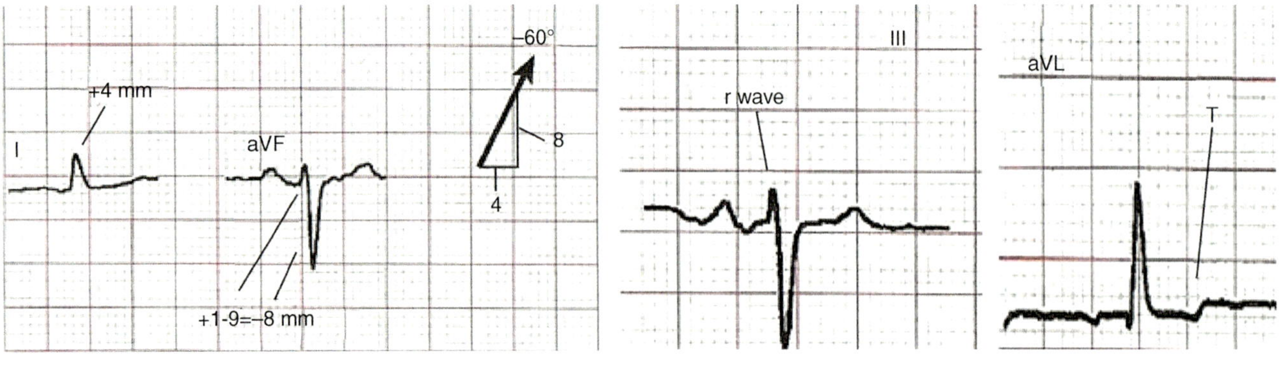

Fig. 52.54 Left anterior fascicular block

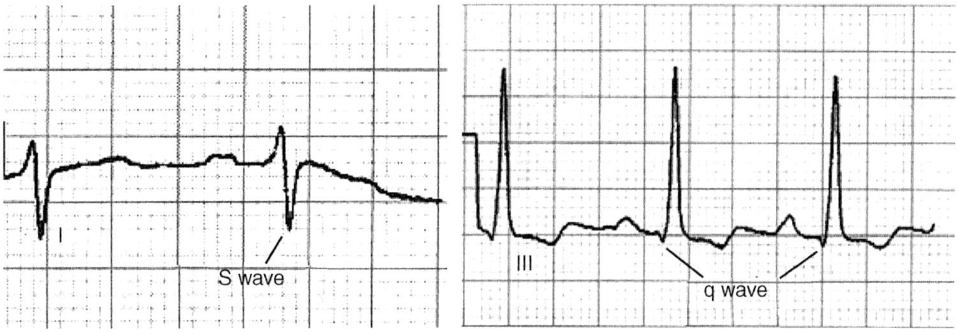

Fig. 52.55 Left posterior fascicular block

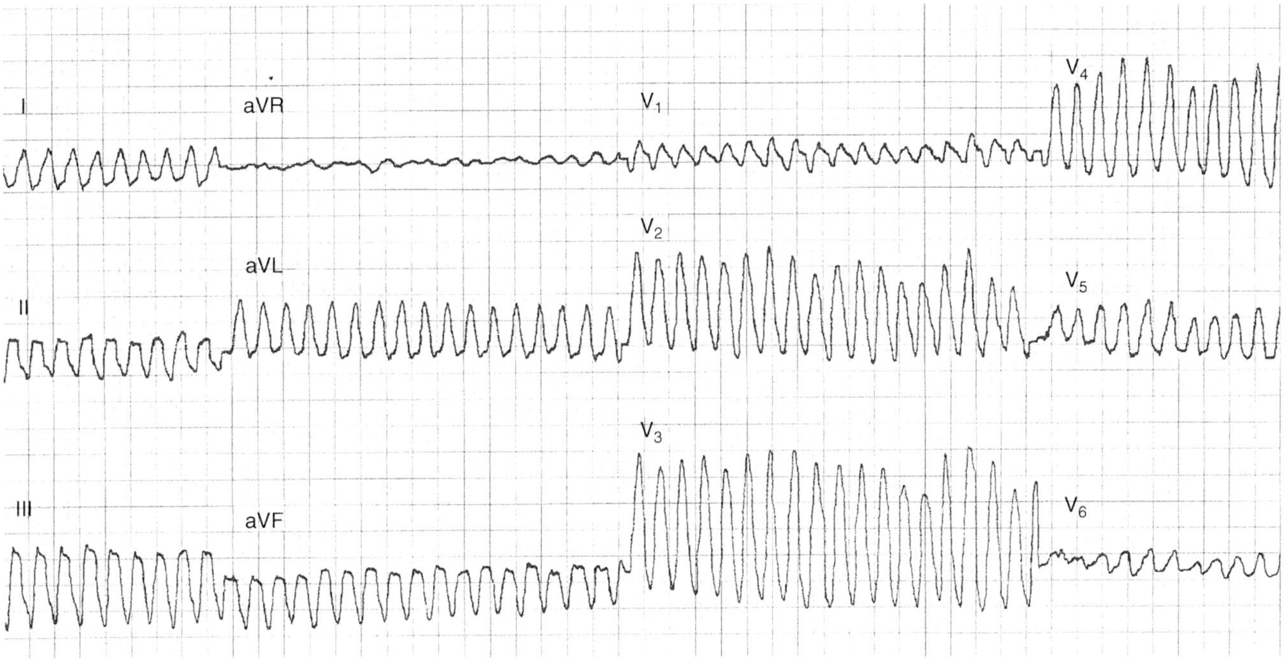

Fig. 52.56 Ventricular flutter

52.4.3 Absence of QRS Complex

52.4.3.1 Ventricular Flutter

ECG Recognition (Fig. 52.56)

1. P wave is absent in all leads.
2. No identifiable QRS-T complex, but sine wave-like *flutter waves* are present.
3. Frequency: 200–250 bpm.

52.4.3.2 Ventricular Fibrillation

ECG Recognition (Fig. 52.57)

1. No visible QRS-T complex.
2. Rapid, coarse and irregular fibrillation waves are present.
3. Frequency of fibrillation waves: 250–500 bpm.

52.5 Section 5: Analyze ST Segment

ST segment refers to the line connecting the end of QRS complex and the beginning of T wave. Pathologically, ECG tracing may show ST segment elongation or shortening, but more often the elevation and depression, such as the ST pattern in myocardium ischemia (MI).So in MI, as the ST vector points from normal myocardial cells to abnormal ones, ST segment elevation could be seen on patients with subepicardial ischemia (transmural myocardial ischemia), and the direction of vector is from endocardium to epicardium and ST segment depression on those with subendocardial ischemia, with the direction of vector from epicardium to endocardium. Besides, it is worth noting that MI can generally disturb the normal depolarization of ventricular myocardium, which may lead to some other ST abnormal signs on ECG tracing.

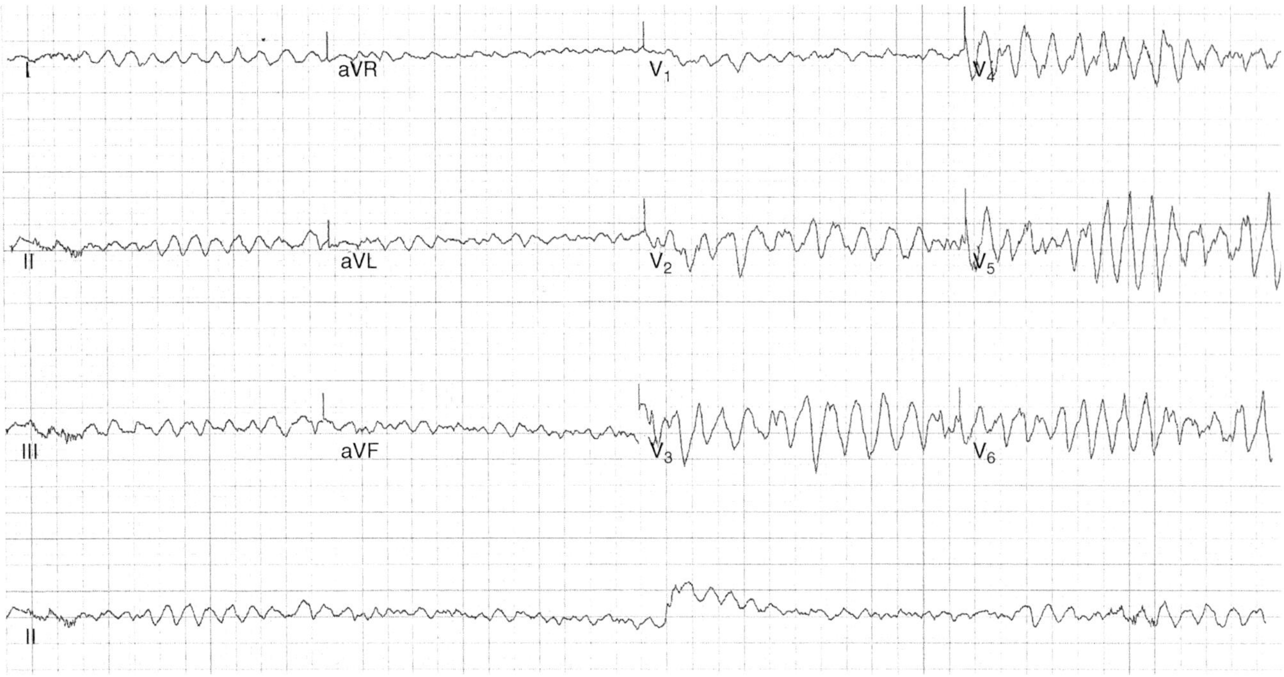

Fig. 52.57 Ventricular fibrillation

However, these changes are not specific for MI, and they could also be attributed to organic cardiac disease, electrolyte disturbances or effect of drugs. It is even seen on some normal people. **Therefore, it's important to consider clinical symptoms when analyzing ECG tracing and be cautious to dynamic changes.**

52.5.1 Normal ST Segment

52.5.1.1 ECG Recognition

1. ST segment at baseline without deviation.
2. Deviation within normal range:
   - Depression of ST segment is less than 0.05mv in all leads.
   - Elevation of ST segment is less than 0.1 mv in all limb leads and leads V_4 to V_6, while less than 0.3 mv in leads V_1 and V_2, less than 0.5 mv in lead V_3.

52.5.2 Abnormal ST Segment

52.5.2.1 ST Segment Elevation

ST segment elevation can be caused by many reasons, among which acute myocardial infarction (AMI), early repolarization syndrome, acute pericarditis, ventricular hypertrophy and bundle branch block are more common. We have already learned ventricular hypertrophy and bundle branch block, here we focus on acute myocardial infarction.

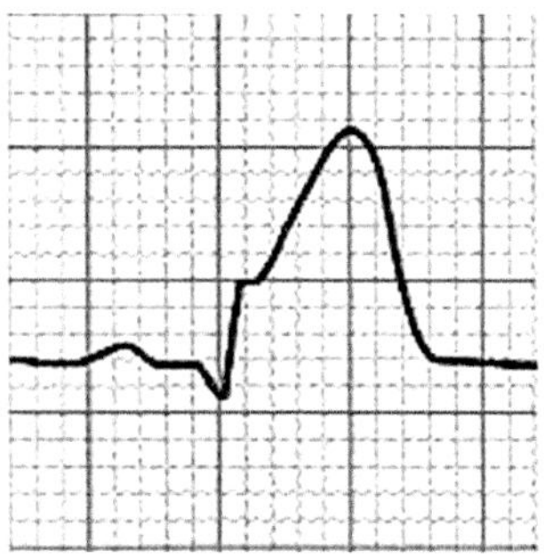

Fig. 52.58 ST segment changes in superacute phase

Acute Myocardial Infarction

AMI is a severe and common cardiac disease showing as ST elevated myocardial infarction. And the ECG tracing of such patients can be very regular, thus providing meaningful ECG proof for clinical physicians. We could also divide MI into four phases by their ECG tracings (Figs. 52.58, 52.59, 52.60, 52.61). However, these phases are defined artificially, and these typical changes do not appear on everyone. One should always consider individual variation and be flexible about interpretation of the tracing. Typical ECG changes of AMI are as follows:

Superacute Phase (Early Phase, Minutes to Hours)

ECG Recognition (Fig. 52.58)

1. Tall, upright and symmetrical T wave.
2. ST elevation with obliquely straight morphology.
3. No pathological Q wave.

Acute Phase (Hours/Days to Weeks)

ECG Recognition (Fig. 52.59)

1. Inverted T wave.
2. ST elevation with obliquely straight morphology/convex.
3. Pathological Q wave.

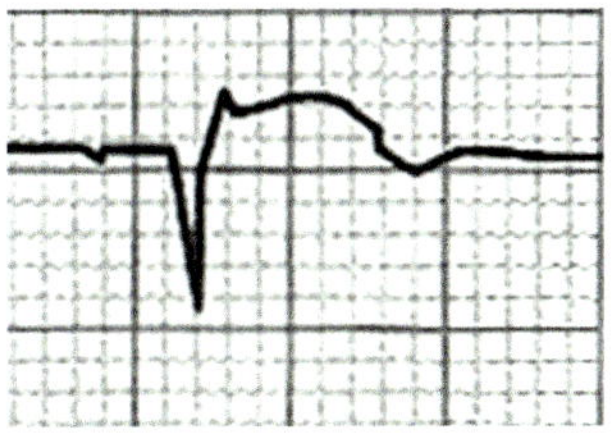

Fig. 52.59 ST segment changes in acute phase

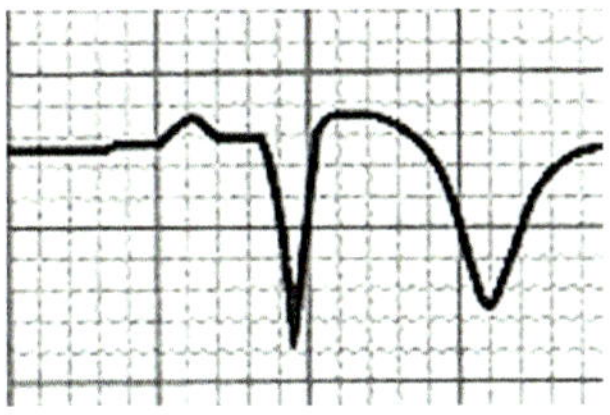

Fig. 52.60 ST segment changes in subacute phase

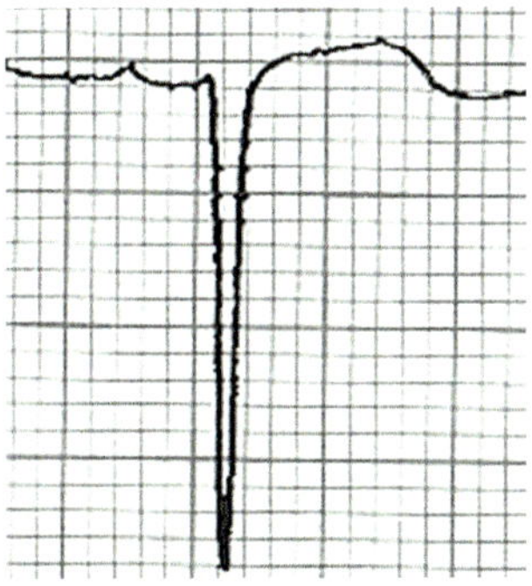

Fig. 52.61 ST segment changes in recovery phase

Subacute Phase (Weeks to Months)

ECG Recognition (Fig. 52.60)

1. Inverted T waves but smaller, ST segment at baseline.
2. Pathological Q wave.

Recovery Phase (Several Months Later)

ECG Recognition (Fig. 52.61)

1. T wave upright without changes anymore.
2. ST segment at baseline.
3. Pathological Q wave.

Besides, the ECG can tell the location of myocardial infarction based on the leads in which the basic patterns of myocardial infarction present.

- Inferior wall: leads II, III, aVF
- Anterior wall: leads V_1, V_2, V_3, V_4, V_5, V_6
- Lateral wall: leads V_5, V_6, I, aVL
- Posterior wall: leads V_7, V_8, V_9, or V_1, V_2 with tall R waves and peaked T waves.
- Right ventricle: leads V_{3R}, V_{4R}, V_{5R}, V_{6R}.

The hexaxial reference system and axes of the chest leads may help us memorize the location of myocardial infarction (Fig. 52.62).

Using what you learned above, analyze the following practice strips and find out the location and phase of myocardial infarction (Figs. 52.63, 52.64, 52.65, 52.66).

52.5.2.2 ST Segment Depression

Many diseases can cause ST Segment depression, such as myocardial ischemia, ventricular hypertrophy and bundle branch block. Ventricular hypertrophy and bundle branch block have already been learned before, here we put our mind on myocardial ischemia.

Myocardial Ischemia

ECG Recognition (Fig. 52.67)

1. PR segment is usually used as the baseline to compare and judge the ST segment depression.

Fig. 52.62 The hexaxial reference system and the axes of chest leads

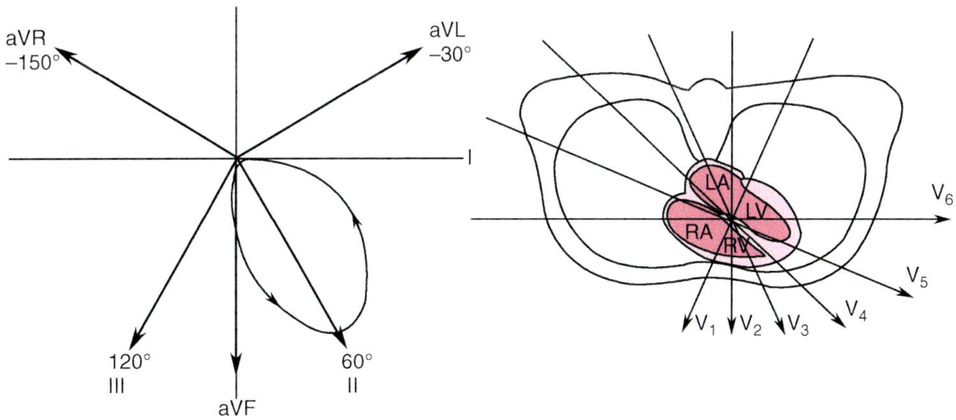

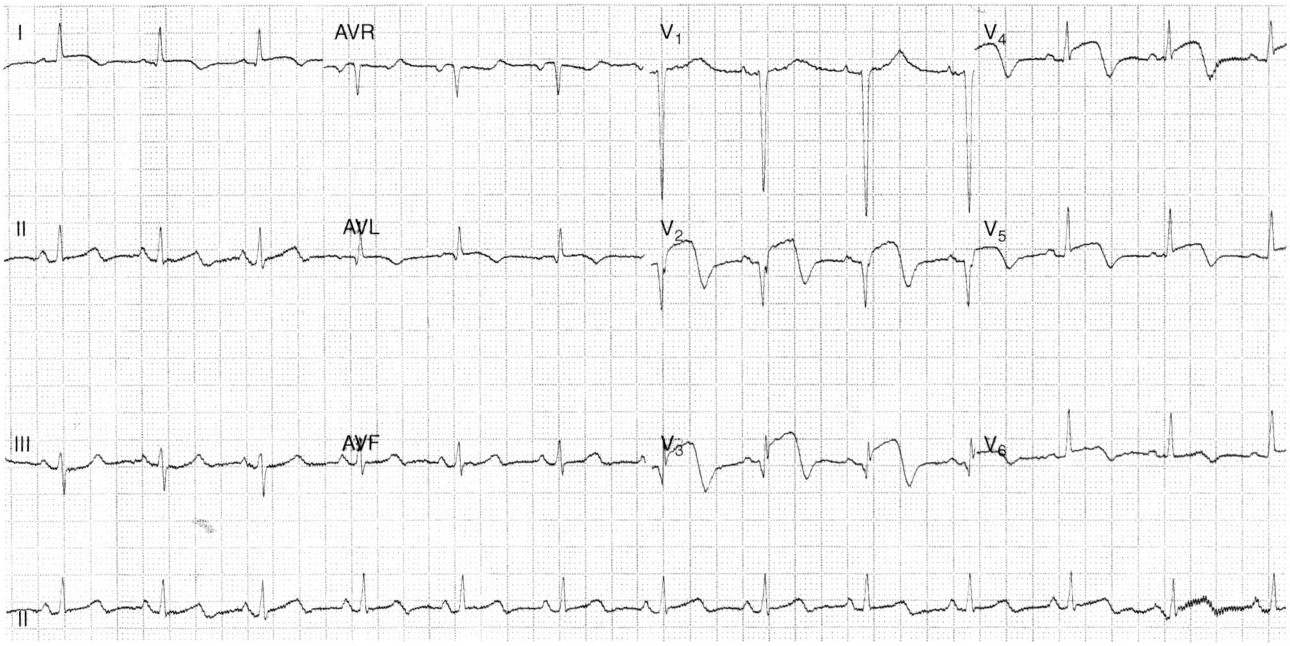

Fig. 52.63 Acute anterior infarction (ST segment elevation in leads V_2 to V_6)

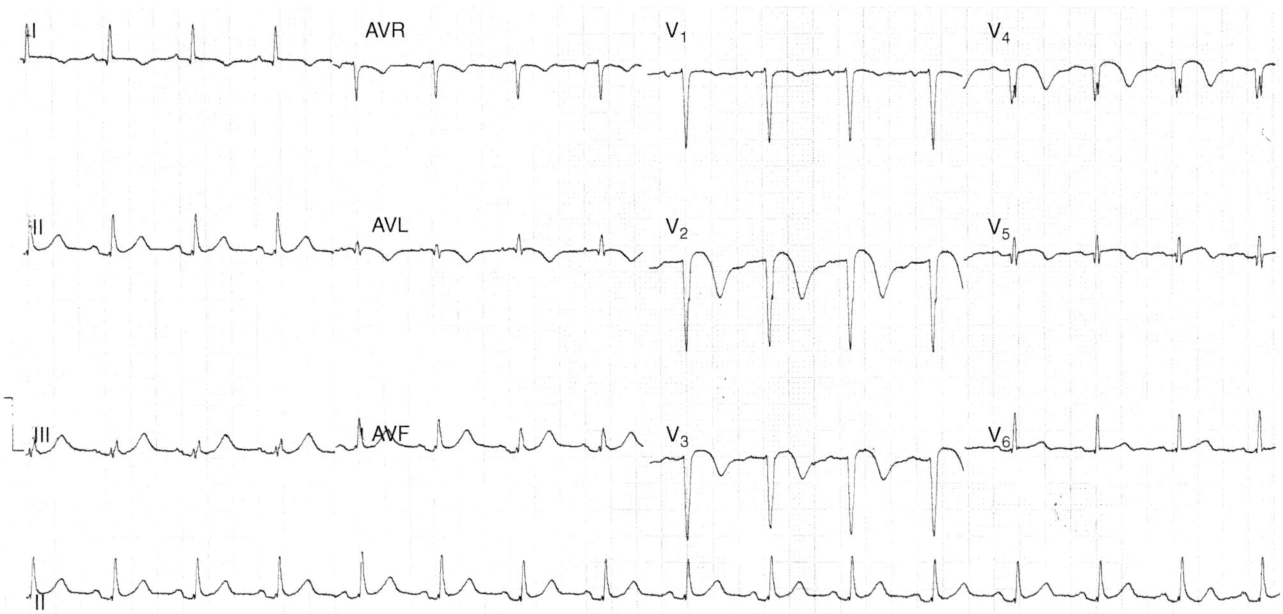

Fig. 52.64 Subacute anterior myocardial infarction (Inverted T wave, ST segment at baseline, pathologic Q wave in leads V_2 to V_5)

2. ST segment depression are various, such as J point depression, up-sloping depression, horizontal depression and down-sloping depression, the specificity for ST segment to diagnosis of myocardial ischemia improves gradually (Fig. 5-12).

Using what you learned above, analyze the following practice strips and find out the location of myocardial infarction (Figs. 52.68 and 52.69):

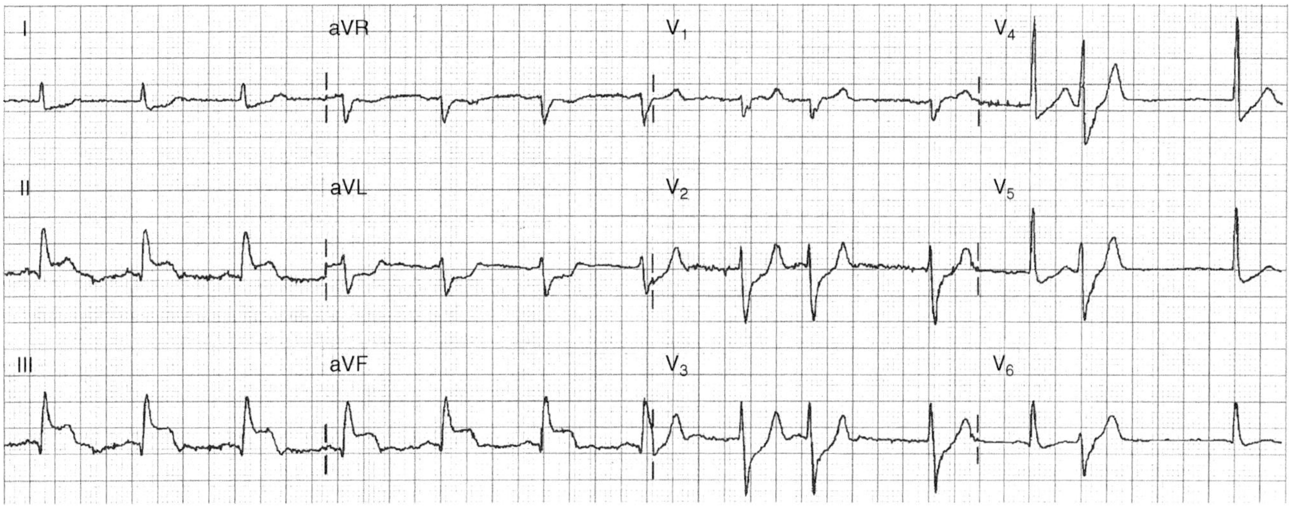

Fig. 52.65 Superacute inferior myocardial infarction (ST segment elevation in leads II, III, and aVF, tall and peaked T wave, no pathologic Q wave)

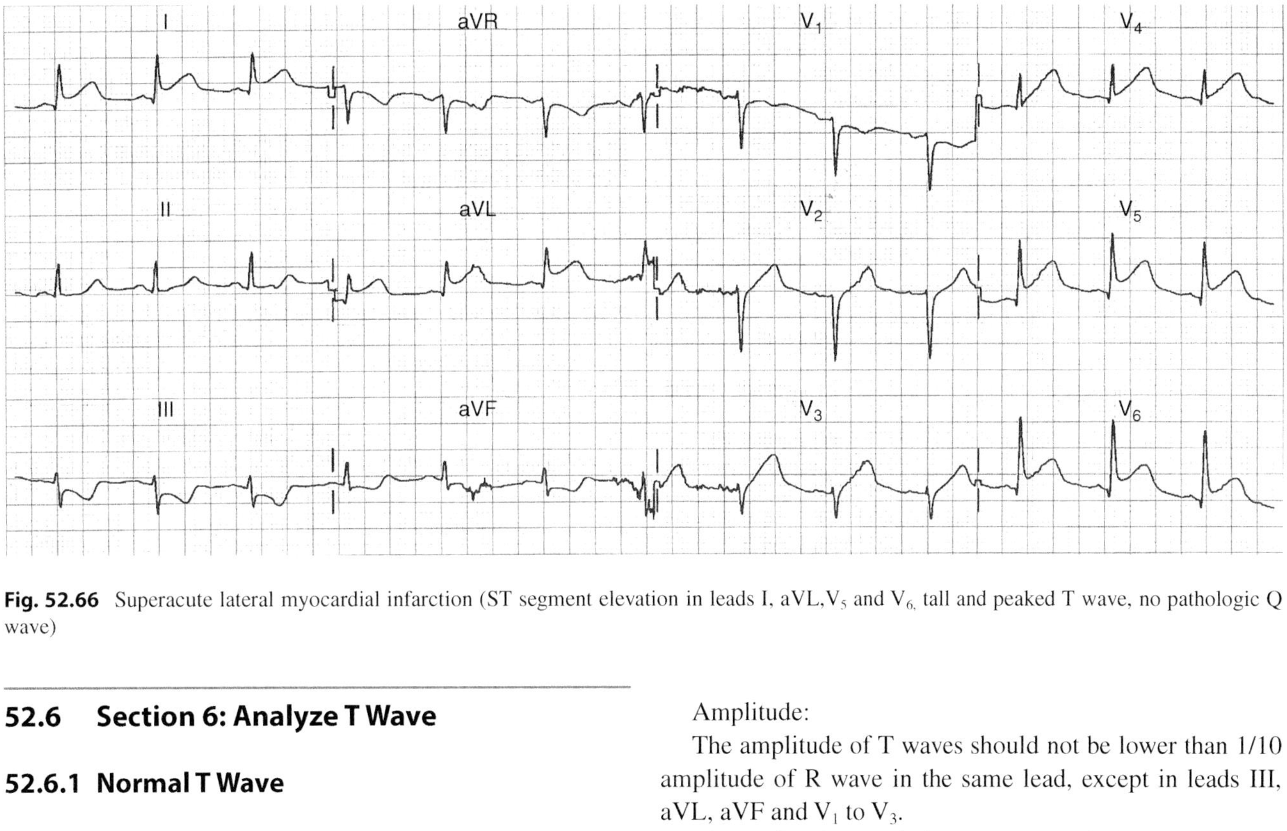

Fig. 52.66 Superacute lateral myocardial infarction (ST segment elevation in leads I, aVL,V_5 and V_6, tall and peaked T wave, no pathologic Q wave)

52.6 Section 6: Analyze T Wave

52.6.1 Normal T Wave

T wave represents the rapid ventricular repolarization, also as known as the ventricular recovery phase.

52.6.1.1 ECG Recognition (Fig. 52.70)

Direction:

1. T waves is usually upright in leads I, II, V_4 to V_6.
2. The morphology of T waves is variable in leads III, aVF, aVL and V_1 to V_3.
3. T wave is always inverted in lead aVR.

Amplitude:

The amplitude of T waves should not be lower than 1/10 amplitude of R wave in the same lead, except in leads III, aVL, aVF and V_1 to V_3.

Above all, when analyzing T wave, the judgment should be based on the patient's history and clinical manifestation, not only the ECG, because various factors can change the morphology of P wave, and T wave change lacks specificity for diagnosis.

52.6.2 Useful Methods for Analyzing T Wave

Analyze T wave according to its morphology (peaked, flat or inverted) (Fig. 52.71).

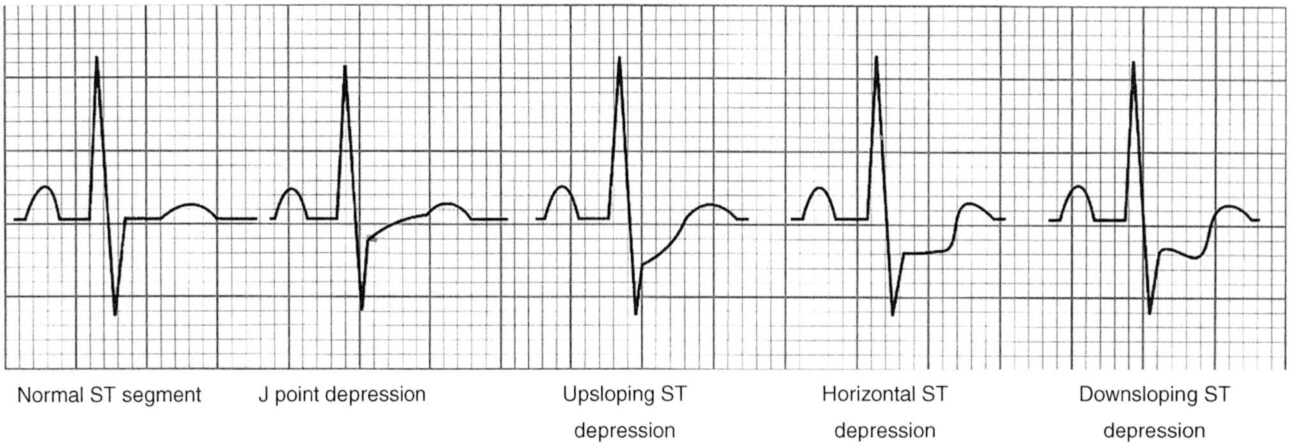

Fig. 52.67 The specificity for ST segment to diagnosis of myocardial ischemia

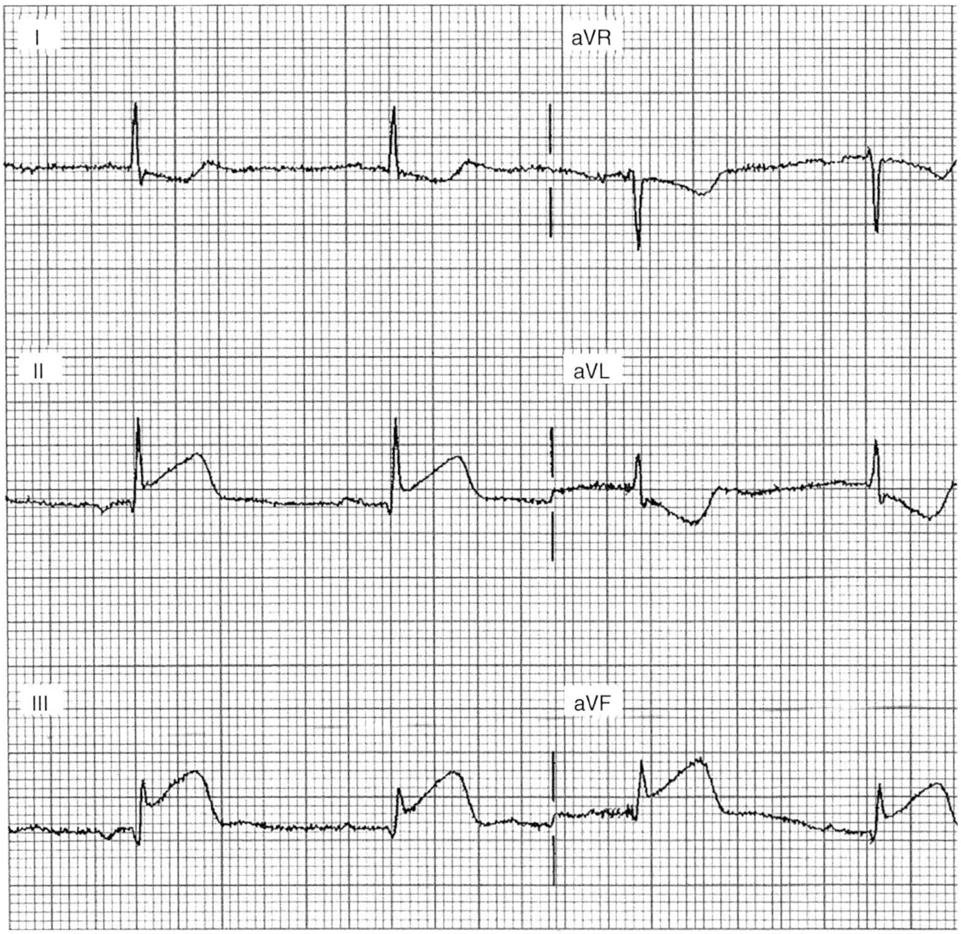

Fig. 52.68 Acute inferior myocardial infarction and lateral myocardial ischemia (ST segment elevation in leads II, III, and aVF, and ST segment depression in leads I and aVL)

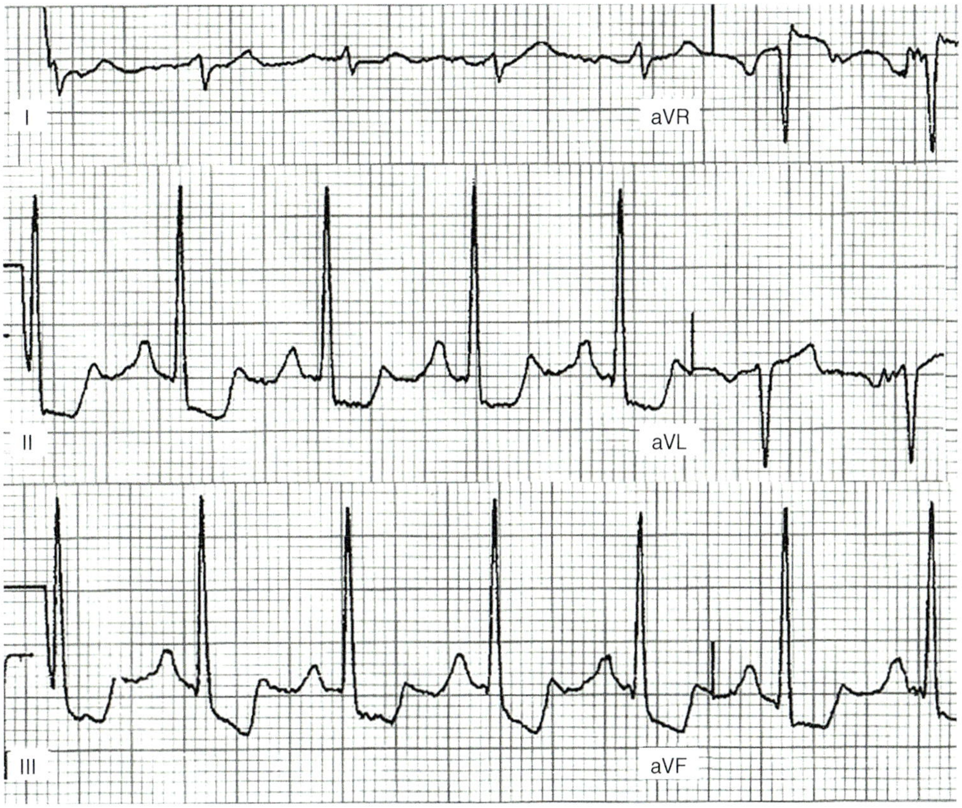

Fig. 52.69 Inferior myocardial ischemia (ST segment depression in leads II, III, and aVF)

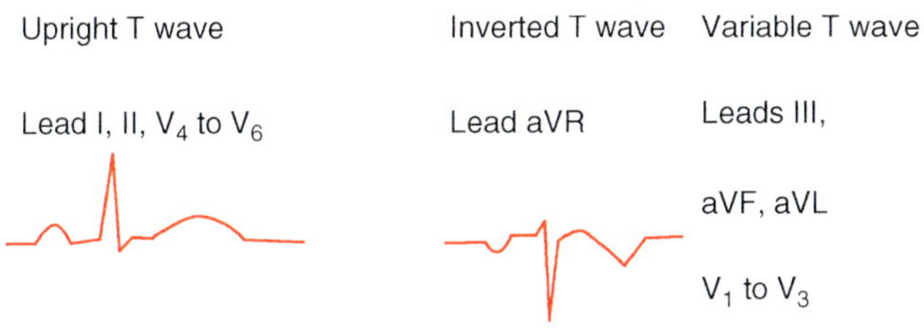

Fig. 52.70 Normal T wave

52.6.3 Analysis of Abnormal T Wave

52.6.3.1 Inverted T Wave

Common causes:

1. In leads I, II, V_4 to V_6, inverted T wave is usually abnormal.
2. If T wave is inverted with apparent change in ST segment (horizontal or downsloping ST segment depression >1 mm, Fig. 52.72), then you can consider myocardial ischemia; Inverted T wave with ST segment depression <1 mm or downsloping depression is non-specific, which can be caused by cardiac disease and non-cardiac disease.
3. Simple T wave inversion without apparent ST segment changes is non-specific under most circumstances (Fig. 52.73),but the prospect for myocardial ischemia can not be totally eliminated.
4. 4.Widespread deep inverted T wave without apparent ST segment elevation or depression is not specific for diagnosis, and can be attributed to following causes (Fig. 52.74): myocardial ischemia, dynamic evolution of myocardial infarction, Adams-Stroke syndrome attack, ventricular and superventricular tachycardia attack, myocarditis, pericarditis, cardiomyopathy, pulmonary embolism, medications (cocaine, tricyclic antidepressants, etc.), alcoholism, electrolyte disturbances, subarachnoid hemorrhage, acute pancreatitis, gallbladder disease, pheochromocytoma, etc.
5. Symmetrical inverted T wave: the proportion of female to male is 4:1, and the common cause is myocardial ischemia, but the causes mentioned above should also be taken into consideration.
6. Slightly inverted T wave without ST segment change can be caused by the following factors, apart from aforementioned conditions: hyperventilation, feeding or cold drinks (fasting ECG is normal),mitral valve prolapse, ventricular block, pneumothorax. Besides, slight changes in T wave, without apparent ST segment changes, can still be normal variant.

52.6.3.2 Peaked T wave

Normally, the height of T wave in limb leads are usually <5 mm, and <10 mm in any chest leads. If the height of T wave is >5 mm in limb leads and >10 mm in chest leads, it is defined as peaked T wave. This ECG variant is always seen under the following circumstances:

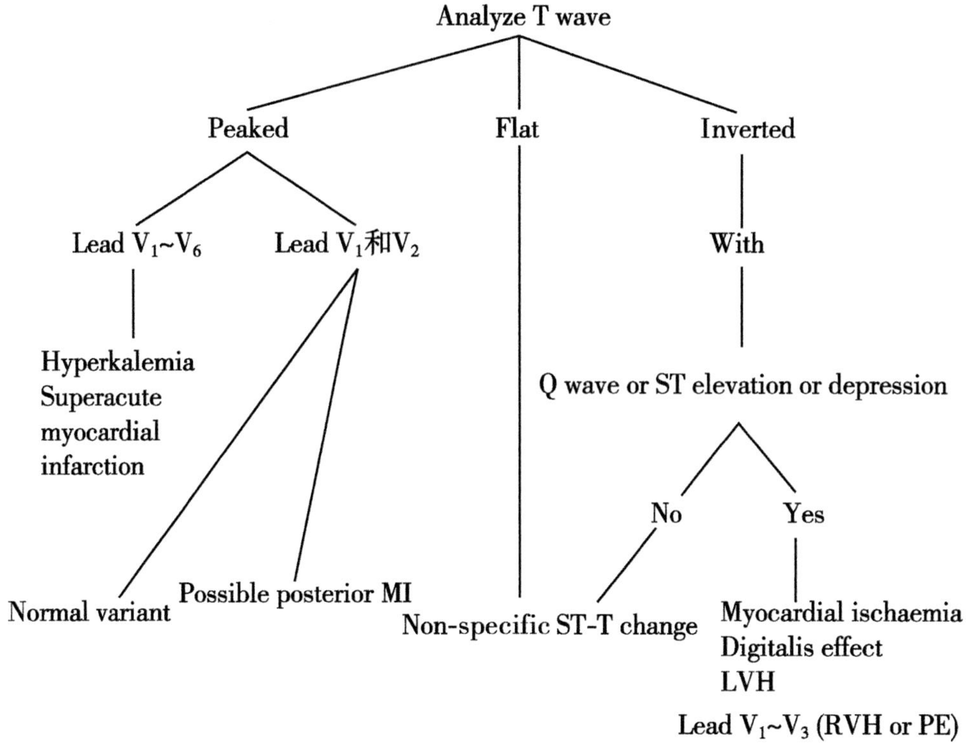

Fig. 52.71 Algorithm for T wave morphology analysis

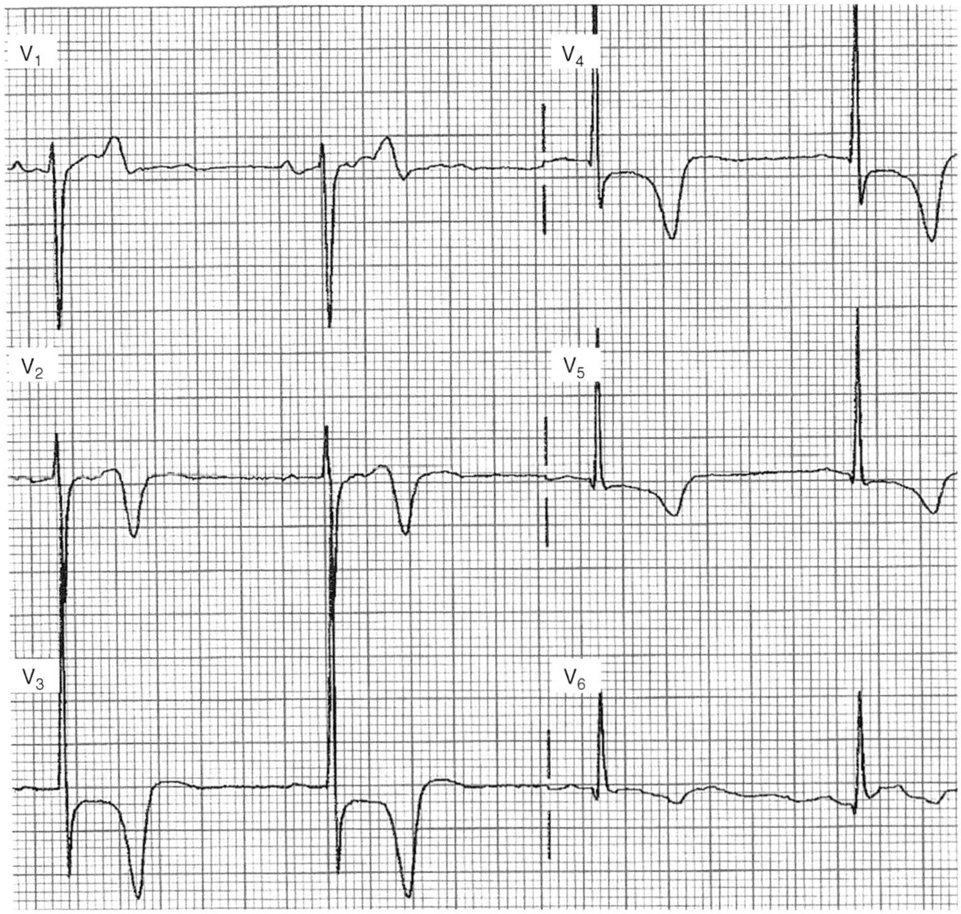

Fig. 52.72 Female patient, aged 53, unstable coronary syndrome onset 1 week before. Notable deep inverted T wave with horizontal ST depression in leads V_2 to V_6. ECG indicates myocardial ischemia

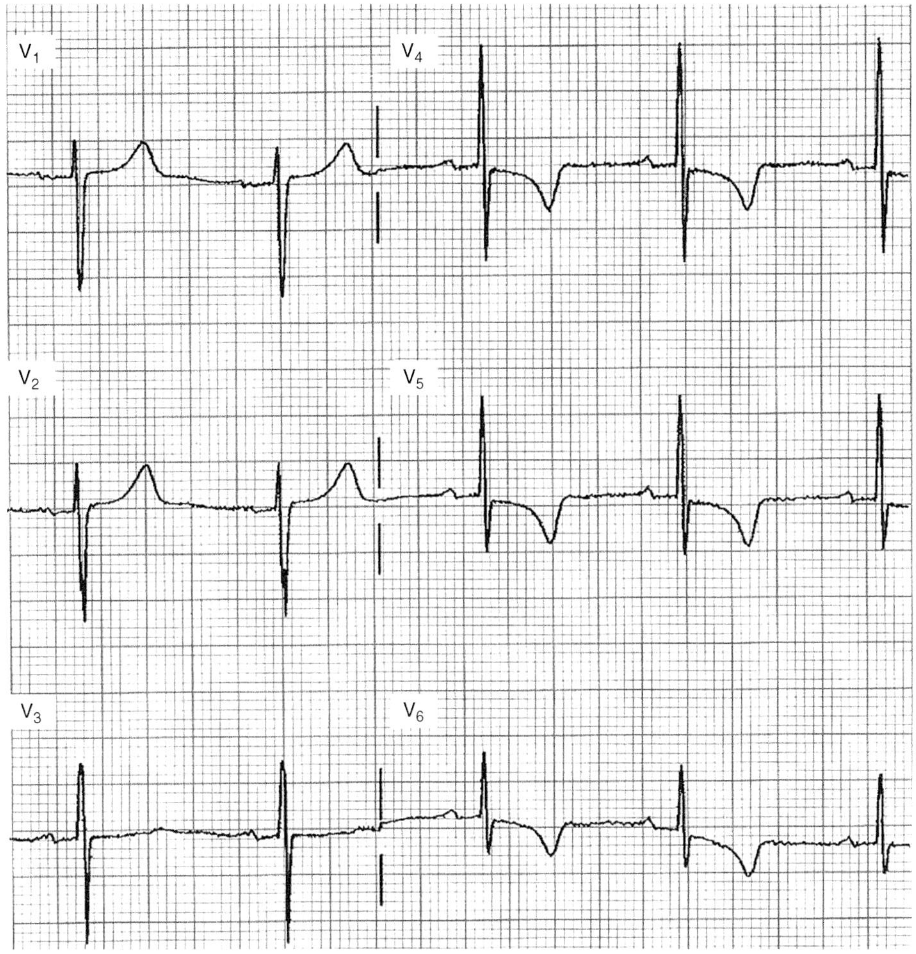

Fig. 52.73 Male patient, aged 35, ECG in conventional health examination. Notable inverted T wave with non-specific ST change in leads V_4 to V_6

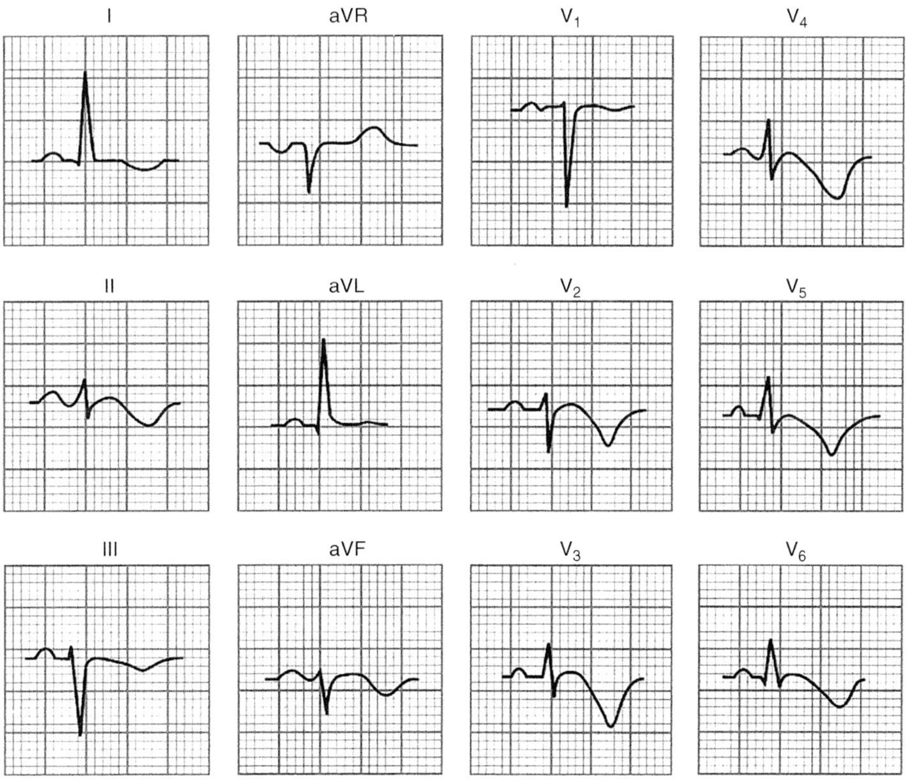

Fig. 52.74 Male patient, aged 48, severe brain hemorrhage in trauma. Notable inverted T wave in most leads

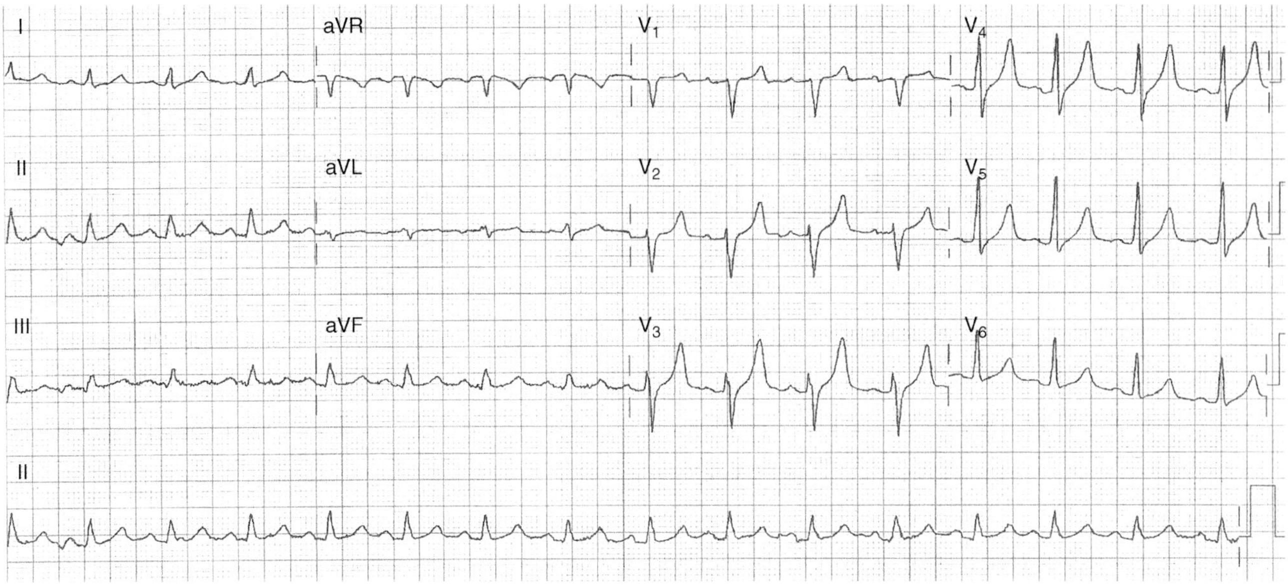

Fig. 52.75 Healthy Male, aged 30, ECG in health check. Notable peaked T wave in leads V_3 to V_5

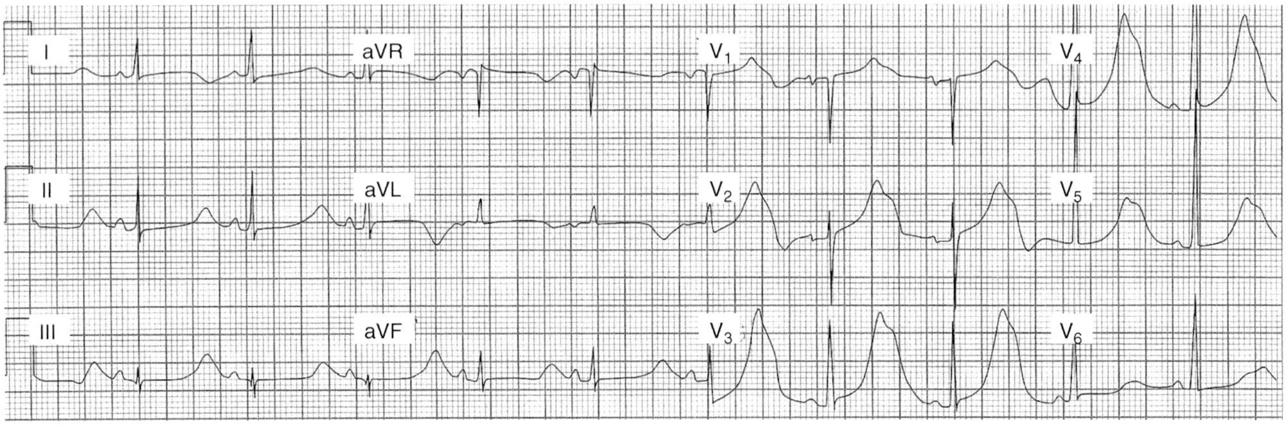

Fig. 52.76 Male patient, aged 70, acute myocardial infarction. Notable abnormal huge peaked T wave is present in chest leads

1. In V_2 to V_5leads, the base of normal peaked T wave is narrow. And if T wave is peaked, usually seen in healthy people, it is also a normal variant (Fig. 52.75).
2. Acute myocardial ischemia or myocardial infarction (Fig. 52.76, superacute phase).
3. Hyperkalemia (Fig. 52.77).
4. Patients with overloaded left ventricle, such as severe mitral regurgitation.
5. Patients with cerebrovascular events such as subarachnoid hemorrhage.

52.7 Section 7: Other Common Abnormal ECG

52.7.1 QT Interval Prolongation

QT interval represents the total time from ventricular depolarization to repolarization. The prolongation of QT interval indicates the prolongation of ventricular repolarization, and entrant arrhythmia such as torsade de pointes is likely to take place during this interval.

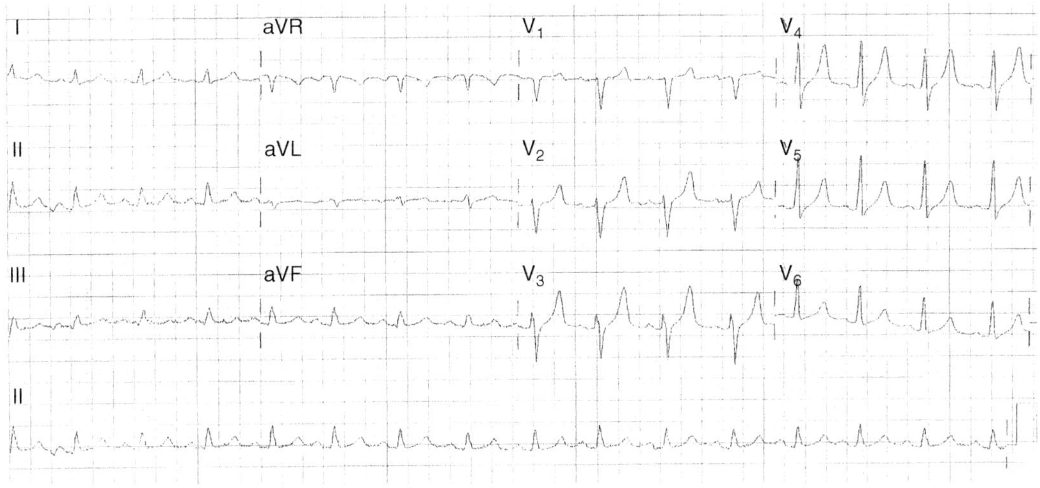

Fig. 52.77 Female patient, aged 65, toxuria without regular hemodialysis, serum potassium 7.5 mmol/L during ECG examination. Notable abnormal narrow peaked T wave could be found in chest leads

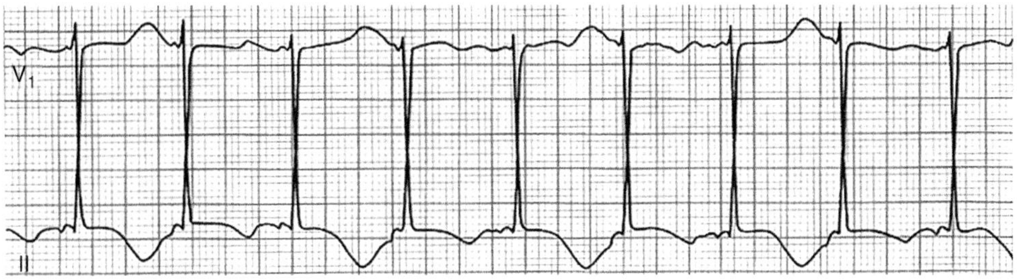

Fig. 52.78 Prolonged QT interval

52.7.1.1 Common Causes of QT Interval Prolongation

- Congenital long QT interval syndrome
- Acquired long QT interval syndrome

Non-drug-related reasons: Myocardial ischemia, central nervous conditions, severe bradyarrhythmia, hypokalemia.

Drug-related reasons: Type Ia, Ic and III antiarrhythmia medications, erythromycin, non- sedative antihistamines (e.g. astemizole and terfenadine).

ECG Recognition (Fig. 52.78)

1. QT interval is affected by heart rate; QTc needs to be calculated, which represents the actual QT interval when the rate is 60 bpm; $QTc = QT/\sqrt{RR}$.
2. The normal heart rate is between 60 and 100 bpm, and normal QT interval is between 0.32 and 0.44 s.

52.7.2 Hyperkalemia

52.7.2.1 ECG Recognition (Fig. 52.79)

1. Mild Hyperkalemia: when the serum potassium level is approximately between 5.7 and 6.5 mmol/L, P wave widens; tall, peaked, narrow-base and tented T waves occur in many leads; PR interval prolongs, and first-degree AVB can happen.
2. Severe Hyperkalemia: when serum potassium level is over 6.5 mmol/L, the latter portion of the QRS complex is significantly widened, which shows marked notching or slurring. As a result, the widened QRS will merge with tall and tented T wave, and ST segment will be elevated.
3. High-degree AVB: P wave disappears.
4. Ventricular tachycardia, ventricular fibrillation or autonomous ventricular rhythm.
   (a) Serum potassium >6.0 mmol/L: the earliest change is that T wave tends to be tall, narrow-based and tented, and PR interval may be prolonged.
   (b) Serum potassium >7.0 mmol/L: P wave flattens or disappears; QRS complex widens; and prominent S wave can be seen.
   (c) Serum potassium >8.0 mmol/L: S wave widens and deepens progressively, and the ST segment is steeper; no ST segment is isoelectric.

52.7.3 Hypokalemia

52.7.3.1 ECG Recognition (Fig. 52.80)

1. Mild Hypokalemia: when the serum potassium level is approximately between 3.0 and 3.5 mmol/L, the amplitude of T wave decreases progressively, and the amplitude of U wave is as small as T wave.

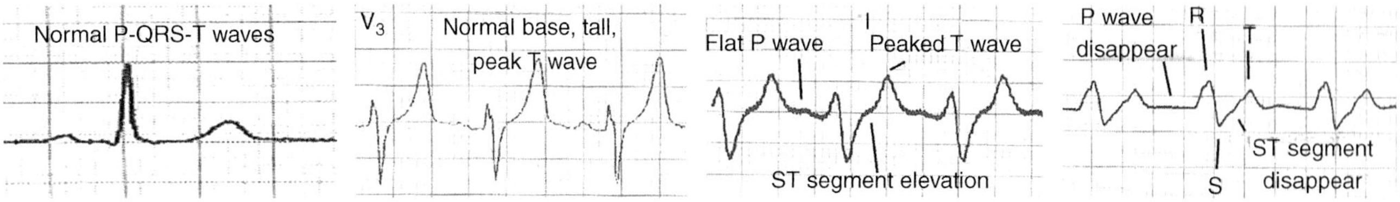

Fig. 52.79 ECG manifestation of increased levels of hyperkalemia

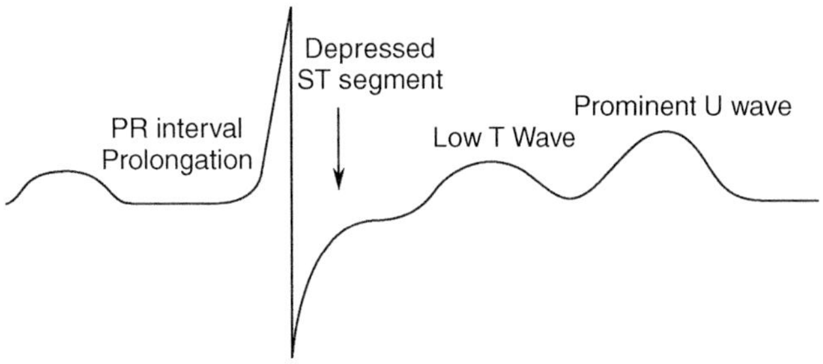

Fig. 52.80 ECG manifestation of hypokalemia

2. Severe Hypokalemia: when the serum potassium level is less than 3.0 mmol/L, there is an apparent increase in the amplitude of U wave, and U wave grows taller than T wave. When the serum potassium level is less than 1.5 mmol/L, T wave and U wave can merge, which is most obvious in leads V_2 to V_5.
3. ST segment depresses progressively.
4. QRS complex duration is prolonged.
5. PR interval slightly is prolonged.

53 Common Types of Tachycardia

Rui Zeng

53.1 Section 1: Tachycardia with Narrow QRS Complex

Tachycardia with narrow QRS complex have a QRS interval less than or equal to 120 ms, and a frequency greater than or equal to 100 bpm. 95% of the cases are supraventricular tachycardia, which originates from above the division of the bundle branches; 5% are ventricular tachycardia, particularly idiopathic ventricular tachycardia in children which can have a QRS interval less than 120 ms. Common types of narrow QRS complex tachycardia include atrioventricular nodal reentrant tachycardia (AVNRT), atrioventricular reentrant tachycardia (AVRT) and atrial tachycardia.

53.1.1 Atrioventricular Nodal Reentrant Tachycardia

The structural basis of AVNRT is the two types of conduction pathways with different properties in the AV node, which is called dual atrioventricular nodal pathway. One of the pathways has a slow conduction rate and short refractory period, called slow pathway (α pathway). The other pathway has a fast conduction rate, but longer refractory period, and is known as fast pathway (β pathway). Normally, an excitation originating in the SA node reaches the ventricle via the fast pathway. On reaching the end of the circuit, the excitation go in retrograde via the slow pathway, offsetting the excitation that went in anterograde fashion through the same pathway (Fig. 53.1a); when atrial pacemaker discharges an impulse, as fast pathway has a longer refractory period than slow pathway, the impulse more than often pass along the slow pathway which has recovered from the refractory state, resulting in a long P′-R interval. At this time, if the excitation through the fast pathway already nears the end of the circuit and the cells in the fast pathway has recovered from the refractory state, the impulse can go in retrograde via the fast pathway back to the atria, but as the same impulse proceed again toward the ventricle, the slow pathway is still in the refractory period, stopping the impulse from passing through again. Therefore, a small pseudo r wave appears on ECG (retrograde p′ wave, Fig. 53.1b); The earlier the atria is excited, the slower the excitation pass through the slow pathway, as the impulse reaches the start of the circuit again via the fast pathway as the retrograde limb, the slow pathway has recovered from the refractory state, enabling the impulse to pass through again, forming a continuous reentrant excitation and causing what we call AVNRT (Fig. 53.1c). This is the most common mechanism of AVNRT, also known as "slow-fast" AVNRT.

There is another type of AVNRT which is more uncommon. Its fast pathway has a refractory period shorter than the slow pathway. The anterograde conduction of the reentrant excitation is through the fast pathway, and retrograde conduction via the slow pathway, forming "fast-slow" AVNRT. This type of AVNRT is very rare and makes up approximately 10% of all cases. It is more commonly seen in children. We will focus on the "slow-fast" AVNRT (Fig. 53.2) in this chapter and will not go over the details of the uncommon type (Fig. 53.3).

53.1.1.1 Slow-Fast Atrioventricular Nodal Reentrant Tachycardia

ECG Recognition (Fig. 53.2)

1. Tachycardia is usually induced by premature atrial contraction, frequency at 160–200 bpm.
2. RR interval is even, heart rhythm is regular.
3. In most cases there are no P waves because the retrograde p wave is buried in QRS complex. In a few cases there might be a retrograde p′ wave after QRS complex, some of which appear at the J point on QRS, forming a pseudo s wave in leads II, III, aVF and a pseudo r wave in lead V_1.
4. R-P′ interval < P′-R interval, R-P′ interval < 70 ms.

R. Zeng (✉)
Department of Cardiology, Sichuan University, Chengdu, China

X.-H. Wan, R. Zeng (eds.), *Handbook of Clinical Diagnostics*, https://doi.org/10.1007/978-981-13-7677-1_53

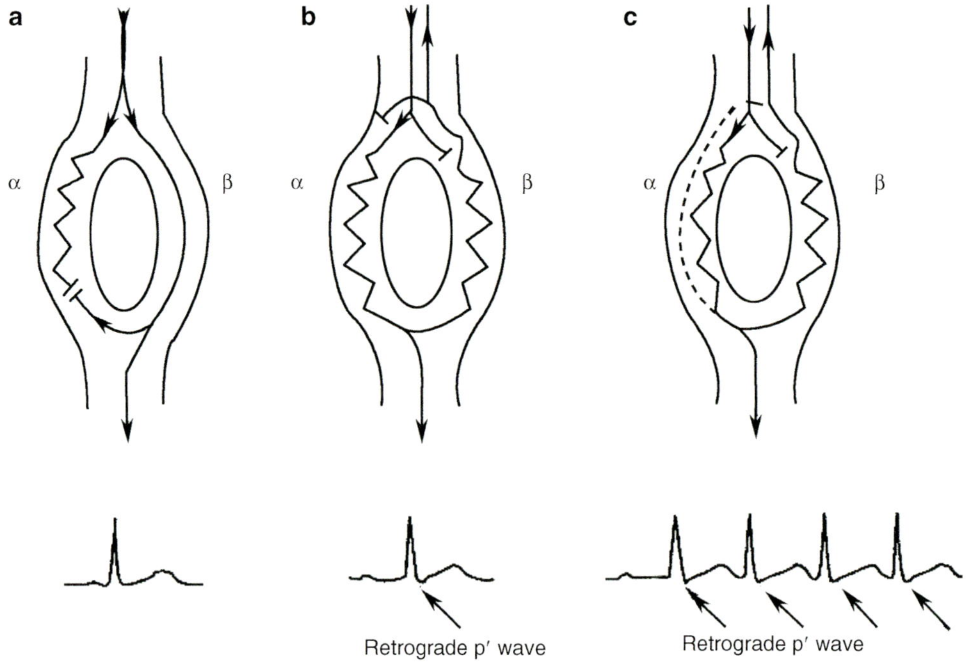

Fig. 53.1 Mechanism of slow and fast AVNRT. (**a**) An excitation originating in the SA node reaches the ventricle via the fast pathway and go in retrograde via the slow pathway; (**b**) Retrograde p′ wave appears on ECG; (**c**) How to form a continuous reentrant excitation and causing what we call AVNRT

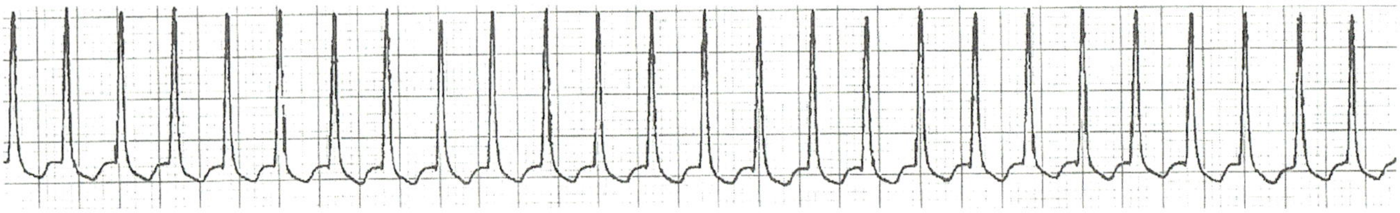

Fig. 53.2 Slow-fast atrioventricular nodal reentrant tachycardia

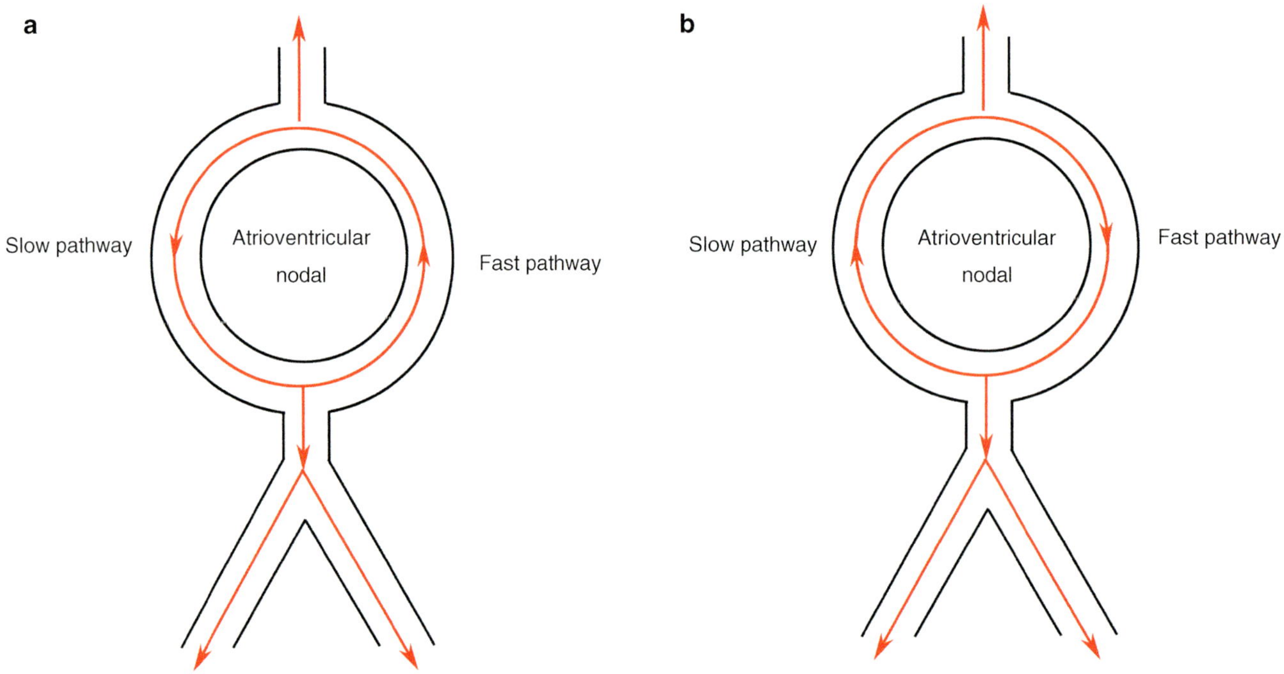

Fig. 53.3 Two types of AVNRT. (**a**) atrioventricular nodal reentrant tachycardia (common type); (**b**) atrioventricular nodal reentrant tachycardia (rare type)

5. QRS complex usually have a normal appearance. If there is aberrant ventricular conduction or existing bundle branch block, QRS complex may appear to be widened. In some patients electrical alternans in the QRS complex might be seen.

53.1.1.2 Atrioventricular Reentrant Tachycardia

Under normal circumstances, AV node-His-Purkinje system is the only conduction pathway between the atria and the ventricles. The atrioventricular ring surrounding the system are insulated, functioning as a barrier. In some patients with congenital developmental anomalies, there are additional conduction bundles (also known as accessory pathways) beside the normal conduction pathway. Excitation from the atria can reach the ventricles through the original pathway or the accessory pathway. Because of the unique electrophysiological characteristics of the accessory pathway, atrioventricular reentrant conduction is more likely to occur as the atria, the original atrioventricular conduction pathway, the ventricles as well as the accessory pathways join to form a big reentrant circuit, resulting in AVRT.

There are two types of accessory atrioventricular pathways that cause AVRT

1. **Concealed accessory pathway:** there can only be retrograde conduction through the pathway and no anterograde conduction, so during a sinus rhythm or tachycardia, impulse is conducted in the normal manner to the ventricles, and passes back through the accessory pathway. Its ECG features include a normal QRS complex with no delta wave (Refer to pre-excitation syndrome related material). This is called orthodromic AVRT.
2. **Dominant accessory pathway:** There can be both anterograde and retrograde conduction through the pathway. During a sinus rhythm, the sinus excitation can either be conducted in the normal manner down to the ventricles or pass through the accessory pathway and reach some parts of the ventricles at a faster rate, causing associated cardiac muscles cells to depolarize earlier. Its manifestation on the ECG is a delta wave before the QRS complex; When tachycardia occurs, the excitation can spread downward through the normal pathway, go in reverse through the accessory pathway, causing orthodromic AVRT, with normal QRS complex on ECG tracing without any delta wave (Fig. 53.4a);The excitation can also spread downward through the accessory pathway and pass back through the normal pathway, causing antidromic AVRT, with wide QRS complex along with delta wave on ECG tracing (Fig. 53.4b).

53.1.1.3 Orthodromic Atrioventricular Reentrant Tachycardia

ECG Recognition (Fig. 53.5)

1. Heart rate during tachycardia is 150–250 bpm, but it's usually >200 bpm.
2. Regular heart rate.
3. Under most circumstances there is no P wave because the retrograde p wave is buried in the QRS complex, but occasionally we can see a retrograde p′ wave after the QRS complex.
4. R-P′ interval < P′-R interval, R-P′ interval > 70 ms.
5. Atrioventricular conduction ratio is 1:1. There shouldn't be atrioventricular block because normal conduction

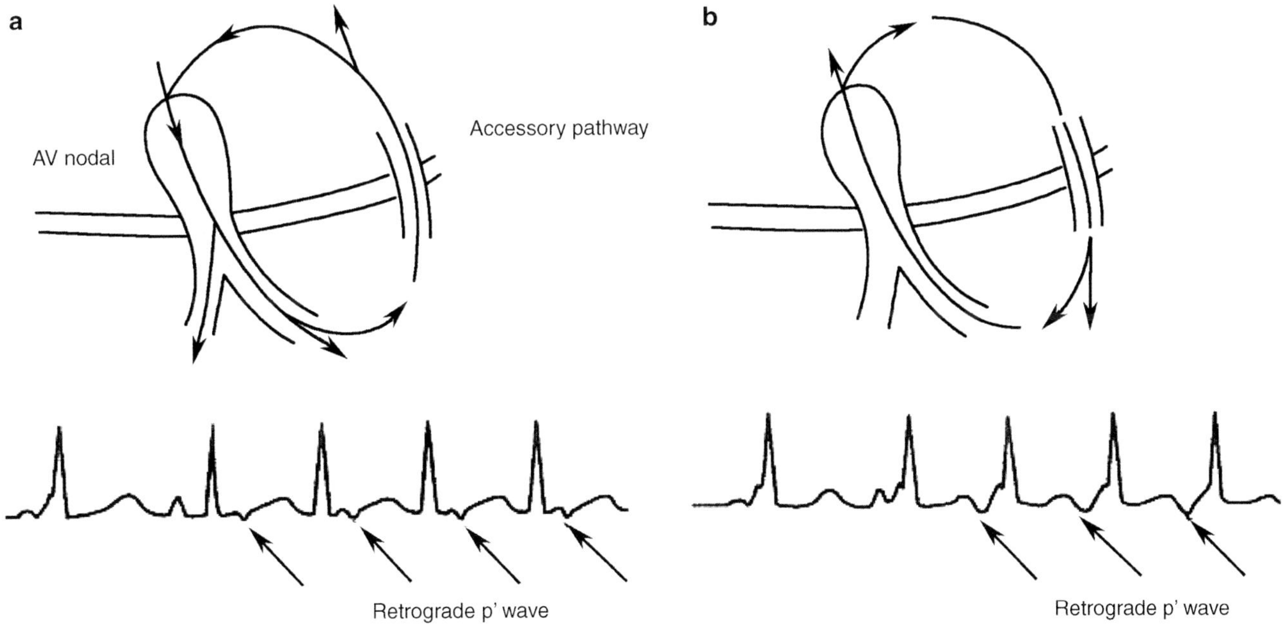

Fig. 53.4 AVRT by dominant accessory pathway. (**a**) Orthodromic AVRT with normal QRS complex without any delta wave on ECG; (**b**) Antidromic AVRT with wide QRS complex along with delta wave on ECG

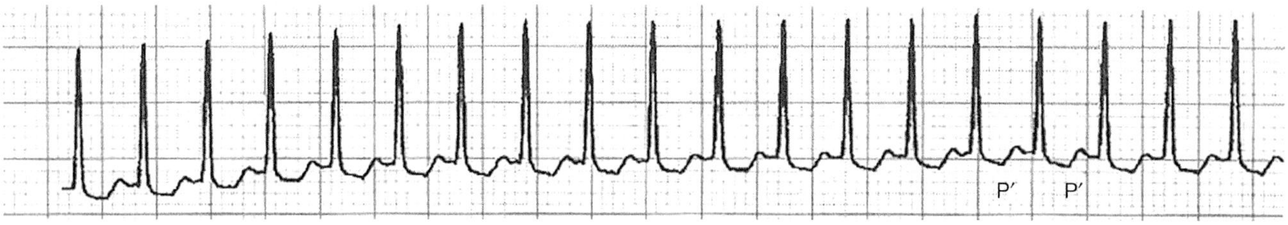

Fig. 53.5 Orthodromic atrioventricular reentrant tachycardia

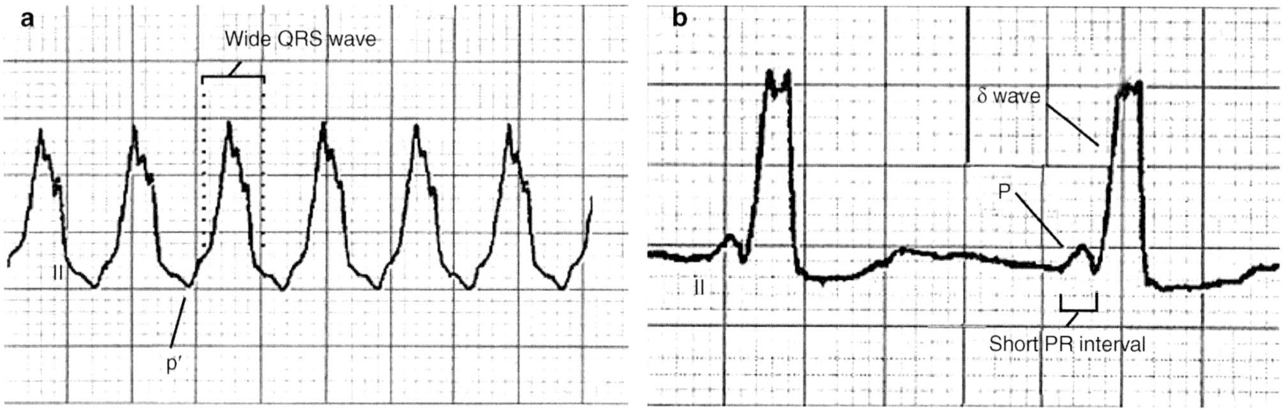

Fig. 53.6 Antidromic atrioventricular reentrant tachycardia. (**a**) During tachycardia; (**b**) during normal sinus rhythm

between the atria and the ventricles is the prerequisite for maintaining reentry. If atrioventricular block occurs, we can eliminate the possibility of AVRT.

6. QRS complex usually have a normal appearance. If there is aberrant ventricular conduction or existing bundle branch block, QRS complex may appear to be widened. In some patients electrical alternans in the QRS complex might be seen.
7. AVRT can often be induced or stopped by premature atrial or ventricular contraction.
8. Tachycardia induced by the dominant pathway can have a normal QRS complex on ECG tracing; During sinus rhythm, ECG tracing shows feature of pre-excitation syndrome.

53.1.1.4 Antidromic Atrioventricular Reentrant Tachycardia

ECG Recognition (Fig. 53.6)

1. Delta wave can be seen at the start of the QRS complex.
2. heart rate during tachycardia is between 150 and 250 bpm, usually it's >200 bpm, with a regular heart rhythm.
3. In most cases there is no P wave, if there is P′ wave, then R-P′ interval > P′-R interval.
4. During a sinus rhythm, QRS complex shows features of pre-excitation syndrome.

53.1.1.5 Atrial Tachycardia

The mechanism of atrial tachycardia is rather different than what we see on ECG, it can be categorized into three types, automatic atrial tachycardia (AT), reentrant atrial tachycardia and multifocal atrial tachycardia (MAT). Its most important characteristic is P waves with altered appearance than those from sinus origin.

ECG Recognition (Fig. 53.7)

1. Atrial rate is usually 150–200 bpm, ventricular rate is usually between 100 and 150 bpm.
2. P wave alter in appearance from those in a normal sinus rhythm(upright in leads II, III, aVF, inverted in aVR); it can also become a retrograde p′ wave(inverted in leads II, II, aVF and upright in aVR), those with uneven P′-P′ or P′-R intervals are called multifocal atrial tachycardia (MAT).
3. Often, second-degree AV block type I or type II can be seen, with a conduction ratio of 2:1, but it does not affect the state of tachycardia.
4. The isoelectric line still exist between P waves(which is distinct from atrial flutter, when the isoelectric line disappears).
5. Stimulation of the vagus nerve cannot stop tachycardia, instead it can aggravate AV block.
6. Heart rate gradually increases at the onset of atrial tachycardia.

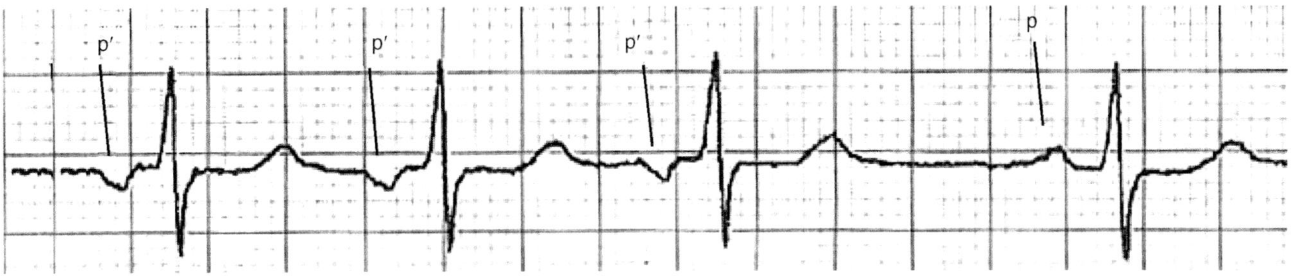

Fig. 53.7 Atrial tachycardia

Fig. 53.8 Algorithm For differential diagnosis Of QRS narrow tachycardia

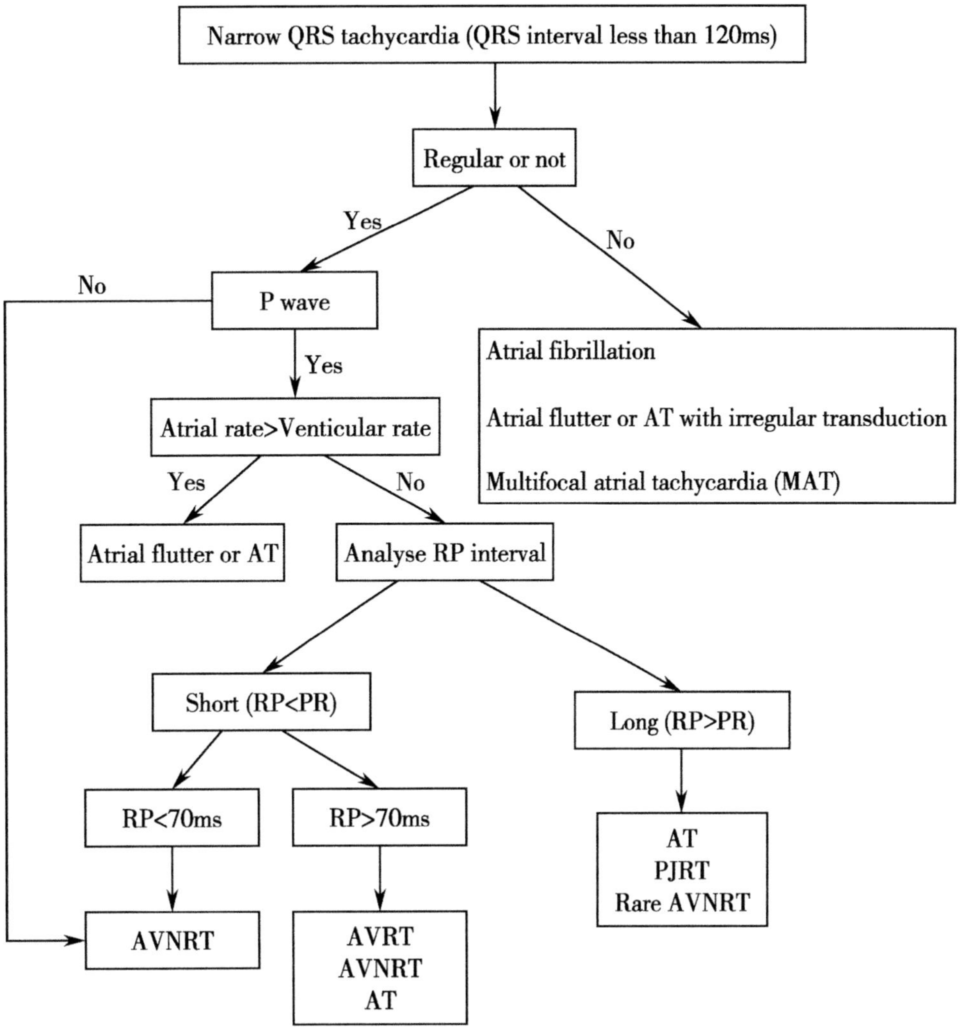

Addendum: Algorithm For Differential Diagnosis Of QRS Narrow Tachycardia (Fig. 53.8)

53.2 Section 2: Tachycardia with Wide QRS Complex

Wide complex tachycardia refers to tachycardia with the duration of QRS complex ≥0.12 s and HR > 100 bpm. The following types of wide complex tachycardia are common in clinical practice:

1. Ventricular tachycardia (accounting for about 70–80% of wide complex tachycardia).
2. Supraventricular tachycardia with any of the followings:
   - With aberrant intraventricular conduction (including bundle branch blocks or other types of intraventricular blocks, accounting for 15%).

- With accessory pathway conduction (accounting for 1–5%).
- With effect of medication or electrolyte disturbances.
- With slow ventricular conduction (postoperative).

3. Ventricular pacing

Diagnosis of wide QRS complex SVT requires the ECG before the onset of tachycardia as reference, but we are not going into further details on this in this section. Here we will focus on differential diagnosis of VT versus wide complex tachycardia.

53.2.1 Ventricular Tachycardia(VT)

53.2.1.1 ECG Recognition (Fig. 53.9)

1. Continuous wide QRS complexes, duration≥0.12 s and HR > 100 bpm.
2. Frequency: usually 150–200 bpm.
3. Tachycardia can be either paroxysmal or sustained.
4. If all QRS complexes have the same morphology and amplitude, the ECG variant is defined as monomorphic VT (Fig. 53.9a); If three or more QRS complexes with distinct morphology appear in the same lead with a frequency of more than 200 bpm, and such pattern continues for ten or more heartbeats, the variant is defined as polymorphic VT (Fig. 53.9b). Polymorphic VT can be subdivided into two types: sinus rhythm with normal QT intervals; sinus rhythm with prolonged QT intervals, which is usually torsade de pointes (Fig. 53.9c).

53.2.2 Differential Diagnosis of Wide Complex Tachycardia

53.2.2.1 Ventricular Rate and Ventricular Rhythm

1. Ventricular rate: In most VT cases, ventricular rate is between 150 and 200 bpm and ventricular rate more than 180 bpm rarely happens. If this rate is too high, then it is more likely a SVT or atrial flutter with 1:1 AV conduction rather than VT.
2. Ventricular rhythm: In VT, ventricular rhythm can be either regular or a bit irregular. However, in SVT the rhythm is strictly regular.

53.2.2.2 Atrioventricular Dissociation (AV Dissociation), Ventricular Capture and Ventricular Fusion Wave

If AV dissociation is present and ventricular rate is faster than atrial rate, the diagnosis of VT can be confirmed. In addition, ventricular capture and the appearance of ventricular fusion wave are important evidence for the diagnosis of VT.

53.2.2.3 Duration of the QRS Complex

In general, the wider the QRS complex, the greater possibility of VT. A RBBB-like morphology with duration more than 0.14 s, or a LBBB-like morphology with duration more than 0.16 s is highly suggestive of VT. In a few cases, the duration of QRS complex in VT can be normal, such as in idiopathic left ventricular tachycardia (IVT).

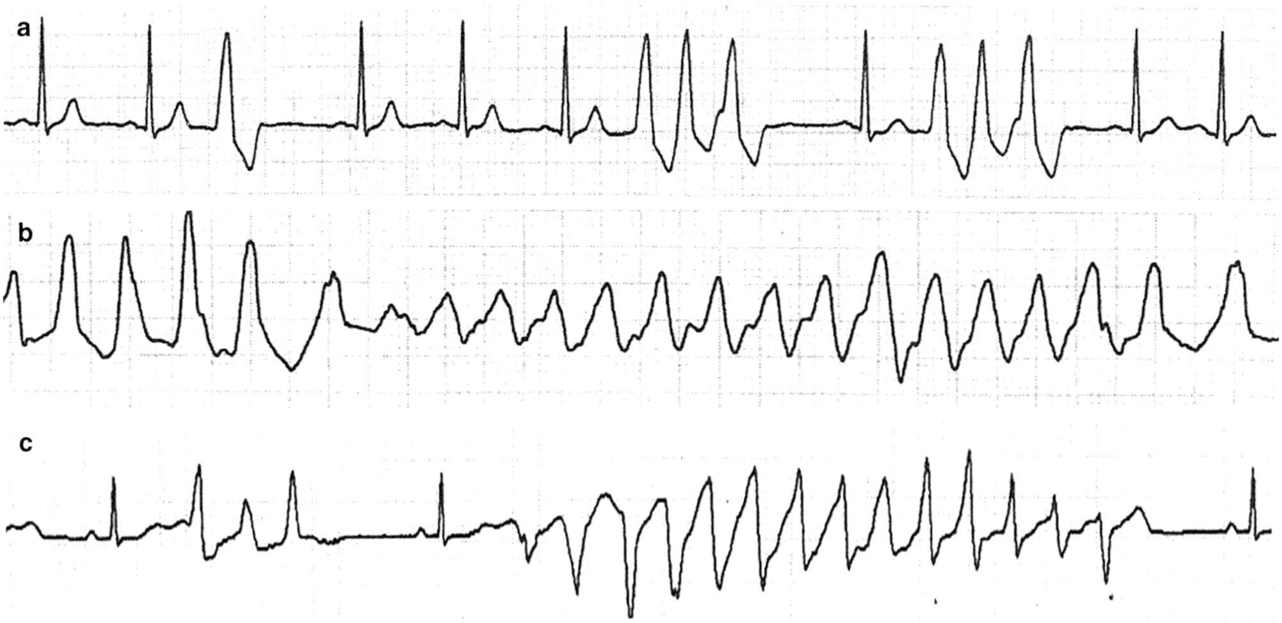

Fig. 53.9 Morphology of VT. (**a**) Monomorphic VT; (**b**) Polymorphic VT; (**c**) Torsades de pointes

53.2.2.4 Mean QRS Axis

If mean QRS axis lies between −90° and −180° (also known as extreme right axis deviation, northwest or no man's land), in most cases it's VT.

53.2.2.5 QRS Complex in Chest Leads

1. Concordant negative QRS complex pattern in chest leads indicates VT; concordant positive QRS complex pattern in chest leads, in most cases indicates VT and in a few cases is suggestive of atrioventricular reentry tachycardia (AVRT) involving a left accessory pathway.
2. When tachycardia occurs, if QR, QS or qR pattern rather than RS pattern (including RS, rS and Rs complex) is present in leads V_1 to V_6, diagnosis of VT can be clearly confirmed; If RS pattern is present in leads V_1 to V_6 with the duration of any RS waveform (the interval between the onset of R wave and the lowest point of S wave) is more than 0.1 s, VT can also be confirmed (Fig. 53.10).
3. Characteristics of QRS complex in leads V_1 and V_6: Could be divided into RBBB-like morphology (positive mean electrical axes of QRS Complexes in lead V_1, Fig. 53.11) and LBBB-like morphology (negative mean electrical axes of QRS Complexes in lead V_1, Fig. 53.12).

53.2.2.6 Others

1. A wide complex tachycardia with LBBB morphology and obvious right axis deviation indicates the diagnosis of VT. Negative mean electrical axis in leads II, III and aVF is very likely to be an indication of VT.
2. Precipitating factors of tachycardia: In most cases, tachycardia triggered by supraventricular premature contraction is SVT; Tachycardia evoked by ventricular premature contraction is usually VT.
3. Comparing ECG taken before onset of tachycardia: If the QRS complex is consistent in morphology with the complex in sinus rhythm, it usually indicates SVT, if not, then it is likely to be VT.

According to clues above to diagnosis of VT, we can summarized the ECG recognition under the condition of definitive diagnosis of VT and probable VT, and hoped it could be helpful for clinical practice:

You can make a definitive diagnosis of VT if:

- The mean electrical axes of QRS complexes in leads V_1 to V_6 are negative.
- No RS pattern is in leads V_1 to V_6.

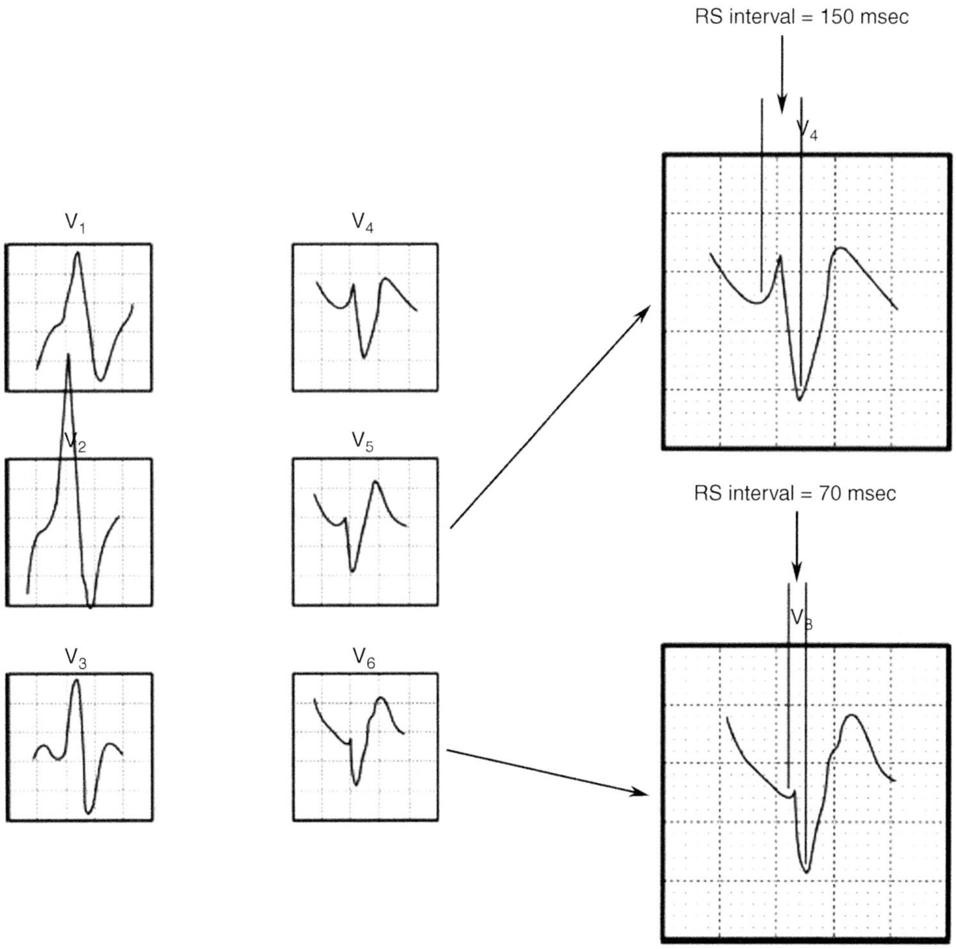

Fig. 53.10 RS pattern in leads V_1 to V_6 and measuring duration of RS complex

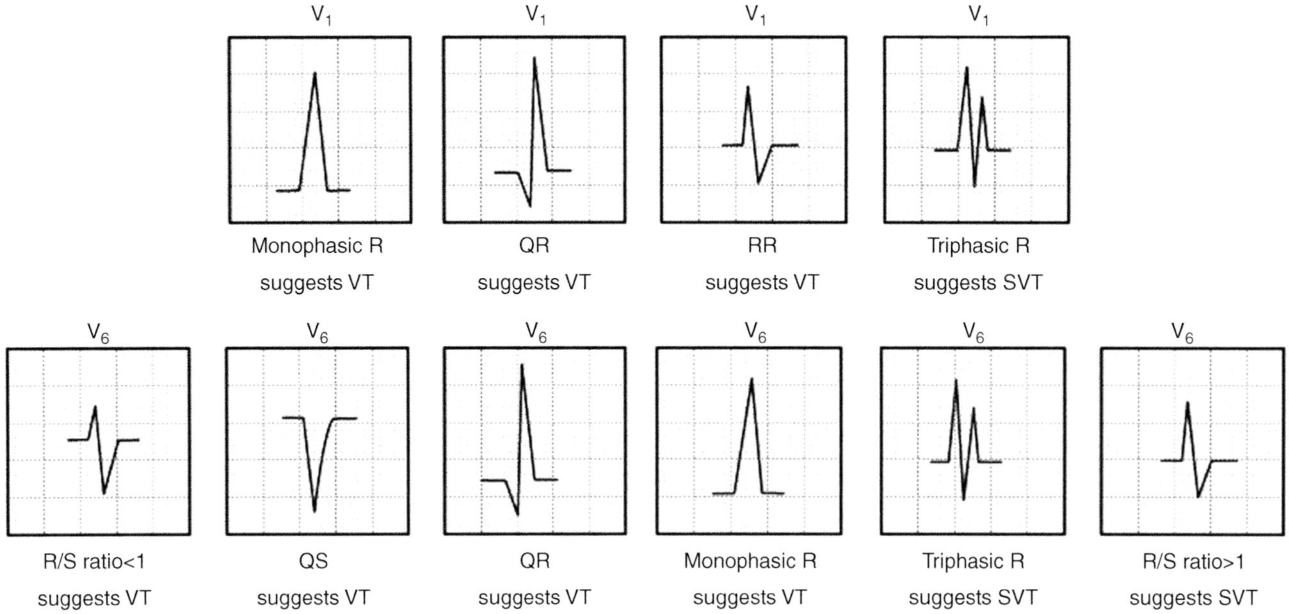

Fig. 53.11 QRS complex in RBBB-like morphology

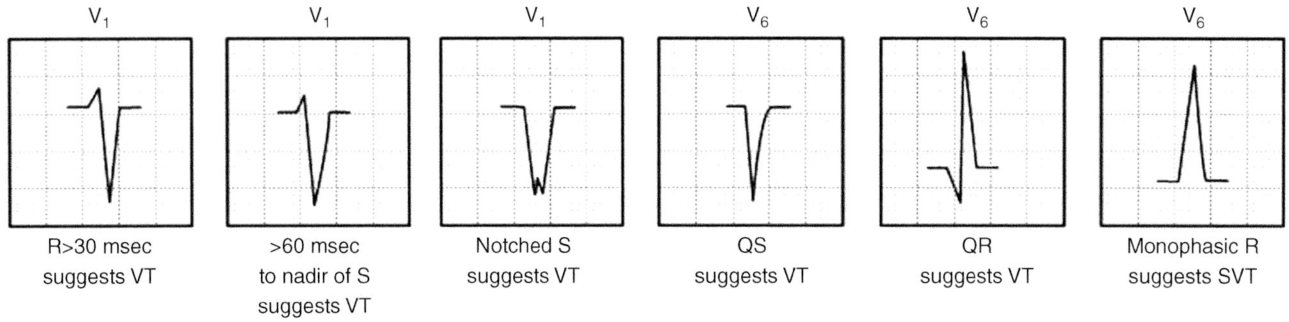

Fig. 53.12 QRS complex in LBBB-like morphology

- RS pattern is present in leads V_1 to V_6, but RS duration is more than 0.1 s.
- Evident AV dissociation with ventricular rate greater than atrial rate.
- LBBB variant with right axis deviation.
- Concordant ECG tracing with ventricular premature contraction before the onset of tachycardia.
- Presence of tall positive R wave in lead aVR.

VT highly probable if:

- All the mean electrical axes of QRS complexes in leads V_1 to V_6 are positive.
- Severe right axis deviation.
- The duration of QRS complex is more than 0.16 s in LBBB-like morphology or more than 0.14 s in RBBB-like morphology.
- All the mean electrical axes of QRS complexes in leads II, III and aVF are negative.

54 Arterial Blood Gas Analysis and Determination of Acid and Alkali

Ke Wang and Rui Zeng

The suitable power of hydrogen (pH) of the internal environment is essential for the organism's metabolism. The value of PH is 7.35–7.45 and the mean is 7.40. The process of maintaining a relatively stable internal environment is called the acid-base balance. However the acid-base disorders usually occur in the pathological state, in which the acid or base overloads or is severely inadequate. The judgment of acid-base state based on the arterial blood gas analysis has been the basic method in the clinical diagnosis and treatment.

54.1 Section 1: The Values and Clinical Significance of the Common Indices

54.1.1 Power of Hydrogen

Power of hydrogen (PH) is the index which reflects the concentration of H+. Because the concentration of H+ is difficult to measure, PH is represented by the negative log of the concentration.

- Reference Value: 7.35–7.45 (the mean, 7.40), the pathologically maximum range is 6.80–7.80.
- Clinical significance: PH<7.35 is called academia or acidosis, PH>7.45 is called alkalemia or alkalosis. The normal PH is commonly seen in these conditions: no acid-base disorders, compensatory acid-base disorders and mixed acid-base disorders. However the types of acid-base disorders, metabolic, respiratory or mixed can not be distinguished just relying on PH, therefore other indices are also need to be measured.

54.1.2 Arterial Partial Pressure of Oxygen

Arterial partial pressure of oxygen (PaO_2) is the pressure of physically dissolved oxygen in the blood.

- Reference Value: 80–100 mmHg (10.6–13.3 kPa), the computational formula: 100–0.33 × age ± 5 mmHg.
- Clinical significance: It is defined hypoxemia when PaO_2 is lower than normal or below limit of the peers. PaO_2<60 mmHg is the standard of respiratory failure. PaO_2<40 mmHg represents severe hypoxia. If PaO_2<20 mmHg, it usually means a failed aerobic metabolism and the life can not be maintained.

54.1.3 Arterial Oxygen Saturation

The arterial blood oxygen saturation (SaO_2) is defined as the percentage of the oxyhemoglobin concentration to the total hemoglobin concentration.

- Reference Value: 95–98%
- Clinical significance
  (a) Indicator of hypoxia
  SaO_2 is an index to judge the lack of oxygen in blood stream, however it is not sensitive. Because the oxygen dissociation curve (ODC) changes as an 'S' curve (Fig. 54.1), which means the curve reaches plateau when PaO_2 > 60 mmHg and SaO_2 may change little while PaO_2 significantly changes in the plateau stage. Therefore, when mild hypoxia happens, SaO_2 may not change significantly even though PaO_2 drops obviously. On the other hand, the ODC appears steep when PaO_2 < 57 mmHg and SaO_2 will drop significantly even though PaO_2 decreases slightly.

K. Wang
Department of Respiratory, Jilin University, Changchun, China

R. Zeng (✉)
Department of Cardiology, Sichuan University, Chengdu, China

X.-H. Wan, R. Zeng (eds.), *Handbook of Clinical Diagnostics*, https://doi.org/10.1007/978-981-13-7677-1_54

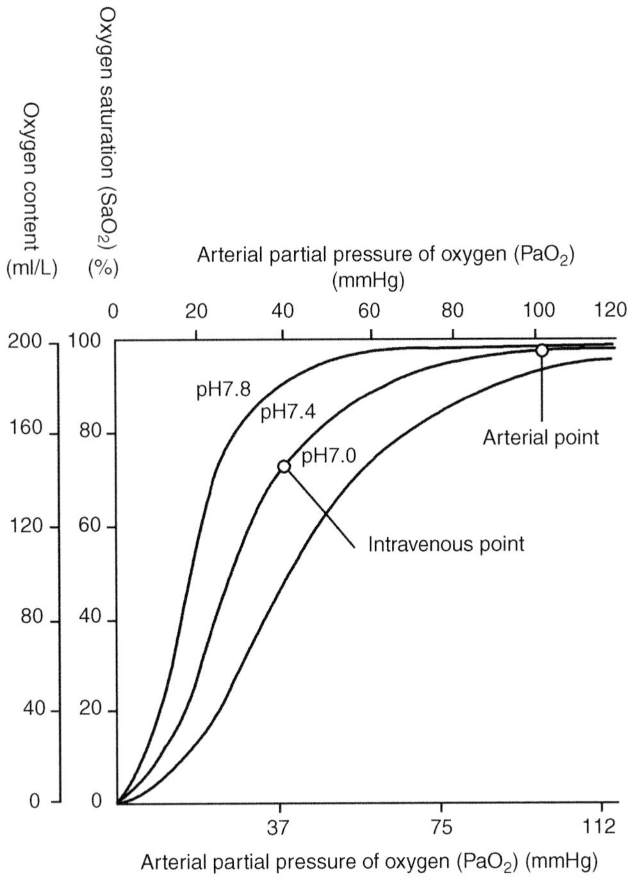

Fig. 54.1 Oxygen dissociation curve (ODC)

(b) Influencing factors of ODC
ODC is affected by many factors, for example the PH value, PCO_2, the temperature, and the content of 2,3-DPG in red blood cells. ODC will fluctuate when the PH value changes, which is called 'Bohr effect'. ODC will shift to the right if the PH value decreases, which leads to more oxygen released from oxyhemoglobin while SaO_2 just decreasing slightly. On the contrary, ODC will shift to the right if the PH value rises, resulting in more severe hypoxia.

54.1.4 Arterial Partial Pressure of Carbon Dioxide

Arterial partial pressure of carbon dioxide ($PaCO_2$) is defined as the pressure caused by the physically dissolved CO_2 in the arterial blood. Because CO_2 diffuses fast through the respiratory membrane, the arterial partial pressure of carbon dioxide ($PaCO_2$) is equivalent to the alveolar partial pressure of carbon dioxide (P_ACO_2). Alveolar ventilation can be reflected by $PaCO_2$.

- Reference Value: 35–45 mmHg (the mean = 40 mmHg)
- Clinical significance

(a) Judgment of alveolar ventilation
PCO_2 is in inversely proportional to alveolar ventilation. PCO_2 will rise when alveolar ventilation is insufficient. On the contrary, PCO_2 will decrease in the condition of hyperventilation.

(b) Judgment of respiratory acidosis or alkalosis
PCO_2 is an important index to reflect the respiratory acidosis or alkalosis. $PCO_2 > 50$ mmHg means the retention of carbon dioxide. $PCO_2 < 35$ mmHg means exhaling too much carbon dioxide.

54.1.5 Bicarbonate

Bicarbonate (HCO_3^-) is an index to reflect the metabolic acidosis or alkalosis, including actual bicarbonate (AB) and standard bicarbonate (SB). AB refers to the measured HCO_3^- content under the condition of actual body temperature, PCO_2 and SaO_2in the arterial blood specimen isolated from the air; SB refers to the measured HCO_3^- content under the condition of 38 °C, $PCO_2$40mmHg and $SaO_2$100% in the arterial blood specimen. There is no difference between AB and SB in health people.

- Reference Value: 22–27 mmol/L (the mean = 24 mmol/L)
- Clinical significance
  (a) SB is not affected by the respiratory factors, therefore it is treated as an index to reflect metabolic acidosis or alkalosis. SB>27 mmol/L implies metabolic alkalosis, SB<22 mmol/L implies metabolic acidosis.
  (b) AB is affected by both of the respiratory and metabolic factors.

AB=SB and $PaCO_2 = 40$ mmHg implies normal status.

AB > SB and $PaCO_2 > 40$ mmHg implies respiratory acidosis or compensatory metabolic alkalosis.

AB < SB and $PaCO_2 < 40$ mmHg implies respiratory alkalosis or compensatory metabolic acidosis.

AB=SB > 27 mmol/L implies the increase of HCO_3^- and metabolic alkalosis.

AB=SB < 22 mmol/L implies the decrease of HCO_3^- and metabolic acidosis.

54.1.6 Buffer Base

Buffer base (BB) is defined as the total anion with buffered effect in the blood, including HCO_3^-, Hb^-, HbO_2^-, Pr^- and HPO_4^-.

- Reference Value: 45–55 mmol/L (the mean = 50 mmol/L)
- Clinical significance

BB is also an index to reflect the metabolic acid-base disorder, and is not affected by the respiratory factors. BB will decrease when metabolic acidosis occurs and increase when metabolic alkalosis occurs.

54.1.7 Base Excess

Base excess (BE) is the base concentration as measured by titration with acid to PH 7.40 at a PCO_2 of 40 mmHg at SaO_2 of 100% at 38 °C. Acid is required to titrate when excess base exists in the blood, then BE is expressed as a positive number. For negative value of BE, the titration must be carried out with base.

- Reference Value: −2.3–+2.3 mmol/L
- Clinical significance

More negative values of base excess may indicate metabolic acidosis while more positive base excess may indicate metabolic alkalosis.

54.1.8 Anion Gap

Anion Gap (AG) is the difference between the unmeasured anion (UA) and the unmeasured cation (UC) in serum.

The common cation in serum includes Na^+, H^+, K^+, Ca_2^+, Mg_2. The primary cation Na^+ and K^+(about 145 mmol/L) is called measured cation, and the rest is unmeasured cation. The common anion includes Cl^-, PO_4^{3-}, SO_4^{2-}, HCO_3^-.The primary anion Cl^- and HCO_3^- (about 128 mmol/L) is called measured anion, and the rest is unmeasured anion. Generally the total cation charge and anion charge has equal amount: $Na^++K^++UC=Cl^-+HCO_3^-+UA$, that is to say, $Na^++K^+-(Cl^-+HCO_3^-) = UA-UC$. Because the content of K^+ in serum is very low and does not change obviously, it's charge amount can be ignored. Generally, $AG = Na^+-(Cl^-+HCO_3^-) = UA-UC$.

- Reference Value:8–16 mmol/L
- Clinical significance

AG can help distinguish the types of metabolic acidosis.

The increased AG is commonly seen in (1) high AG metabolic acidosis (AG > 16 mmol/L), such as lactic acidosis, diabetic ketoacidosis and salicylism; (2) the mixed acid-base disorders, such as a combination of high AG metabolic acidosis and metabolic alkalosis, triple acid-base disorders. Sometimes the increased AG also appears in some circumstances such as dehydration and myeloma without metabolic acidosis.

Normal AG metabolic acidosis, also known as hyperchloremic acidosis, is due to the reduce of HCO_3^- or the application of overmuch chloric acid.

54.1.9 Carbon Dioxide Combining Power

Carbon dioxide combining power (CO_2-CP) is defined as the difference between the total content of CO_2 in the venous plasma which has been balanced with 5.5% CO_2 or normal alveolar gas ($PCO_2$40mmHg, $PO_2$100mmHg) at room temperature and the content of physically dissolved CO_2in the plasma. In a word, it refers mainly to the combinative state of CO_2 in the plasma.

- Reference Value: 22–31 mmol/L (the mean = 27 mmol/L)
- Clinical significance: CO_2-CP reflects the base reserve in vivo.

54.2 Section 2: The Clinical Application of Blood Gas Analysis

54.2.1 To Confirm the Type and Degree of Respiratory Failure

Respiratory failure exists when PaO_2<60 mmHg with or without $PaCO_2 \geq 50$ mmHg under the conditions that a person breathes the room air in a quiet state under the atmospheric pressure at sea level, excluding left heart failure and the abnormal shunt in the heart or between large vessels. Type I respiratory failure is defined as PaO_2<60 mmHg and $PaCO_2$in normal level or $PaCO_2$<35 mmHg. Type II respiratory failure is defined as PaO_2<60 mmHg and $PaCO_2 \geq 50$ mmHg. Mild hypoxia makes the mental activity weakened, however the increased $PaCO_2$ may lead to intracranial hypertension, lethargy, deliration even coma. The classification of respiratory failure is shown in table below (Table 54.1).

54.2.2 To Judge the Types and Classification of Acid-Base Disorders

The judgement of acid-base disorder types is based primarily on PH, $PaCO_2$, HCO_3^-,Siggaard-Andersen card (Fig. 54.2)

Table 54.1 The classification of respiratory failure

Degree	PaO_2 (mmHg)	$PaCO_2$ (mmHg)	SaO_2 (%)
Mild	<60	>50	>80
Moderate	<50	>70	80–40
Severe	<40	>90	<40

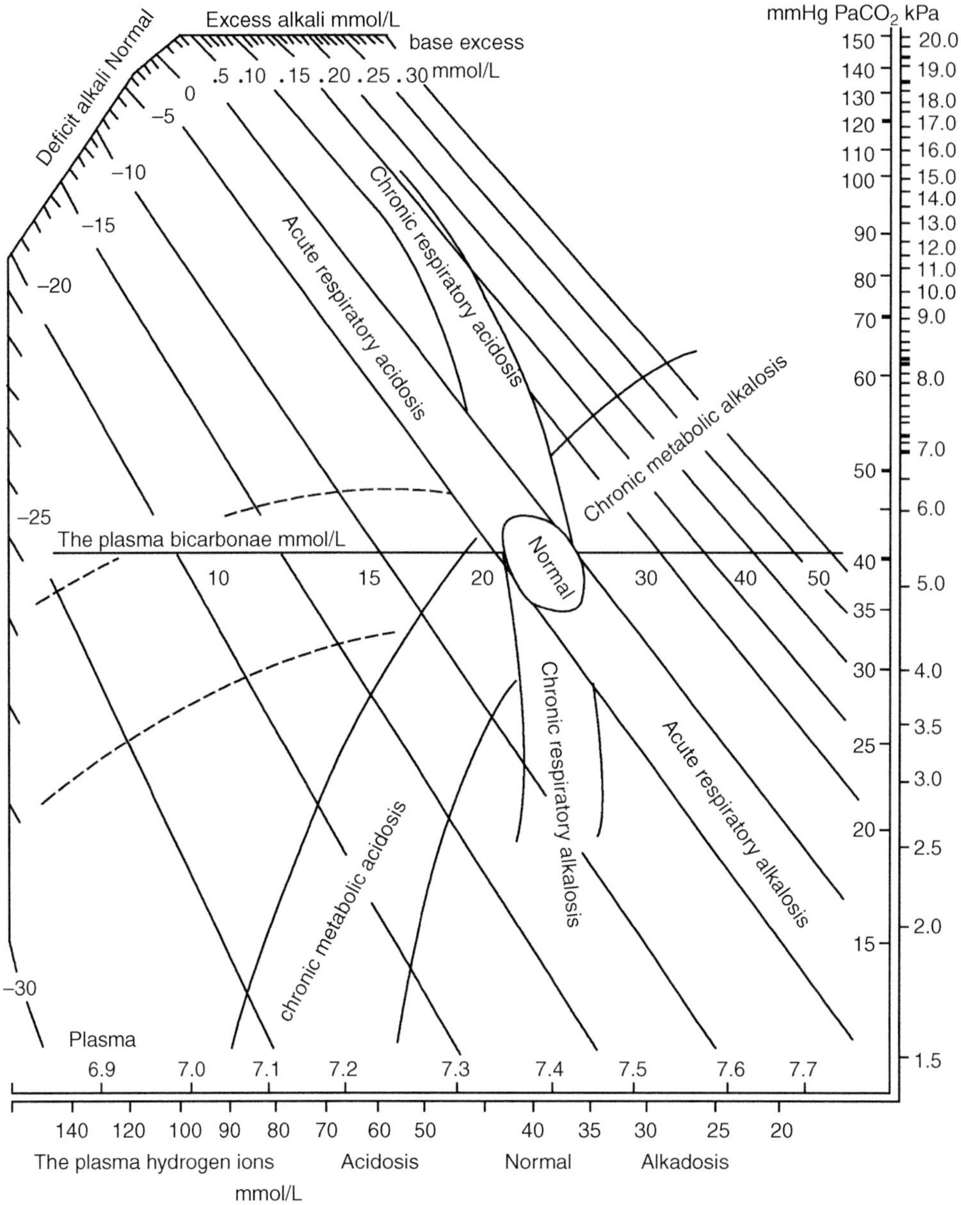

Fig. 54.2 Siggaard-Andersen card

Table 54.2 Expected changes in primary acid-base disorders

Primary disorders	Primary change	Compensatory change	Compensatory formula	Compensatory limitation
Respiratory acidosis	$PaCO_2$↑	HCO_3^-↑	Acute$\triangle HCO_3^- = \triangle PaCO_2 \times 0.07 \pm 1.5$	30 mmd/L
			Chronic$\triangle HCO_3^- = \triangle PaCO_2 \times 0.35 \pm 5.58$	45 mmol/L
Respiratory alkalosis	$PaCO_2$↓	HCO_3^-↓	Acute$\triangle HCO_3^- = \triangle PaCO_2 \times 0.2 \pm 2.5$	18 mmol/L
			Chronic$\triangle HCO_3^- = \triangle PaCO_2 \times 0.5 \pm 2.5$	12 mmol/L
Metabolic acidosis	HCO_3^-↓	$PaCO_2$↓	$PaCO_2 = HCO_3^- \times 1.5 + 8 \pm 2$	10 mmHg
Metabolic alkalosis	HCO_3^-↑	$PaCO_2$↑	$\triangle PaCO_2 = \triangle HCO_3$- $\times 0.9 \pm 5$	55 mmHg

and estimated compensation formula (Table 54.2), however, the clinic features also need to be considered.

54.2.2.1 Siggaard-Andersen Card

How to use the card? Firstly, find the corresponding value of PH and $PaCO_2$ in the card, secondly, judge the types of acid-base disorders according to the actual value of $HCO3^-$ and the corresponding range of $HCO3^-$ in the card. For example, if PH is 7.2 and $PaCO_2$ is 40 mmHg, with a value of 15 mmol/L actual $HCO3^-$ indicates simple acute base deficit. Another example, when PH is 7.2 and $PaCO_2$ is 70 mmHg, with a value of 15 mmol/L actual HCO_3^- indicates a combination of acute hypercapnia and acute base deficit.

54.2.2.2 The Steps of Analyzing Acid-Base Disorders

- To verify the accuracy of the results

The changes of pH, $PaCO_2$, and HCO_3^- values should conform to Henderson formula ($[H^+] = 24 \times PaCO_2/[HCO_3^-]$),otherwise the results may be misleading.

1. To discern the primary and secondary changes
   Respiratory alkalosis is defined as the primary decrease of $PaCO_2$. Metabolic alkalosis is defined as the primary increase of HCO_3^-. Metabolic acidosis is defined as the primary decrease of HCO_3^-.When the simple acid-base disorder appears, the body will initiate compensatory mechanism to keep $[HCO_3^-]/[H_2CO_3]$ in normal range. As long as the ratio is 20:1, PH will be in normal range, and this is called compensatory patterns in acid-base disorder. Otherwise, it is called decompensated acid-base disorder.
2. To analyze the simple or mixed disorders
   (a) The opposite changing tendency of $PaCO_2$ and HCO_3^- usually indicates the mixed acid-base disorders.
   (b) The mixed acid-base disorders exist when the actual value is greater or less than the predicted one which is calculated by the equation (Table 54.2).

54.2.2.3 The Common Types of Acid-Base Disorders

- Metabolic acidosis

Metabolic acidosis is defined as the pathophysiological procedure caused by the decrease of HCO_3^- primarily. It happens when overmuch acid is produced, acid excretion is dysfunctional or overmuch alkali is lost. Common causes of metabolic acidosis include diabetes, alcoholism and fasting, etc.

Arterial blood gas analysis: PH is decreased or almost normal. HCO_3^-, CO_2-CP, AB, SB and BB are decreased, the negative value of BE becomes larger. $PaCO_2$ is decreased or normal.

- Metabolic alkalosis

Metabolic alkalosis is defined as the pathophysiological procedure caused by the increase of HCO_3^- primarily and related to the decrease of H^+. Generally, the loss of gastric juice due to vomiting and severe hypochloremia or hypokalemia will lead to metabolic alkalosis.

Arterial blood gas analysis: PH is increased or almost normal. HCO_3^-, CO_2-CP, AB, SB and BB are increased. The positive value of BE becomes larger. $PaCO_2$ is increased or normal.

- Respiratory acidosis

Respiratory acidosis is defined as the pathophysiological procedure caused by the increase of $PaCO_2$ primarily. Respiratory acidosis usually associated with the respiratory function disorders, such as chronic obstructive pulmonary disease, chronic pulmonary heart disease, asthma. Carbon dioxide retention due to the alveolar ventilation decline is the primary cause of respiratory acidosis.

(a) Acute respiratory acidosis: $PaCO_2$ is increased, PH may be decreased, normal or increased, $HCO_3^-$is normal or increased slightly (3–4 mmol/L), BE is normal.
(b) Chronic respiratory acidosis: $PaCO_2$ is increased, PH is decreased or normal,

$HCO_3^-$is increased, AB>SB, the positive value of BE becomes larger. In addition, the serum chlorine is reduced and potassium may increase.

- Respiratory alkalosis

Respiratory alkalosis is defined as the pathophysiological procedure caused by the decrease of $PaCO_2$ primarily. Respiratory alkalosis is usually caused by hyperventilation, which include craniocerebral injury, hysteria, hypoxia and improper mechanical ventilation, et al.

Arterial blood gas analysis: $PaCO_2$ is decreased, PH is normal or increased. $HCO_3^-$is normal or decreased slightly in acute respiratory alkalosis. However HCO_3^- is decreased obviously in chronic respiratory alkalosis, AB<SB and the negative value of BE becomes larger.

- Mixed respiratory acidosis and metabolic alkalosis

Mixed respiratory acidosis and metabolic alkalosis are due to combination of primary respiratory acidosis with disproportional high HCO_3^- or primary metabolic alkalosis with disproportional high $PaCO_2$. The decrease of alveolar ventilation and the retention of CO_2 in chronic obstructive pulmonary disease patients may lead to respiratory acidosis, meanwhile, hypokalemia or hypochloremia caused by the improper application of diuretic usually lead to metabolic alkalosis.

Arterial blood gas analysis: $PaCO_2$, $HCO_3^-$and CO_2-CP are all increased obviously. HCO_3^-may exceed the limitation of expected compensation(the actualHCO_3^->24 + $\triangle PaCO_2 \times 0.35 + 5.58$). The positive value of BE becomes larger, PH may be normal, increased or decreased.

- Mixed respiratory acidosis and metabolic acidosis

Mixed respiratory acidosis and metabolic acidosis are due to the combination of acute or chronic respiratory acidosis with the improper decrease of HCO_3^- and the metabolic acidosis with the improper increase of $PaCO_2$. In addition to the hypoventilation, the increased production of unvolatile acid, the decreased elimination of fixed acid and the excess loss of alkali are more important reasons. For example, lactic acid increases when peripheral circulatory failure or severe hypoxia occurs, and the loss of alkali increases from diarrhea.

Arterial blood gas analysis: $PaCO_2$ is increased obviously, HCO_3^-may be decreased, normal or increases slightly. Therefore, PH is decreased obviously. AG is increased.

- Mixed respiratory alkalosis and metabolic acidosis

Mixed respiratory alkalosis and metabolic acidosis occur when respiratory alkalosis combines with an improper decrease of HCO_3^- or metabolic acidosis combines with an improper decrease of $PaCO_2$. The hyperventilation diseases such as pneumonia, fever and interstitial lung disease may lead to respiratory alkalosis. Meanwhile, renal failure and under-excretion of acid may lead to metabolic acidosis.

Arterial blood gas analysis: $PaCO_2$ and $HCO_3^-$is decreased, the negative value of BE becomes larger, AG is increased, PH is increased or almost normal.

- Mixed respiratory alkalosis and metabolic alkalosis

Mixed respiratory alkalosis and metabolic alkalosis are due to the increase of $HCO_3^-$and decrease of $PaCO_2$ at the same time, which makes PH increased obviously and always suggests a bad prognosis. It is commonly caused by the improper treatment of chronic pulmonary heart disease. Mechanical ventilation or the application of excessive respiratory stimulant always brings about the excessive or over-quick discharge of carbon dioxide and the rapid decrease of $PaCO_2$ in patients with chronic pulmonary heart disease. However, with the renal compensation for the primary respiratory alkalosis, the discharge of excessive HCO_3^- becomes relatively slow, and the content of $HCO_3^-$is still high. Therefore, this acid-base disorder is also called hypercapnic alkalosis.

Arterial blood gas analysis: $PaCO_2$ is decreased, HCO_3^- may be increased, normal or decreased, PH is increased apparently, the positive value of BE becomes larger.

The common changes of blood-gas indices in acid-base disorders could be seen in Table 54.3.

Table 54.3 The changes of blood-gas indices in common acid-base disorders

Types	pH	$PaCO_2$	HCO_3-	BE	AG	CO_2-CP
Metabolic acidosis	↓/—	—/↓	↓	(−)↑	—/↑	↓
Metabolic alkalosis	↑/—	—/↑	↑	(+)↑		↑
Acute respiratory acidosis	↓	↑	—/↑	–		
Chronic respiratory acidosis	↓/—	↑	↑	(+)↑		
Respiratory acidosis+ Metabolic alkalosis	↑/↓/—	↑	↑	(+)↑		↑
Respiratory acidosis+ Metabolic acidosis	↓↓	↑/↓/—	↓/—/↑	(−)↑	↑	
Respiratory alkalosis	↑/—	↓	↓	(−)↑		
Respiratory alkalosis+ Metabolic alkalosis	↑↑	↓	↑	(+)↑		
Respiratory alkalosis+ Metabolic acidosis	↑/—	↓	↓	(−)↑	↑	

Notes:
↑: increased; ↑↑:increased obviously
↓:decreased; ↓↓: decreased obviously
—: normal
(+)↑:the positive value becomes larger
(−)↑: the negative value becomes larger

Pulmonary Function Test

55

Ke Wang and Rui Zeng

Pulmonary function test is an important method to check the respiratory diseases. The aims of pulmonary function test include: (a) judgment whether the respiratory symptoms such as dyspnea, cough and cyanosis are caused by respiratory diseases; (b) management and monitoring of severity, progression and therapeutic reaction of the established respiratory diseases; (c) assessment of potential risks of respiratory failure or other respiratory complications after surgery or drug therapy; (d) quantitative evaluation of labor capacity of occupational pulmonary disease patients; (e) conduction of the epidemiological investigation of respiratory diseases caused by smoke or dust; (f) clinical evaluation of health.

55.1 Section 1: Common Test Items

The items of pulmonary function test include: lung volume test, ventilation function test, gas exchange function test, pneodynamics test etc. How to choose the items for the certain subjects depends on the purpose of diagnosis, however, no matter which item is chosen, the interpretation of the pulmonary function test results needs to be combined with the clinical and radiological data of the patients.

55.1.1 Lung Volume Test

Lung volume is defined as the gas volume change in one breath at resting state. It is not limited by time and has statically anatomic significance. The gas volume inside the lung always changes corresponding to the expansion and retraction of the lung, forming four types of basal lung volume and four types of basal lung capacity (Fig. 55.1).

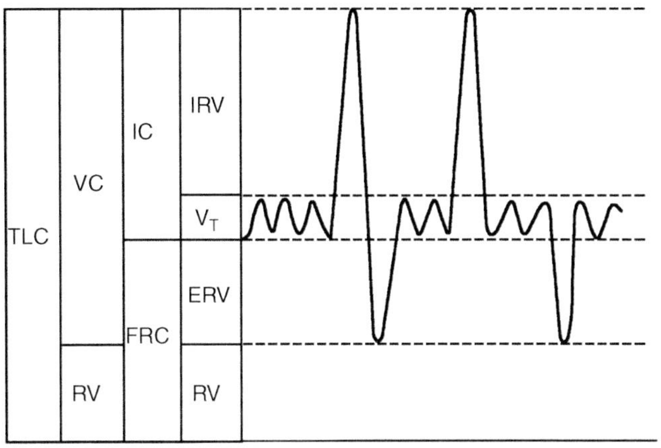

Fig. 55.1 Basal lung volume and capacity

55.1.1.1 Basal Lung Volume

Basal lung volume includes tidal volume, expiratory reserve volume, inspiratory reserve volume and residual volume.

Tidal Volume (V_T)

Tidal volume is defined as the gas volume breathed in and out of the lung in each breath at resting state. The normal reference is about 10 mL/kg body weight. The main influence factor of V_T is the inspiratory muscle function. 75%of the V_T depends on the movement of diaphragm, and the rest is from the contraction of intercostal muscles.

Expiratory Reserve Volume (ERV)

ERV is defined as the gas volume exhaled as much as possible at the end of the normal expiration. ERV has a wide range of fluctuation, and it is related to the body position, for example, ERV drops by 600–900 mL from standing to supine.

K. Wang
Department of Respiratory, Jilin University, Changchun, China

R. Zeng (✉)
Department of Cardiology, Sichuan University, Chengdu, China

X.-H. Wan, R. Zeng (eds.), *Handbook of Clinical Diagnostics*, https://doi.org/10.1007/978-981-13-7677-1_55

Inspiratory Reserve Volume (IRV)
IRV is defined as the gas volume inhaled as much as possible at the end of the normal inspiration.

Residual Volume (RV)
RV is defined as the residual gas volume contained in the lung at the end of the maximal expiration. It depends on the balance between the contraction strength of respiratory muscles and the stiffness of thoracic wall. In clinic, RV/TLC% is a critical determinant for emphysema. V/TLC% $\leq$ 35% is defined as normal, however, RV/TLC% $\geq$ 40% suggests emphysema.

55.1.1.2 Basal Lung Capacity

Basal lung capacity, which includes inspiratory capacity, functional residual capacity, vital capacity and total lung capacity, is consisted of at least two types of basal lung volume.

Inspiratory Capacity (IC)
IC is defined as the gas capacity inhaled as much as possible at the end of the normal expiration, that is, IC = VT + IRV. The normal IC accounts for 2/3 or 4/5 of the vital capacity. The main influence factor of IC is the inspiratory muscle strength, and when the function of respiratory muscle is impaired, IC will drop. In addition, when the thoracic mobility decreases, the lung elastic recoil increases or the airway is obstructed, IC will also drop.

Functional Residual Capacity (FRC)
FRC is defined as the gas capacity contained in the lung at the end of the normal expiration, that is, FRC = ERV + RV.

Vital Capacity (VC)
VC is defined as the maximal gas capacity exhaled as much as possible following the maximal inspiration, that is, VC = VT + ERV + IRV. VC is the main index to determine the severity of restrictive ventilation dysfunction. The measured value of VC/ the predicted value of VC < 80% is defined ad abnormal, 60–79% is slightly decreased, 40–59% is moderately decreased, <40% is severely decreased.

Total Lung Capacity (TLC)
TLC is defined as the gas capacity contained in the lung after the maximal inspiration, that is, TLC = VC + RV.

55.1.2 Ventilation Function Test

Pulmonary ventilation function means the gas volume and flow velocity in and out of the lung with the breathing in unite time. All the physiological or pathological factors influencing the respiratory rate, breath extent and flow velocity can influence the ventilation function.

55.1.2.1 Minute Ventilation (V_E)

V_E is defined as the gas volume exhaled or inhaled in the resting state in 1 min.

V_E = Tidal volume (V_T) × Respiratory rate(RR).

The normal reference value: (6.7 ± 0.2)L/min in male, (4.2 ± 0.2) L/min in female. V_E > 10 L/min suggests hyperventilation which may lead to respiratory alkalosis; V_E < 3 L/min suggests hypoventilation which may lead to respiratory acidosis.

55.1.2.2 Maximum Voluntary Ventilation (MVV)

MVV means the exhaled gas volume in the fastest rate and the deepest extent in 1 min. In clinic, MVV is usually used to evaluate the reserve capacity of pulmonary ventilation before the thoracic or abdominal operations and forecast the pulmonary complication risks. When the measured value of MVV/ the predicted value of MVV < 80%, it suggests pulmonary ventilation dysfunction.

55.1.2.3 Forced Vital Capacity (FVC)

FVC is defined as the exhaled gas capacity with the maximum expiratory force and at full speed in the state of total lung capacity. FVC, which is influenced by respiratory muscle function, airway resistance and lung tissue elasticity, is a common index to reflect the ventilation function.

55.1.2.4 Forced Expiratory Volume in 1 s (FEV_1)

FEV_1 is defined as the exhaled gas volume of FVC in the first second. It is the most common index to reflect the severity of ventilation function impairment and the reversibility of airway obstruction and to guide operations.

55.1.2.5 FEV_1/FVC%

FEV_1/ FVC% is the most common index for distinguishing obstructive ventilation dysfunction and restrictive ventilation dysfunction. Even though obstructive ventilation dysfunction exists, the patients may breath out sufficiently if their expiratory time is long enough, therefore FVC will stay normal or decrease slightly, however FEV_1/ FVC% will decrease due to the obviously slow speed of the expiration. When the obstruction becomes ingravescent, FEV_1/ FVC% will decrease more significantly. However in the circumstance that the airway obstruction is apparent and the patients can not exhale fully, FEV_1/ FVC% will increase instead. The decrease of lung elasticity and thoracic compliance may lead to restrictive ventilation dysfunction, but it will not limit the expiration. Therefore FEV_1 drops less than FVC, and FEV_1/ FVC% stays normal or increases.

55.1.2.6 Maximal Expiratory Flow-Volume Curve (MEFV)

The curve is recorded according to the exhaled gas volume and the corresponding expiratory gas flow when exhaling

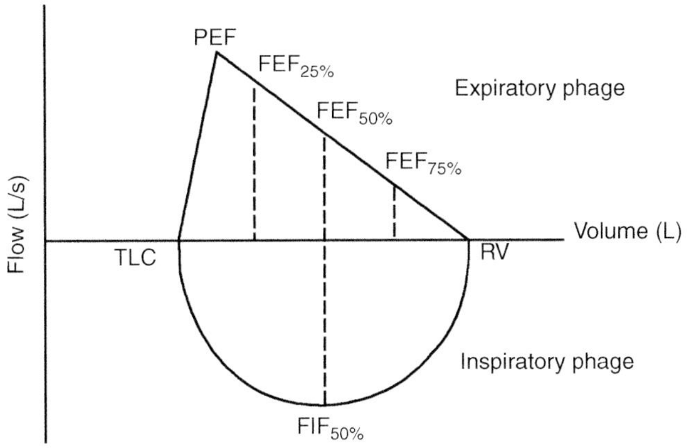

Fig. 55.2 Flow-volume curve

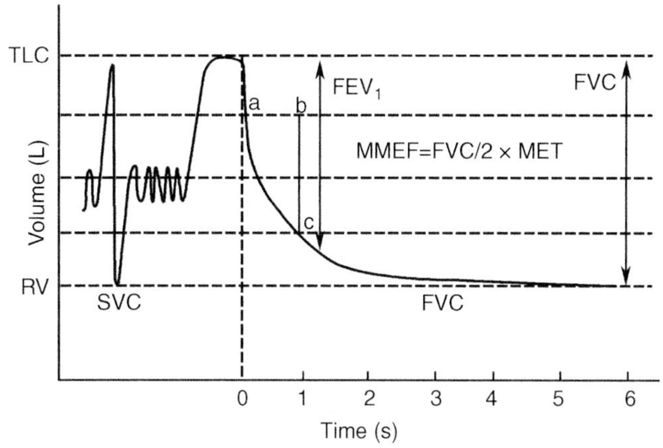

Fig. 55.3 Time-volume curve

with the greatest effort and at full speed from TLC. It is also called flow-volume curve (F-V curve, Fig. 55.2) which is the most common way to judge the types of airflow limitation. The involved parameters include peak expiratory flow (PEF), forced expiratory flow at 25% of FVC exhaled ($FEF_{25\%}$), $FEF_{50\%}$ and $FEF_{75\%}$.

- PEF: It is referred to the fastest instantaneous airflow exhaled with the greatest effort and at full speed from TLC. It reflects the strength of respiratory muscles and helps judge if airway obstruction exists. Besides, it is always used in the follow-up of asthma.
- $FEF_{25\%}$:$FEF_{25\%}$ is the index to reflect air flow in the early stage of expiration. $FEF_{25\%}$ is slightly below PEF in normal, however it will decrease significantly when the major airways is obstructed.
- $FEF_{50\%}$:$FEF_{50\%}$ is the index to reflect air flow in the middle stage of expiration. It approximates maximum mid-expiratory flow (MMEF) and evaluates small airway function together with MMEF and $FEF_{75\%}$. It will prompt small airway diseases or obstruction if there are more than two of the three indexes.
- $FEF_{75\%}$: $FEF_{75\%}$ is the index to reflect air flow in the late stage of expiration and also an important parameter to evaluate the small airway function.

Above all, PEF and $FEF_{25\%}$ depend on the expiratory strength, the unobstructed degree of airway as well as the thoracic and pulmonary elasticity, while $FEF_{50\%}$ and $FEF_{75\%}$ more depend on the unobstructed degree of small airway.

55.1.2.7 Maximum Mid-Expiratory Flow (MMEF)

MMEF is defined as the forced expiratory flow at 25–75% of FVC exhaled, therefore it is also called $FEF_{25-75\%}$. It is calculated by time-volume curve (T-V curve) (Fig. 55.3), which describes the relationship between expiratory time and lung volume in forced expiration. FVC, FEV1 and MMEF are all common indexes of T-V curve.

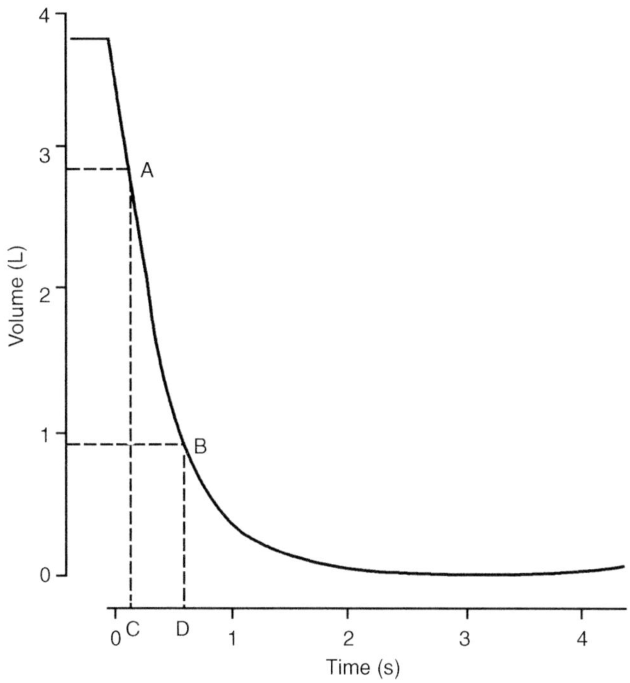

Fig. 55.4 Maximum mid-expiratory flow

Divide FVC into four parts equally in the curve, and analyze the relationship between the second and third parts (that is $FEF_{25-75\%}$) and the corresponding expiratory time (mid-expiratory time, MET) (Maximum mid-expiratory flow, Fig. 55.4).

MMEF which depends mainly upon the non-forced part of FVC will descend while FEV1, FEV1/ FVC% and the airway resistance may be still normal when small airway lesion occurs.

55.1.3 Gas Exchange Function Test

Effective gas exchange requires not only adequate ventilation and blood flow, but also the normal distribution of inspiratory gas, ventilation/perfusion ratio and diffusing function. In clinic, diffusion function is a very common and convenient way to test the gas exchange function.

55.1.3.1 Diffusion Function

Diffusion function of lung is defined as the ability of gas diffusion from alveolus to capillary through the alveolar-capillary membrane and to combine with hemoglobin. Diffusing capacity of lung (DL) is an important parameter for diffusion function, which is defined as the amount of gas transferring through the alveolar membrane in every minute when the gas pressure difference on both sides of the membrane is 1 mmHg.

The Detection Method

In general, the detection of the diffusion capacity of O_2 (D_LO_2) is difficult in technology. Diffusion coefficient through alveolar-capillary membrane and reaction rate with hemoglobin of CO are similar to O_2, and the CO content in normal plasma is almost zero, therefore CO is considered as the target gas to measure the diffusion capacity of lung (D_LCO). D_LCO is defined as the amount (mL or mmol) of CO which is transferred from alveoli to capillary and combines with hemoglobin under 1 mmHg in 1 min. It's in unit of mL/(min·mmHg) or mmol/(min·kPa). In clinic, the most common detection method of diffusion function is D_LCO single-breath method.

The Outcome Assessment

The normal range of D_LCO is 80–120% of the predicted value; 60–80% suggests mild diffusion dysfunction; 40–60% suggests moderate diffusion dysfunction; <40% suggests severe diffusion dysfunction.

It is important to note that the lung volume and ventilation function should also be taken into account when assessing the results of diffusion function test. When the lung volume and ventilation function are normal, the declined D_LCO may prompt anemia, pulmonary vascular disease, the early stage of interstitial pulmonary disease or emphysema. If the restrictive ventilation dysfunction exists but the diffusion function is normal, it prompts thoracic wall disease or neuromuscular disease. If the restrictive ventilation dysfunction and the declined D_LCO coexist, it prompts interstitial pulmonary disease. If the obstructive ventilation dysfunction and the declined D_LCO coexist, it prompts emphysema.

55.2 Section 2: Clinical Application

55.2.1 The Types of Ventilation Dysfunction

55.2.1.1 Obstructive Ventilation Dysfunction

Obstructive ventilation dysfunction is featured by the declined respiratory flow. The features include: (a) FEV_1 is normal or decreased; (b) FEV_1/FVC is decreased; (c) expiratory time is longer than normal in V-T curve; (d) the descending limb which represents the expiratory phase in F-V curve sinks to horizontal axis (Fig. 55.5).

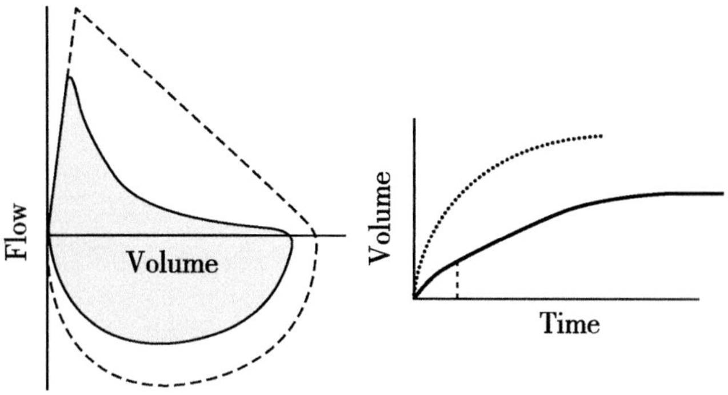

Fig. 55.5 Normal ventilation function and obstructive ventilation dysfunction

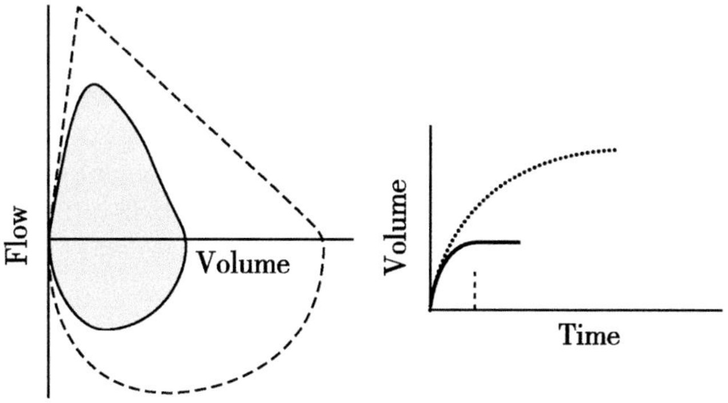

Fig. 55.6 Normal ventilation function and restrictive ventilation dysfunction

Small airway impairs in the early stage of airway obstruction when MMEF, $FEF_{50\%}$ and $FEF_{75\%}$ are decreased obviously. If two of these three indices are lower than 65% of the predicted values, small airway disease is diagnosed definitely.

55.2.1.2 Restrictive Ventilation Dysfunction

Restrictive ventilation dysfunction is featured by the declined expiratory volume. The features include: (a) FEV1 is normal or decreased; (b) VC and FVC is decreased; (c) the part of V-T curve in vertical axis descends and the exhale platform appears in advance; (d) the shape of F-V curve becomes narrow (Fig. 55.6).

Restrictive ventilation obstruction can be found in many diseases including: (a) interstitial lung diseases; (b) pulmonary inflammatory diseases; (c) pleural diseases, such as pleural effusion; (d) diseases of chest wall, such as thoracocyllosis, ankylosing spondylitis.

55.2.1.3 Mixed Ventilation Dysfunction

Mixed ventilation dysfunction is featured by the declined expiratory volume and flow at the same time. The features include: (a) TLC, VC, FVC, FEV1 and FEV_1/FVC% are declined; (b) the part of V-T curve in vertical axis descends and the expiratory time is longer than normal; (c) the shape

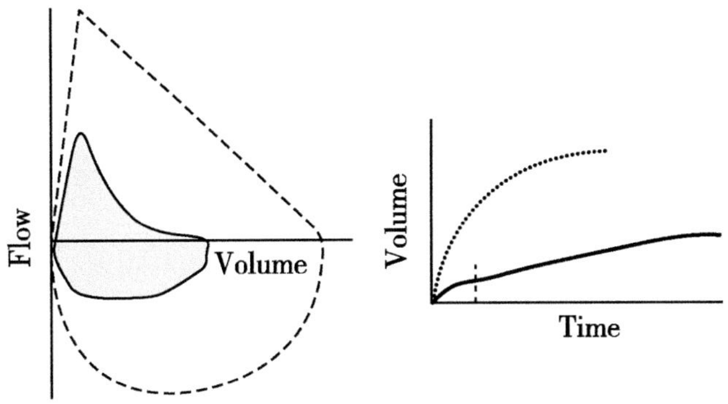

Fig. 55.7 Normal ventilation function and mixed ventilation dysfunction

of F-V curve becomes narrow, and the descending limb which represents the expiratory phase in F-V curve sinks to horizontal axis (Fig. 55.7).

55.2.2 Assess the Airway Responsiveness

Airway responsiveness means the spasmodic contraction of airway smooth muscle when all kinds of stimulates (e.g. the physical, chemical or biological agents) act on the airway.

55.2.2.1 Peak Expiratory Flow Rate (PEFR)

The PEF at each interval within 1 day may be different, and PEFR can be calculated by the PEFs which are continuously measured at every morning and afternoon in 1 week by the mini peak flow meter.

$PEFR = 2 \times (PEF_{max} - PEF_{min})/(PEF_{max} + PEF_{min}) \times 100\%$

PEFR < 20% is normal.

PEFR ≥ 20% suggests the bronchial hyperresponsiveness and is helpful to diagnose asthma.

55.2.2.2 Bronchialdilation Test

Bronchial dilation test is applied to observe the dilation reaction of airway and assess the reversibility of airway obstruction after the inhalation of salbutamol. It is appropriate for the suspected asthma patients whose $FEV_1 < 70\%$.

Detection Method

Pulmonary function test should be tested after stopping usage of the bronchial dilation medicine for 24 h. When FEV_1 or FEV_1/FVC declines, the patient is enjoined to inhale salbutamol 0.2 mg. Then measure FEV_1 or FEV_1/FVC again after 15–20 min and calculate the change rate of FEV_1 according to the formula below.

$\triangle FEV_1\%$ = (the latter FEV_1-the basal FEV_1)/the basal $FEV_1 \times 100\%$.

Evaluation of the Results

If the change rate of FEV_1 is greater than 12% and the increased absolute value of FEV_1 is more than 200 mL at the same time after the application of bronchial dilation medicine, the bronchial dilation test is positive.

55.2.2.3 Bronchial Provocation Test

If the bronchial dilation test is negative, and the doctor still suspects the patient with asthma, bronchial provocation test can be selected for the diagnosis of asthma. During the test, bronchoconsitriction can be induced by certain stimulants (e.g. methacholine or histamine) and the extent of airway spasm can be reflected by the pulmonary function parameters. The severity of the bronchial hyperresponsiveness can be judged subsequently. Bronchial provocation test is applied to the suspected asthma patients with normal lung function or mild obstructive ventilation dysfunction ($FEV_1 \geq 70\%$ of the predicted value).

- Detection method

The stimulants (e.g. methacholine or histamine) are diluted with the physiological saline to 0.03–16 mg/mL in a method of double ratio increasing, and then stored at 4 °C. Firstly, test the basal FEV_1 of the subject, then repeat FEV_1testing after aerosol inhalation of the physiological saline by the subject for 2 min. Aerosol inhalation of the physiological saline is aimed to familiarize the subject with the method of inhalation and make sure there is no airway reaction. If the latter FEV_1 does not decrease obviously than the former, the stimulants will be inhaled from low to high concentrations in tidal breathing by the subject. Each FEV_1 will be tested after each concentration of the stimulant inhale until the FEV_1 value is lower by≥20% than the one which is tested after the atomization inhale of the physiological saline.

- Evaluation of the results

Provocation concentration (PC) and accumulated provocation dose (PD) are the most common parameters to evaluate the test. PC_{20}-FEV_1 is defined as the concentration when FEV_1 decreases by 20% than the basic value. Methacholine PC20-FEV_1 < 8 mg/mL is the positive criteria in bronchial provocation test, while PC20-FEV_1 > 8 mg/mL is considered to be negative (PC_{20}-FEV_1 > 16 mg/mL in normal adults). PD_{20}-FEV_1 is defined as the accumulated dose of the stimulants when FEV_1 decreases by 20% than the basic value. Methacholine PD_{20}-FEV_1 < 12.8umol/L or histamine PD_{20}-FEV_1 < 7.8umol/L suggests bronchial hyperresponsiveness or bronchial provocation test is positive.

Bronchial provocation test is mainly applied for the diagnosis of asthma, however the test in patients with allergic rhinitis or bronchiectasis may also be positive.

Contraindications for the test include absolute contraindications and relative contraindications. Absolute contraindications: (a) there is a definite hypersensitivity to the stimulants; (b) the basal pulmonary ventilation function is severely impaired (FEV1 < 60% of the predicted value); (c) cardiac insufficient, the recent cardiac infarction, the severe arrhythmia; (d) the severe hypertension; (e) the recent cerebrovascular accident; (f) the severe hyperthyroidism; (g) the inexplicable urticarial; (h) the situations in which FVC testing is inhibited such as pulmonary bullous and pneumothorax. Relative contraindications include: (a) the basal pulmonary ventilation function is moderate impaired ($FEV_1 < 70\%$ of the predicted value); (b) airway spasm exists in the pulmonary ventilation function test; (c) the recent respiratory tract infection; (d) the seizure need to be controlled by drugs; (e) asthma in the stage of attack; (f) the pregnant women.

55.2.3 Evaluation of the Tolerance and Security in Operation

FVC, FEV1, MVV are indices to help evaluate the security of thoracic or abdominal operations and the life quality after the operations (Table 55.1).

Table 55.1 Evaluation of the risk in operation by pulmonary function test

Parameters	Increased risk	High risk
FVC	<50%	≤1.5 L
FEV1	<2 L or < 50%	<1 L
MVV		<50%
PaCO2		≥45 mmHg

Basic Information of Endoscopy

56

Zhijun Duan, Ke Wang, and Rui Zeng

56.1 Section 1: Gastrointestinal Endoscopy

The electronic endoscope has become an advanced instrument for diagnosis and treatment of stomach and colon diseases (Fig. 56.1), and many types have been developed. For example, the endoscopic ultrasonography can be used to assess the visceral walls of the digestive tract or surrounding organs under the guidance of an endoscopic ultrasound probe. Narrow band image and magnifying endoscopes can be used to discover fine mucosal lesions and identify benign or malignant diseases. The confocal endoscope guides the confocal microscope into the gastrointestinal lumen to achieve optical biopsy. Capsule endoscopy can capture regular video images by using swallowed wireless capsules, and can be used as a tool to diagnose intestinal lesions. At present, endoscopies are applied not only to diagnosis of digestive diseases, but also for the treatment of the diseases in the gastrointestinal tract, bile duct and pancreatic duct.

56.1.1 Upper Gastrointestinal Endoscopy

Upper gastrointestinal endoscopy, usually known as gastroscopy, includes examinations of the esophagus, stomach and duodenum. The gastroscope was the first of the endoscopes to appear and is developed the most rapidly.

56.1.1.1 Indications

The indications of upper gastrointestinal endoscopy are widely ranged, including diseases in the esophagus, stomach, and duodenum, and routine physical checkup. The main indications are as follows:

1. Dysphagia, retrosternal pain, burning sensation, upper abdominal pain, discomfort, fullness, loss of appetite, and other unexplained upper gastrointestinal symptoms.
2. Acute and chronic gastrointestinal bleeding. Upper gastrointestinal endoscopy is not only available for etiological diagnosis, but also allows treatment.
3. Upper gastrointestinal lesions that cannot be diagnosed or explained by a barium swallow examination, especially mucosal lesions and suspected tumors.
4. Diseases that require follow-up observation, such as peptic ulcer, atrophic gastritis, reflux esophagitis and Barrett esophagus.
5. Upper gastrointestinal disease follow-up after medical or surgical treatment.
6. Conditions that require endoscopic treatment, such as foreign body extraction, hemostasis for upper gastrointestinal bleeding including sclerotherapy and ligation of esophageal varices, dilation treatment of esophageal stricture, removal of upper gastrointestinal polyps, endoscopic mucosal resection (EMR), endoscopic submucosal dissection (ESD), peroral endoscopic myotomy (POEM), and natural orifice transluminal endoscopic surgery (NOTES).

56.1.1.2 Contraindications

With the advances in equipment and improvement of technology, contraindications are greatly reduced nowadays, but still require close attention. The contraindications of gastroscopy are as follows:

1. Serious heart and lung diseases, such as severe arrhythmia, heart failure, acute stage myocardial infarction, severe pulmonary insufficiency and asthma attack. Mild cardiopulmonary dysfunction is not a contraindication. When necessary, the procedure should be carried out under electrocardiographic monitoring.
2. Critical conditions such as shock and coma.

Z. Duan
Department of Gastroenterology, Dalian Medical University, Dalian, China

K. Wang
Department of Respiratory, Jilin University, Changchun, China

R. Zeng (✉)
Department of Cardiology, Sichuan University, Chengdu, China

X.-H. Wan, R. Zeng (eds.), *Handbook of Clinical Diagnostics*, https://doi.org/10.1007/978-981-13-7677-1_56

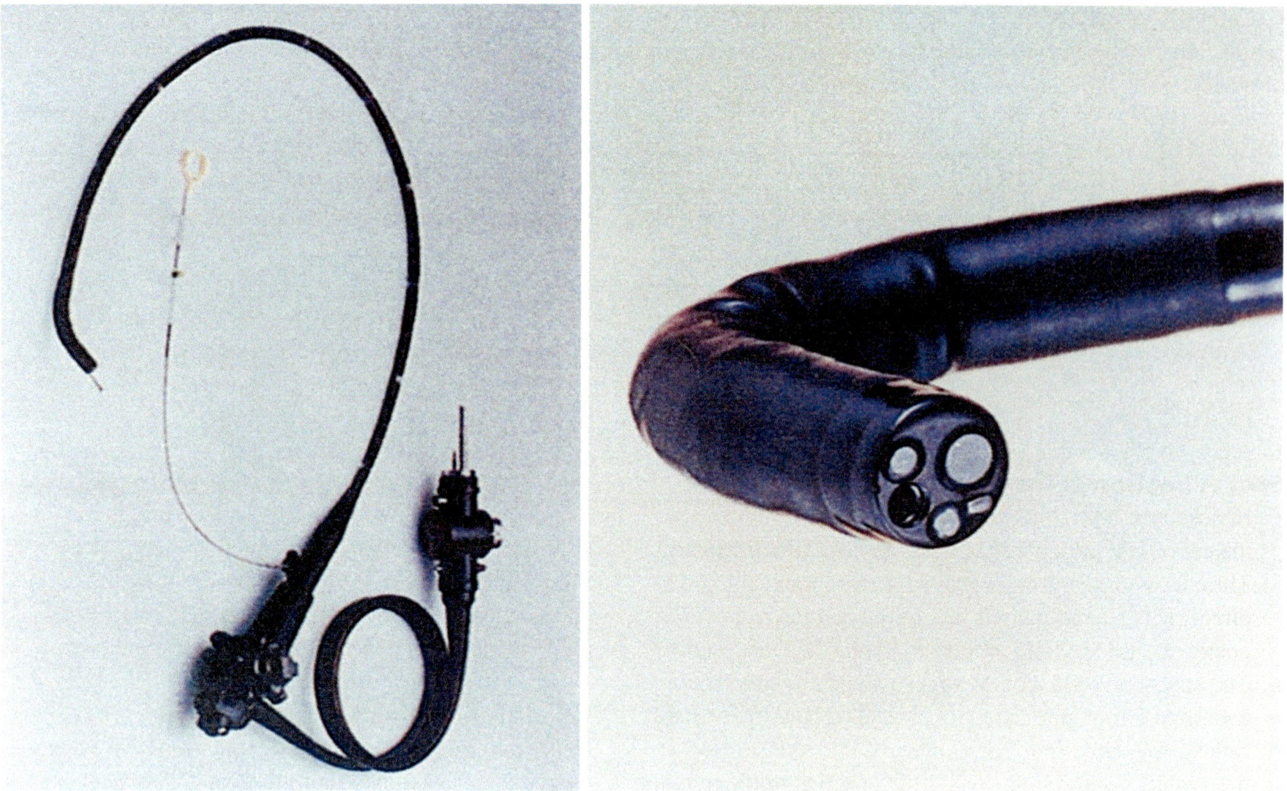

Fig. 56.1 Gastrointestinal endoscopy system

3. Uncooperative patients or those with unstable conditions due to delirium and mental disorders.
4. Acute perforations of the esophagus, stomach and duodenum. Perforations caused by endoscopic examination or treatment do not always require surgery if the diagnosis and management are performed in a timely manner under endoscopy. Therefore, under such circumstances, perforation is not a contraindication.
5. Severe throat disease, erosive esophagitis, erosive gastritis, huge esophageal diverticulum, aortic aneurysm and severe cervical thoracic spinal malformations.
6. The examination for acute infectious hepatitis or gastrointestinal infectious diseases can be postponed. Special sterilization should be provided for patients with positive hepatitis B and C, surface antigen and HIV.

56.1.1.3 Methods

Preparation Before Examination

- Require patients to be fasting for 6 h before examination. Those with delayed gastric emptying should prolong the duration of fasting. Patients with pyloric obstruction should be given gastric lavage before examination.
- Review application for gastroscope, obtain a brief medical history, necessary physical examination, and check for indications or contraindications. Determine whether there are any risks.
- Doctor-patient communication. Doctors introduce themselves to patients and explain the examination in detail to minimize fear and explain the necessity and safety of the inspection to obtain mutual cooperation.
- Sedation and anesthesia. Sedatives are seldom required. For severely anxious patients, intramuscular injection of midazolam (1–2 mg) may be administered. Recently, gastroscopy has been conducted under general anesthesia in some institutions with intravenous injections of fentanyl citrate (0.6–1.0 μg/kg), combined with propofol (1.0–2.0 mg/kg). Midazolam can also be used for enhancing the sedative effect. Endoscopy under general anesthesia should be performed under professional administration and observation; carefully monitored to prevent cardiac accident, respiratory depression and other complications; and followed by optimal postoperative treatment. For local anesthesia, 2% lidocaine throat spray should be used two or three times, or 1% lidocaine glue (10 mL) should be swallowed 5–10 min before the examination. The latter has the function of anesthesia and lubrication.
- Oral defoamers. Foaming can be suppressed by adding a diluted emulsion of simethicone so better visualization can be obtained.

- Carefully check the gastroscope and accessories including light, water supply, threshold of air supply, suction device, and the bending angle operated by the control knob. Be aware of the performance and quality of the endoscope. Check the lines of the electronic gastroscope, power switch, and screen. In addition, the endoscopy room should be equipped with monitoring devices, oxygen and first aid supplies.

Key Points of the Procedure

- Patients are placed in a left lateral position, with the neck relaxed, head resting on a pillow, and collar and belt loosened.
- A curved plate or disposable bag is placed around patients' mouths. Patients are asked to bite down on a dental pad.
- Endoscopist holds the control knob with the left hand, and the endoscope at 20 cm from the tip with the right hand. The endoscope is inserted gently into the esophagus under direct visualization, with careful observation. Avoid rough operation and entry into the trachea.
- The endoscope can be advanced easily through the cardia and into the fundus of the stomach. The endoscope is rotated slightly towards the left and upward to observe the gastric body cavity. Followed by slow advancement of the endoscope to the pyloric region, enter into the duodenal bulb. The tip of endoscope is turned right and upward, then rotate "right", while adjusting the depth of gastroscope to visualize the descending part of the duodenum and papilla. Observation should be done with a careful combination of air insufflation and suction during withdrawal of the gastroscope. Each part of the duodenum, stomach and esophagus are examined sequentially. Pay attention to the size and shape of the gastrointestinal cavity, gastrointestinal wall, mucosal, submucosal capillary, secretions and gastric motility. When the gastroscope is located in the gastric antrum, the gastric angle and its vicinity may be observed. After that, the inferior part of the gastroscope is inverted to detect the cardia and fundus. After straightening the gastroscope, examine carefully and sequentially to avoid blind areas. Pay close attention to lesions in the gastric angle, vertical portion and posterior wall of the gastric body, and the area below the cardia.
- For significant lesions, image capture, biopsy, and extraction of gastric contents are necessary for diagnosis.
- Expel as much gas as possible after the procedure to prevent bloating. Patients with biopsy are not allowed to eat hot or rough food immediately.

56.1.1.4 Complications and Managements

1. **General complications:** Include throat spasms, temporomandibular joint dislocation, throat injury, parotid gland swelling, Mallory-Weiss Syndrome.
2. **Serious complications:** The following complications are rare but serious, and should be prevented.
   - Bleeding: May occur as a result of endoscopic manipulation, biopsy or inappropriate hemostasis after endoscopy. Hematemesis, melena and hypovolemia may occur, and supplement and hemostasis should be administered. Endoscopic hemostasis may be performed if necessary.
   - Perforation: Caused by rough and blind operation of the gastroscope. Esophageal perforation often leads to intense pain in the chest and back or immediate subcutaneous emphysema in the mediastinum near the neck. Gastric perforation may cause intense abdominal pain and pneumoperitoneum. Endoscopy should be conducted in a timely manner to clarify the diagnosis and to close the perforation in order to avoid surgery.
   - Hypoxemia: Caused by ventilation disorders or nervous suffocation. More common in endoscopy examinations performed under anesthesia. This complication can be improved by immediately terminating examinations and supplying oxygen.
   - Infection: Aspiration pneumonia can occur in some cases. To prevent the transmission of hepatitis B and C, a blood virus test is needed before gastroscopy. For hepatitis-positive patients, a special instrument is required and thorough sterilization should be done after endoscopy.
   - Cardiac arrest, myocardial infarction, and angina: Most are caused by stimulation of the vagus nerve and hypoxemia induced by endoscopy. When encountered, the examination should be terminated immediately, and emergency treatment should be performed.

56.1.1.5 Endoscopic Diagnosis of Upper Gastrointestinal Disease

Endoscopy is very important for diagnosing superficial mucosal lesions, early tumors and etiologies of upper gastrointestinal bleeding. It is reported that inflammatory diseases account for about 70–80% of upper intestinal diseases, peptic ulcers for about 10–20%, and tumors for about 3–5%. Additionally, endoscopy can also be used for diagnosing polyps, esophageal varices, vascular malformations, Mallory-Weiss syndrome, diverticulitis, foreign bodies and parasites.

1. **Inflammation:** Chronic inflammation is the major indication for gastroscopy, while it is seldom indicated in cases of acute inflammation.
   - Chronic non-atrophic gastritis (superficial gastritis) Mucosal hyperaemia and reddening are manifested as rash and erythema with a striped or clustered distribution. Mucosal edema makes the contours more obvious. Surface erosion can be seen in the mucosa of flat or raised pimples. Submucosal bleeding can be spotty

or patchy. Fresh bleeding is dark red, whereas old bleeding is brown. Chronic non-atrophic gastritis is commonly associated with Helicobacter pylori infection, bile reflux, and recent application of non-steroidal anti-inflammatory drugs (NSAIDs).

- Atrophic gastritis appears as pale or versicolor (mainly white) changes in the mucous membranes. There are no mucosal folds and blood vessels are easily seen through pale atrophic mucosa. In addition, the lesion also appears as rough nodule or granule with focal hyperplasia and intestinal metaplasia. The manifestation also includes loss of surface luster, fewer secretions, and a small quantity of mucus. Biopsy samples should be taken to confirm the diagnosis.
- Special types of gastritis are extremely rare, including infectious gastritis, chemical gastritis, eosinophilic gastritis, lymphocytic gastritis, non-infectious granulomatous gastritis, and radiation gastritis.

2. **Ulcers**: Most are duodenal ulcers and gastric antral ulcers. Under a gastroscope, ulcers appear as relatively round or oval defects with diameters of about 0.5–1.5 cm, and may have a white or dirty fur coating at the base. They are usually symmetrical with smooth margins and clean bases. Congestion, edema and mucosa concentration indicates an active ulcer and scarring process. According to the ulcer morphology, it can be divided into active phase (A period), healing phase (H phase) and scarring phase (S phase) under an endoscope.

   Malignant ulcers (ulcerative carcinoma) are larger and more irregular than benign ulcers, with irregular peripherals and uneven bases. They are hard in texture and bleed easily when touched. Sometimes, they are difficult to distinguish from benign ulcers, requiring tissue diagnoses.
3. **Tumors**: Upper gastrointestinal tumors, such as gastric cancer and esophageal cancer are very common in China, and are the main indications for gastroscopy. In Japan and other countries, with the help of endoscopy-based cancer screening programs, the detection rate of early gastric cancer is over 50%, allowing patients to receive early treatment. Doctors are required to pay close attention to inflammation, polyps, ulcers, bumps and other pathological changes under an endoscope, and accurately identify the lesions in order to improve the detection rate of early cancer.

Early gastric cancer that involves the mucosa or submucosa with no lymph node metastasis can be treated and cured via endoscopic methods. Therefore, timely and accurate diagnosis is of great significance. Tumors are characterized by a small polyp or a defect no more than 1 cm in diameter. A diagnosis should be determined by careful observation in combination with staining, fluorescence, magnifying endoscopy and biopsy. Borrmann classification of advanced gastric cancers according to morphology: Type I: polypoid fungating, Type II: ulcerative with elevated distinct borders, Type III: ulcerative with indistinct borders, and Type IV: diffuse, indistinct borders. Borrmann I-III are not difficult to identify. Usually, Bowman IV type cannot be found in the stomach under gastroscopy, but the stomach wall may become stiff and thickened, with limited distension and absent peristalsis, called linitis plastica, which may be easily overlooked. The gross type of esophageal cancer is similar to that of gastric cancer, but is mainly derived from the squamous epithelium. A few adenocarcinomas are associated with chronic esophagitis and esophageal mucosa columnar metaplasia.

56.1.2 Lower Gastrointestinal Endoscopy

Lower gastrointestinal endoscopies include colonoscopy and enteroscopy. Colonoscopy can be used to detect lesions from the anus to the ileocecus, including the terminal ileum, the entire colon and the rectum, for the diagnosis of diseases in the lower gastrointestinal tract. Equipments and technologies of enteroscopy are rapidly developing. However, only colonoscopy (used more frequently) will be discussed in this chapter.

56.1.2.1 Indications

1. Symptoms and signs of diarrhea, hemafecia, hypogastralgia, anemia, and abdominal masses with unknown etiologies.
2. Colorectal diseases, including stenosis, ulcers, polyps, carcinomas, and diverticula. Unexplained diseases by barium enema.
3. Diagnosis and follow-up for inflammatory bowel disease.
4. Preoperative diagnosis and follow-up examination of colon cancer, surveillance of precancerous lesion, and postoperative follow-up of post-polypectomy.
5. Patients who need hemostasis and polypectomy.

56.1.2.2 Relative Contraindications

1. Serious stenosis of the anus or rectum.
2. Acute severe colitis such as severe dysentery, ulcerative colitis and diverticulitis.
3. Acute diffuse peritonitis and abdominal viscera perforation.
4. Pregnant women.
5. Severe heart-lung failure, psychiatric disorders and coma.

56.1.2.3 Methods

Preparation

Bowel preparation is of vital importance for the endoscopy examination.

- Patients should consume semifluid food 1–2 days before endoscopy and fast during the day of the exam.

- There are many methods to cleanse the entire colon. Saline is the most convenient and effective. Three hours before colonoscopy, patients are required to drink an intestinal lavage solution (3000–4000 mL) containing sodium chloride or phosphate buffer solution, no more than 1000 mL. The solution of polyethylene glycol is highly recommended and produces a good cleansing effect. Mannitol is a useful way of achieving rapid bowl preparation. There is a potential explosion hazard following mannitol usage, because colonic bacteria possess enzymes that metabolize mannitol to form an explosive concentration of hydrogen. Therefore, electrosurgery is hazardous.
- The endoscopist needs to take a brief medical history, perform a complete physical examination, and recognize indications and contraindications for endoscopy. The necessity and safety of the operation should be carefully explained to minimize patients' fears.
- Premedication for adults includes diazepam (2.5–5 mg) or pethidine (50 mg) via intramuscular injection. To facilitate the operation, a spasmolytic agent can be given to reduce bowel peristalsis. An intramuscular injection of atropine (0.5 mg) or scopolamine (10 mg) is administered 5–10 min before the operation. For patients with mental illness or young patients less than 12 years of age, intravenous anesthesia has to be administered by an expert anesthesiologist during endoscopy. If an endoscopist is experienced and a cooperative patient can fully understand information regarding the procedure, anesthesia will not be required.

Key Points of the Procedure

- Currently most endoscopists perform colonoscopy independently. In fact, colonoscopy is more difficult to perform than gastroscopy, so an endoscopist needs standardized training before he or she operates alone.
- Patients are advised to put on pants with a hole that exposes the anus and lay in the left lateral position with legs bent.
- Endoscopist should perform a digital rectal exam first, followed by endoscopy to identify the presence of tumors, stenosis, haemorrhoids, fissures, etc. Lubricant fluid should be used to lubricate the distal end of endoscope (silicone oil is commonly used, while liquid paraffin has been largely abandoned). Patients should be told to relax the anal sphincter. The right index finger is used to press the objective lens, then smoothly slide the endoscope into the anus.
- The colonoscope is pushed gently along the lumen. Suction is used to shorten and straighten the sigmoid and transverse colon. Hook and rotate the colonoscope moderately at the splenic flexure and hepatic flexure. Minimize the turning angle and decrease the distance of the examination in coordination with the patient's breathing pattern and position.
- According to the requirement of the endoscopist, an assistant can press on the abdomen using the appropriate manipulation to decrease intestinal luminal curvature and to prevent the sigmoid flexure and transverse colon from convolving, which is helpful for examination.
- The ileocecal valve is the only definite anatomical landmark in the colon. The signs that one has reached the ileocecal junction are the appearance of the crescent-shaped appendix orifice, the Y-shaped fold of the ileocecal junction, and the fishmouth-shaped ileocecal valve. Advance the endoscope into the ileocecal valve to observe the gut cavity and mucosa of the terminal ileum ranging from 15 to 30 cm.
- When the colonoscope is withdrawn, the endoscopist manipulates the up/down or left/right control knobs of the colonoscope to flexibly rotate its anterior segment. Inspect the walls of the intestine by insufflating or sucking out the appropriate amount of gas in the intestines to observe the lumen, intestinal wall and haustra of the colon. Adjusting the angle, or changing the patient's position may also be helpful. Repeated observation is necessary to avoid any blind areas.
- For significant lesions, image capture, biopsy, and cytologic examination are needed for further diagnosis.
- When finishing the examination, the endoscopist should exhaust the air in the lumen to alleviate abdominal distention and allow patients to rest for 15–30 min before leaving.
- Patients who have received hemostasis and polypectomy should consume liquid or semiliquid food for 4–5 days following the procedure to prevent complications.

56.1.2.4 Complications and Management

1. **Perforation:** Occurrence may be attributed to abnormal structure such as diverticulum, conglutination, intestinal reverse, improper operation, etc. Patients usually have signs of abdominal distension and pain, pneumoperitoneum, and peritonitis. A deep fissure can be seen through enteroscopy. X-ray is helpful to confirm the diagnosis.
2. **Hemorrhage:** It is mostly caused by colonoscopy-induced iatrogenic injury, excessive biopsy, lack of proper coagulation and hemostasis management, etc. Precautions for these causes of bleeding are necessary. The methods chosen for hemostasis depend on the amount of bleeding. Endoscopic hemostasis can be performed when necessary.
3. **Mesenteric injury:** May be caused by extensive operation and can result in abdominal pain and intraperitoneal hemorrhage. Minor hemorrhage should be treated conservatively, while exploratory laparotomy should be considered for massive hemorrhage or after failure of more conservative treatments.

4. **Cardiac arrest, myocardial infarction, and angina:** Provoked by intense vagal stimulus due to forceful or prolonged colonoscopy, arrhythmia or hypoxemia. Endoscopy should be terminated immediately when encountered, and doctors should rescue in a timely manner.
5. **Gas explosion:** It is reported that when used for intestinal cleaning, mannitol may produce flammable gas such as methane, resulting in intestinal gas explosion during polypectomy. Since the consequences of intestinal gas explosion are serious, mannitol should be avoided for bowel preparation.

56.1.2.5 Endoscopic Diagnosis of Colonic Disease

Colonic diseases share similar basic pathological changes with upper gastrointestinal diseases, such as inflammation, ulceration and tumors. Inflammation in the colonic mucosa can be caused by multiple diseases. Non-specific inflammation mainly involves ulcerative colitis and Crohn's disease. Diagnoses can be made by combining morphological changes with the etiology, biopsy pathology, and clinical manifestation. Ulcerative colitis has a variety of manifestations such as erosions or superficial ulcers. Morphology, size, and distribution of the lesion are helpful for the diagnosis and treatment of the disease. Aphthous ulcer is another ulcerative disease which may be caused by infection and allergic reaction. In addition, it is very important to diagnose Crohn's disease at its early active stage by combining clinical data with pathological biopsy. Patients with benign or malignant colonic tumors are common, and these tumors are the main indications for colonoscopy. Colonic adenoma is a common benign tumor. It is a type precancerous lesion, so the size, form, and pedunculus are important features for evaluating its characteristics and prognosis.

Malignant tumors, including colon cancer, rank fourth in incidence for malignant tumors in certain areas of China, which requires great attention. Pathological types of colon cancer are similar to those of gastric cancer. Polypoid type and mass type, produced by canceration of adenoma, are major types of colon cancer, followed by ulcerative type and infiltrative type. Laterally spreading early cancers have gradually increased in recent years, which should be alerted in clinical settings. Colon cancer occurs mainly in the rectosigmoid colon, which is the main location for differential diagnosis and further colonoscopy follow-ups. Colonoscopy can provide valuable evidence for clinical diagnosis of colonic vascular lesions, colonic diverticula, and other colonic diseases caused by organ transplantation, acquired immune deficiency syndrome, etc.

56.2 Section 2: Electronic Bronchoscopic Examination

Electronic bronchoscopic examination which belongs to an endoscopic technology has been applied to the diagnosis and treatment of the diseases of trachea or bronchi, the deep-seated lesions in lung and e mediastinal lesions. Electronic bronchoscope can get into trachea, bronchus, segmental bronchi and even subsegmental bronchi where tissue biopsy, puncture, brush biopsy or bronchoalveolar lavage for the lesions can be accomplished. Transbronchial lung biopsy (TBLB) and transbronchial needle aspiration (TBNA) may help diagnosis and treatment of pleural diseases in place of medical thoracoscopy, and the biopsy of lung tissue, mediastinal masses or enlarged lymph nodes as well. In addition, the interventional therapy technology has been applied to resect the masses in trachea or bronchi and treat the airway stenosis by the technique of freeze, laser, argon plasma coagulation and stents. The routine examination of electronic bronchoscope is simple and practicable, and always applied in the assessment of pulmonary diseases and research teaching.

56.2.1 Indications

56.2.1.1 For Diagnosis

- Unknown chronic cough.
- Unknown hemoptysis or bloody sputum for which the position and cause of bleeding need to be identified.
- Unknown partial wheezing rale for which the cause, position and character of airway obstruction need to be identified.
- Unknown hoarseness.
- Cancer cells or the suspicious cancer cells are found.
- Abnormal changes in chest X-ray or CT, such as pulmonary atelectasis, lung nodules or masses, obstructive pneumonia, non-absorbing inflammation, the diffuse lesions in lung, hilar nodes or mediastinal nodes enlargement, tracheostenosis or bronchial stenosis, and unknown pleural effusion.
- Preoperative examination for directing the position and range of the resection and assessing the prognosis.
- The etiology diagnosis of pulmonary or bronchial infection.
- Definite diagnosis for the tracheal or bronchial fistula.

56.2.1.2 For Treatment

- Taking out the foreign body of trachea or bronchi.
- Clearing away the abnormal secreta in airway, including sputum, suppurative sputum emboli and thrombus.

- Realizing local hemostasis by the lavage of ice physiological saline or the injection of thrombin after the identification of the bleeding position in patients with hemoptysis.
- Injecting chemotherapeutic drug locally by electronic bronchoscope in patients with lung cancer.
- Intubating with the electronic bronchoscope.
- Resecting the masses in trachea or bronchi and treating the airway stenosis on the assist of freeze, laser, argon plasma coagulation and stents.

56.2.2 Contraindications

In the following status, the decision of taking bronchoscopy inspection is made only in the situation of life-saving or imperative diagnosis

- The active massive hemoptysis.
- The severe hypertension and arrhythmia.
- The newly-occurring myocardial infarction or unstable angina pectoris.
- The severe cardiac or pulmonary insufficiency.
- The remediless coagulation disorders.
- The severe superior vena caval obstruction syndrome.
- The suspected aortic aneurysm.
- Multiple pulmonary bullae.
- The extreme weakness of the body.

56.2.3 Inspection Method

56.2.3.1 Preoperative Preparation

- Illustrating the purpose, process and method to patients before the inspection to comfort the patients.
- Inquiring the medical history, measuring blood pressure and testing the cardiac and pulmonary functions.
- Taking chest X-ray or CT to identify the lesion position.
- Fasting for solids 4 h and fasting for liquids 2 h before the inspection.
- Establishing the vein passage if sedative is in demand and keeping the passage until the end of convalescence.
- Detecting the platelet count, prothrombin time and activated partial thromboplastin time for patients who need biopsy.

56.2.3.2 Local Anaesthesia

Two percent lidocaine aerosol is always applied in the nasal or laryngopharyngeal anesthesia, and the amount of lidocaine injected into the bronchi should be reduced as less as possible.

56.2.3.3 Intraoperative Monitoring

- Have all the patients inhale oxygen in order to keep oxyhemoglobin saturation above 90% to reduce arrhythmia genesis during and after the inspection.
- Electrocardiography monitoring is not regularly applied, however it is necessary for the patients who suffer from severe myocardial diseases and hypoxemia even in the case of continuous oxygen inhalation.
- At least two assistants are required for the inspection, and one of them must be special nurse.
- Tracheal intubation, related drugs and facilities should be prepared.

56.2.3.4 Operation Steps

- Patients are maintained in the supine position. The inspector stands by the head of the patient, and hold the control section of the bronchoscope with two hands, then insert the endoscope into the patients' oral cavity to find the epiglottis and glottis by sliding the angle demodulator, and to observe the activity of glottis.
- Insert the bronchoscope into the patients' trachea quickly when the glottis is open, and move the bronchoscope forward until the carina while observing the lumen of trachea and the form of carina.
- After observing the opening of bilateral main bronchi, insert the bronchoscope into main bronchus, lobar bronchi and segmental bronchi sequentially by sliding the angle demodulator. The principle of inspection is checking the contralateral side first and the affected side second.
- Observe the surface flatness and color of the bronchial mucosa, and pay attention to the abnormalities such as congestion, edema, exudation, bleeding, erosion, anabrosis, hyperplasia, nodule and neoplasma. Judge whether the ridge is broadening, the bronchial wall is pressed and the lumen is narrow or not.
- Biopsy, brush biopsy and bronchoalveolar lavage of the visible lesions are common methods to get the cytological and etiological specimen.

56.2.3.5 Postoperation Management

- Some patients, especially the ones with impaired pulmonary function, still need oxygen inhalation for a period of time after the electronic bronchoscopic examination.
- Fast for 2 h after the examination to avoid aspiration.
- Some patients may have temporary fever after the examination for the inflammatory mediators released by the pulmonary macrophage. The fever may be not required to deal with, but should be distinguished from the postoperative infection.

56.2.4 Clinical Application

56.2.4.1 Assisting Diagnosis of Diseases

- Diagnosis of lung cancer: A variety of sampling method such as needle biopsy, forceps biopsy, brush biopsy and lavage by electronic bronchoscope may improve the diagnosis rate of lung cancer.
- Etiological diagnosis of pulmonary atelectasis: Cancer, non-specific inflammation, tuberculosis and some special causes (e.g. foreign body, thrombus) can lead to pulmonary atelectasis, while electronic bronchoscopic examination is of great importance to the differentiation of the causes.
- Etiological diagnosis of hemoptysis: To hemoptysic patients with a normal chest radiograph, electronic bronchoscopic examination may help determine the bleeding site, clear the blood clot and stanch bleeding.
- Diagnosis of pulmonary infection: Bacterial culture of the bronchoalveolar lavage fluid may provide etiological diagnosis basis for the infection, especially for the atypical tuberculosis or endobronchial tuberculosis.
- Diagnosis of diffused parenchymal lung diseases: Biopsy or alveolar lavage by electronic bronchoscope can help exclude other diseases.
- Diagnosis of pleural diseases: The application of electronic bronchoscope replacing thoracoscopy can help implement the pleural biopsy and improve the diagnostic rate of pleural diseases.
- Diagnosis of mediastinal diseases: The biopsy of mediastinal neoplasm or swollen lymph nodes through transbronchial needle aspiration (TBNA) can help confirm the diagnosis of primary mediastinal tumors or mediastinal lymph node metastasis of lung cancer.

56.2.4.2 Assisting Treatment of Diseases

- Removing the secretion in airway: When the thick secretion obstructs air passages, sputum aspiration and bronchial lavage with electronic bronchoscope are effective and safe treatment for patients with severe lung infection.
- Treatment of complications after the thoracic trauma and the thoracic or abdominal surgery: The limited tussis action after the trauma or surgery brings to the retention of sputum and the corresponding complications such as pulmonary infection and atelectasis. However the suction of secretion in airway by the electronic bronchoscope may avoid or reduce the occurrence of the complications above.
- Removal of foreign bodies from airway.
- Treatment of pulmonary infectious diseases: The suction of secretion in airway and topical administration of drugs by the electronic bronchoscope are conductive to treat the patients with the diseases of much purulent secretion in airway such as pulmonary abscess and bronchiectasis.
- Interventional therapy for central airway stenosis.

56.2.5 Complications

The major complications during the electronic bronchoscopic examination include bleeding, pneumothorax, pyrexia, laryngospasm and anesthetic reaction.

56.2.5.1 Laryngospasm

Laryngospasm which belongs to a kind of serious complication is always caused by anesthetic drugs, or occurs during the examination in asthma or COPD patients. Tic, respiratory depression and even sudden cardiac arrest may also appear with laryngospasm. The detailed inquest of the patients' history of drug allergy and common diseases before the examination may help avoid laryngospasm.

56.2.5.2 Hypoxemia

It is known that the PaO2 of nearly 80% patients during the examination will decrease about 10 mmHg, and the longer the examination takes, the more decline in PaO2 value will be. Hypoxemia may induce arrhythmia, cardiac infarction and sudden cardiac arrest.

56.2.5.3 Intraoperative and Postoperative Bleeding

Biopsy, brush biopsy or intense coughing during the electronic bronchoscopic examination all will cause bleeding of varying degree. Mild bleeding can stop spontaneously or by hemostatics injection locally. While for the massive bleeding, the continuous negative pressure suction by electronic bronchoscope and injection of diluted epinephrine or thrombin locally may be the effective way to hemostasis. When these methods are not successful, intravenous hemostatics and suction through tracheal intubation or rigid bronchoscope replacing electronic bronchoscope in time are necessary.

56.2.5.4 Pneumothorax

Pneumothorax, the incidence of which is 1–6%, is mainly caused by lung biopsy.

56.2.5.5 Postoperative Fever

After excluding the fever induced by the inflammation mediators released by alveolar macrophages, the secondary pulmonary infection or bacteremia should be considered reasons for the postoperative fever.

56.2.6 Bronchoalveolar Lavage

Bronchoalveolar lavage (BAL) is a safe and effective way to investigate the pulmonary immunopathogenesis by obtaining the pulmonary immune effector cells directly. For some diseases, especially the diffuse interstitial lung diseases (such as idiopathic pulmonary fibrosis, sarcoidosis, extrinsic allergic alveolitis and pulmonary alveolar proteinosis), lung tumors and pulmonary specific pathogen infection, BAL has been the important detection means of assisting clinical diagnosis and judging the prognosis.

56.2.6.1 Indications

- Evaluate the inflammatory degree of the diagnosed diffuse interstitial lung diseases.
- Diagnose the pulmonary infectious diseases and some kinds of diffuse interstitial lung diseases.
- Collect data for the differential diagnosis and formulating effective therapeutic plan for the pulmonary infectious diseases and diffuse interstitial lung diseases.
- Therapeutic lavage for pulmonary alveolar proteinosis.

56.2.6.2 Relative Contraindication

- Patients are non-cooperative.
- FEV1 < 1000 mL.
- Asthma with airway obstruction, hypercapnia and irreformable hypoxemia.
- Severe cardiopulmonary disorders.
- Obvious bleeding tendency.

56.2.6.3 Inspection Method

Preoperative Preparation

The section is the same as that in the basic bronchoscopic examination. BAL is taken before the biopsy or brush biopsy in normal. Two percent lidocaine is applied as the local anesthetic.

Operation Procedure

Hold the bronchoscope in the opening of the lesions bronchial and inject 2% lidocaine to anaesthetize the corresponding pulmonary segment. Then inject 25–50 mL of physiological saline every time by the biopsy hole of the bronchoscope to total 100–250 mL of but not more than 300 mL. After every injection of the physiological saline, the lavage must be recovered by the 50–100 mmHg vacuum aspiration and insure the recovery surpasses 40%. At least 5 mL (10–20 mL is appropriate) lavage should be sent to the laboratory immediately.

56.2.6.4 Cell Components of the Lavage

BALF of the Healthy Non-smokers

- Total number of the cells: (5–10) × 106/L, alveolar macrophages >85%, lymphocytes 10–15%, neutrophils ≤3%, eosinophils ≤1%, squamous cells ≤5%, the cilium columnar epithelia ≤5%.
- T cell subsets

T lymphocytes account for about 70% of all the lymphocytes. CD4+ T lymphocytes account for about 50% of T lymphocytes, and CD8+ T lymphocytes account for about 30%. Therefore the normal ratio of CD4+/CD8+ is about 1.5–1.8.

BALF of the smokers

The total number of the cells, the numbers of the alveolar macrophages and neutrophil in the BALF of the smokers are all increased obviously. The number of the lymphocytes is not significantly different from that in the healthy non-smokers, but the proportion of CD8+ is increased and the ratio of CD4+/CD8+ is decreased.

56.2.6.5 Clinical application

The cytology, chemistry, enzymology and immunology of the BALF are all important basis of exploring the etiology, pathology and diagnosis, evaluating the efficacy and judging the prognosis.

1. **The diseases for which BALF may provide diagnosis basis and therapeutic means are listed below.**
   - Non-infectious diseases: sarcoidosis, idiopathic pulmonary fibrosis, allergic pneumonia, eosinophilic pneumonia, idiopathic pulmonary hemosiderosis disease, asbestosis(Table 56.1).
   - Infectious diseases: viral pneumonia, bacterial pneumonia, aspergillosis, pulmonary candidiasis, pulmonary cryptococcosis.

Table 56.1 The cell components changes of BALF in interstitial lung diseases

				T cell subsets			
Diseases	Total number of cells	Lymphocytes	Neutrophils	$CD4^+$	$CD8^+$	$CD4^+/CD8^+$	IgG/albumin
Idiopathic pulmonary fibrosis	↑	–	↑	–	–	↓	–
Extrinsic allergic alveolitis	↑	↑	–	↓	↑	↓	>1
Sarcoidosis	↑	↑	–	↑	↓	↑	<1

Table 56.2 The characteristic changes of BALF in pulmonary non-infectious diseases

Diseases	Characteristic changes
Pulmonary alveolar proteinosis	Coloration PAS is positive and lamellar bodies can be found in alveolar macrophages.
Pulmonary histiocytosis X	CD_1^+ cells accounts for 4% and X bodies (cytoplasmic inclusions) or Birbeck particles can be found by electron microscope.
Beryllіosis	The lymphocytes transformation test is positive, CD4+/CD8+ >4.0, and the proportion of alveolar macrophages is increased.

2. **The diseases which can be diagnosis by BALF are listed below.**
   - Non-infectious diseases: pulmonary alveolar proteinosis (PAP), pulmonary histiocytosis X (PHX), berylliosis (Tables 56.2 and 56.3).
   - Infectious diseases: pneumocystis pneumonia (PCP), legionella pneumonia, mycoplasmal pneumonia, chlamydia pneumonia, tuberculosis, influenza virus pneumonia, respiratory syncytial virus pneumonia.

Table 56.3 The characteristic changes of BALF in pulmonary infectious diseases

Diseases	Characteristic changes
Sarcoidosis	The lymphocytes account for more than 18%, CD4+/CD8+ >4.0, and the proportion of alveolar macrophages is increased
Idiopathic pulmonary fibrosis	The neutrophils, eosinophils and lymphocytes are increased, however lymphocytes decrease prompts a bad prognosis
Allergic pneumonia	Neutrophils infiltrate in the lung tissue in the acute stage, while lymphocytes >80% in the BALF in the subacute or chronic stage with CD4+/CD8+ decreasing
Eosinophils pneumonia	Eosinophils >60% in the BALF accompanied by neutrophils increasing slightly
Idiopathic pulmonary hemosiderosis disease	The typical iron particles can be seen in alveolar macrophages

Part V

Common Diagnostic Techniques

Common Diagnostic Techniques

Diagnostic techniques are medical procedures that every clinical doctor should master. They not only play an important role in making the diagnosis, but also have therapeutical effect by administering medicines.

Therefore, when starting to learn diagnostics, every doctor should master common diagnostic techniques, including indications, contraindications, procedures, and improve the accuracy and proficiency of these techniques in clinical practice. Meanwhile, mastering common diagnostic techniques is necessary for a doctor to be certified.

Prior to the procedure, every doctor should be familiar with the patients' medical history, talk to the patients and their relatives about the reason to perform this diagnostic test in order to make them fully understand the procedure and cooperate with the clinicians. Clinicians should make sure the basic information including bed number, admission number and name is correct and obtain informed consent if necessary.

The procedures should be performed in the treatment room, or in the ward or at the bedside if needed but the bed should be seperated from the surrounding environment with a curtain.

Prior to the procedure, operators must check all the equipments are assembled and wash hands following the instructions of hand hygiene. If necessary, wear isolation gown, mask, gloves and follow strictly the rules of sterile operation. Watch for any changes in the patient during the procedure and handle the contaminated equipments appropriately.

57 Thoracentesis

Rui Zeng

57.1 Indication

This procedure, which can be used diagnostically or therapeutically, is indicated when unexplained fluid accumulates or patients complain of symptoms associated with pulmonary effusion.

57.2 Procedure

1. **Position:** Thoracentesis is usually performed with the patient in a sitting position (facing the back of the chair), sitting upright with arms resting on the back of the chair and the forehead resting on the arms. The lateral recumbent position can be used if the patient is unable to sit upright, with arms hugging the back of the head.
2. **Site selection:** Puncture site should be located where the dullness to percussion is most apparent. In case of large amount of pleural effusion, puncture site is usually selected in seventh to eighth intercostal space along the scapular or posterior axillary line and sometimes in sixth to seventh intercostal space on the mid axillary line or the fifth intercostal space on the anterior axillary line. For patients with encapsulated effusions, ultrasound can guide the direction and depth of the needle, also the optimal entry location on skin.
3. **Site preparation with antiseptic and anesthetic:** Skin surrounding the puncture site should be cleaned with antiseptics. The operator should wear sterile gloves and cover the puncture site using drape with fenestration. Next, local anesthetic is administered (2% lidocaine) at the upper border of the rib from epidermis to the visceral pleura.
4. **Puncture:** The operator should press and hold the skin in place surrounding the puncture site using left index and middle finger and close the three-way stopcock with right hand. Next, slowly advance the puncture needle at the anesthetic site. When resistance disappears suddenly, rotate the stopcock to let it communicate with pleural cavity and aspirate the fluid. The assistant helps stabilize the puncture needle with haemostatic forceps in order to avoid injury to lung tissue. When the syringe is filled with fluid, rotate the stopcock to let it communicate with outside environment and remove the fluid.
5. **If a thick long puncture needle is used instead of the needle discussed above**, the plastic tube attached to the needle should be clamped first with a haemostatic forceps before doing the procedure. After the needle is advanced into the pleural cavity, loosen the forceps and then start aspiration. After the syringe is full, clamp the tube again and withdraw the syringe, immediately place the fluid in a kidney basin to record the fluid volume or sent it to the laboratory for analysis.
6. **Compression and fixation:** After the fluid is removed, withdraw the puncture needle and cover the puncture site with sterile gauze. Compress the site for a few seconds and fix the gauze with adhesive plaster. The patient should lie still after the procedure.

57.3 Attention

1. The reason for thoracentesis should be explained in details to the patients prior to puncture in order to relieve their anxiety. For anxious patients, clinicians can administer 10 mg diazepam 30 min prior to the procedure or 30 mg codeine.
2. Closely observe the patients' reaction during the procedure. Fluid removal should be discontinued when the following symptoms occur: dizziness, pallor, sweating, palpitation, pressing or severe pain in the chest, syncope or continuous coughing, shortness of breath. Treatment include subcutaneous administration of 0.1% epinephrine 0.3–0.5 mL or other symptomatic treatment.

R. Zeng (✉)
Department of Cardiology, Sichuan University, Chengdu, China

X.-H. Wan, R. Zeng (eds.), *Handbook of Clinical Diagnostics*, https://doi.org/10.1007/978-981-13-7677-1_57

3. Clinicians should neither aspirate too much or too fast at one time. The volume of fluid removed during diagnostic thoracentesis is 50–100 mL. During therapeutic thoracentesis, the maximum volume of the fluid removed is 600 mL initially and 1000 mL later on in order to avoid pulmonary edema. For patients with pulmonary empyema, the fluid should be removed as much as possible.

   If the patient is suspected with pyogenic infection, the assistant should take the specimen with a sterile tube in order to make Gram-stains for microscopic examination and perform bacterial culture as well as drug sensitivity test. When evaluating for malignancy, the minimum amount of fluid needed is 100 mL in order to increase the diagnostic yield. Specimen should be sent immediately in order to avoid autocytolysis.
4. Aseptic technique is required in order to avoid pleural infection.
5. Operators should avoid air from going into the pleural cavity and maintain its negative pressure during the procedure.
6. The puncture site should be above the ninth rib to avoid injury to diaphragm and abdominal organs.
7. For patients with malignant pleural effusion, antineoplastic drugs and sclerosing agent can be injected into the pleural cavity to induce chemical pleuritis, which causes pleural adhesion and subsequent closure of the pleural cavity to avoid re-accumulation of the fluid.

Procedure: After removing 500–1200 mL fluid, lidocaine 150 mg + normal saline 50 mg is injected into the pleural cavity first. Next, drugs (e.g. minocycline, talcum powder, erythrocin, hypertonic glucose, Staphylococcal enterotoxin C) diluted with 20–30 mL normal saline is administered. Then, the patient is told to lie in bed and change his or her position in order to let the medicines evenly distribute inside the pleural cavity. The fluid is removed 24 h later.

If a drainage tube is inserted by using a catheter, the drugs above are injected after a proper amount of fluid is removed. Continuous suction device is placed 24 h later and will work for 24 h with a negative pressure of 11–30 mmHg until the drainage amount is less than 150 mL per day.

58 Abdominal Paracentesis

Rui Zeng

58.1 Indication

The procedure is indicated for diagnostic or therapeutic purpose in patients with ascites.

58.2 Contraindication

1. Patients at risk for hepatic encephalopathy. Fast removal of a large amount of ascitic fluid may induce hepatic encephalopathy.
2. Patients with tuberculous peritonitis and subsequent adhesive mass.
3. Patients without ascites. For instance, patients with huge ovarian cyst, hepatic echinococcosis.
4. Patients with severe abnormal coagulation.

58.3 Procedure

1. **Patient preparation:** Patients should empty the bladder prior to the procedure in order to avoid puncturing the bladder. Abdominal circumference, pulse, blood pressure, abdominal signs should be recorded to examine changes during the procedure.
2. **Position:** Abdominal paracentesis can be performed with the patient in supine, lateral decubitus or sitting position.
3. **Common puncture site**: (a) Lateral one-third of the distance from the anterior superior iliac spine to the umbilicus. (b) 1.0 cm above the midpoint between umbilicus and pubic symphysis and 1.5 cm leftward or rightward to that point. (c) In lateral decubitus position, diagnostic puncture site is often where the horizontal line passing the umbilicus intersects the anterior axillary line or mid axillary line. (d) Small amount of ascites, especially encapsulated effusions, can be removed under the guidance of ultrasound.
4. **Site preparation with antiseptic and anesthetic:** Routine cleaning is performed at the puncture site. The operator should wear sterile gloves and cover the puncture site with sterile drapes. Next, local anesthesia is performed from epidermis to parietal peritoneum with 2% lidocaine.
5. **Puncture and fluid removal:** Operator stabilize the skin with left hand, and using the right hand to insert the needle perpendicular to the abdominal wall. Sudden disappearance of the resistance is an indication that the needle has passed through parietal peritonium. The operator can then aspirate fluid and send the specimen to laboratory. Diagnostic paracentesis can be performed directly with a 20 mL or 50 mL syringe as well as a proper needle. Recently, corresponding paracentesis kit is usually used when large volumes of fluid is removed. Common paracentesis kit include various-sized syringes, paracentesis needles and drainage tubes. The vacuum bottles have scales making the procedure easier and safer.
6. **Compression and fixation:** Remove the needle after drainage. Cover the puncture site with a sterile gauze. After few minutes compression with fingers, fix the gauze with adhesive plaster.
7. **After fluid removal**. Abdominal girth, pulse, blood pressure and abdominal signs should be recorded again.

58.4 Attention

1. Closely observe the patients' general condition during the procedure. The procedure should be discontinued if patients complain of dizziness, palpitations, nausea, shortness of breath, tachycardia as well as pallor, etc. and proper treatment should be performed.
2. Removal of the fluid should not be too fast. However, most scholars believe that large amount of fluid can be removed if albumin is administered continuously (40–60 g/L ascites).

R. Zeng (✉)
Department of Cardiology, Sichuan University, Chengdu, China

X.-H. Wan, R. Zeng (eds.), *Handbook of Clinical Diagnostics*, https://doi.org/10.1007/978-981-13-7677-1_58

In the above setting, up to four to six liters or even all of the ascitic fluid can be removed within 1–2 h.

3. If a poor flow of fluid is encountered, the operator can adjust the paracentesis needle slightly or let the patient change the position a little bit.
4. For patients with a large volume of fluid, a Z-track technique can be used. The skin can be punctured by approaching the chosen entry site tangentially with the needle. Once the needle is subcutaneous, it is then placed perpendicular to the abdominal wall and advanced to the abdominal cavity. Obvious fluid leakage after fluid removal is an indication that patients still have large volumes of fluid and the abdominal pressure is too high. If this is the case, fluid removal should be continued. When the abdominal pressure drops and the patient feels comfortable, no fluid leakage will occur after the paracentesis.
5. When the fluid is collected for cell count, differential, chemical testing, bacterial culture and cytological testing, the specimen should be sent for examination as soon as possible to achieve a high quality.

Bone Marrow Puncture

59

Rui Zeng

59.1 Indication

1. Hepatomegaly, splenomegaly and lymphadenopathy of undetermined origin, fever, cachexia.
2. Immature blood cells in peripheral blood.
3. Increase or decrease of single and/or multiple lineage of blood cells in the peripheral blood.

59.2 Contraindication

1. Patients with hemophilia and hemorrhagic tendency.
2. Diagnosis already confirmed by peripheral blood test.
3. Bone marrow puncture should be done with caution in women in the second and third trimester of pregnancy.

59.3 Procedure

1. **Choose the site of puncture:**
   - Puncture site at anterior superior iliac spine: 1–2 cm posterior to the anterior superior iliac spine where the bone surface is flat and easily fixed. It is convenient to operate on and has minimal risk.
   - Puncture site at posterior superior iliac spine: The puncture site is on both side of the sacral vertebra where the bone protrudes superior to the hip.
   - Sternum puncture site: located in the midline of sternal body at the second intercostal space. The sternum is the thinnest at this site posterior to which large vessels and atria is found. Extreme caution is to be taken during puncture to avoid penetrating the sternum. Abundant bone marrow is found at this site therefore when it is an option when puncture at other sites fail.
   - Puncture site at lumbar vertebra: The protuberance of spinous process of the lumbar vertebra.
2. **Position**: When puncturing at anteriorsuperior iliac spine and sternum, patients are maintained at supine position; when puncturing at posterior superior iliac spine, patients are maintained at lateral decubitus position; when puncturing at lumbar vertebra, patients are sitting or in lateral decubitus.
3. **Anesthesia**: After routine cleaning of local skin with antiseptic, operators should wear sterile gloves and cover the site with sterile drape with fenestration. Then use 2% lidocaine for local anesthesia of the skin, subcutaneous tissue and periosteum.
4. **Fixation:** The needle is fixed at a proper depth using the apparatus at the end of the needle. It is usually 1.5 cm for iliac puncture and 1.0 cm for sternum puncture.
5. **Puncturing**: The operator should fix the puncture site with left thumb and index finger while advancing needle perpendicular to bone surface with the right hand. When doing sternum puncture, the needle should be at a 30–40° angle to the sternum. After reaching the bone surface, the operator should spin the puncture needle along the longitudinal axis and slowly advance into the bone. Sudden disappearance of resistance indicate that the puncture needle has reached the bone marrow. If the needle is not fixed in place, push it in a little bit until it stabilizes within the bone.
6. **Aspiration of bone marrow**: Remove the stylet and connect a sterilized syringe (10 mL or20 mL) and start aspiration of the bone marrow with appropriate force. When puncture needle is in the bone marrow cavity, patients can feel an acute aching pain during aspiration, followed by red bone marrow entering into the syringe. We usually aspirate 0.1–0.2 mL bone marrow. Dilution of the bone marrow is likely to occur if too much force is used during aspiration or too much is extracted. If bacteria culture is needed, 1–2 mL can be aspirated after bone marrow is

R. Zeng (✉)
Department of Cardiology, Sichuan University, Chengdu, China

X.-H. Wan, R. Zeng (eds.), *Handbook of Clinical Diagnostics*, https://doi.org/10.1007/978-981-13-7677-1_59

withdrawn for cytology and smears. If efforts to aspirate the bone marrow fails, it may be due to obstruction of the needle by tissue or dry tap. The stylet should be put back in place with slight adjustment of needle depth. Pull out the stylet again. If blood is found on the stylet, a second aspiration is most likely to yield red bone marrow.

7. **Bone marrow smear:** Drip a few drops of bone marrow on a slide for cytology and smear preparation.
8. **Compression**: After aspiration, replace the style. Place a sterile gauze at the puncture site with left hand and pull out the puncture needle with right hand. Compress for 1–2 min and finish the dressing with plaster.

59.4 Attention

1. The bleeding time and coagulation time should be checked and special attention should be paid to patients with hemorrhagic tendency, hemophilia is a contraindication for bone marrow puncture.
2. The puncture needle and syringe should be kept dry in order to avoid hemolysis.
3. After piercing into the bone, movement of the needle should be avoided to prevent breaking it. When doing sternum puncture, the operator shouldn't overexert or advance too deep to prevent serious complications after penetration.
4. If the bone is too hard to puncture into, the operator should not pierce with the brute force to avoid breaking the needle. Osteopetrosis should be suspected and X-ray should be done to determine the diagnosis.
5. When aspirating for cytological testing, avoid extracting too much bone marrow which will hinder judgement of degree of hyperplasia, cell count and differential.
6. When aspirating for culture, extraction of 1–2 mL bone marrow after smear preparation is needed.
7. When there are too many immature cells in the bone marrow, it is prone to coagulation. Smears should be prepared immediately after aspiration.
8. When sending the bone marrow smear for examination, two or three blood smears should be sent at the same time.
9. Lidocaine skin test should be done before anesthesia.

Lumbar Puncture

60

Rui Zeng

60.1 Indication

1. Patients with meningeal irritation sign.
2. Patients suspected with intracranial hemorrhage, meningeal leukemia and intracranial tumor metastasis.
3. Severe headache with unknown cause, coma, seizures or paralysis.
4. Patients with demyelinating diseases.
5. CNS diseases which require intrathecal administration, anesthesia and myelography.

60.2 Contraindication

1. Patients with high intracranial pressure or mass in the posterior fossa.
2. Patients with shock or systemic failure.
3. Pyogenic infection at the puncture site.
4. Patients with coagulation disorders.

60.3 Procedure

1. **Position.** Patients are put in lateral decubitus position on the bed, with back vertical to the bed surface, chin bent towards the chest, hugging both knees to the stomach, making a curve with his or her spine; the assistant can help by holding the patient's head and popliteal fossa and bringing them as close together to increase the intervertebral space, making it easier for needle advancement. For patients who are obese, or those who have arthritis or scoliosis, puncture can be done in a sitting position where the patient bends forward with arms crossed on the back of the chair to form a curve in the spine.
2. **Choosing the puncture site.** Puncture site is the intersection of the line running through both posterior superior iliac spines and the posterior midline, which is the third or fourth lumbar interspace. Sometimes the interspace above or below can also be used.
3. **Site preparation with antiseptic and anesthetic.** After routine cleaning of local skin, the operator should wear sterile gloves and put down drape with fenestration. 2% lidocaine is used for local anesthesia from the skin to ligamenta intervertebralia.
4. **Puncturing.** The operator should press and hold the puncture site with left thumb and index finger while using the right hand to advance the needle perpendicular to skin surface. The tip of the needle is tilted toward the cranial direction and the depth is around 4–6 cm in adults, 2–4 cm in children. When the needle pierces through the ligament and the dura, there is a sudden disappearance of resistance. The stylet then can be withdrawn slowly (prevent rapid leakage of CSF resulting in cerebral hernia) to see if there is fluid return.
5. **Measuring opening pressure.** Before collection of cerebrospinal fluid, opening pressure should be measured first using the manometer. Reference range is 70–180 mm H_2O.
6. **Queckenstedt Test.** This test is used to check the patency of subarachnoid space. After measuring the initial pressure, the assistant presses the jugular vein for 10s, then press the other side, finally press both sides. If the cerebrospinal pressure goes up twice as high after pressing and goes down immediately 10–20s after releasing, the result is negative which indicates no obstruction. If the pressure doesn't go up after exerting pressure, the test is positive which indicates obstruction of the subarachnoid space. Increased intracranial pressure is a contraindication of this procedure.
7. **Collection of sample.** Remove the manometer and collect 2–5 mL cerebrospinal fluid for examination. Use aseptic technique to collect specimen if culture is needed.
8. **Dressing and fixation**. After collection, insert the stylet and remove the needle. Apply a sterile gauze at puncture site and fix it with adhesive plaster. Patients should lie for 4–6 h afterwards and drink normal saline water to prevent headache caused by low intracranial pressure.

R. Zeng (✉)
Department of Cardiology, Sichuan University, Chengdu, China

X.-H. Wan, R. Zeng (eds.), *Handbook of Clinical Diagnostics*, https://doi.org/10.1007/978-981-13-7677-1_60

60.4 Attention

1. Aseptic technique should be strictly performed. Avoid damaging the capillary while puncturing.
2. Master contraindication of lumbar puncture. If the patient has high intracranial pressure, fundus examination is required before puncturing. Patients who have papilloedema or risk of cerebral hernia are refrained from this procedure. Shock, systemic failure, local skin inflammation, space occupying lesion in the posterior cranial fossa are also contraindications. If lumbar puncture needs to be carried out in patients with the last two conditions, the cerebellomedullary cistern route can be taken.
3. If any abnormality is found in respiration, pulse and complexion, the procedure should be stopped immediately and symptomatic treatment should be administered.
4. Equivalent amount of cerebrospinal fluid should be withdrawn before intrathecal administration.

61 Urethral Catheterization

Rui Zeng

61.1 Indication

1. To relieve urinary retention (including urinary retention caused by prostatic hypertrophy, coma and other reasons) and overflow urinary incontinence.
2. To obtain an uncontaminated sample of urine for bacterial culture.
3. To perform indwelling catheterization or measure urinary output per hour.
4. To drain the bladder prior to, during and after the abdominal and pelvic surgeries
5. For patients with bladder, urethral surgery or injury; measure bladder pressure, inject drugs and contrast agent or detect urethrostenosis, etc.

61.2 Procedure

1. **Genital area cleaning.** Clean genital area with soap water; retract the foreskin and clean it if non-circumcised in male patients.
2. **Disinfection.** Put a pad under hip and place the patient in supine position with knees bent and hips flexed. Sterilize with cotton balls with 0.1% benzalkonium bromide (or 0.1% Chlorhexidine, 0.5% iodophor) on it, from the inside outward, from top to bottom Move cotton balls from inside to the outside, from the top down towards the bottom of mons pubis and the upper 1/3 of inner thigh. Female disinfection area is the vulva, and male disinfection area is penis and scrotum. Each cotton ball should be used only once and vulva should be covered with aseptic drape with fenestration. Penis should be wrapped around with a towel and the urethral meatus needs to be exposed.
3. **Disinfection of urethral meatus.** Wear sterile gloves and stand on the patient's right side, lift the penis with the left thumb and index finger in men. For female patients, separate the labia and expose urethral meatus to clean them with benzalkonium bromide cotton ball from top-down. Use a circular motion from the meatus to the base of the penis and swap for several times. Then, hold the penis and form a 60° angle with the abdomen.
4. **Insert catheter.** Use right hand to slowly insert the sterile lubricated catheter into the urethral meatus, clip the external catheter with a hemostatic forceps and put the outer end of the catheter in the sterilized kidney basin. Insert about 15–20 cm into the urethral meatus in male patients and about 6–8 cm in female patients. Loosen the hemostatic forceps for the urine to flow. If there's a need for bacterial culture, mid-portion urine should be obtained in a sterile test tube.
5. **Removal of urinary catheter.** Withdraw the catheter after the catheter is clipped as to avoid contamination of clothes by urine flowing out of the foley.
6. **Indwelling catheter.** Secure the catheter to the thigh with plaster, inflate the balloon slowly with liquid to the volume recommended on the catheter, and gently withdraw the catheter slightly until resistance is felt. Clip the tube with the hemostatic forceps and wrap the end with a sterile gauze to prevent urine flow and contamination; or connect a sterile drainage bag hanging on the side of the bed.

61.3 Attention

1. Use aseptic techniques strictly to prevent urinary tract infection.
2. Insertion of the catheter should be gentle to prevent damage of the urethral mucosa. If resistance is felt, gently rotate the catheter in other directions [male urethra has two bendings (prepubic curvature, subpubic curvature) and three sites of stenosis, transform the position of penis according to the anatomical characteristics in order to

R. Zeng (✉)
Department of Cardiology, Sichuan University, Chengdu, China

X.-H. Wan, R. Zeng (eds.), *Handbook of Clinical Diagnostics*, https://doi.org/10.1007/978-981-13-7677-1_61

insert], insert another 2 cm after urine begins to flow. It should neither be inserted too deep nor too shallow. Avoid repeatedly withdrawal and insertion the catheter.

3. Select the proper size of the catheter. Choose the fine catheter for children and those suspected of urethrostenosis.
4. For patients with over-filling bladder, urine outflow should be slow so as not to cause bleeding or syncope by sudden fall of pressure.
5. Ask the patient to urinate prior to measuring residual urine volume, and then perform urethral catheterization. The residual urine volume is usually 5–10 mL. Volume exceeding 100 mL suggests urinary retention.
6. Check if the catheter is fixed regularly in patients with indwelling catheter, and wash the bladder with aseptic liquid every day if necessary. Replace the catheter every 5–7 days. Let the urethra relax for a few hours prior to reinsertion.
7. Ensure the duration of indwelling catheter: the necessity of indwelling catheters should be assessed, withdraw the catheter as early as possible to prevent urinary tract infection. Deflate the balloon and clip the tube before withdrawing the catheter.

62 Gastric Tube Implantation

Rui Zeng

62.1 Indication

1. Diagnosis and disease monitoring, gastric juice collection.
2. Gastric lavage for overdose or poisoning
3. Nutrition: coma patients or those who are unable to swallow due to a variety of reasons, such as swallowing dysfunction (bulbar paralysis) caused by neurological diseases, patients with severe oral disease, or patients undergoing oral and throat surgery; patients who are unable to open the mouth, such as tetanus patients; premature infants and critically ill patients and those refusing to eat. Esophageal or cardiac obstruction patients.
4. Decompression: acute dilatation of the stomach; upper digestive tract perforation or gastrointestinal obstruction; acute abdomen with obvious flatulence or prior to and after a major abdominal surgery.

62.2 Contraindication

1. Nasopharyngeal tumor or nasal obstruction.
2. Patients with esophageal varices.
3. Esophageal and cardiac stenosis or obstruction.
4. Esophagostenosis caused by taking corrosive drugs, or those at risk of esophageal perforation.

62.3 Procedure

1. Preparation
   - Train the patient to coordinate movements with intubation for a smooth procedure.
   - Required equipments: nasogastric tube, kidney basin, tweezers or pliers, 10 mL syringe, gauze, drapes, lubricant, cotton swabs, plaster, clip and stethoscope.
   - Check the patency of nasogastric tube and whether the marking is clear.
   - Check the ventilation of nasal cavity before intubation and select the patent nostril.
2. Method
   - Wash hands and bring the prepared materials to the bedside of the patient, check the patient, explain to the patient and their families the purpose and procedure of operation, wear mask and gloves.
   - Help the patient get in semi Fowler's position or supine position, place drape and kidney basin near the patient's mouth, choose the patent side of the nostril. Open the pack and take the tube out to estimate insertion distance. There're two methods: one is the distance from the hairline to the xiphoid process at base of sternum; the second is the distance from lips, around ear, and to xiphoid process at base of sternum. Adult insertion length is about 45–55 cm.
   - Lubricant the tip of gastric tube, use left hand to hold the gastric tube with gauze and use the right hand to grip the tip of the tube, place the tip of the catheter inside the chosen nostril and advance it gently into the throat (about 14–16 cm), and have the patient swallow when advancing the catheter into the esophagus at a predetermined distance. Fix the tube with tape and check if the tube is coiled in the mouth.
   - There are usually three methods to determine the place of nasogastric tube: Extraction of gastric juice: which is the most reliable method for determining if the gastric tube is in the stomach. Gas acoustic: place the stethoscope at the stomach area, a gurgling sound can be heard over the fast injection of 10 mL air through the tube into the stomach. Place the distal end of the tube in the water, and there are no bubbles escaping.
   - Confirm that the tube is in the stomach, wipe mouth secretions with gauze, withdraw kidney basin and

R. Zeng (✉)
Department of Cardiology, Sichuan University, Chengdu, China

X.-H. Wan, R. Zeng (eds.), *Handbook of Clinical Diagnostics*, https://doi.org/10.1007/978-981-13-7677-1_62

remove the gloves, use the plaster to fix the tube on the cheek. Fold back the end of the tube and wrap it with gauze, remove the drape, use a pin to fix the tube on the pillow or patient's collar.

- Ask how the patient is feeling, position the patients comfortably.
- Corresponding operation, such as connecting suction device, enteral nutrition, gastric lavage.

62.4 Attention

1. Intubation should be gentle to avoid injury of esophageal mucosa. It should be noted that a timely insertion should be performed during swallowing.
2. It is necessary to analyze the reasons of resistance during intubation, have the patient swallow as you further advance the catheter, blindly using force will lead to folding or coiling of the tube in the oropharynx.
3. Intubation should pause if nausea occurs and ask the patient to take a deep breath to relieve patient's nervousness. Symptoms such as cough, dyspnea indicate that catheter is misplaced in the pharynx, which needs immediate extubation; if the insertion is not smooth, check gastric tube to see if it's folded or coiled in the oropharynx instead of using force, pull out the tube a little and then insert again.
4. During intubation of comatose patient, the patient's head should be leaned back. Hold the patient's head when the gastric tube feeds in 15 cm, and hold the lower jaw close to the manubrium to increase the curvature of the pharyngeal channel, let the tube slide along the posterior wall and advance it to the required distance.

63 Skin Allergy Test

Rui Zeng

In the course of clinical diagnosis and treatment, some drugs including penicillin, streptomycin and cephalosporin may cause allergic reactions, manifesting as hypotension, pharyngeal edema, bronchial spasm, even death. Therefore, skin allergy tests should be done before the administration of these drugs. The technique and result of cephalosporin and streptomycin allergy skin test are basically the same as that of penicillin, so we use penicillin as an example.

63.1 Section 1: Penicillin Skin Test

For those expected to be treated with penicillin, the skin test must be carried out if the patient hasn't used penicillin within three days. Special attention should be paid when switching to different batches, skin test should be carried out again using the same batch of penicillin.

63.1.1 Procedure

1. **Skin test solution preparation:**
   - Dissolve 800 k units of penicillin with 4.0 mL normal saline to a concentration of 200 k units of penicillin per mL.
   - Extract 0.1 mL solution with 1.0 mL syringe, add normal saline to 1.0 mL reaching the concentration of 20 k units of penicillin per mL.
   - Remove 0.9 mL and add normal saline to 1.0 mL again, ending with 2000 units of penicillin per mL.
   - Repeat the last step to reach the final concentration of 200 units per mL.
2. **Intradermal injection:** inject 0.1 mL (containing 20 units) in flexion side of lower 1/3 forearm (after cleaning with 75% alcohol), and make a 5 mm wheal. Ask the patient not to squeeze it, the results can be interpreted after 20 min in bright natural light.
3. **Interpretation of results:**
   - Negative: no changes of the wheal diameter and no swelling of the skin around, no redness and no symptoms.
   - Positive: wheal diameter increases over 10 mm with redness, pseudopods around and local itching. Blisters, dizziness, chest tightness palpitations, shortness of breath, sweating, nausea, irritability indicates a strong positive result. Anaphylactic shock occurs in severe cases.

63.1.2 Attention

1. Medical history or history of allergy should be carefully asked before the skin test, and it should not be carried out if there is a history of penicillin allergy.
2. Positive skin test should not only be recorded, but also told to the patient or their families to prevent the use of similar drugs.
3. For patients going into or about to go in allergic shock, emergent rescue should be performed. Place the patient in supine position, and rapidly inject subcutaneously 0.1% epinephrine 0.5–1.0 mL, start oxygen inhalation with direct intravenous injection of dexamethasone 10 mg if necessary.
4. Those with a negative skin test can also develop allergic reactions in the course of administration, so patients should be closely observed for 20 min after the injection of medication.

63.2 Section 2: Procaine Allergy Skin Test

Procaine, which is also known as novocaine, is a commonly used local anesthetic. Occasionally mild to severe allergic reactions occur, so skin test should be done before application. The concentration of solution for skin test is 0.25% and the

R. Zeng (✉)
Department of Cardiology, Sichuan University, Chengdu, China

X.-H. Wan, R. Zeng (eds.), *Handbook of Clinical Diagnostics*, https://doi.org/10.1007/978-981-13-7677-1_63

injection volume of the solution is 0.1 mL. The method and the interpretation of the results is same as penicillin skin test.

63.3 Section 3: Iodine Allergy Test

At present, the commonly used iodine contrast agents are angiografin, cholografin, iohexol and iotrolan. Allergic reactions are common adverse reactions, severe anaphylactic shock and convulsions can be seen sometimes, allergy skin test is needed before using.

Intradermal skin test: inject 0.1 mL of iodine contrast agent into the skin at flexor side of the forearm. Results are interpreted after 20 min in the same way as a penicillin skin test. In addition to intradermal test, there're eye test and intravenous injection test as well.

1. **Eye test:** Drop 1 to 2 drops of iodine contrast agent into the eye and watch for 10 min. A positive test result involves conjunctival injection and edema.
2. **Intravenous injection test:** it's most commonly used clinically. Take 1.0 mL of 30% meglumine and inject slowly after local disinfection, observe for 15 min. A positive test is followed by nausea, vomiting, numbness of limbs or urticaria.

63.4 Section 4: Tetanus Antitoxin Skin Test

Tetanus antitoxin (TAT) is a product containing tetanus toxin serum from the cattle, and are given to patients with suspected exposure to tetanus, such as trauma patients and treatment of patients with tetanus. TAT is a heteroantigen with antigenicity, which can cause allergic reactions and even anaphylactic shock, so skin test should be done before use.

63.4.1 Procedure

1. **Preparation of skin test solution:** extract 0.1 mL of TAT (1500 units/mL) with 1.0 mL syringe and dilute with normal saline to 1.0 mL.
2. **Intradermal injection:** inject 0.1 mL of the solution (15 units) into the skin at flexor side of the forearm, and interpret results after 20 min.
3. **Positive result:** redness of the wheal, induration>15 mm, or diameter of redness>40 mm, pseudopods, local itching. A strong positive result involves nasal itching, sneezing, urticaria and other systematic symptoms.

63.4.2 Attention

1. If the result is negative, preventive medication is needed, which means subcutaneous or intramuscular injection of 1500 units to 3000 units.
2. If the result is positive, but according to the condition the injection of TAT is necessary, then desensitization is required. According to Table 63.1, subcutaneous injection is required every 20 min. Complete the total injection (1500 units) if there is no abnormal reaction according to the desensitization plan.

Table 63.1 Desensitization plan

Time	TAT volume (mL)	NS volume (mL)
1	0.1	0.9
2	0.2	0.8
3	0.3	0.7
4	Rest of the amount	Dilute to 1.0

Tuberculin Test

64

Rui Zeng

Tuberculin test is type IV hypersensitivity reaction to tuberculin, typically used to identify *Mycobacterium tuberculosis* infection, do tuberculosis epidemiological research, assist diagnosis and differential diagnosis, identify those who need the Bacillus Calmette Guerin (BCG) vaccination and to evaluate the effect of inoculation, so as to judge the state of cellular immunity.

64.1 Antigen

There are two types, namely old tuberculin (OT) and purified protein derivative (PPD):

- OT is a brown, transparent liquid concentrate that is made from *Mycobacterium tuberculosis* var. hominis. After culturing for 2 months, mycobacteria is killed by heating and filtered, whereas the product containing autolyzed agents and culture medium is concentrated to 1/10 of the original volume. In 1952, the technique was standardized by WHO, each milliliter contains 1000 mg, or ten million TU (tuberculin units).
- PPD is a protein chemically extracted from filtrate of *Mycobacterium tuberculosis* cultures, which is purer than OT. It has strong specific reactions and high diagnostic value. National PPD-C (80–1) has completely replaced OT and been widely used clinically (Table 64.1).

64.2 Procedure

There're three methods, namely scratch, prick and intradermal injection. The latter is the most widely used because of accurate results:

R. Zeng (✉)
Department of Cardiology, Sichuan University, Chengdu, China

Table 64.1 Comparison of the titer (unit) and content between OT and PPD

TU	OT [mg/0.1 mL (dilution ratio)]	PPD (mg/0.1 mL)
1	0.01 (1 : 10,000)	0.00002
5	0.05 (1 : 2000)	0.0001
10	0.10 (1 : 1000)	0.0002
100	1.00 (1 : 100)	0.005

Table 64.2 Results of PPD skin test

Reaction	Result
Diameter of induration<5 mm	Negative (−)
Diameter of induration 5–9 mm	Weak or general positive (+)
Diameter of induration 10–19 mm	Positive or medium positive (++)
Diameter of induration ≥20 mm or blisters, necrosis, or lymphatic inflammation	Strong positive (+++) (++++)

1. **Site selection**. Flexor region of left forearm without scar. If the test was done again recently (within 2 weeks), the second skin test should be done 3–4 cm diagonally from the first injection site, or at the right forearm to avoid complex strong effect (push effect).
2. **Intradermal injection**. Disinfect local skin with 75% alcohol, use 1.0 mL syringe and the 4.5th needle (needle bevel should not be too long), extract 0.1 mL (5TU) of the dilution and inject intradermally to form a 6–8 mm orange peel-like bump.
3. **Results**. Read the result 48 h after injection and then a second time at 72 h. Measure transverse diameter and longitudinal diameter of local redness and induration (generally the redness and induration have the same diameter, so the results are easily determined), take the average as the diameter. The tuberculin test results are interpreted in Table 64.2.

64.3 Clinical Significance

1. Positive
   - It suggests infection by *Mycobacterium tuberculosis*, which has produced allergic reactions.

X.-H. Wan, R. Zeng (eds.), *Handbook of Clinical Diagnostics*, https://doi.org/10.1007/978-981-13-7677-1_64

- Urban residents and the majority of adults are positive, which has no significant meaning in diagnosis.
- If the result turned positive recently, the person should be closely observed for there may be possibility to develop TB.
- Children under 3 years old who are not vaccinated with Bacillus Calmette Guerin (BCG), regardless of presence of clinical symptoms, there may be active tuberculosis (even with a normal chest X-ray) inside the body.
- Strong positive: Adults: may have active TB and detailed examination should be done; Children: It is of diagnostic significance. Tuberculosis detection rate of children is about 20%, so they should be treated with medication.

2. Negative
   - It indicates that the body has not been infected with *Mycobacterium tuberculosis*, or body allergic reaction has not yet been established (4–8 weeks) although the body has been infected; redo the skin test 1 week after with 5TU, considering tuberculin strong effect, if it is still negative, then *Mycobacterium tuberculosis* infection can be ruled out.
   - The negative rate in the elderly is significantly increased, and the rate of people over 80 years old (OT test) reaches 50%.
   - Allergic reactions are suppressed in children with measles or pertussis, but it will gradually recover after about 3 weeks.
   - Severe tuberculosis (even if the body has active TB, 5% of the result are negative), when there's improvement of the illness after treatment, the tuberculin reaction can turn positive.
   - Sarcoidosis (positive rate is only 10%, and mostly the result is weakly positive), patients with lymphoma and other malignancies.
   - Patients treated with corticosteroids or immunosuppressive agents.
   - Malnutrition and AIDS patients.

64.4 Attention

1. The reagent should be stored in shade and at 4 °C.
2. The skin test time needs to be rearranged if there's forearm skin injury or during menstruation.
3. Glass and plastic can absorb tuberculin. Shaking should be avoided after preparation of the diluted reagent which should be used within 2 h, otherwise the reduction of titer can influence the results.
4. Use a specialized 1 mL syringe with disposable needles. Do not mix with BCG syringe. Before extraction, use diluted PPD to damp the needle to avoid reduction of titer caused by absorption
5. Some adverse reactions may occur after tuberculin test, and it should be handled properly.
   - Local reactions: blisters or ulcers. The skin should be kept clean and coated with 2% gentian violet. Use syringes to extract blister fluid when necessary.
   - Systemic reactions: (a) Fever: mostly it is associated with nonsterile equipments. Generally, it will recover within a few hours. (b) Syncope and shock: related to tension or fear. Ask the patient to lie in supine position and keep the patient warm. The subcutaneous injection of 0.1% epinephrine 0.5–1.0 mL is necessary sometimes. (c) Focal reaction: hypersensitive perilesional inflammation can develop hours after injection, caused by expansion of capillaries in the lung, increased permeability and exudation. Generally special treatment isn't necessary and it can subside on its own in 2–5 days.
6. Older people respond to PPD more slowly than young people, it may take 72 h to interpret the results of the reaction.
7. Approximately 20% of patients with active pulmonary tuberculosis can manifest as false negative. It's suggested that a repeated PPD test be done 1–3 weeks after initial test, the result may be positive due to the effect of multiple strong positive reaction.
8. Patients with the followings conditions are temporarily unfit for tuberculin test: (a) fever (body temperature of 37.5 °C or above). (b) Recovery period of infectious disease, organic heart disease, kidney disease, psychological disease, epilepsy, cellular immunity defect, immunoglobulin deficiency and menstruation.

Part VI

Medical Record

65 Significance

Shiming Liu and Rui Zeng

Medical records are the collection of data of characters, symbols, tables, images, sections, etc., including outpatient, emergency and inpatient medical records. They record medical activities by summarizing, analyzing, and sorting relative data obtained from inquiries, physical examinations, auxiliary examinations, diagnoses, treatments, nursing, etc. They are the comprehensive records of clinical practices, reflecting onsets, progresses, outcomes, diagnoses, and treatments of the patient's illness. Clinical physicians use medical records as scientific evidences to diagnose, treat, and prevent diseases. Medical records can reflect hospital management, medical quality, and professional skill. They are basic data of clinical teaching, scientific research, and information management, as well as important basis for qualification evaluation of medical service. They are medical files of legal effects and important basis for medical disputes and litigation. Recently, medical records have been required to be in accordance with strict standards and requirements by the (National Health and Family Planning Commission). They are forbidden to be forged, hidden, destroyed, or seized. The patient has the right to cope some part of medical records, including some medical notes, body temperature sheets, medical order sheets, test reports, medical imaging data, special examination consent forms, surgery consent forms, surgery and anesthesia records, pathological data, nursing records, etc. So, it is a basic clinical skill for each physician to write medical records correctly and carefully.

S. Liu
Department of Cardiology, Guangzhou Medical University, Guangzhou, China

R. Zeng (✉)
Department of Cardiology, Sichuan University, Chengdu, China

X.-H. Wan, R. Zeng (eds.), *Handbook of Clinical Diagnostics*, https://doi.org/10.1007/978-981-13-7677-1_65

66 Basic Requirement of Medical Record

Shiming Liu and Rui Zeng

66.1 Contents Are Truthful and Written on Time

Medical records must reflect the patient's illness and treatment processes objectively, without surmise or fiction. This is not only related to the quality of medical records, but also shows the physician's morality.

1. Contents of medical records should be objective, authentic, accurate, integrated, well arranged, brief, and focused.
2. Individual document in the medical records should be completed on time according to their requirements. Outpatient medical record should be completed instantly, and emergency medical record should be completed instantly or right after treatments. Complete medical record or admission record (*re- or multi-admission record*) should be completed within 24 h after the patient's admission. Admission and discharge record within 24 h should be completed within 24 h after the patient's discharge, and admission and death record within 24 h should be completed within 24 h after the patient's death. Medical records for emergency or critical patients should be completed on time. If resuscitation delays their completion, they should be completed within 6 h after resuscitation, with data of when the resuscitation was completed, when the record was written, the patient's original status, the resuscitation process, etc.
3. All kinds of records should be marked with the year, month, and day, while records for emergency or resuscitation should extra include the hour and minute, according to the 24-hour time system, for example, 2012-08-28, 16:08.

S. Liu
Department of Cardiology, Guangzhou Medical University, Guangzhou, China

R. Zeng (✉)
Department of Cardiology, Sichuan University, Chengdu, China

66.1.1 Standard Formats and Integral Items

Medical records have special formatting requirements. Complete medical record is classified as traditional and tabular format, with both having almost the same items. The following should be noted.

1. All blanks should be carefully filled in, with "/" or "-" for no content.
2. National standard units of measurement should be used.
3. All kinds of examination reports should be placed in the medical record after grouped and sorted by date.

66.1.2 Accurate Expressions and Proper Words

Medical records should be written in standard Chinese (or other standard nation-recognized languages in other countries, and same principles in the following), with accurate expressions, clear sentences, and correct punctuation.

1. Standard Chinese words should be used, with simplified and variant words subjected to the Xinhua Dictionary. Double-digit or higher numbers should be recorded as Arabic numerals, while one-digit numbers should be presented as Chinese words.
2. Medical records should be written in Chinese medical terms. Foreign languages can be used only for common-used foreign abbreviations as well as symptoms, signs, disease names, and drug names of no formal Chinese names.
3. The names and codes of disease diagnoses, surgeries, and all kinds of treatments should be recorded in accordance with the requirements of the "International Classification of Diseases" (ICD-10, ICD-9-CM-3).

X.-H. Wan, R. Zeng (eds.), *Handbook of Clinical Diagnostics*, https://doi.org/10.1007/978-981-13-7677-1_66

66.1.3 Neat Handwriting and Clear Signatures

Medical records should be written clearly and neatly. All modification should be marked with the date and time, as well as the relevant doctor's signature.

1. Medical records should be written with blue-black or carbon ink.
2. The physician should sign his full name clearly at the bottom right corner of the end of individual records.
3. The patient or his legal representative should sign the informed consent form for some special medical activities if necessary.

66.1.4 Strict Review and Normative Modification

Medical records written by a resident or an intern should be strictly reviewed, modified, and signed by a certified physician. It should be carried out according to correction standards required by the National Ministry of Health. Generally, medical records should be modified within 72 h, with the modified time marked and the original records clear, as well as the physician's signature at the left of the resident or intern, separated by a slash.

66.1.5 Obeying Legislation and Respecting Rights

The patient's rights of being informed and choices provided should be presented in the medical records. The patient or his relatives should have a strong understanding of treatments, prognoses, possible adverse effects, and pretreatment protocols available for the patient. And these should be recorded in detail and signed by the patient or his relatives to indicate that the patient has been informed about his illness. Some special medical activities, such as blood transfusion, anesthesia, surgeries, etc., can be performed only after relevant informed consent form is signed by the patient himself. Informed consent form can be signed by the patient's legal representative if the patient is not at full capacity for civil conduct, or by his close relative if he cannot sign due to his illness. If there's no close relative, it may be signed by a friend. If the patient needs resuscitation but informed consent form cannot be signed on time by his legal representative, close relative, or friend, a responsible staff member in the medical institution or another authorized person can provide the consent by signature.

67 Denomination, Format, and Content of Medical Record

Shiming Liu and Rui Zeng

67.1 Section 1: Inpatient Medical Record

The broad *inpatient medical record* includes all kinds of inpatient data regarding the medical activities for the patient, while the narrow one is medical files that summarize, analyze, and sort the relevant data obtained from inquiries, physical examinations, auxiliary examinations, diagnoses, treatments, etc., mainly including complete medical record, admission record, re- or multi-admission record, admission and discharge record within 24 h, admission and death record within 24 h, general and special *progress records*, all kinds of informed consent forms, and *critical illness notice*.

67.1.1 Complete Medical Record

Complete medical record is a detailed admission record and the most complete model of medical records. It is generally written by an intern or a resident, and must be completed within 24 h after the patient's admission.

67.1.1.1 The Format and Content for Complete Medical Record

Complete Medical Record

1. **General data:** It includes the patient's name, sex, age, marital status, birth place (including the province, city, and county), nationality, occupation, work unit, address, medical history informant (marked with his relationship to the patient), reliability, date of admission (marked with detailed time including hours and minutes, if the patient is in critical condition), and the record date. All items should be completed, with no omissions.

S. Liu
Department of Cardiology, Guangzhou Medical University, Guangzhou, China

R. Zeng (✉)
Department of Cardiology, Sichuan University, Chengdu, China

2. **Chief complaint:** It is the main reason for the patient's admission, including symptoms (or signs) and their persisting time. It should be concise, generally described in 1–2 sentences, about 20 words.
3. **History of present illness:** It is the main content of complete medical record. Its main contents should include the following:
   - Onset and duration of the disease, including the time of onset, prodrome, possible etiologies and precipitating factors, etc.
   - Main symptoms and their characteristics, including their locations, nature, duration, and the factors increasing or reducing the symptoms. Some negative symptoms should be included for differential diagnoses.
   - Development and evolution of the illness, including changes of the main symptoms and new symptoms.
   - Accompanying symptoms, including their occurrence time, characteristics, and evolution process, as well as their relationship main symptoms.
   - Processes and effects of treatments. Drug names, diagnoses, and surgeries provided by a patient should be recorded in quotation marks ("").
   - General situation since the disease onset, including changes of the patient after the disease onset, such as the mental status, sleep, appetite, urine, stool, weight, etc.
4. **Past history:** It include the following: (a) the history of general health and disease; (b) the history of vaccination and infectious diseases; (c) the history of surgeries, trauma, and blood transfusions; (d) the history of food or drug allergies; etc.
5. **System review:** Common symptoms should be recorded, including those of the head and its organs, respiratory system, circulatory system, digestive system, urogenital system, hematopoietic system, endocrine and metabolic system, musculoskeletal system, nervous system, and the mental state.
6. **Personal history:** It should include the following: (a) social experiences including the birthplace, residence,

X.-H. Wan, R. Zeng (eds.), *Handbook of Clinical Diagnostics*, https://doi.org/10.1007/978-981-13-7677-1_67

visiting some affected area of epidemic diseases or not, etc.; (b) life habits and hobbies, including cigarette smoking, alcohol intake, narcotic drug use, etc.; (c) professional and working conditions; (d) sexual history; (e) history of mental trauma.

7. **Menstrual history:** The following should be recorded, including menarche age, menstrual period, menstrual cycle, and last menstrual period (or menopause age), as well as the menstrual blood volume, color, etc.

   The record format is as follows: Menarche age last menstrual period or menopause age
8. **Marital history:** The following should be recorded, including the patient's marital status (single or married), marriage age, health status of the spouse, and sexual life.
9. **Childbearing history:** It is stated in the following order: number of term births, number of preterm births, number of miscarriages or abortions, and number of survival.
10. **Family history**
    - It should be recorded for the health status of parents, brothers, sisters, and children, especially for some members suffering from the same illness as the patient.
    - It should be recorded for whether some family members suffer from any infectious diseases, such as tuberculosis, hepatitis, sexually transmitted diseases, etc.
    - It should be recorded for whether some family members suffer from some familial hereditary diseases, such as diabetes, hemophilia, etc.

Physical Examination

1. **Vital signs:** Temperature °C, pulse beats/min, respiration times/min, blood pressure/mmHg.
2. **General appearance:** Development (normal, abnormal); nutrition (well, fairly, poor); height; body weight; body type (thin, fat); consciousness (clear, indifference, fuzzy, lethargy, delirium, coma);body position (active, passive, forced); face and expression (quiet, anxiety, fretful, painful, with acute or chronic diseases, special); whether the patient is cooperative to examine.
3. **Skin, mucosa:** Color (normal, red, pale, cyanosis, yellow, pigmentation); temperature;moisture; elasticity; with or without edema, skin rashes, petechiae, purpura, subcutaneous nodules, lumps, spider angioma, hepatic palm, ulcers and scars; hair growth and distribution.
4. **Lymph node:** With or without swelling systemic or local lymph nodes (location, size, number, rigidity, adhesion, mobility); with or without local skin red, volatility, tenderness, fistula, scar, etc.
5. **Head and its organs**

   Head: size; shape; with or without lumps, tenderness, scarring; hair (density, luster, distribution).

   Eyes: eyebrows (exutive, thin); eyelashes (trichiasis); eyelids (edema, activity, prolapse, contracture); eyes (convex, concave, activity, tremor, strabismus); conjunctiva (congestion, edema, pallor, bleeding, follicular);with or without yellow sclera; cornea (nebula, white spot, softening, ulcers, scarring, reflection, pigment ring); pupils (size, shape, symmetric or asymmetric, light reflex and convergence reflex).

   Ears: auricle with or without deformity, secretion, mastoid tenderness; listening ability.

   Nose: with or without deformity, nasal ala flap, secretions, bleeding, obstruction; with or without nasal sinus (frontal sinus, ethmoid sinus, maxillary sinus) tenderness.

   Mouth: smell; with or without mouth breathing; lip (deformity, color, herpes, fissure, ulcers, pigmentation); tooth (caries, edentulous, dentures, residual roots, position, fluorosis teeth); gums (color, swelling, ulcer, overflow pus, bleeding, lead wire); tongue (morphology, quality, covering, ulcers, activity, tremor, deflection); mucosa (rashes, bleeding, ulcers, pigmentation); pharynx (color, secretions, reflex, uvula location);tonsils (size, hyperemia, secretions, pseudomembrane); larynx (articulate, hoarseness, stridor, aphonia).
6. **Neck:** Symmetry; resistance; with or without nuchal rigidity, jugular vein distention, hepatojugular reflux, carotid artery abnormal pulse; trachea position; thyroid (size, rigidity, tenderness, nodules, tremor, bruits).
7. **Chest**: Topography (symmetry, deformity, with or without local bulging, retraction or tenderness); respiration (frequency, rhythm, and depth); breast (size, symmetry, nipples, with or without mass, red, swelling, or tenderness); with or without varicose vein or subcutaneous emphysema in the chest wall, etc.
8. **Lung and pleura**

   Inspection: movement of respiration (both sides contrasted); type of respiration; with or without intercostal space wide or narrow.

   Palpation: chest expansion ratio; tactile fremitus (both sides contrasted); with or without pleural friction feelings, subcutaneous crepitus, etc.

   Percussion: percussion note (resonance, hyperresonance, dullness, flatness, tympany and their position); lower borders of lungs and their range of mobility.

   Auscultation: breath sound (feature, strong or weak, abnormal breath sounds and their position); with or without rhonchi or moist rales, or pleural friction rubs; vocal resonance (increased, decreased, undetected), etc.
9. **Heart**

   Inspection: bulging in precordial region; position, area and strength of apex impulse.

Palpation: nature and position of apex impulse; with or without thrills (position period) or pericardial friction feelings.

Percussion: both cardiac dullness borders, presented by the distance from left or right intercostal space of the second, third, fourth and fifth to the midline (cm). The distance (cm) should be marked from the left clavicular midline to the anterior midline.

Auscultation: heart rate; cardiac rhythm; strength of heart sounds; P2 and A2 strength comparison; with or without heart sound split, extra heart sound, murmur (location, feature, systolic or diastolic or continuous, strength, conduction direction as well as its relationship with activity, body position and breath), pericardial friction rub, etc.

10. **Radial artery**: Pulse rate; rhythm (regular, irregular, pulse deficit); with or without paradoxical pulse, etc.; pulse strength; arterial wall elasticity; tensity (both sides contrasted).
11. **Peripheral vascular sign**: With or without capillary pulse, pistol shot, water hammer pulse or abnormal arterial pulse.
12. **Abdomen:** Abdominal perimeter (measured when the patient with ascites or abdominal mass).

    Inspection: shape(symmetric, flat, distention, scaphoid);movement of breath; gastrointestinal peristalsis wave; upper abdominal wave; with or without skin rashes, pigment, purple striae, scars, abdominal venous distention (and its blood flow direction);position, size and shape of hernia and local distention (organs or masses); abdominal hair.

    Palpation: abdominal wall tension; with or without tenderness, rebound tenderness, fluid thrill, succussion splash, masses (position, size, shape, rigidity, tenderness, mobility, surface conditions, pulse).

    Liver: size (presented in cm for right lobe by distance between right liver lowest edge and cross point of right clavicular midline and right lowest rib edge, and for left lobe by distance between left liver lowest edge and cross point of anterior midline and inferior edge of xiphoid process); quality(first-degree: soft; second-degree: toughness; third-degree: hard); surface (smoothness); edge; with or without nodules, tenderness, pulse, etc.

    Gallbladder: size; shape; with or without tenderness, Murphy's sign.

    Spleen: size;quality; surface; edge; mobility; with or without tenderness, friction feelings; presented by three-line measurement for obviously enlarged spleen.

    Kidney: size; shape; rigidity; mobility; with or without tenderness.

    Bladder: with or without distention, tenderness point for kidney or ureters.

    Percussion: upper border of liver; borders of liver dullness (shrink, obliteration); with or without tenderness in liver region, shifting dullness, high-degree tympany, tenderness in renal region, etc.

    Auscultation: borborygmus (normal, increased, decreased, unheard, metallic sounds); with or without gurgling, vessel bruits, etc.
13. **Anus and rectum**: Examine or not depending on the illness. With or without anal fissure, anal fistula, haemorrhoid, rectocele, etc.; digital rectal examination (sphincter tension; with or without narrowness, masses, tenderness, blood on fingerstall, etc.; size and rigidity of prostate; with or without nodules or tenderness in prostate, etc.).
14. **Genitalia:** Examine or not depending on the illness

    Male: foreskin; scrotum; testis; epididymis; spermatic cord; with or without malformations or hydrocele.

    Female: female staff member must be present when examining, and a gynaecologist can be consulted to help examine if necessary. Its contents include external genitalia (pubic hair, labia majora, labia minora, clitoris, mons pubis) and internal genitalia (vagina, uterus, fallopian tubes, ovaries).
15. **Musculoskeletal system**

    Spine: activity; with or without deformity (lateral, anterior or posterior protruding), tenderness, percussion pain, etc.

    Extremities: with or without deformity, acropachy (drumstick toe), venous distention, edema, fracture.

    Joints: with or without red, swelling, pain, tenderness, effusion, limit of mobility, deformity, rigidity, and edema.

    Muscles: with or without atrophy, limb paralysis, increased or decreased muscle tone.
16. **Nerve system:** Tests for cranial nerve, sensory, motor, and nerve reflexes can be performed depending on illness.

    Physiological reflex: superficial reflex (corneal reflex, abdominal wall reflex, cremasteric reflex); deep reflex (biceps, triceps, knee tendon, Achilles tendon reflexes).

    Pathological reflex: Babinski sign, Oppenheim sign, Gordon sign, Chaddock sign, Hoffmann sign.

    Meningeal irritation sign: nuchal rigidity, Kernig sign, Brudzinski sign.

    Other examinations may be performed for motor, sensory or other nerve system, if necessary.
17. **Specialized situation:** Different contents should be recorded according to requirements of different department, such as surgery, gynecology (gynecology/obstetrics), ophthalmology, otolaryngology, dental, neurology, psychiatry, etc.

Auxiliary Examination

Auxiliary examinations refer to the main examinations and their results associated with the patient's disease before admission. They should be classified and sorted by the time order. The name of the institute and the examination number should be provided.

Summary

Main data of medical histories, physical examinations, and auxiliary examinations are collected in this part. Its main contents include important positive results that help to make diagnoses, and negative results that help to make differential diagnose.

Preliminary diagnosis.

Physician's signature.

Diagnosis

Diagnoses should be listed clearly and orderly, including etiological, pathoanatomical and functional diagnoses to the greatest extent. If the diagnosis is uncertain, a question mark (?) can be added after the disease name. If the etiology cannot be found in a short time, the patient can be diagnosed temporarily with a certain symptom of unknown origin followed by one or two probable diseases, such as "left pleural effusion of unknown origin: tuberculosis? tumor?"

1. **Preliminary diagnosis:** It is made with comprehensive analysis of the patient's situation on admission by the physician. It should be written on the right side of the midline at the end of complete medical record or admission record.
2. **Admission diagnosis:** It is made by the attending physician after his first ward-round. It should be written beneath the preliminary diagnosis and marked with the date. The superior physician can provide his signature to regard the preliminary diagnosis as the admission diagnosis, when the two diagnoses are the same.
3. **Corrected diagnosis (containing supplemental diagnosis):** The superior physician should make it for uncertain, incomplete or incorrect diagnosis. It should be written on the left side of the midline at the end of complete medical record or admission record, marked with the date, and provided with the superior physician's signature.

67.1.2 Example of Complete Medical Record

67.1.2.1 Complete Medical Record

- Name: XXZhang; Birth place: Shanghai city.
- Gender: Female Race: Han.
- Age: 40 yrs. Date of admission: 2008/8/6.
- Marital status: Married Date of record: 2008/8/6.
- Occupation: Housewife Informant: Patient herself Address: 3740 Heping Street, Changchun city, Jilin province.
- Reliability: Reliable Workunit: None.
- Tel.: 0431–27,344,388.

67.1.2.2 Medical History

1. **Chief complaint:** Heart palpitation, dyspnea on exertion for 7 years, and lower limbs edema for 4 days
2. **History of present illness:** The patient experienced heart palpitation and dyspnea on exertion or climbing stairs that could be relieved by rest 7 years ago. She visited a doctor in a certain Chongqing hospital. The chest fluoroscopy examination showed "cardiomegaly". This did not affect her from doing household chores, so she did not choose further diagnosis or treatment. Five years ago, she came to Changchun city. Because of the cold weather, she often caught a cold and coughed, felt heart palpitation and dyspnea even at rest, and chose to sleep in the semi-recumbent position. She visited doctors in the Changchun First Hospital because of a fever. She felt recovered after injections of "penicillin" (unknown dosage) and "glucose", and staying in the bed for 2 weeks. She started experiencing a gradually swelling abdomen in the recent 2 years, but did not experience any lower extremity edema. No diagnosis or treatment was made. One month ago, after exertion and catching a cold, the patient suffered from a sore throat, cough, expectoration, blood in phlegm, heart palpitation and dyspnea, and could not lie down in horizontal position. She visited a doctor at a local health center, receiving some "cough medicine" and intravenous injections of "penicillin". However, there was no relief for her symptoms. In the recent 4 days, she experienced lower extremities edema and abdominal distention, but did not receive "digitalis" treatment. She came to our hospital for further diagnoses and treatments, and was admitted in the hospital with the impression of "heart failure". Since onset of illness, the patient is in poor spirits, lack of appetite and sleep, has less but deep-color urine with normal stool once per day, and does not obviously lose her body weight.
3. **Past medical history:** The patient was in a weak status, and often had a sore throat since childhood. Eleven years ago, she suffered from "malaria", but recovered after 1 week of oral "quinine". No history of acute or chronic infectious diseases, such as hepatitis, tuberculosis, etc. No history of other chronic diseases, such as hypertension, diabetes, etc. No history of wandering joint pain. No history of drug or food allergies. No history of blood transfusion. No history of trauma or surgery. The history of immunizations is not available.
4. **Review of systems**

   Head and its organs: no history of visual impairment, deafness, tinnitus, dizziness, nose bleeding, toothache, gum bleeding, or hoarseness.

Respiratory system: no chest pain or night sweats, but with the above described history of sore throat, cough, expectoration, blood in phlegm, dyspnea and fever.

Circulation system: see the history of present illness. No history of high blood pressure or syncope.

Digestive system: no history of belching, sour regurgitation, dysphagia, abdominal distention, abdominal pain,diarrhea, vomiting, jaundice, haematemesis, or melena.

Urinary system: no history of frequency of urination, urgency of urination, odynuria, lumbago, hematuria, dysuria, abnormal urine volume, facial edema, or external genital ulcer.

Endocrine system and metabolism: no history of fear of cold, fear of heat, hyperhidrosis, tiredness, headache, palpation, abnormal appetite, excessive thirst, polyuria, edema, or obesity.

Hematopoietic system: no history of ochrodermia, dizziness, giddiness, hemorrhagic spot or ecchymosis in the skin, swelling lymph nodes, hepatosplenomegaly, or skeletal pain.

Neural system: no history of headache, syncope, hypomnesis, abnormal skin sensitivity or convulsion, language disorder, or disturbance of consciousness.

Muscle and bone joint system: there was paroxysmal pain in bilateral knee joints during cold weather or weather changes 3 years ago, without migratory pain, local red or swelling, or physical inactivity. No history of muscular atrophy or limb weakness.

Mental state: no history of hallucination, delusion, disorientation, or abnormal emotion.

5. **Personal history:** Birth place is Shanghai. She came to Changchun city 5 years ago. No history of visiting epidemic area. She graduated from middle school with no job after marriage. No history of alcohol or tobacco use. No history of feculent coitus. No history of close contact with a patient with tuberculosis.
6. **Menstrual history:** 15 LMP July 26. No history of blood clots and dysmenorrhea. Her menstruation has a normal amount, without abnormal smell.
7. **Marital history:** She was married at a proper marriageable age. Her spouse is healthy, without a history of sexually transmitted diseases.
8. **Childbearing history:** Married and childless.
9. **Family history**: Her parents are alive. She has two older sisters and two younger brothers, who are in good health except for her oldest sister suffering from sore knee joints. No similar case and no history of any other genetic diseases in her family.

67.1.2.3 Physical Examination

Temperature 38 °C, pulse 70 beats/min, respiration 30 times/min, blood pressure 100/70 mmHg.

General appearance: Development normal; nutrition poor; body type tall and thin; facial features with chronic diseases; consciousness clear; facial expression indifferent; lazy and slow to answer; resting in semi-sitting position; shortness of breath.

Skin and mucosa: A little high temperature and slightly dry; furfures found on both arms and back; without rashes or hemorrhagic spots in the skin.

Lymph node: A lymph node with a diameter of about 1.5 cm can be separately palpated under the both jaws; both nodes are soft, moveable, and of mild tenderness.

Head: Normocephalic; hair black, shiny and well distributed; no scars on head; both cheeks flushing.

Eyes: no edema of the eyelids; conjunctiva with mild congestion but without hemorrhagic spot; sclera mild yellow; cornea normal; pupils of the same size and circle, with normal light and collective reflexes.

Ears: normal hearing; no pus present; no tenderness detected over mastoid process.

Nose: clear; no runny nose; no tenderness detected over frontal and maxillary sinuses.

Mouth: lip cyanotic; teeth are present in fair condition; no obvious caries; no swelling gingivae or gingival pus; bilateral tonsils enlarged (class II), with mild congestion and clear fossulae; three to four white pinhead-sized exudates present on the right tonsil; throat mild congestion, with no hoarseness of voice.

Neck: No resistance; bilateral symmetry; abnormal jugular vein distention with normal carotid artery pulse; hepatojugular reflux positive; trachea midline; no thyroid enlargement.

Chest: Symmetry; mainly thoracic breathing; shortness of breath but with regular rhythm; both breasts flat and loosen, without scleroma.

- Lungs: (a) Inspection: symmetric respiratory motion bilaterally. (b) Palpation: the same range of respiratory motion bilaterally; no different tactile fremitus bilaterally; no pleural friction feeling. (c) Percussion: clear; the bottom of left lung lies at the sixth intercostal space of the left midclavicular line and that of right lung at the fifth intercostal space of the right midclavicular line, meanwhile the bottom of both lungs lie at the tenth intercostal space of scapular lines and at the ninth intercostal space of midaxillary lines. The distance of excursion is about 4 cm. (d) Auscultate: ronchi rales present bilaterally; moist rales present in the bilateral inferior lungs, especially in the right lung.
- Heart: (a) Inspection: dispersive apex impulse; the point of maximal impulse lies at the fifth intercostal space and 2.5 cm external to midclavicular line. (b) Palpation: the position of apex impulse as above; palpable thrill. (c) Percussion: both cardiac borders enlarged bilaterally; the

Table 67.1 Cardiac relative dullness

Right (cm)	Intercostal space	Left (cm)
2	II	5
4	III	7.5
5	IV	9.5
	V	11

The distance between the left midclavicular line and the anterior midline is 8.5 cm

relative cardiac dullness could be seen in Table 67.1. (d) Auscultation: heart rate is 100/min; absolutely irregular rhythm; pulse deficit; heart sounds inequality; the mid-diastolic rumbling murmur and a grade 5/6 systolic blowing murmur can be heard at the apex, with systolic murmur conducting towards left armpit; accentuated S2 can be heard in the pulmonary valve area.

Peripheral vessels sign: No capillary pulse, pistol-shot sound, water-hammer pulse, or abnormal arterial pulse.

Abdomen: (a) Inspection: slight distention; abdominal vein distension with blood flowing upwards; no intestinal pattern or peristaltic wave. (b) Palpation: soft; no tenderness; liver is palpable at 5 cm under the rib edge of the right midclavicular line; palpable liver is hard, with clear edge, smooth surface, and slight tenderness; spleen not palpated. (c) Percussion: percussion note is tympanitic at the middle abdomen, but dull on both sides; shifting dullness positive. (d) Auscultation: bowel sounds present at a rate of 2 times/min.

External genitalia and anus: Pubic hairs distribution normal; vulva development normal; no scar or ulcer; no archoptoma or haemorrhoids.

Spine: Curvature normal; no malformation; activity normal; no tenderness or percussion pain.

Extremities: Fingertips mild cyanotic; bilateral lower limbs moderate pitting edema; no acropachy; no atrophy muscle or varicose vein; joints without red, swelling, tenderness, or malformation; joints with normal motor function.

Nervous system: Abdominal wall reflex normal; biceps, patellar tendon and Achilles tendon reflexes normal; Hoffmann sign (−), Babinski sign (−), Oppenheim sign (−), Kerning sign (−), and Brudzinski sign (−).

67.1.2.4 Auxiliary Examination

Blood routine test (2008/08/06, outpatient department in our hospital): Red blood cells 3.9×10^{12} /L, hemoglobin 110 g/L, white blood cells 14.0×10^{9} /L, neutrophilic granulocytes 82%, eosinophilic granulocyte 1%, lymphocyte 16%, and monocyte 1%.

Urine routine test (2008/08/06, outpatient department in our hospital): Dark yellow, slight turbidity, acidness, specific gravity 1.019, protein (+), glucose (−). White blood cells 3–5/high power field, and transparent tubes (+)/low power field found in the sediments.

67.1.2.5 Example

The patient, XX Zhang, is a 40 year old housewife. She was admitted to the hospital with chief complaints of heart palpitation, dyspnea on exertion for 7 years, and lower limbs edema for 4 days. The patient experienced heart palpitation and dyspnea on exertion 7 years ago. No detailed diagnosis or treatment was made. In the recent 1 month, her symptoms became more serious with blood in phlegm, and she could not lie down in horizontal position in the evening. Lower limbs edema and less urine occurred in the recent 4 days. She was admitted to the hospital with the impression of "heart failure" on August 6, 2008. She never received "digitalis" treatment during the whole course of the disease.

Physical examination: T 38 °C, P 70 beats/min, R 30 times/min, BP 100/70 mmHg. General appearance bad. The patient is in semi-sitting position, with shortness of breath. Sclera mild yellow. Lip cyanotic. Fingertips mild cyanotic. Abnormal jugular vein distention. Hepatojugular reflux positive. Ronchi rales present bilaterally. Moist rales present at the bilateral inferior lungs. Thrill can be palpated at apex. Both cardiac borders enlarged bilaterally. Fast heart rate, absolutely irregular rhythm, pulse deficit and heart sounds inequality. The mid-diastolic rumbling murmur and a grade 5/6 systolic blowing murmur can be heard at the apex, with systolic murmur conducting towards left armpit. Accentuated S2 can be heard in the pulmonary valve area. Enlarged liver is palpable at 5 cm under the rib edge, with slight tenderness. Shifting dullness positive. Bilateral lower limbs with moderate pitting edema.

Outpatient examination: Blood routine test: red blood cells 3.9H $\times 10^{12}$ /L, hemoglobin 110 g/L, white blood cells 14.0×10^{9} /L, and neutrophilic granulocytes 82%. Urine routine test: protein (+), a little white blood cells and transparent tubes found in the sediments, and others normal.

Preliminary Diagnosis

1. Rheumatic heart disease, Mitral stenosis and incompetence, Atrial fibrillation

   Heart failure class IV∗ (∗New York Heart Association classification).
2. Chronic tonsillitis, acute attack

   Physician's signature: Xin Zheng.

67.1.3 Other Medical Records

Admission record is a focused, concise, and a brief form of complete medical record. It should be completed within 24 h by the resident after the patient's admission. Chief complaints and the history of present illness are the same as those of complete medical record. The other medical histories (such as past history, personal history, menstrual history, childbearing history and family history) and physical examination can be recorded concisely. Summary is not necessary.

Some certain records are used for patients' admission in some special situations or some departments, such as re- or multi-admission record, *tabular admission record*, admission and discharge record within 24 h, as well as admission and death record within 24 h. They have almost the same format and content as admission record, while for the latter two, some extra contents should be included, such as the process of diagnosis and treatment (or resuscitation), discharge (or death) diagnoses, etc.

Different kinds of progress record and informed consent form are used for different phages or targets after a patient is admitted to the hospital.

1. **Progress record:** It refers to frequent and successional records of the illness development, diagnosis, and treatment during the whole process of the patient's hospitalization. It is written by a physician or an intern with the physician's signature. The content should be true and include the patient's illness changes, important auxiliary examination results, ward-round opinions of superior physicians, consultation opinions, physicians' discussion, treatments and their effects, changes of therapeutic schedule, etc. For a patient with critical illness, progress record should be written at any time according to the illness changes, updated at least once a day, and marked with detailed time including minutes. It should be updated at least every 2 days for a patient with serious illness, and at least every 3 days for a patient in stable condition. Its detailed contents and requirements are as follows:
   - First progress record. It should be completed within 8 h after the patient's admission by a physician on duty. Its contents should include the following: (a) characteristics of the case: it should be described after comprehensive analysis of the medical history, physical and auxiliary examination, including positive findings, important negative symptoms and signs that help in differential diagnosis, etc.; (b) discussion about the probable diagnosis (diagnostic bases and differential diagnoses): raise the preliminary diagnosis and diagnostic bases, make differential diagnoses, and analyze feasibility of next treatment; (c) the plan for treatment and examination.
   - Daily progress record Its contents include the following: (a) some pointed situation, such as the patient's subjective symptoms, emotional state, diet, etc.; (b) illness changes, changes or new findings of symptoms and signs, auxiliary test results, as well as their analysis, judgment and evaluation; (c) all kinds of operation records, such as thoracentesis, abdominocentesis, bone marrow puncture, etc.; (d) supplementation or correction of the clinical diagnosis and their bases; (e) therapeutic effect, reasons for drug use, reasons for changes of prescription, etc.; (f) feedback and comments from the patient's relatives or other relevant persons, etc.; (g) record time and signature.
   - Others Some other progress records are used in different situations, including the superior physician ward-round record, intractable cases discussion record, log record, department-transferal record, invasive operation record, consultation record, emergency-treatment record, stage summary, preoperative summary, preoperative discussion, visit record before anesthesia, anesthesia record, operation record, surgical safety inspection record, postoperative record for the first time, visit record after anesthesia, discharge record, death record, death discussion record, etc.
2. **Informed consent form:** According to the series of documents entitled "The Professional Medical Practitioners Law of the People's Republic of China", etc., all the patients should be informed about their treatments and provide signature for their consent, before receiving surgical treatment, special inspection and treatment, experimental clinical medical care, or medical cosmetology. Common-used consent forms in clinical practice include operation consent form, anesthesia consent form, consent form for special examination and treatment, blood transfusion informed consent form, critical illness notice, etc.

67.2 Section 2: Outpatient and Emergency Medical Records

67.2.1 Requirements

Outpatient and emergency medical record should be brief, concise, and focused.

1. It should be carefully recorded about the patient's general data on the coversheet of the medical note, including name, gender, date of birth, race, marital status, occupation, address, work unit, history of allergies, etc.
2. It should be recorded for the patient's visiting data and department at each time. The detailed time should be recorded for an emergency patient, including hours and minutes.
3. When using common-used medical notes, a stamp should be provided next to the last outpatient record consisting of "XX year XX month XX day XX hospital XX department outpatient", the space of which should be filled in by the physician on duty.
4. The person, who accompanies a pediatric patient, a patient without consciousness, or a patient with trauma or mental disorder, should provide his name and relationship with the patient. If necessary, the working

organization, address, and telephone number should also be provided.

5. Examinations performed in another hospital should be marked with the date and the hospital's name.
6. Important information should be recorded for emergency and critical patients, including the body temperature, pulse rate, respiratory rate, blood pressure, state of consciousness, diagnosis, emergency treatment, etc. For a patient who dies after unsuccessful resuscitation, the physician on duty should record in the medical note the resuscitation processes, names and titles of the medical staff participating in the resuscitation, detailed time of death, death diagnosis, etc.
7. Outpatient diagnosis should be made at the first or at a subsequent visit. If it is difficult to make a definite diagnosis, a symptomatic diagnosis can be made with one or several suspicious diseases.
8. The physician should provide the signature of full name in the outpatient or emergency medical record, regardless of the first or subsequent visit. The physician's signature should be at the bottom right corner of the medical record, while prescriptions at the left side of the medical record.
9. The notifiable disease should be marked with whether epidemiological report has been issued.
10. An admission certificate should be issued for the outpatient's admission.

67.2.2 Content

67.2.2.1 First-Visit Medical Record

1. **Chief complaint:** It concludes the main symptoms (or signs) and their persisting time.
2. **History of illness:** It concludes history of present illness, past history related to the present illness, personal history, family history, etc.
3. **Physical examination:** It mainly includes positive signs and negative signs to help make a differential diagnosis. For an emergency patient, body temperature, pulse rate, respiratory rate, and blood pressure should be recorded routinely.
4. **Auxiliary examination.**
5. **Preliminary diagnosis:** It should be written at the bottom right corner of the medical record.
6. **Prescription:** It includes drug administration, further examinations, epidemiological reports, etc.
7. **The physician's signature.**

67.2.2.2 Example of First-Visit Outpatient Medical Record

Sep. 15, 2008 Department of Digestive System.

The patient complains of upper abdominal dull pain for 3 years and getting worse in the recent 3 months.

- Three years ago, the patient experienced a dull pain in the upper abdomen, with sour regurgitation and belching. It usually occurred before a meal and was relieved after a meal. There was no fever, jaundice, hematemesis, or melena. For the recent 3 months, he has suffered from the above abdominal pain frequently, with the pain getting worse, no regularity and no relief after a meal.
- No diseases in the past. No history of hepatopathy or gastropathy. No history of drug allergies.
- Physical examination: P 75 beats/min, BP 120/80 mmHg. No yellow sclera. No supraclavicular lymphadenectasis. No abnormalities of the heart or either lung. Abdomen is flat and soft. Slight tenderness in middle of upper abdomen. Liver and spleen untouched. Murphy's sign is suspiciously positive. No masses. No shifting dullness. Borborygmus is normal.

Preliminary diagnosis
Epigastric pain of unknown origin

1. Chronic gastritis?
2. Peptic ulcer?
3. Chronic cholecystitis?

Treatment

1. Blood routine test, stool routine test, coagulation function examination, and electrocardiogram.
2. Making an appointment for gastroscopy and Hp test.
3. Ultrasound scan for cholecyst.

Mingli Li (signature).

67.2.2.3 Subsequent-Visit Medical Record

1. It is emphasized to record illness changes and therapeutic effect after the patient's first visit, record modified medical history, signs, and test results, and prescribe further auxilary examinations if necessary.
2. Physical examination, mainly including changes of previously positive signs and new positive signs.
3. Supplemental laboratory tests or other special examinations.
4. Diagnoses, including supplemental or corrected diagnoses.
5. Prescription.
6. Physician's signature.
7. Write medical record for the subsequent-visit patient with a common-used medical note as a new one according to the requirement of the first visit, when he visits a doctor in another hospital, in another department or when he comes for a different disease.

Appendix

Electronic Medical Record

Concept and Content

Electronic medical record (EMR) is to have paperwork of traditional medical record filled out electronically by computer software and hardware. It records all information related to the patient's diagnoses and treatments, and has data functions of gathering, recording, processing, storing, managing, transferring, etc. It is a digitalized medical service for outpatients and inpatients, used as a type of clinical resource to record the complete and detailed information of patients. It is an inevitable product of the application of information and internet technology in medical field. Moreover, it has become an irresistible trend to have EMR in the computer network administration system in hospitals. The paper medical record has been named as a traditional medical record after introduction of the concept of EMR. The main contents of EMR, according to its basic concept and framework, include several parts of basic medical service, such as abstract of medical record, outpatient and emergency medical record, inpatient medical record, health examination, referral record, legal medical certification and report, messages from the medical institution, etc.

Basic Requirement

EMR must conform to requirements of all kinds of legislations and regulations in China. All information of objective contents and integral data must be inputted by medical staff, with traces left for all modified and deleted data. EMR system should have functions of data ultilization, such as (a) reviewing previous medical records of inpatients, outpatients, and emergency patients; (b) printing all kinds of contents of medical records; (c) supporting statistical analyses and automatically outputting statistical forms; (d) connected to other systems to form an integral hospital information system; etc. In addition, this system should be high-efficiency, secure and reliable, with all processes in accordance with the requirements of medical regulations.

Development Trend

Compared with traditional medical record, EMR has a lot of advantages, such as information integration, information sharing and interaction, information intellectualization, saving resources, etc. However, there are still many problems that need resolved, such as EMR standardization, legal responsibility and system security. "Basic Framework and Data Standards for Electronic Medical Records" (exposure draft) was issued by The National Health and Family Planning Commission of China in August 2009, which established the basic framework and data standards for EMR for the first time. Six parts are included: preface, basic concepts and systemic framework, basic contents and information sources, information models, standards for data sets and elements, as well as basic models and data standards. These have preliminarily solved problems related to the national standardization of EMR. However, individual standard in EMR still requires continuous supplementation and improvement. Only when problems are continuously explored, discovered and solved, can EMR have a greater effect on clinical practice.

68 Content and Method for Medical Case Report

Shiming Liu and Rui Zeng

In routine clinical practice, the physician needs to orally report a patient's medical record to the superior physician or the consultant for advice. A written medical report needs to be issued when the patient needs referral treatment in a superior or academic hospital, or a medical case discussion is needed.

68.1 Oral Medical Case Report

When ward-round by a superior physician or consultation by a physician from different department, a resident or an intern should orally report the medical record briefly, with contents outlined as follows:

1. **First ward-round or consultation**:
   - General data: the patient's name, gender, age, occupation, and date of admission.
   - Medical History: chief complaint, history of present illness, past history, positive or important negative history in system review, personal history, important history related to the present illness, menstrual and childbearing history if related to history of present illness, and brief family history.
   - Physical examination: positive signs and important negative signs that help differential diagnoses.
   - Auxilliary examination: positive results and negative results that help differential diagnoses.
   - Preliminary diagnosis.
   - Plans for treatment and further examination.
   - Raise problems needed to be solved and ask for advice of the superior physician or the consultant.
2. **Repeated ward-round or consultation:** Changes of illness should be emphasized to report, such as new or changed symptoms and signs, new results of auxilliary examinations and therapeutic effects. In addition, problems needed to be solved can be raised for advice of the superior physician or the consultant.

68.2 Written Medical Case Report

A written medical case report should be issued when a patient needs referral treatment, or a medical case discussion is needed. The report should briefly summarize changes of the illness and the entire process of diagnosis and treatment before referral treatment or discussion, with contents outlined as follows:

1. **Abstract of complete medical record:** General data (name, gender, age, occupation), chief complaint, history of present illness, past history, system review, personal history, female menstrual and childbearing history, marital history, family history, physical examination, and auxilliary examination.
2. **Process of diagnosis and treatment:** The progress of the illness, processes of diagnoses and treatments, therapeutic effects, laboratory tests, special examinations, consultation, and present diagnoses.
3. **Raising problems:** Reasons and purposes of the referral should be demonstrated clearly. Problems needed to be solved should be written to obtain advice when discussion.
4. **Physician's signature**.

Key Terms

1	Medical record	病历
2	Outpatient medical record	门诊病历
3	Emergency medical record	急诊病历
4	Complete medical record	完整病历
5	Admission record	入院记录
6	Re- or multi-admission record	再/多次入院记录
7	Admission and discharge record within 24 h	24小时出入院记录

S. Liu
Department of Cardiology, Guangzhou Medical University, Guangzhou, China

R. Zeng (✉)
Department of Cardiology, Sichuan University, Chengdu, China

X.-H. Wan, R. Zeng (eds.), *Handbook of Clinical Diagnostics*, https://doi.org/10.1007/978-981-13-7677-1_68

8	Admission and death record within 24 hours	24小时内入院死亡记录
9	Informed consent form	知情同意书
10	Inpatient medical record	入院病历
11	Progress record	病程记录
12	Critical illness notice	病危通知书
13	Tabular admission record	表格式入院病历
14	Electronic medical record	电子病历

Study Questions

1. List major items of admission record.
2. What are major contents for history of present illness?
3. Briefly state significance of medical records.
4. Briefly state major contents for oral medical case report.

Part VII

Clinical Reasoning

Clinical Reasoning

Diagnosis-making is a basic practice for any doctor. It is a process in which doctors draw conclusions by making analyses, summaries, judgements and reasoning based on the information acquired through inquiry, physical examination and auxiliary examinations. A diagnosis is the foundation and precondition for the treatment of a disease. This is why we usually say that "a correct treatment relies on a correct diagnosis", and "the top priority for clinical medicine is diagnosis". When a doctor does not take the diagnosing process seriously, he will not be able to explore the nature of the disease; what he can do at most is "treat the head when the head aches, and treat the foot when the foot aches". Therefore, clinicians, in their clinical practice, must establish a correct diagnosis after identifying the nature of the patient's disease through meticulous inquiries and examinations, careful observations and thorough thinking, and comprehensive analyses based on the combination of medical knowledge and experience. The improvement of clinical competence is a process of lifetime learning, starting from the study of clinical diagnosis to practical application of theories; and "there is no best, but only better".

69 The Importance of Clinical Reasoning

Xuehong Wan and Rui Zeng

Before learning to diagnose, medical students have already studied various medical foundation courses, obtained theoretical knowledge and practiced skills of inquiry and physical examination. These are particularly important for clinical diagnosis; but such knowledge and skills alone are insufficient. Medical students must learn and apply the methods of clinical reasoning, and they must study clinical knowledge on diseases of different systems in the human body thoroughly. If theoretic knowledge is likened to a walking stick for students, just having the stick is not enough: they must be taught on how to use the stick, guided to take correct paths and directions and instructed on how to apply such knowledge and skills with scientific reasoning in clinical diagnosis. Only by doing so can such knowledge and skills truly work. With the rapid progress of medical technologies, new diagnostic technologies keep emerging, but the importance of clinical reasoning by the doctor will not fade. It is irreplaceable.

X. Wan
Department of Internal Medicine, Sichuan University, Chengdu, China

R. Zeng (✉)
Department of Cardiology, Sichuan University, Chengdu, China

X.-H. Wan, R. Zeng (eds.), *Handbook of Clinical Diagnostics*, https://doi.org/10.1007/978-981-13-7677-1_69

Procedures of Diagnosis-Making

70

Xuehong Wan and Rui Zeng

Generally, diagnosis-making consists of a few procedures: information gathering, analysis and summary, primary diagnosis and verification or correction of diagnosis.

1. **Information gathering**
   - A detailed and complete medical history can usually provide the bulk of information on the disease. History taking does not mean a mechanical inquiry. In fact, it is a continuous process of data-driven reasoning, continuous analysis and judgements, and adjustments between details and omissions. The wider range of knowledge and the richer experience the doctor has, the more effectively he can identify the key points of the medical history and approach the nature of the disease revealed by such a history.
   - Based on the history, a comprehensive physical examination with intensive focuses on key problems should be able to identify important evidence for the diagnosis of a disease. During the physical examination, the doctor may complement and verify the medical history. When doing so, the doctor may take an approach of checking and asking, and doing and thinking, to verify the facts and ultimately ensure the integrity, authenticity and accuracy of the information.
   - Laboratory examination and other necessary auxiliary examinations are conducted on the basis of inquiry and physical examination. Based on data-driven reasoning and the diagnostic hypothesis hereby made, doctors should prescribe appropriate examinations to verify the hypothesis. To some extent, the wide application of various modern technologies in medicine embodies the capacity of modern clinical diagnosis. However, it is the doctor who decides what examinations to be done and for what purpose(s). Therefore, instead of relying on auxiliary examinations only, the doctor must combine the examination results with the clinical information when making a diagnosis.
2. **Analysis and summary:** Based on the information acquired from medical histories, physical examinations, laboratory examinations and other various auxiliary examinations, doctors make analyses, evaluations and summaries; they discard the dross and select the essential, eliminate the false and retain the true, and proceed from one point to another and from the exterior to the interior. Then, they categorize the information; using knowledge on pathology and diseases, they summarize groups of symptoms and signs, extract the main problems of the patient and make comparisons to see which symptoms, signs or conditions of the problems are similar to or the same as those of the suspected diseases. Then, drawing from their theoretical knowledge and clinical experience, the doctors list the problems with high likelihoods to make diagnostic hypotheses continuously; and they keep searching further information for confirmation or negation. Thus, although "analysis and summary" is listed as the second step following "information gathering", it is actually overlapped with "information gathering", and it is continually proceeded with improvements.
3. **Primary diagnosis:** After analyzing, evaluating and summarizing the acquired and relatively integrated clinical information in various categories, and exerting medical knowledge and clinical experience, the doctor lists the diseases with high likelihoods. Following the diagnostic principles and using various ways of reasoning, the doctor selects the most probable disease that can best explain all the clinical findings to make a primary diagnosis.
4. **Confirmation or correction of diagnosis:** Recognition cannot be completed once and for all. Instead, it is a repetitive and dynamic process. There should be further clinical practice to confirm whether the primary diagnosis is correct or needs a correction.

X. Wan
Department of Internal Medicine, Sichuan University, Chengdu, China

R. Zeng (✉)
Department of Cardiology, Sichuan University, Chengdu, China

X.-H. Wan, R. Zeng (eds.), *Handbook of Clinical Diagnostics*, https://doi.org/10.1007/978-981-13-7677-1_70

When prescribing an examination, doctors need to take the following questions into consideration: (a) Which examinations are the most suitable? What is the normal range for reference? (b) How are the sensitivity, specificity and accuracy of the examinations? (c) What is the frequency distribution for examination results of various diseases? (d) What is the probability of a confirmed diagnosis? (e) What are the pros and cons and security of the examinations for the patient? (f) Cost-effective analysis. For instance, when doctors consider examination on AFP for a patient with a chronic liver disease, such are the questions they should ask themselves to identify the rationality, security and clinical value of the examination.

With regard to difficult diseases that cannot be diagnosed even through various examinations, the doctor may follow the diagnostic guidelines formed in long-term practice by numerous clinical departments, or conduct diagnostic treatments, also known as experimental treatments. Such is also a viable solution.

The diagnostic process diagram illustrates the four basic procedures and their relations among each other (Fig. 70.1).

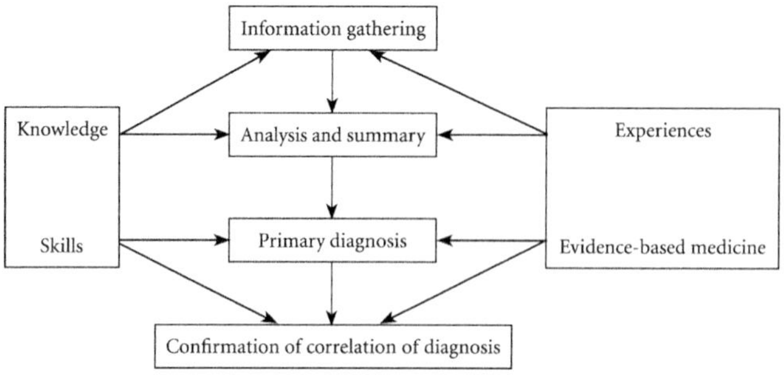

Fig. 70.1 Procedures for making a diagnosis

Clinical Reasoning

71

Xuehong Wan and Rui Zeng

Clinical reasoning refers to a way of logical thinking to recognize diseases and conclude diagnoses based on a series of mind activities during the process of probe and study, analysis and summary, and judgement and inference on the disease phenomena of the patient.

1. **Two major factors of clinical reasoning:**
   - Clinical practice is also known as "bedside". It is a practice in which doctors obtain firsthand information through multiple clinical activities such as inquiries and physical examination. With the help of laboratory and other auxiliary examinations, the doctors observe closely the changes of patient conditions to identify, analyze and solve problems; and they keep asking further questions that they try to answer through practice. Sufficient practice and detailed firsthand information serves not only as the foundation for a correct diagnosis but also as the source for clinical reasoning.
   - Scientific reasoning is a reasoning process where the general rules of maladies are applied to identify the disease of a particular individual. It is also a process of sorting, analyzing and summarizing practical materials, as well as a process of comprehensive evaluation, logical association, judgement and reasoning. Only after going through such a process, can the doctor make a diagnosis.
2. **Basic principles of reasoning for clinical diagnosis:**
   - Seeking truth from facts. Doctors must try their best to obtain first-hand information and handle the objective clinical information with a down-to-earth spirit. They cannot accept or reject the information discretionarily based on their own range of knowledge and limited experience, or place it into their own understanding framework or mind track in a far-fetched manner; they should avoid subjectivity and one-sidedness.
   - Monism, namely the singular pathological principle, refers to the principle of using one disease to explain multiple clinical manifestations. In clinical practice, it is very unlikely that multiple diseases co-exist but are little relevant to each other. When facing numerous and complicated clinical manifestations, doctors should try to select one disease to generalize or explain the multiple manifestations of the patient. For instance, when a patient has a long-term fever and shows multiple pathological manifestations in his skin, joints, heart, liver and kidneys, the doctor should not diagnose him with concurrent diseases such as rheumatism, tuberculosis, skin disease, arthritis, heart disease and hepatitis. Instead, systemic lupus erythematosus (SLE) is probably the correct choice. However, if it is confirmed that several diseases do exist concurrently, the doctor does not have to be constrained by "the pathological monism"; rather, he should draw a clear distinction between the primary and the secondary and decide on priorities.
   - The principle that common diseases should be considered first. The morbidity of diseases is influenced by multiple factors. The spectrum of human diseases varies by time, region and environmental condition. When several diagnostic possibilities exist simultaneously, common and frequently-occurring diseases should be considered first, and then rare and uncommon diseases.
   - The principle that organic diseases should be considered first. This principle could best help doctors avoid missing the good opportunities for treating organic diseases. For instance, a patient of colon cancer with a manifestation of abdominal pain can be cured by means of surgery if diagnosed early. Nevertheless, the golden chance for treatment may be lost if the disease is diagnosed as functional. Certainly, doctors should be aware that an organic disease may have functional

X. Wan
Department of Internal Medicine, Sichuan University, Chengdu, China

R. Zeng (✉)
Department of Cardiology, Sichuan University, Chengdu, China

X.-H. Wan, R. Zeng (eds.), *Handbook of Clinical Diagnostics*, https://doi.org/10.1007/978-981-13-7677-1_71

symptoms and may even co-exist with functional diseases. If so, the diagnosis of an organic disease should be considered with priority.

- The principle that curable diseases should be considered first. This principle can facilitate an early and timely treatment. For instance, when the X-ray results of a patient with hemoptysis show shadows in the upper part of the right lung that cannot secure a confirmed diagnosis, the diagnosis of tuberculosis should be considered first to avoid delay in treatment.
- The principle of human-oriented, comprehensive assessment. The doctors need to bear in mind that the subject of a disease is a human being. The patient's age, sex, physique, living conditions, occupation, nutritional conditions, psychological status and education level would all have impacts on the occurrence and clinical manifestations of a disease. When making a diagnosis, if the doctor focuses only on the name of the disease while ignoring the human factors, it is difficult for them to make a comprehensive and accurate diagnosis, let alone develop a reasonable diagnostic plan and therapeutic regime.

3. **Procedures and contents of clinical reasoning:** The process of clinical reasoning of a doctor begins from the early stage of clinical practice. This process is not only active, but also orderly. It can be divided into ten procedures, which are to be considered in the following sequence:
   - From an anatomic point of view, consider any structural abnormality that may exist.
   - From a physiological point of view, consider any functional change that may have taken place.
   - From a pathophysiological point of view, propose possibilities of pathological changes and pathogenesis.
   - Consider a number of possible pathogenic factors.
   - Consider the severity of the disease and avoid missing severe conditions.
   - Propose 1–2 particular hypotheses.
   - Verify the hypothesis by judging and weighing the symptoms and signs that may or may not support the hypothesis.
   - Seek particular assemblages for differentiated diagnosis.
   - Narrow down the diagnostic range and decide on the most possible diagnosis; and
   - Suggest further examinations and treatments.

   This process of clinical reasoning seems tedious and mechanical. As a matter of act, however, it represents good order. Such a process in which a doctor learns to diagnose resembles that in which a beginner learns to dance. The dance learner studies the divided movements first and then bring them together until the final mastery of all of them. Likewise, the doctor achieves proficiency in his trade through frequent and repeated practice on each and every one of the ten procedures.
4. **Commonly-used methods of clinical diagnosis:**
   - Direct diagnosis: This method is employed when the disease conditions are simple and evident. For diseases like nettle rash, traumatic hematoma, acute tonsillitis and acute gastroenteritis, just to name a few, the doctor may confirm the diagnosis based on medical history and signs and with the help of some simple laboratory examinations; in some cases, he may not even need any laboratory or other auxiliary examinations at all.
   - Exclusion diagnosis: When clinical symptoms and signs are not specific, and multiple diseases may co-exist, the doctor needs to make in-depth examinations and comprehensive analyses to identify doubtful points. After excluding the diagnosis of multiple possibilities and keeping one or two possibilities for further confirmation, the doctor should be able to propose a confirmed diagnosis.
   - Differentiated diagnosis: The main symptoms and signs of a disease may suggest multiple possibilities. Therefore, it is still difficult to differentiate them or conclude a diagnosis even after comprehensive analysis. Under such a circumstance, the doctor needs to make continual comparisons and judgements, and gather various kinds of information to differentiate diagnoses. If the new information does not support the existing diagnosis, the original possibilities should be eliminated; or a new diagnosis should be proposed. Such diagnostic reasoning over multiple possibilities, a method through continuous differentiation and comparisons for a final diagnosis, is a commonly used method of diagnosis-making for difficult and complicated diseases.

Common Reasons for Misdiagnoses and Omitted Diagnoses

72

Xuehong Wan and Rui Zeng

Simply put, a misdiagnosis is an incorrect or partly true judgement on a disease. A misdiagnosis means concluding a wrong diagnosis of a disease rather than a correct one; and usually the diseases is treated based on the wrong diagnosis. An omitted diagnosis may occur when a patient has two or more concurrent acute diseases, usually due to uncomprehensive diagnosis or because of the symptoms of one disease covering up those of another. A misdiagnosis often leads to therapeutic errors.

Therefore, it will more or less take some toll, regardless of how serious the errors may be: it will prolong the disease course, to say the least. An omitted diagnosis is usually a cognitive problem during the diagnostic process; and for this reason, it usually does not lead to therapeutic errors as the misdiagnosis does, except for special situations where death or severe disabilities result from the omission of major diseases, for example. Despite the good wish of both doctors and patients though, misdiagnosis and omitted diagnosis do exist as an objective reality.

Viewed from different angles, misdiagnoses can be divided into different categories, non-faulty misdiagnoses and faulty misdiagnoses, for instance. The former refers to the misdiagnosis caused by the limitations of human being's cognition on diseases, the complexity of diseases and the constraints of diagnostic conditions. For faulty misdiagnosis, however, the aforementioned constraints do not apply; instead, all kinds of conditions are available, but the doctor is still unable to make a correct diagnosis because of personal reasons. According to the degree of errors, misdiagnoses can be divided into complete misdiagnosis, partial misdiagnosis and delayed misdiagnosis. Based on the consequences, misdiagnoses can be divided into lethal misdiagnosis, harmful misdiagnosis and ordinary misdiagnosis. Misdiagnoses can also be divided into two categories using human and non-human factors as a criterium. Human factors include the patient such as erroneous medical history, or the doctor, such as insufficient professional knowledge, lack of experience and wrong reasoning methods. Non-human, or called as objective factors, such as complicated disease conditions, early stage of disease, overly divided clinical departments, and misleading by auxiliary examinations, etc. In a word, although misdiagnoses can not be avoided completely, doctors should try to minimize misdiagnoses by keeping learning and improving themselves.

From the perspective of clinical reasoning, the reasons for common clinical misdiagnoses and omitted diagnoses are as follows:

1. **Basic information is insufficient**. For instance, the medical history is incomplete or inexact; it fails to reflect the course of disease and characteristics of the patient as an individual. The physical examination is not comprehensive or systematic.
2. **Observations are not meticulous**. Key signs in clinical observation are ignored and examination results are inaccurate.
3. **The doctor does not take clinical manifestations into consideration**. Instead, he depends on examination results without analysis or misinterpret the examination results.
4. **The doctor has problems of preoccupation and subjective assumption**. His experience and incorrect impressions of certain cases may have dominated his reasoning, thus preventing him from making objective and thorough considerations.
5. **The doctor lacks medical knowledge and clinical experience**.
6. **The doctor inappropriately applies or sticks to a few principles of diagnostic reasoning**. Such as the

X. Wan
Department of Internal Medicine, Sichuan University, Chengdu, China

R. Zeng (✉)
Department of Cardiology, Sichuan University, Chengdu, China

X.-H. Wan, R. Zeng (eds.), *Handbook of Clinical Diagnostics*, https://doi.org/10.1007/978-981-13-7677-1_72

"monism", by which they use the diagnosis of one disease to arbitrarily explain all clinical manifestations of the patient, thus possibly leading to an omitted diagnosis.

7. **The doctors does take into consideration factors.** Include early stage, rare and difficult cases, unconspicuous clinical manifestations, or poor diagnostic conditions.

Key Terms

1	Clinical reasoning	临床思维
2	Diagnosis-making	做临床诊断
3	Clinical diagnosis	临床诊断
4	Misdiagnose	误诊
5	Omitted diagnoses	漏诊

Study Questions

1. What are the procedures of diagnosis-making?
2. What are the basic principles of reasoning for clinical diagnosis?
3. What are the common reasons for misdiagnoses and omitted diagnoses?

Suggested Readings and Websites

1. Bickley LS. Bates' guide to physical examination and history taking. 10th ed. Philadelphia: Lippincott Williams & Wilkins; 2009.
2. Swartz MH. Textbook of physical diagnosis. 7th ed. Amsterdam: Elsevier; 2014.

References

1. Wan X, Chen H. Clinical diagnostics. 3rd ed. Beijing: People's Medical Publishing House; 2015.
2. Wan X, Lu X. Diagnostics. 8th ed. Beijing: People's Medical Publishing House; 2013.
3. Ministry of Health, People's Public of China. Basic requirement for medical record. No 11. legislation. [Accessed 1/3/2010]. http://www.nhfpc.gov.cn/
4. Ministry of Health, People's Public of China. Requirement for electronic medical record system (trial). No 24. Legislation. [Accessed 1/4/2010]. http://www.nhfpc.gov.cn/
5. Ministry of Health, People's Public of China. Measures for management of medical cosmetology service. No 19. Legislation. [Accessed 22/1/2002]. http://www.nhfpc.gov.cn/
6. The ninth session of Committee of National People's Congress. Law of the People's Republic of China on medical practitioners. [Accessed 1/5/1999]. http://www.npc.gov.cn/

Index

X.-H. Wan, R. Zeng (eds.), *Handbook of Clinical Diagnostics*, https://doi.org/10.1007/978-981-13-7677-1

J

K

L

M

N

O

P

R

Printed by Printforce, the Netherlands